COMMUNITY MEDICINE

Solved Question Papers

COMMUNITY MEDICINE
Solved Question Papers

(With PG Entrance Points)

SIXTH EDITION

Singi Yatiraj
Kalaburagi, Karnataka
India

PG Entrance Points by
Roopali Somani
Kalaburagi, Karnataka
India

Foreword
G Ajaykumar

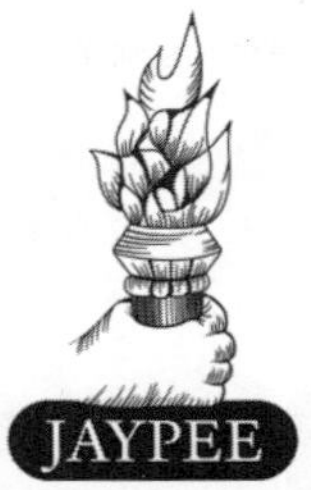

JAYPEE BROTHERS MEDICAL PUBLISHERS
The Health Sciences Publisher
New Delhi | London

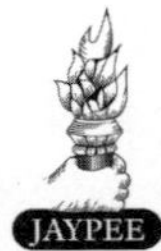

Jaypee Brothers Medical Publishers (P) Ltd

Headquarters
EMCA House, 23/23-B
Ansari Road, Daryaganj
New Delhi 110 002, India
Landline: +91-11-23272143, +91-11-23272703
+91-11-23282021, +91-11-23245672
e-mail: jaypee@jaypeebrothers.com

Corporate Office
4838/24, Ansari Road, Daryaganj
New Delhi 110 002, India
Phone: +91-11-43574357
Fax: +91-11-43574314
e-mail: jaypee@jaypeebrothers.com

Overseas Office
JP Medical Ltd.
83, Victoria Street, London
SW1H 0HW (UK)
Phone: +44-20 3170 8910
e-mail: info@jpmedpub.com

EU GPSR Authorised Representative
Logos Europe, 9 rue Nicolas Poussin
17000, La Rochelle, France
Phone: +33 (0) 6 67 93 73 78
e-mail: contact@logoseurope.eu

Website: www.jaypeebrothers.com
Website: www.jaypeedigital.com

Community Medicine Solved Question Papers

First Edition: 2009
Second Edition: 2010
Third Edition: 2011
Fourth Edition: 2013
Fifth Edition: 2015
Sixth Edition: 2018

Reprint : **2025**

ISBN: 978-93-5270-296-1

Printed at: Sterling Graphics Pvt. Ltd.

।। ॐ श्री फलौदी ब्रम्हाणी देवी नमः ।।
Om Shri Falaudi Brahmani Devi Namah

Dedicated to

That person
Who has brought happiness in my life;
Who has given me a reason to smile;
Who has trusted me all the time; and
Showed me that I can do it.

This book is a tribute to my respectable
Late Sister Anupama
and
Grandmother Rajubai

Foreword

Community Medicine Solved Question Papers by Dr Singi Yatiraj is a marvelous piece of work for the undergraduate students of community medicine. His efforts reflect in the number of papers and quality of answers provided from various sources including standard textbooks in the field of public health.

His style of presentation especially the National Health Programs has simplified the subject content for the undergraduates.

This book is a good companion for examination preparation for 3rd year students.

I wish Dr Singi Yatiraj and his books a great success.

G Ajaykumar MD
Professor and Head
Department of Community Medicine
Gulbarga Institute of Medical Sciences
Kalaburagi, Karnataka, India

Preface

Dear students,

Examinations are very crucial event in a student's life. They decide whether one would pass and go to the next phase or not. Every student tries his best to clear their examinations but call it bad fate; few fail. Not because they did not study, but because they could not revise at the eleventh hour or could not impress the examiners with their presentation.

With increasing competition, it is becoming imperative to score well in the university examinations. After strenuous night out and hard work, it is the right of the student to farewell in examinations, but he may be denied this just for lack of experience in presenting the answer in an excellent manner. Though he may know every nook and corner of a textbook, but it may happen that he may waste his time writing some answers more than needed and find it difficult to meet both ends of rope on the last bell during an examination.

During my examinations time, I could not have access to such book and wasted a lot of time procuring the syllabus, pattern of question papers, previous years question papers and searching answers for the questions in them; so this thought struck to me to prepare such a book, which combines all these into one and help the students. As they say *Necessity is the Mother of Invention*.

Therefore, book which will solve all the worries of the students during preparation of any examination, is in your hands right now. It includes the question papers of Rajiv Gandhi University of Health Sciences (RGUHS) in solved format as to reduce the workload on a student to refer numerous books for a single question. Also needed for perfect preparation are the Course Contents and the University Examination Pattern. Students should not waste time procuring these materials, as it is also included in this book. In short, I can say that this is a comprehensive manual for preparation of any examinations.

The most common suggestion received by me was to make this book chapterwise, so that it could be used even during college internals which have limited syllabus. But from updating point of view, this suggestion is impracticable. For every university examinations, three question papers are generated (including Revised Scheme 3). So in a year, 6 question papers have to be added to the book which will benefit the students only. Therefore, I always refuted this suggestion. Moreover, as the title of the book suggests, these are the solved question papers; so it looks ridiculous to make it chapterwise with the same title. However, considering infinite requests and suggestions, a new system of *Chapterwise Page References* were devised after considerable thinking, permutations and combinations, which has the following advantages:

- The questions are arranged in chapterwise format
- Under each chapter, they are further subclassed in *Long Essays, Short Essays* and *Short Answers*
- The next column has page number from this book only on which the answer for the question is located
- Final column has the list of examination in which this question is appeared
- The originality of the questions is maintained, thus it also serves as an index
- Overall, a chapterwise question bank with solved answers.

This book is presented in a handy form for easy handling during examinations. The books referred to write the answers are the ones that are commonly read by the students; so as not to cause confusion and avoid perpetuation of the tension at eleventh hour. The questions that are repeated have been referred. The emphasis is on the revised scheme 3, as it is applicable to the present batches.

My loyal readers would have found that by purchasing my books, they made no mistake during these examinations. Such is importance of such books because they let you revise in nick of time. They also help you understand the various modes of presenting answers to score well. But by far and large and also in the opinion of the students, the significance of this book lies in 3 marks questions which they are answered schematically and precisely.

Another important aspect of this book is that it contains a combination of different authors in a particular answer. A student cannot afford to read numerous books on a single subject in the prescribed time of one year for the first phase. So, this book will help the students prepare answers to the bouncer questions or answer the questions which are not there in the textbook opted by the students.

I have tried to provide all the necessary and latest information as possible. But let me make it clear that the book can never be a substitute to a textbook.

I sincerely solicit your valuable comments to improve this book and make it more useful. So please do write your comments to my mail *singi_yatiraj@yahoo.com* or contact me in Facebook on my page *Singi Yatiraj*.

I hope, even this edition, would receive same warm response as the previous ones and my other books.

In conclusion, I would like to thank my readers for their overwhelming support and wish my new readers *Best Wishes* for upcoming examinations.

Singi Yatiraj
www.drsingiyatiraj.5u.com

Acknowledgments

I would like to thank:

- Dr B Mallikarjun, Former Dean, MR Medical College, Kalaburagi, Karnataka, India, for his encouragement and support.
- Dr Ajay Guddur, Proferssor and Head, Department of Community Medicine, Gulbarga Institute of Medical Sciences, Kalaburagi, for his precious time for going through entire script and suggesting necessary corrections and being there whenever I needed him.
- Dr Rajshekhar Kapate, Dr S Nigudagi, Sri Srinivas, Dr Reshmi, Dr Jayashree Pattankar, and Dr Sharad Tenglikar, former staff members and rest of the staff members, and Postgraduates of Department of Community Medicine, MR Medical College, Kalaburagi, for their selfless excellent teaching.
- Mr Kalburgi and *Late* Sri Puranik of Computer Section, for providing me with the question papers of latest examinations.
- My teachers, for they are the ones who made me this capable.
- My friends Kiran, Nagaraj and Wali, for their help, support, suggestions and encouragement throughout the project.
- Mr Md Bari, Mr Yousuf Patel and Mr Rashid, Star Computers, for all the assistance in time and neat computer printing of the manuscript.
- My all friends and well-wishers, for their best wishes.
- Mr Santosh Patil, M/s SS Patil Medical Book Sellers, for his cooperation.
- Shri Jitendar P Vij (Group Chairman) and Mr Ankit Vij (Group President) of M/s Jaypee Brothers Medical Publishers (P) Ltd, New Delhi, India, for publishing the book in the same format as wanted well in time.
- Ms Sunita Katla (Publishing Manager), Ms Samina Khan (Executive Assistant to Director–Publishing), Mr KK Raman (Production Manager), Ms Uma Adhikari, Mr Laxmidhar Padhiary, Ms Seema Dogra and others at the M/s Jaypee Brothers Medical Publishers (P) Ltd, Typesetting Unit, for their painstaking effort to make this book this attractive and lucid.
- Mr Venugopal (Associate Director–South)) and other staff members of M/s Jaypee Brothers Medical Publishers (P) Ltd, Bengaluru, for taking this book to every corner of Karnataka.
- Mr Tarun, Mr Gopal and Mr Balaji, for introducing me to this publication house and being a close associate.
- All the students, for their overwhelming response and support to my prior endeavors.
- All those who have helped me directly or indirectly.
- Most important of all, my parents, sister, uncles and aunties, for their eternal love, care and support.

Thank you all of you,

Without you, this book would not have been a reality.

Contents

Course Contents

THEORY

I. Evolution of Public Health and Concepts of Health

Must Know

- Evolution of public health
- Definition of health, holistic concept of health, appreciation of health as a relative concept, determinants of health
- Characteristics of agent, host and environmental factors in health and disease and the multifactorial etiology of disease
- Understanding the natural history of disease and application, interventions at various levels of prevention with appropriate examples
- Indices used in measurement of health
- Health profile in India.

II. Environment and Health

Must Know

- Water:
  - The concept of safe and wholesome water
  - The requirement of sanitary sources of water
  - Understanding the methods of purification of water on small scale and large scale
  - Various biological standards including WHO guidelines for third world countries
  - Principles and methods for assessing quality of water
- Sources, health hazards and control of environmental pollution
- Problems in the disposable of refuse, sullage, human excreta and sewage and its remedies
- Awareness of standards of housing and the effect of poor housing on health
- Role of vectors in the causation of diseases
- Identifying features and mode of transmission of vector-borne diseases.

Desirable to Know

- Methods of vector control with advantages and limitations of each
- Modes of action, dose and application cycle of commonly used insecticides and rodenticides.

III. Health Education

Must Know

- Communicate effectively with individuals, family and community using tools and techniques of information, education and communication. To do so, the students should know:
  - Principles of communication, methods and evaluation of health education and understand and apply adult education methods
  - Appreciate barriers of effective communication
  - List various methods of health education with their advantages and disadvantages
  - Select and use of appropriate media (simple audiovisual) for effective health education
  - Practice of health education
- Use every opportunity for health education of the individual, family and the community.

IV. Nutrition and Dietetics

Must Know

- Common sources of various nutrients and special nutritional requirements according to age, sex, activity, physiological condition
- Nutritional assessment of individual, families and the community by selection and using appropriate methods such as anthropometry, clinical, dietary and laboratory techniques
- Plan and recommend a suitable diet for the individuals and families bearing in mind the local availability of foods, economic status, etc.
- Common nutritional disorders—protein-energy malnutrition, vitamin A deficiency, anemia, iodine deficiency diseases, fluorosis, food toxin disease, and the control and management
- National programs in nutrition
- Nutritional surveillance, education and rehabilitation.

V. Occupational Health

Must Know

- Relate the history of symptoms with the specific occupation including agriculture
- Employees State Insurance Scheme
- Identification of the physical, chemical, biological and social hazards to which workers are exposed while working in a specific occupational environment
- Influence of physical factors like heat, humidity, cold, radiation and noise on the health of the individual and community
- General preventive measures against these diseases including accident prevention.

Desirable to Know

- Various legislation in relation to occupational health.

VI. Medical Sociology and Community Mental Health

Must Know

- Conduct of a clinico-social evaluation of the individual in relation to social, economic and cultural aspects, educational and residential background; attitude to health, disease and to health services, the individuals, families and communities
- Assessment of barriers to good health, recovery from sickness and to lead a socially and economically productive life
- Development of good doctor-patient and community relationship
- Identification of sociocultural factors related to the health and disease in the context of urban and rural societies
- Impact of urbanization of health and disease
- National Mental Health Program.

Desirable to Know

- Community psychiatry.

VII. Fundamentals of Biostatistics

Must Know

- The scope and uses of biostatistics
- Collection of data, common sampling techniques, simple statistical method for the analysis, classification, interpretation and presentation of data, frequency distribution, measures of central tendency, measures of variability and laws of probability
- Analyze and interpret data
- Obtaining health information, computing indices (rates and ratio) and making comparisons.

Desirable to Know

- Apply statistical methods in designing of studies
  - Choosing appropriate controls
  - Applying tests of significance (large sampling tests)
  - Use of statistical tables.

VIII. Basic Epidemiology

Must Know

- Epidemiology
  - Definition, concept and role in health and disease
- Use of basic epidemiological tools to make a community diagnosis of the health situation in order to formulate appropriate intervention measures
- Definition of the terms used in describing disease transmission and control
- Modes of transmission and measures for prevention and control of communicable and noncommunicable diseases
- Principal sources of epidemiological data
- Definition, calculation and interpretation of the measures of frequency of diseases and mortality
- Need and uses of screening tests
- Accuracy and clinical value of diagnostic and screening tests (sensitivity, specificity, predictive values)
- Planning, collecting, analyzing and interpreting data with community participation to reach a community diagnosis
- General principles of epidemiology of communicable and noncommunicable diseases of public health importance and their control
- Awareness of programs for control of noncommunicable diseases
- Planning and investigation of an epidemic of communicable disease in a community setting
- Institution of control measures and evaluation of the effectiveness of these measures.

Desirable to Know

- The derivation of normal values and the criteria for intervention in case of abnormal values
- Applications of computers in epidemiology.

IX. Epidemiology of Specific Communicable and Noncommunicable Diseases

Must Know

- The specific objectives of selected communicable and noncommunicable diseases of public health importance for which National Disease Control/Eradication Programs have been formulated are described here. For other diseases, the individual teacher would formulate the objectives while drawing the lesson plans. The idea of formulation objectives for a few diseases here is to highlight their importance and emphasize certain learning outcomes.
  a. *Communicable diseases*
    - Intestinal infections
      * Poliomyelitis, viral hepatitis, diarrheal disease, cholera, helminthiasis including dracunculiasis
    - Respiratory infections
      * Acute respiratory infections, measles, diphtheria, whooping cough, tuberculosis
    - Vector-borne infections
      * Malaria, filariasis, kala-azar, dengue
    - Surface infections
      * Sexually transmitted diseases, HIV and AIDS, tetanus, leprosy
    - Zoonosis
      * Rabies, Japanese encephalitis, plague, Kyasanur forest disease
  b. *Noncommunicable diseases*
    - Coronary heart disease, hypertension, rheumatic heart disease, cancers, diabetes, blindness and accidents
    - Extent of the problem, epidemiology and natural history of the disease

- Relative public health importance of particular disease in a given area
- Influence of social, cultural and ecological factors on the epidemiology of the disease
- Prevention and control of communicable and noncommunicable diseases by:
  * Diagnosis and treating a case and in doing so demonstrate skills in:
    ⇒ Clinical methods
    ⇒ Use of essential laboratory techniques
    ⇒ Selection of appropriate treatment regimes
    ⇒ Follow-up of cases
  * Principles of planning, implementing and evaluating prevention and control measures for the disease at the community level bearing in mind the relative importance of the disease
- Institution of programs for the education of individuals and communities
- Investigating the epidemic disease and the principles of measures of controlling it
- Awareness of National Disease Control Program.

Desirable to Know

- Level of awareness of causation and prevention of disease amongst individuals and communities
- Control of communicable and noncommunicable diseases by diagnosing and treating a case and in doing so demonstrate skills in:
  - Instituting measures, where necessary, for preventing disabilities/deformities
  - Rehabilitation of the patient.

X. Demography

Must Know

- Definition of demography and family welfare program
- Stages of the demographic cycle and their impact on the population, concept of demographic gap and population explosion
- Definition, calculation and interpretation of demographic indices like birth rate, death rate, fertility rates
- Reasons for rapid population growth in India and population dynamics
- Need for population control measures and the National Population Policy.

XI. Reproductive and Child Health

Must Know

- Need for specialized services for these groups
- Magnitudes of morbidity and mortality in these groups in the local area and different regions
- Local customs and practices during pregnancy, childbirth, lactation and complementary feeding
- Concepts of reproductive child heath (RCH), components including Child Survival and Safe Motherhood, Universal Immunization Program, Integrated Child Development Scheme and other existing programs.
- Handicapped child
- Organization, implementation and evaluation of reproductive child health program components
- Identify and describe the different family planning methods and their advantages and shortcomings
- Demonstrate skills in motivating a couple for selecting an appropriate family planning method
- Medical Termination of Pregnancy (MTP) Act.

Desirable to Know

- Organization, technical and operational aspects of the National Family Welfare Program and participate in the implementation of the program.

XII. School Health

Must Know

- Objectives of the school health program
- Activities of the programs like:
  - Carrying out periodic medical examination of the children and the teachers

- Immunization of the children in the school
- Health education
- Mid-day meals.

Desirable to Know

- Obtaining participation of the teachers in the school health programs including maintenance of the records, defining healthy practices, early detection of abnormalities, national school health programs.

XIII. Urban Health

- Common health problems (medical, social, environmental, economical, psychological) of urban slum dwellers
- Organization of health services for slum dwellers
- Organization of health services in urban areas.

XIV. Health System in India

XV. Health Planning and Management Including Disaster Management

- Awareness regarding important health legislation in India such as Birth and Death Registration Act, Prevention of Food Adulteration (PFA) Act and MTP Act
- Awareness regarding important health legislation in India such as Child Labour Act, Consumer Protection Act, Prenatal Diagnostic Act, Human Organ Transplantation Act, etc.

XVI. International Health

XVII. Geriatrics

PRACTICAL

- Spotters from nutrition, environmental health and entomology, helminthes and parasites, occupational health, immunization, MCH and FP devices, etc.
- Problem-solving exercises including epidemiology and biostatistics
- Clinicosocial case studies of common communicable diseases, noncommunicable conditions and MCH and FP beneficiaries.

UNIVERSITY EXAMINATION PATTERN

Eligibility for Writing the University Examination

The candidate should have at least 35% aggregate in the two of the three internals conducted by the college and should also have minimum 75% attendance in Theory and Practical classes conducted.

Criteria for Passing the University Examination

The candidate should secure minimum 50% in the university theory examination (University theory + Viva voce) and the university practical examinations separately. Internal assessment marks would not be considered for passing criteria, however, they would be added to final marks to determine class of passing.

Distribution of Marks

	Internal Assessment		*University Examination*	
	Maximum marks	*Minimum marks to qualify*	*Maximum marks*	*Minimum marks to pass*
Theory examination	60 marks	21 marks	200 marks	120 marks
Viva voce	—	—	40 marks	
Practical examination	20 marks	14 marks	80 marks	40 marks

Distribution of Marks for University Examination

Theory Examination

It is of 300 marks in total, which consists of:

University Examination	200 Marks
University Viva Voce	40 Marks
Theory Internals	60 Marks

Pratical Examination

It is of 100 marks in total, which consists of:

University Practical	80 Marks
Practical Internals	20 Marks

Theory Examination

There shall be 2 theory papers carrying 100 marks each. The pattern of questions would be of three types:

2 Long Essay Questions	2 × 10 Marks	20 Marks
10 Short Essay Questions	10 × 5 Marks	50 Marks
10 Short Answer Questions	10 × 3 Marks	30 Marks
	Total	**100 Marks**

Distribution of chapters in paper I and II for university examination with weightage of marks

Paper I	*Paper II*
Evolution of public health and concepts of health	Epidemiology of specific diseases—communicable and non-communicable diseases
Environment and health	Demography
Health education	Reproductive and child health, school health, geriatrics, urban health
Nutrition and dietetics	Health system in India
Occupational health	Health planning and management including disaster management
Medical sociology and community mental health	International health
Biostatistics	
Basic epidemiology	

Practical Examination

Practical examination will carry 80 marks

10 Spotters	10 Marks
2 Problem Solving Exercises	35 Marks
1 Clinicosocial Case Discussion	35 Marks

Viva Voce Examination

Viva voce carries 40 marks and encompasses all aspects of syllabus.

CHAPTERWISE PAGE REFERENCES

Contd...

Contd...

Questions	Page No.	Examination
25. Carrier state in disease—salient features, classification with examples.	108	J08(RS2), D08(RS2), J09(RS2), D11(RS2), J13(RS3), J14(RS3)
26. Write the various modes of disease transmission with examples and control measures based on each.	108	D17(RS3)
27. Write a short note on biological transmission of arthropod borne disease.	110	J12(RS2)
28. Herd immunity and its importance.	319	J12(RS2)
29. Live vaccines.	446	J14(RS3)
30. Cold chain.	20	D15(RS3)
31. Cold chain equipment (present in PHC).	20	D07(RS2), J15(RS3), J17(RS3)
32. Methods for control of "reservoir of infection".	112	J08(RS2)
33. Quarantine.	605	D16(RS3)
34. Methods for disinfection for control of communicable diseases.	238	J08(RS2)
Short Answers		
1. Difference between and epidemic and outbreak.	271	J11(RS2)
2. Differentiate between endemic and epidemic.	246	D10(RS2)
3. International quarantine.	41	D07(RS2), D08(RS2)
4. Difference between quarantine and isolation.	517	J15(RS3)
5. Mode of action of handwash gels.	272	J11(RS2)
6. Aims of epidemiology.	298	D11(RS2), J14(RS3)
7. Tools of measurement of disease magnitude.	547	D07(RS2)
8. Crude death rate.	8	D08(RS2)
9. Write briefly on case fatality rate.	9	D10(RS2)
10. Standardized death rate.	10	D09(RS2)
11. Relationship between incidence and prevalence (difference).	446	D07(RS2)
12. What are the different types of epidemics?	603	D09(RS2)
13. Migration studies.	199	J10(RS2)
14. Odds ratio.	440	J12(RS2), D13(RS3), J14(RS3), J16(RS3)
15. Relative risk—define, calculations.	599	J11(RS2), D11(RS2), D15(RS3)
16. Attributable risk—calculations.	600	J10(RS2), D12(RS3)
17. Advantages and limitations of animal experiments.	26	D07(RS2)
18. What is blinding in randomized controlled trials?	545	D12(RS3)
19. Spurious association.	634	J09(RS2)
20. Epidemic.	603	J16(RS3), D17(RS3)
21. Sporadic diseases.	270	J11(RS2)
22. Exotic diseases with examples.	127	J09(RS2)
23. Secondary attack rate and its calculations.	517	J15(RS3)
24. Herd immunity.	319	D17(RS3)
25. Killed vaccines.	609	D16(RS3)
26. Toxoids.	550	D15(RS3)
27. What is vaccine vial monitor (VVM)?	408	J13(RS3)
28. Hazards of immunization (adverse events following immunization).	601	D07(RS2)
29. Quarantine.	605	D11(RS2)
30. National immunization schedule (for under-5).	42	D07(RS2), J16(RS3)
31. Disinfection of air.	553	D15(RS3)
32. Epidemiological case sheet for investigation of an epidemic.	546	J08(RS2)

Contd...

Contd...

Questions	Page No.	Examination
Short Answers		
1. Epidemiological basis for eradication of smallpox.	372	D12(RS3)
2. Describe rash in measles.	313	D11(RS2)
3. Prevention of measles.	252	J10(RS2)
4. Measles vaccine.	252	D14(RS3), J17(RS3)
5. Congenital rubella.	277	D12(RS3), D14(RS3), D17(RS3)
6. Influenza vaccine.	228	J10(RS2)
7. Influenza A (H1N1).	466	D17(RS3)
8. DPT—common side effects.	283	J11(RS2)
9. Vaccine for meningococcal meningitis.	148	J09(RS2)
10. Severe acute respiratory syndrome (SARS)—preventive measures.	593	J16(RS3)
11. Define new case, relapse, failure with reference to tuberculosis.	264	D10(RS2)
12. Mantoux test.	162	J11(RS2)
13. Directly observed treatment short course chemotherapy (DOTS)—strategy, components.	362	J08(RS2), J13(RS3)
B. Intestinal Infections		
Long Essays		
1. Describe in detail the strategies for polio eradication in India.	457	J14(RS3)
2. Discuss polio eradication in the light of epidemiological factors influencing poliomyelitis.	67	J08(RS2)
3. Discuss the epidemiology, clinical course and prevention of hepatitis B infection.	491	D14(RS3)
4. What are the epidemiological factors contributing to acute diarrheal diseases? Discuss briefly about its prevention and control measures.	420	D13(RS3)
Short Essays		
1. Describe the intensified pulse polio program (IPPI).	146	J09(RS2), J10(RS2)
2. Chandler's index and its public health importance.	612	D16(RS3)
3. What is acute flaccid paralysis surveillance?	458	D14(RS3)
4. Mention the steps involved in eradication of poliomyelitis.	457	J12(RS2), J17(RS3)
5. Hepatitis B—modes of transmission/prevention and control.	491	D09(RS2), J12(RS2), J15(RS3), J17(RS3)
6. Hepatitis B vaccine—schedule.	494	J14(RS3)
7. Oral rehydration therapy—indications.	470	J14(RS3)
8. Write briefly about measures to be taken to control a cholera outbreak.	496	D14(RS3)
9. Typhoid fever—epidemiological features/prevention and control (of carriers).	218	J10(RS2)
10. Anti-typhoid vaccine.	221	J16(RS3)
11. Steps of investigation of food poisoning in a boy's hostel.	511	J15(RS3)
12. Differential diagnosis of cholera and food poisoning.	174	D09(RS2)
13. Prevention and control of food poisoning.	527	J15(RS3)
14. Primary prevention of amoebiasis.	172	D09(RS2)
15. Enumerate the soil transmitted helminthes and diseases caused by them.	255	D10(RS2)
16. Prevention of hookworm infestation.	645	D17(RS3)
Short Answers		
1. Define acute flaccid paralysis.	458	D16(RS3)
2. What is Chandler's index?	612	J12(RS2), J17(RS3)
3. Salk polio vaccine.	538	J15(RS3)
4. Oral polio vaccine.	371	D12(RS3)
5. Mopping up in polio eradication.	458	D17(RS3)
6. Rotavirus.	539	J15(RS3)
7. Diarrheal disease control program.	148	J09(RS2)

Contd...

Contd...

Questions	Page No.	Examination
Short Essays		
1. Control of trachoma.	558	D15(RS3)
2. Tetanus neonatorum—prevention.	403	J13(RS3)
3. Write about the treatment strategy of leprosy eradication (multidrug therapy in leprosy).	96	D08(RS2), J15(RS3)
4. Epidemiology of STD's.	613	D16(RS3)
5. Syndromic management of vaginal discharge.	560	D15(RS3)
6. Management of genital ulcers.	472	J14(RS3)
7. What are the measures for control of sexually transmitted diseases?	333	J12(RS2), J17(RS3)
8. Clinical manifestation of HIV infection.	527	J15(RS3)
Short Answers		
1. HAART (human AIDS antiretroviral therapy).	592	J16(RS3)
2. Prevention of neonatal tetanus.	403	D11(RS2), D14(RS3), J15(RS3)
3. Fernandez reaction.	284	J11(RS2)
4. Objectives of multidrug therapy in leprosy.	96	D16(RS3)
5. Treatment for leprosy.	96	J12(RS2), J17(RS3)
6. What are the deformities occurring in the leprosy?	178	D09(RS2)
7. Syndromic management of urethral discharge.	590	J16(RS3)
8. Window period.	179	D09(RS2)
9. Case definition used for diagnosis of AIDS.	531	J12(RS2), J17(RS3)
10. Western blot test.	480	J14(RS3)
F. Emerging and Re-emerging Infectious Diseases		
Short Essay		
1. Ebola fever.	587	J16(RS3)
Short Answers		
1. Preventive measures in ebola virus disease (EVD)—disease transmission.	587	J17(RS3)
2. Control of ebola virus disease (EVD).	587	D16(RS3)
G. Hospital-acquired Infections		
Short Answer		
1. What are nosocomial infections? Give examples.	387	J13(RS3)
CHAPTER 6		
EPIDEMIOLOGY OF CHRONIC NONCOMMUNICABLE DISEASES AND CONDITIONS		
Long Essays		
1. Describe the natural history of stroke. What measures can be taken at the community level to control it?	68	J08(RS2)
2. Write about risk factors (multicausation) and complications of diabetes mellitus. Add a note on control and prevention of diabetes mellitus (in district)/add a note on self-care in diabetes.	201	J10(RS2), D11(RS2)
3. Define accident. Enumerate the types of accident. Give an account of primary factors associated with accidents.	639, 585	D17(RS3)
4. Describe the epidemiology of road traffic injury. Describe the prevention and control of accidents in India.	585	J16(RS3)
Short Essays		
1. Domestic accident prevention.	474	J14(RS3)
2. How do you measure the burden of coronary heart disease in the community.	311	D11(RS2)
3. Risk factors in coronary heart disease (coronary risk factors).	536	J15(RS3)
4. Prevention of coronary heart disease.	538	D15(RS3)
5. "Rules of Halves" in hypertension.	102	D08(RS2), D10(RS2), J14(RS3)
6. What are the risk factors for hypertension? Discuss briefly its preventive measures.	368	D12(RS3)
7. Prevention of rheumatic fever (heart disease).	616	D16(RS3)

Contd...

Contd...

Questions	Page No.	Examination
6. What is blood safety? How do you ensure blood safety? What is the current policy regarding blood donation?	278	J11(RS2)
7. Briefly discuss "National Program for Prevention of Blindness"—strategies.	554	D07(RS2), D13(RS3)
8. Vision 2020.	398	J13(RS3), D15(RS3)
9. Essential obstetric care for ensuring safe motherhood.	89	J08(RS2)
10. National Cancer Control Program.	144	J09(RS2)
11. Write salient features of National Mental Health Program.	310	D11(RS2)
12. Integrated disease surveillance project.	588	J16(RS3)
Short Answers		
1. Measures for control of urban malaria.	78	J08(RS2)
2. DOTS agents.	594	J16(RS3)
3. Sentinel surveillance for HIV in India.	39	D07(RS2)
4. Voluntary counseling and testing center.	521	J08(RS2)
5. Social marketing of condoms.	77	J08(RS2)
6. Vision 2020: The right to sight.	398	D08(RS2)
7. Reproductive and child health (RCH)—package/components.	88	J15(RS3)
8. Essential newborn care.	90	D07(RS2)
9. Nutrition rehabilitation center—concept.	482	J14(RS3)
10. Enumerate the illnesses managed under Integrated Maternal and Neonatal Childhood Illnesses (IMNCI).	75	D15(RS3)
11. Adolescent Reproductive and Sexual Health (ARSH) or SNEHA clinics.	564	D15(RS3)
12. Integrated disease surveillance system.	588	J08(RS2)
CHAPTER 8		
MILLENNIUM DEVELOPMENT GOALS TO SUSTAINABLE DEVELOPMENT GOALS		
Long Essay		
1. What are the millennium development goals (MDG's)? Critically analyze India's progress in achieving the goals with respect to maternal and child health.	424	D13(RS3)
Short Essays		
1. Millennium development goals.	424	D08(RS2)
2. How many millennium development goals are related to the health of the community? What are they? Write about any one of them.	425	J11(RS2)
CHAPTER 9		
DEMOGRAPHY AND FAMILY PLANNING		
Long Essay		
1. Define population explosion. What are the demographic trends in India? What measures do you suggest for the control of population explosion?	273	J11(RS2)
Short Essays		
1. Demographic cycle and its stages.	175	D09(RS2), D14(RS3), D16(RS3)
2. What is sex-ratio? Add a note on PNDT Act.	400	J13(RS3)
3. Write briefly about effects of urbanization on health.	351	D12(RS3)
4. Factors influencing fertility in a community/factors responsible for higher fertility in India.	70	J08(RS2)
5. List out fertility-related statistics.	99	D08(RS2)
6. Salient features of the National Population Policy.	33	D07(RS2), D17(RS3)
7. Enumerate national demographic goals to be achieved by 2010.	33	D10(RS2)
8. Barrier (Spacing) methods of family planning/conventional contraceptives—benefits.	255	D10(RS2)
9. Intrauterine device—ideal candidate, advantages, contraindications and side effects.	138	J09(RS2), D17(RS3)
10. Hormonal contraceptives—classify, mode of actions, method of administration, effects, contraindications, adverse effects and complications.	328	J12(RS2), D12(RS3), J17(RS3)

Contd...

Contd...

Contd...

Contd...

Questions	Page No.	Examination
17. Differentiate between monitoring and surveillance with examples.	123	J15(RS3)
18. What is pasteurization of milk? What are the tests used to check for the efficiency of pasteurization (methylene blue test)?	153	J11(RS2), J13(RS3), J14(RS3)
19. Write short notes on aflatoxins.	246	D10(RS2)
20. Epidemic dropsy.	609	D16(RS3)
21. Endemic ascites.	355	D12(RS3)
22. Food fortification and food enrichment.	321	J12(RS2)
23. What is food adulteration? Give examples.	199	J10(RS2), D13(RS3), D14(RS3)
24. Classify and list national (community) programs in nutrition.	247	D10(RS2)
25. Balwadi Nutrition Program.	610	D16(RS3)
26. School (Mid-day) Meal Program—principles, composition.	264	D10(RS2)
CHAPTER 12		
SOCIAL SCIENCE AND HEALTH		
Long Essay		
1. What is social security? Describe the benefits under ESI scheme.	151, 348	D09(RS2)
Short Essays		
1. How would you do counseling for a newly married couple for family planning?	32	D07(RS2)
2. Define family. What are the functions of a family?	383	J13(RS3), J17(RS3)
3. Role of family in health and disease.	292	D11(RS2)
4. Social and cultural factors affecting health and diseases.	242	D10(RS2), D13(RS3)
5. What is social stratification? Discuss how social class affects health and utilization of health services.	510	J15(RS3)
6. Diseases of poverty.	83	D08(RS2)
7. Social security.	151	J14(RS3)
Short Answers		
1. Modified Prasad's classification.	86	D08(RS2)
2. Social security available for elderly population.	151	D11(RS2)
3. Acculturation.	321	J12(RS2), J13(RS3)
4. Nuclear family.	384	J08(RS2)
5. What are the functions of the family?	384	D14(RS3)
6. Broken family—define, reasons.	197	J10(RS2)
7. Write about medicosocial worker.	356	D12(RS3)
8. Social security.	151	D17(RS3)
CHAPTER 13		
ENVIRONMENT AND HEALTH		
Long Essays		
1. Define safe water. Enumerate the sources of water. What are the various methods of purification of water on small scale?	410	D13(RS3)
2. Enumerate the vector-borne diseases and add a note on "prevention and control".	441	J14(RS3)
3. Explain the chemical control of arthropods of public health importance.	6	D07(RS2)
Short Essays		
1. What should be the thickness of plastic bags should they be permitted? Why?	268	J11(RS2)
2. Prevention of indoor air pollution in India.	631	D17(RS3)
3. Measures for safe disposal of sullage (in village).	84	D08(RS2)
4. Chlorination of water—principles.	579	J16(RS3)
5. Write in brief about break point chlorination.	605	D16(RS3)
6. What is residual chlorine? Explain free residual chlorine with a diagram. Is it necessary to have residual chlorine (role of residual chlorine in drinking water).	267	J11(RS2)

Contd...

Questions	Page No.	Examination
7. What are the various methods used for purification of water on a small (domestic) scale?	410	J10(RS2), D12(RS3)
8. Methods of household disinfection of water.	410	D11(RS2)
9. Write how you will disinfect a well in a village during an epidemic (steps in well chlorination).	380	J13(RS3)
10. Surveillance of drinking water quality.	575	J16(RS3)
11. What are the methods for determining the bacteriological quality of water (fecal contamination of drinking water).	575	D09(RS2)
12. Describe the different methods for removal of hardness of water.	512	J15(RS3)
13. Indices of thermal comfort.	11	D07(RS2)
14. Thermal comfort zone—define, range of corrected effective temperatures for evaluating comfort zone.	298	D11(RS2), D15(RS3)
15. Air pollutions—major 'air pollutants,' sources and adverse health effects/prevention and control/ monitoring (indices of air pollution).	483	J10(RS2), D14(RS3)
16. Ventilation—standards of ventilation/types.	322	J12(RS2)
17. Lighting standards.	606	D16(RS3)
18. Noise pollution—effects on health (noise-induced hearing loss)/control and prevention.	82	D08(RS2), D15(RS3)
19. Radiation—hazards (biological effects).	241	D10(RS2)
20. Criteria for healthful housing.	12	D07(RS2)
21. Housing standards for rural areas.	84	D08(RS2)
22. Why human fecal matter needs to be treated before disposal?	270	J11(RS2)
23. Oxidation pond.	297	D11(RS2)
24. Write about the different methods of control of arthropods.	193	J13(RS3)
25. Integrated vector control (Culex mosquito).	193	J10(RS2), D11(RS2), D13(RS3), D14(RS3), J16(RS3)
26. What are various mosquito control measures?	193	D10(RS2)
27. Write short notes on residual insecticides.	155	D09(RS2)
28. Diseases transmitted by soft ticks.	618	D16(RS3)
29. Cyclops.	16	D07(RS2)
Short Answers		
1. Nalgonda technique.	551	D15(RS3)
2. Soakage pit—define, mechanism of action.	64	J08(RS2)
3. Advantage and limitation of insecticides as method of vector control.	443	D16(RS3)
4. Back washing.	610	D16(RS3)
5. Residual chlorine (significance) and its testing in the community.	267	D13(RS3)
6. What is break point chlorination?	605	D09(RS2), J12(RS2)
7. Residual chlorination.	267	D17(RS3)
8. How do you determine the chlorine in drinking water? Orthotoludine test.	268	D09(RS2)
9. Stabilized bleach.	299	D11(RS2)
10. Horrock's test.	381	J10(RS2)
11. Rain water harvesting.	551	D15(RS3)
12. Indicators of air pollution.	484	J08(RS2), D10(RS2)
13. Effects of air pollution.	484	D07(RS2)
14. Effects and prevention of noise pollution.	82	J15(RS3)
15. Measures for the control of noise pollution.	83	J13(RS3)
16. Biological effects of radiation (effects of radiation on health).	241	J12(RS2), J14(RS3)
17. Effects of atmospheric pressure on health.	126	J09(RS2)
18. Kata thermometer.	552	D15(RS3)
19. Overcrowding and its effect.	418	D13(RS3)

Contd...

Questions	Page No.	Examination
20. What is sanitary barrier?	65	J08(RS2), J13(RS3)
21. What are the methods of sewage disposal.	246	D10(RS2)
22. Integrated vector control measures.	193	J15(RS3)
23. Aedes mosquitoes and disease.	419	D13(RS3)
24. What is aedes egypti index?	404	J13(RS3)
25. Anti-mosquito measures.	194	D15(RS3)
26. Environmental antilarval measures.	194	D08(RS2)
27. Mention tick-borne diseases.	271	J11(RS2)
28. What are rodenticides?	27	D07(RS2)
29. Enumerate the important zoonatic diseases.	263	D10(RS2)
CHAPTER 14		
HOSPITAL WASTE MANAGEMENT		
Long Essay		
1. What are various methods of treatment and disposal technologies for health-care waste?	167	D09(RS2)
Short Essays		
1. Health hazards of health-care waste.	145	J09(RS2)
2. Categories of biomedical waste in India.	167	D17(RS3)
CHAPTER 15		
DISASTER MANAGEMENT		
Short Essays		
1. What is disaster preparedness? List six components of disaster preparedness.	367	D12(RS3), J13(RS3)
2. Disaster management in floods.	643	D17(RS3)
3. Disaster management in India.	474	J14(RS3)
Short Answers		
1. Disaster cycle.	515	J15(RS3)
2. What is 'triage'. Scope of 'triage' in dealing with emergencies/disaster management.	405	J13(RS3), D14(RS3), J16(RS3), D16(RS3), J17(RS3)
3. Disaster mitigation in health sector.	178	D09(RS2), D11(RS2)
4. Earthquake mitigation.	436	D13(RS3)
5. Pre-disaster phase of disaster management.	367	J08(RS2)
CHAPTER 16		
OCCUPATIONAL HEALTH		
Long Essays		
1. Classify occupational diseases. Describe the various measures for the prevention of occupational diseases.	570	J16(RS3)
2. What is pneumoconiosis? What are the factors that influence causation of pneumoconiosis? Describe the various types of pneumoconiosis and their health effects? What measures are taken to prevent it?	316	J12(RS2)
3. What are the health hazards of workers in coal mines? What steps you would take to reduce the hazards?	50, 572	J08(RS2)
4. Describe in detail, the various health problems due to industrialization.	629	D17(RS3)
5. What are the laws meant for the protection of industrial workers? Write in detail about Factories Act, 1948.	286	D11(RS2)
Short Essays		
1. Classify occupational diseases with examples.	570	J10(RS2)
2. Pneumoconiosis (name giving occupation where they occur).	316	D10(RS2), J15(RS3)

Contd...

Questions	Page No.	Examination
3. Silicosis—epidemiology , manifestation and measures of control.	415	D13(RS3)
4. Outline causes, clinical features, management and prevention of lead poisoning (plumbism).	295	D11(RS2), J15(RS3)
5. Occupational cancers.	13	D07(RS2), D10(RS2), J12(RS2)
6. Occupational dermatitis.	451	J14(RS3)
7. Explain the occupation hazards of agriculture workers.	122	J09(RS2)
8. Prevention of industrial accidents.	640	D17(RS3)
9. What is sickness absenteeism. Enumerate the reasons? Explain the significance of sickness absentism.	622	J17(RS3)
10. Health problems due to industrialization.	629	J10(RS2)
11. What (medical) measures can be taken to protect the workers health?	572	D09(RS2), D14(RS3)
12. Provisions under Factories Act, 1948—health promotion/health safety and welfare provisions.	286	J08(RS2)
13. Employees State Insurance Act, 1948—benefits to employees (sickness/medical).	347	D10(RS2), J11(RS2), D12(RS3), J15(RS3)
Short Answers		
1. Occupational hazards of health-care professionals.	636	D17(RS3)
2. Define silicosis. How is it diagnosed?	415	D17(RS3)
3. Asbestosis and control.	385	D08(RS2), J13(RS3)
4. Occupational cancers—enumerate, causes.	13	J10(RS2)
5. Cancer in dye industries.	271	J11(RS2)
6. Occupational risk to farmers.	122	D11(RS2), D12(RS3)
7. Sickness absenteeism—define/measures for prevention.	622	D14(RS3)
8. Preplacement examination and its importance.	572	J08(RS2)
9. Employees State Insurance Act—benefits (medical/sickness/maternity).	348	D09(RS2), J16(RS3)
CHAPTER 17		
GENETICS AND HEALTH		
Short Essays		
1. Chromosomal abnormalities.	19	D07(RS2)
2. Down's syndrome.	432	D13(RS3)
3. Prevention of genetic disorders (Klinefilter's syndrome).	307	D11(RS2), D12(RS3)
Short Answers		
1. Difference between eugenic and euthenics.	455	J14(RS3)
2. Enumerate Mendel's laws of inheritance.	313	D11(RS2)
3. Human genome project.	25	D07(RS2)
4. Population genetics.	300	D11(RS2)
5. Hardy weinberg law.	405	J13(RS3)
6. What is euthenics?	308	D13(RS3)
CHAPTER 18		
MENTAL HEALTH		
Short Essays		
1. What are illusions, delusions and hallucinations.	269	J11(RS2)
2. Warning signals of poor mental health.	122	J09(RS2)
3. Types of mental illness.	453	J14(RS3)
4. Mental health services in India.	607	D16(RS3)
5. Drug dependence/addiction.	17	D07(RS2)
6. Socioeconomic effects of smoking.	586	J16(RS3)
7. Adverse health effects of smoking.	549	D15(RS3)
8. Discuss the effects of tobacco use. What are the preventive measures?	486	D14(RS3)
9. Role of legislation in reducing alcoholism in the society.	632	D17(RS3)

Contd...

Contd...

Contd...

QUESTIONS	PAGE No.	EXAMINATION
Short Essays		
1. Discuss briefly about various levels (three-tier system) of health-care services and in brief its 'characteristics'.	223	J10(RS2)
2. Define "primary health care". Write briefly about the "essential elements" and "guiding principles" of primary health care.	326	J12(RS2), D12(RS3), D14(RS3), J17(RS3)
3. Describe "ASHA"'s role and responsibilities under National Rural Health Mission.	465	D12(RS3)
4. Describe a community health center—functions.	30	D11(RS2)
5. Job description of multipurpose health worker (female).	35	D07(RS2), J09(RS2), J12(RS2), D13(RS3), D14(RS3)
6. Voluntary health agencies in India—define, enumerate and functions.	432	D11(RS2), D13(RS3)
7. Briefly describe the role of NGO's in health care (Non-governmental organization).	262	D10(RS2)
Short Answers		
1. How training of local dais is given?	227	J10(RS2)
2. What is the duration of training of a local dai? What does she learn during her training?	227	J11(RS2)
3. AYUSH in healthcare services for the community.	41	J08(RS2)
4. Describe the different levels of healthcare delivery system in India.	223	D14(RS3)
5. Primary health care—elements (components) and principles.	326	D13(RS3), J16(RS3), D16(RS3)
6. Accredited social health activist (ASHA)—job responsibilities.	465	J09(RS2), J17(RS3), D17(RS3)
7. Community health center.	30	D13(RS3), D17(RS3)
8. Central Government Health Scheme.	314	D11(RS2)
9. Indigenous system of medicine.	41	D07(RS2), J09(RS2)
10. Voluntary health organizations.	432	D09(RS2)
11. Red Cross Society—activities/contribution.	433	J13(RS3)
CHAPTER 23		
INTERNATIONAL HEALTH		
Short Essays		
1. World Health Organization (WHO)—functions/responsibilities.	135	J09(RS2), D11(RS2), J13(RS3), D14(RS3)
2. Expand UNICEF. Describe activities of UNICEF (United Nations Children's Fund) in India—in child nutrition/child health/improving child survival.	216	J08(RS2), J10(RS2), D12(RS3), J16(RS3)
3. Food and agriculture organization (FAO).	615	D16(RS3)
Short Answers		
1. Enumerate functions of UNICEF.	217	D10(RS2)
2. Rockefeller foundation.	147	J09(RS2)
3. International Red Cross Society.	564	D15(RS3)
MISCELLANEOUS		
Short Essays		
1. Ring immunization.	432	D13(RS3)
2. Benefits of forming self-help groups of mothers in villages.	50	J08(RS2)
3. What are the main health problems of urban slum dwellers and factors contributing to it?	351	J08(RS2)
4. Vaccination for international travelers.	35	D07(RS2)
Short Answers		
1. Focus group discussion (FGD).	516	J15(RS3), D16(RS3)
2. Screening for diseases in blood bank.	26	D07(RS2)
3. Attrition.	270	J11(RS2)
4. Institute.	271	J11(RS2)
5. Case definition for malaria.	435	D13(RS3)
6. What are the guidelines for defining "at-risk" groups?	514	J15(RS3)
7. Universal barrier precautions.	40	D07(RS2)
8. Enumerate functions of a manager.	264	D10(RS2)

Contd...

MBBS PHASE III EXAMINATION

DECEMBER 2007

(Revised Scheme 2)

PAPER I

LONG ESSAYS

1. Describe the concept "natural history of disease" with the help of a schematic diagram. Mention the levels of prevention and modes of intervention.

- Natural history of disease is sequence of events in a disease from earliest stage to its termination as recovery, disability or death in absence of any intervention in form of treatment or prevention
- Every disease has an own characteristic history which may vary from individuals to individual.

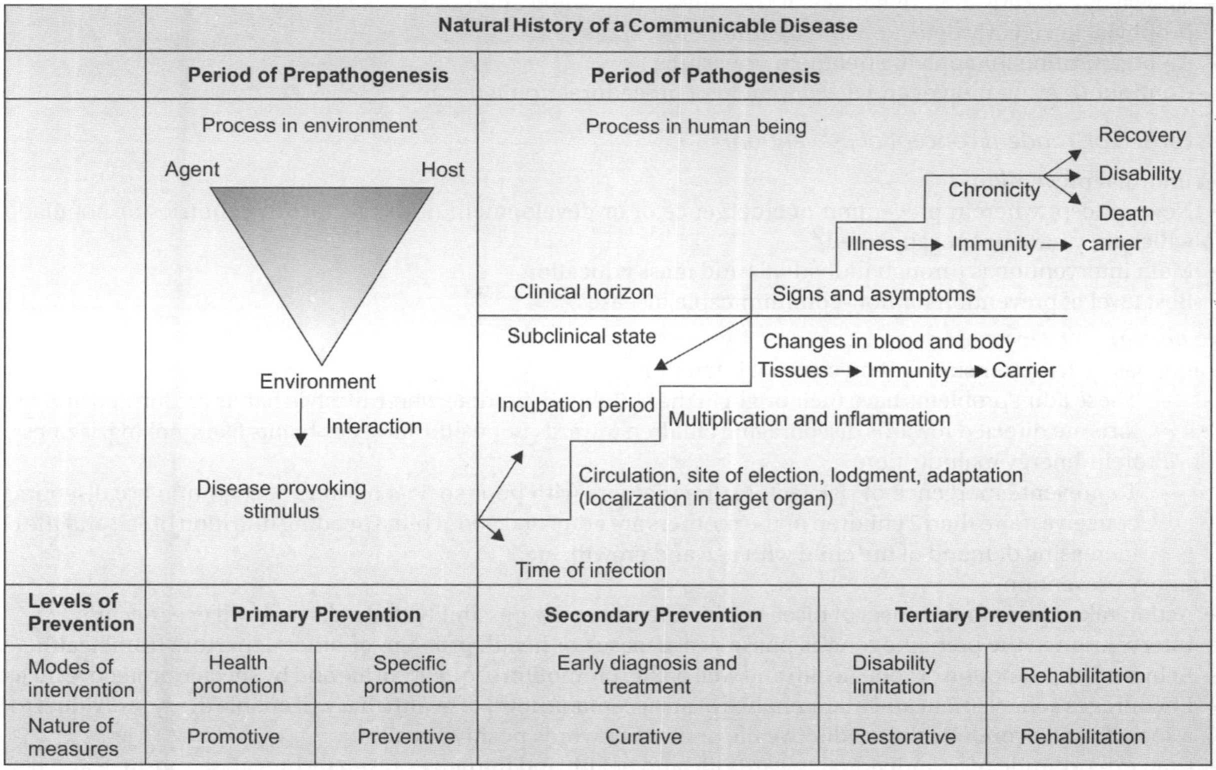

Fig. 1: Natural history of disease

Phases

Prepathogenesis phase (disease process in environment)	*Pathogenic phase (disease process in man)*
▪ Period before onset of disease[Q] in man, i.e. disease agent has not yet entered man ▪ Disease process starts when there is interaction between epidemiological triad, i.e. agent, host and environment[Q] ▪ A man in such scenario which favors this interaction is called man exposed to risk of disease ▪ Primary level of prevention is possible[Q] in this phase	▪ Period after entry of agent in man till disease outcome ▪ Once in man, disease agent multiplies, induces pathological and immunological changes and establishes itself ▪ Disease progresses through a period of incubation and later through early and late pathogenesis resulting in mild, moderate or serves disease depending upon resistance of individual and virulence of agent ▪ Final outcome may be recovery, disability or death ▪ In chronic diseases, early pathogenesis phase is less severe with no manifestations and pathological changes being below level of clinical horizon and is referred as presymptomatic phase. Here clinical stage begins in late pathogenesis phase when sign symptoms appear ▪ In this phase only secondary and tertiary level of prevention is possible[Q]

Levels of Prevention

- Any intervention in this natural history, changes the course of disease and thus the outcome and these interventions are called preventive measures.

Objectives

- To promote health, preserve health, restore health when it is impaired and to minimise suffering and distress
- Successful prevention depends upon
  - Knowledge of causation dynamics of transmission, identification of risk factors and risk groups, availability of prophylactic or early detection and treatment measures
  - An organisation for applying treatment measures
  - Continuous evaluation of and development of procedures applied.

Levels (based on modern concept of prevention)

a. Primordial prevention
   - New concept wherein prevention of emergence of or development of risk factors in countries or population in which they have not yet appeared[Q]
   - Main intervention is through individuals and mass education
   - Best level of prevention for non-communicable diseases[Q].

   Examples

   i. Obesity, hypertension and myocardial infarction[Q]
      - These adult problems have their origin in the childhood, i.e. time where lifestyle habits are formed and thus efforts are directed towards discouraging children towards unhealthy lifestyles habits like smoking, laziness, etc.

   ii. Protein-energy malnutrition
      - To prevent emergence of risk factors, the mothers with poor socioeconomic background are discourage to conceive more than 2 children or the mothers are educated about breastfeeding nutrition of self and the child, increasing demand of the child with age and growth, etc.

b. Primary prevention
   - Action taken prior to the onset of disease which removes the possibility that a disease will ever occur[Q]
   - Intervention in the prepathogenesis phase of a disease[Q] or health problem or other departure from health
   - Achieved by promotion of good health and well being, promotion of quality of life and by specific protective measures
   - Encourages achievement and maintenance of an acceptable level of health that will enable every individual to lead a socially and economically productive life or in other words positive health
   - Concerns attitude of an individual towards life and health and initiatives taken by him about positive and responsible measures for himself, his family and his community
   - Applied when risk factors are present but disease has not yet taken place.

   Examples

   i. Chronic diseases such as coronary heart disease, hypertension and cancer
      - WHO recommends following approaches for primary prevention of chronic diseases

- Population (mass) strategy
  - Directed at whole population irrespective of individual risk level
  - Aims at changing the socioeconomic status behavior and life style pattern[Q]
  - A small reduction in the average blood pressure or serum cholesterol produces large reduction in cardiovascular diseases
- High risk strategy
  - Directed towards individuals at special risk who are detected by optimum use of clinical methods

ii. Protein-energy malnutrition
- WHO expert committee recommends following primary preventive measures
- Health promotion
  - Measures directed to pregnant and lactating women like education, food supplement
  - Promotion of breast feeding
  - Development of low cost weaning food
  - Improving family diet
  - Nutrition education
  - Home economics
  - Family planning and spacing of birth
  - Family environment.
- Specific protection
  - Giving protein and energy rich diet to child possibly containing milk, eggs, fresh fruits
  - Immunization[Q]
  - Food fortification.

Significance
- Primary prevention utilizes knowledge about the prepathogenesis phase of disease including agent, host and environment to promote health or to protect against specific disease agent and hazards in the environment
- It has wide application because of its safety low cost.

c. Secondary prevention
- Action which halts the progress of a disease at its incipient stage and prevents complications[Q]
- Attempts to arrest the disease process restore health by seeking out unrecognized disease and treating it before irreversible pathological changes have taken place and reverse communicability of infections diseases
- Achieves its goal by early diagnosis and adequate treatment
- Largely a domain of clinical medicine
- Applied when disease has already set in
- National programs by Government of India mostly operate at secondary level of prevention[Q]

Examples

i. Health programs initiated by government
- National tuberculosis control program
- National leprosy control program.

ii. Protein-energy malnutrition
- Periodic surveillance
- Early diagnosis of any lag in growth
- Early diagnosis and treatment of infections and diarrhea
- Development of programs for early rehydration of children with diarrhea
- Development of supplementary feeding programs during epidemics
- Deworming of heavily infested children.

iii. Others
- Pap smear[Q]
- Penicillin for rheumatic fever[Q]
- Aminocentesis in early pregnancy[Q]
- Health screening for diabetes mellitus[Q]
- Contact tracing for SITs[Q].

Advantages	Disadvantages
▪ Provides secondary prevention for infected individual and primary prevention for their potential contacts	▪ Patient is already subjected to mental anguish physical pain and community to loss of productivity

Significance

– Secondary prevention is an imperfect tool in control of transmission of disease, is more expensive and less effective

d. Tertiary prevention
– Intervention in late pathogenesis phase
– All measures available to reduce or limit impairment and disabilities, minimise suffering caused by existing departures from good health and to promote the patients adjustment to irremediable conditions
– Encompasses psychosocial vocation and medical fields
– Applied when disease has advanced beyond early stages.

Examples:

i. Rehabilitation of the blind, paralysed or crippled
ii. Protein-energy malnutrition
   - Nutritional rehabilitation services
   - Hospital treatment
   - Follow-up care.

Modes of Intervention

- Intervention is any attempt to intervene or interrupt usual sequence in development of disease.

Modes

a. Health promotion
– Process of enabling people to increase control over and to improve health
– Intended to strengthen the host through a variety of approaches rather than directed against any particular disease.

Ottawa charter for health promotion

5 key action areas	Basic strategies
▪ Public health policy ▪ Supportive environment for health ▪ Strengthen community action for health ▪ Personal skill development ▪ Reorientation of health services	▪ Advocate ▪ Enable ▪ Mediate

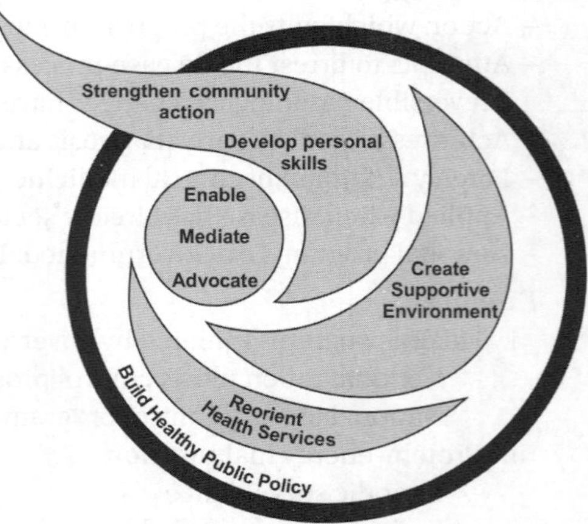

Fig. 2: Ottawa Charter Health Promotion

Approaches

i. Health education (e.g, diarrhea and ORS powder)
   – One of the most cost-effective intervention
   – A large number of diseases could be prevented with little or no medical attention if people were adequately informed and are encouraged to take necessary precautions in time
   – Target groups are general public patients, priority groups, health providers, community leaders and decision makers.
ii. Environmental modification
   – Provision of safe water, installation of sanitary latrines, control of insects and rodents improvement of housing, etc. are essential component of comprehensive environmental modification.
   – Nonclinical and do not involve physicians
   – Have successfully controlled many infections diseases in western countries.
iii. Nutritional interventions
   – Food distribution and nutrition
   – Improvement of vulnerable groups
   – Child feeding programs
   – Nutrition education.

iv. Lifestyle and behavioral changes
   - To bring about life style and behavioral changes is responsibility of the individual and community
   - Even physicians and health workers should work educator rather than therapist
   - Any health promotion program should first identify the target group or at risk individuals and then direct move appropriate message to them
   - Goals must be defined and means and alternative means of accomplishing them should be explored
   - It should involve organizational, political, social and economic interventions designed to facilitate environmental and behavioral adaptations that will improve or protect health.

b. Specific protection
   - Ideal intervention avoid disease altogether but this is possible only in a limited number of cases
   - More concrete and effective

   Interventions
   - Immunization, e.g. smallpox, polio, diphtheria, etc.
   - Use of specific nutrients, e.g. vitamin C for scurvy, iron for anemia, vitamin A for xerophthalmia[Q]
   - Chemophrophylaxis, e.g. malaria[Q]
   - Defluoridation of water in areas with fluoride rich water[Q]
   - Iodiation of salt to prevent iodine deficiency disorders[Q]
   - Usage of condoms for prevention of AIDS/SITs[Q]
   - Protection against occupational hazard
   - Protection from carcinogens
   - Avoidance of allergens
   - Control of specific hazards in the general environment, e.g. air pollution, noise pollution
   - Control of consumer product quality and safely of foods, drugs, cosmetics, etc.

c. Early diagnosis and treatment
   - Detection of disturbances of homeostatic and compensatory mechanism while biochemical, morphological and functional changes are still reversible
   - Should be based on early biochemical, morphological and functional changes that precede the occurrence of manifest signs and symptoms
   - Particular importance in chronic diseases
   - Main interventions of disease control
   - Earlier a disease is diagnosed and treated the better is the prognosis
   - They are not an effective and economical as primary prevention but are critically important in reducing the high morbidity and mortality in diseases, such as essential hypertension, carcinoma cervix and breast cancer
   - For many like STD, leprosy and tuberculosis[Q], it is the only effective mode of intervention
   - Also shortens the period of communicability, considerably and reduces the mortality from acute communicable diseases.

d. Disability limitation
   - Mode of intervention when a patient reports late in the pathogenic phase
   - Aimed to prevent or halt the transition of the disease process from impairment to handicap.
   - Major causes of disability are:
     - Communicable diseases
     - Malnutrition
     - Low quality of perinatal care
     - Accidents.
   - Impairment is any loss or abnormality of psychological, physiological or anatomical structure or function. It may be visible or invisible, temporary or permanent, progressive or regressive. Even one impairment may lead to secondary impairments
   - Disability is any restriction or lack of ability to perform as activity in the manner or within the range considered normal for a human being
   - Handicap is a disadvantage for a given individual resulting from an impairment or a disability that limits or prevents the fulfillment of a role that is normal for that individual[Q]
   - Intervention in disability is social or environmental or medical. The intervention at the earliest stage is mostly medical but at later stage it is mostly social and environmental

– Disability prevention is related to:
  - Reducing the occurrence of impairment
  - Disability limitation by appropriate treatment
  - Preventing transition of disability in handicap.
– Primary prevention is the most effective way of disability limitation.

Example
– Resting of limb in neutral position in polio.[Q]

e. Rehabilitation
– Rehabilitation is combined and coordinated use of medical social educational and vocational measures for training and retraining the individual to the highest possible level of functional ability
– Includes all measures aimed at reducing the impact of disabling and handicapping conditions and at enabling the disabled and handicapped to achieve social integration (active participation of disabled and handicappėd people in the mainstream community life)
– Medical aspects of rehabilitation are physiotherapy, occupational therapy, speech therapy, audiology psychology, etc.
– Areas of rehabilitation
  - Medical rehabilitation: Restoration of function[Q]
  - Vocational rehabilitation: Restoration of capacity to earn a livelihood
  - Social rehabilitation: Restoration of family and social relationships
  - Psychological rehabilitation: Restoration of personal dignity and confidence
– Examples
  - Reconstructive surgery in leprosy
  - Muscle reeducation and graded exercises in neurological disorders like polio,
  - Modification of life in cases of tuberculosis and cardiac patients.
– Purpose of rehabilitation is to make productive people out of nonproductive people.

2. Explain the chemical control of arthropods of public health importance.

- Arthropods comprise the most numerous and varied living things in the environment
- Some of them which live close to the man act as vectors or carriers of the disease and hence are important in public health.

Arthropods of Public Health Importance

Class Insecta					*Class Arachnida*		*Class Crustacea*
Mosquitoes	*Flies*	*Human lice*	*Fleas*	*Bugs*	*Ticks*	*Mites*	
▪ Anophelines ▪ Culicines	▪ Sandflies ▪ Tsetse flies ▪ Black flies	▪ Head and body lice ▪ Crab lice	▪ Rat fleas ▪ Sand fleas	▪ Reduviid bug	▪ Hard ticks ▪ Soft ticks	▪ Leptotrombidium mite ▪ Trombiculid mite ▪ Itch mite	▪ Cyclops

Chemical Control of Arthropods

Principle

- A wide range of insecticides belonging to the organochlorine, organophosphorus and carbmate groups of compounds are available for vector control.

a. **Chemical control of mosquitoes (integrated vector control measures)**
Refer Question No. 11 June 2010 (RS2) Paper I.

b. **Chemical control of house flies**

i. Residual spray	Insecticides based on resistance of flies is sprayed at about 5 liters per 100 m^2 of surface Addition of sugar to insecticide mixture enhances its effectiveness For susceptible flies: 5% DDT, 5% methoxychlor, 0.5% lindane or 2.5% chlordane For resistant flies: 2% diazinon, 2.5% diamethoate, 2.5% fenthion, 5% malathion or 5% runnel
ii. Baits	Solid baits containing 1–2% dianinon, malathion, dichlorvos, runnel and dimethoate or liquid baits containing 0.1–0.2% of the same insecticides along with 10% sugar gives good results Cheapest bait is one that can be made at home also is mixture of 3 teaspoons of commercial formalin with one pint of water or milk along with little sugar

iii. Cords or ribbons	Cords or ribbons impregnated with diazinon, fenthion or diemthoate are hung like festoons from ceilings They offer effective protection for about 1–6 months
iv. Space sprays	Space sprays containing pyrethrin and DDT or HCH are applied indoors or outdoors using hand or power sprays Offers temporary effect on adult fly population and needs repeated application
v. Larvicides	0.5% diazinon, 2% dichlorovos, 2% dimethoate or 1% runnel applied at the rate of 28–56 liters per 100 m^2 is used as larvicides at fly breeding places

c. **Chemical control of Sandflies**

Residual sprays	1–2 g/m^2 of DDT or 0.25 g/m^2 of lindane is used as residual sprays ensure reduction in number of sandflies and offer protection for period of 1–2 years and 3 months respectively

d. **Chemical control of Tsetse flies**

Residual sprays	25% DDT and 18–20% dieldrin are effective in control of Tsetse flies and can be sprayed using aircraft for control measure in large areas.

e. **Chemical control of Blackflies**
   - Blackflies control measure only targets the larvae as range of fly is about 100 miles
   - 0.05–0.1 mg/L of abate is added to river water over a period of 10 minutes weekly

f. **Chemical control of Head and crab lice**
   - 0.5% malathion containing lotion is applied to hair and washed off after 12–24 hours which will kill lice and nits
   - Carbaryl dust is also effective

g. **Chemical control of body lice**
   - 1% malathion powder is method of choice where in powder is applied to inner surface of clothing as well as socks and body of the person and method can be repeated after 7 days to kill late hatching lice
   - Carbaryl dust is also effective

h. **Chemical control of rat fleas**
   - 10% DDT dust is cheapest and most widely used formulation which kills the fleas by getting on fur of rodents when they walk over the dust
   - In areas where rat fleas have developed resistance to DDT, 2% carbaryl or diazinon or 5% malathion is effective when applied to floors and walls up to a height of 1 foot
   - Patch dusting is another technique where powder is applied over rat runs, under gunny bags and other harbourage areas
   - Insecticide dust should also be blown into rodent's burrows in quantity of 30 g per burrow

i. **Chemical control of reduviid bugs**

i. Residual spray	0.5 g/m^2 of HCH or 1 g/m^2 of dieldrin are commonly used

j. **Chemical control of ticks and mites**
   - DDT, chlordane, dieldrin, lindane, malathion and toxaphane at rate of 1-2 lbs per acres applied by dusting or spraying give effective control against ticks and mites

k. **Chemical control of itch mite**
   - Consists of application of sarcopticide to the infested person and also the close contacts such as family members, irrespective of whether they have scabies or not (Blanket treatment)

   Commonly used sarcoticides

– 25% Benzyle benzoate	2 applications 12 hours apart
– 0.5–1.0% Lindane in coconut/vegetable oil or vanishing cream	2 application 2–3 days apart
– 5% Tetmosol	3 applications in a day
– 2.5–10% Sulfur	Daily for 4 days

l. **Chemical control of Cyclops**
   Refer Question No. 9 Jan. 2008 (RS2) Paper I.

Significance

- Chemical control by insecticides being most efficient and most economical control method and unavailability of other alternatives makes it the preferred method of arthropod control.

SHORT ESSAYS

3. What are the advantages of case control study?

Refer Question No. 1 June 2014 (RS2) Paper I.

4. Mortality rates and ratios.

- Mortality indicator (mortality rates and ratios) are indicators of mortality in a community

Commonly used Mortality Indicators

A. Crude death rate
   - Crude death rate is the number of deaths from all causes per 1000 estimated mid year population in a defined geographical area in one year.

$$\text{Crude death rate} = \frac{\text{No. of deaths from all during a given year in a defined geographical area}}{\text{Estimated mid year population}^{Q}} \times 100$$

   - Indicates the rate at which people are dying[Q]
   - It is called crude because it does not specify the age group of death or sex groups of death nor cause of death
   - It these factors are specified then it is called specific death rate.

   Disadvantage
   - Its use for international comparison is restricted because it is influenced by age-sex composition of population.

   Significance
   - Considered a fair indicator of comparative health of people
   - Higher the death rate means poorer health status of the population
   - But decrease in death rate provides a good tool for assessing the overall improvement in a population.
   - Crude death rate in India is 6.4 per 1000 midyear population (SRS September 2017).

B. Specific death rate
   - Death rate in which cause or group is specified.

   Types

   a. Cause specific death rate
      - It indicates number of death due to a particular cause per 1000 estimated mid year population in a defined geographical area in one year.

$$\text{TB specific death rate} = \frac{\text{No. of deaths due to TB during a given year in a defined geographical area}}{\text{Estimated mid year population}} \times 1000$$

   b. Group specific death rate
      - Indicates number of deaths in a particular group per 1000 estimated midyear population in a defined geographical area in one year
      - Groups can be age, sex, race, occupation, social class, etc.

   Examples

   i. Infant mortality rate[Q]
      - Infant mortality rate is number of infant deaths (death below 1 years of age) per 1000 live births in one year in a defined geographical area

$$\text{Infant mortality rate} = \frac{\text{No. of infant deaths during a given year in a defined geographical area}}{\text{Total live births in that year}} \times 1000$$

Significance

- IMR is most universally accepted indicator of health's status of whole population and socioeconomic condition
- Does not include perinatal mortality rate[Q]
- Also a sensitive indicator of availability, utilization and effectiveness of health care particularly perinatal care
- Infant mortality rate in India is 34 per 1000 live births (SRS September 2017).

ii. Under 5 mortality rate

- Under 5 mortality rate is the number of deaths of children below 5 years of age per 1000 live births in one year in a defined geographical area

$$\text{Under 5 mortality rate} = \frac{\text{No. of deaths of children below age of 5 years during a given year in a defined geographical area}}{\text{Total live births in that year}} \times 1000$$

Significance

- Under 5 mortality rate reflects both infant and child mortality rate
- More in communities with poor hygiene
- High rate reflects high birth rates, high child mortality rate and shorter life expectancy.

iii. Maternal mortality rate

- Maternal mortality rate is the number of deaths in females due to puerperal cause per 100,000 live births in one year in a defined geographical area

$$\text{Maternal mortality rate} = \frac{\text{No. of maternal deaths during a given year in a defined geographical area}}{\text{Total live births in that year}} \times 100{,}000$$

Significance

- MMR is one of the indicators used internationally to compare the health status of a nation.

c. Period specific death rate

- It is the number of deaths in a particular period per 1000 estimated mid year population in a particular geographical area.

$$\text{Period specific death rate of May} = \frac{\text{No. of deaths in month of from in a defined geographical area}}{\text{Estimated mid year population}} \times 1000$$

C. Case fatality rate[Q]

- Case fatality rate is ratio of death due to a particular disease to total number of people affected by that disease
- It is a proportion[Q] and is always expressed in %

$$\text{Case fatality rate} = \frac{\text{No. of deaths from due to particular disease}}{\text{Total number of cases of same disease}} \times 100$$

- CFR is complement of survival rate thus CFR = 1 – survival rate

Significance

- Case fatality rate represents killing power (virulence) of a disease[Q]
- Typically used in acute infectious disease like rabies (100% CFR)
- Can be used to measure benefits of new therapy[Q].

Limitations[Q]
- Time interval is not specified[Q]
- Not useful in chronic infections[Q]
- Variable for same disease[Q].

D. Proportional mortality rate (ratio)
- Proportional mortality rate expresses number of deaths due to a particular cause (or in a specific age group) per 100 (or 1000) total deaths.

Examples

$$\text{Proportional nortality from TB} = \frac{\text{No. of deaths from TB in a year}}{\text{Total deaths from all causes in that year}} \times 100$$

$$\text{Under 5 proportional mortality rate} = \frac{\text{No. of deaths under 5 years of age in a year}}{\text{Total number of deaths in that year}} \times 100$$

- Usually computed for a broad disease group or a specific disease of major public health importance
- Used when population data are not available

Disadvantages
- Limited value in making comparison between population groups or different time periods.

Significance
- Useful indicators within any population group of relative importance of specific disease or disease group, as a cause of death
- Proportional mortality rate does not indicate risk of members of population contracting or dying from the disease

E. Survival rate
- Survival rate is proportion of survivors in a group studied and followed over a period.

$$\text{Survival rate} = \frac{\text{Total number of patient alive after 5 years}}{\text{Total number of patients diagnosed or treated}} \times 100$$

- Survival period is usually reckoned from date of diagnosis or start of treatment
- It is a method of describing prognosis in certain disease conditions.

Significance
- Survival experience can be used as a yardstick for assessment of standards of therapy.

F. Standardized death rates (adjusted death rates)
- Death rate corrected for age-sex distribution of population is called standardized death rate[Q]
- It is used to compare death rates of two populations with different age group compositions[Q]
- Besides age, adjustment can be made for sex, race, parity, etc.

Methods

Direct standardization[Q]	*Indirect standardization*[Q]
▪ Standard population is selected ▪ Age specific death rates of the population whose crude death rate is to be standardized is calculated ▪ Expected number of deaths in standard population is then obtained ▪ Total expected deaths is calculated by adding all expected deaths ▪ Standardized age adjusted death rate is calculated by dividing the total expected deaths by total standard population and estimated per 1000 population.	▪ Select a series of standard death rates of different ages ▪ These rates are applied to the population under study to get expected rates ▪ These are then totaled ▪ Dividing the expected deaths by the total population obtains Index death rates ▪ Crude death rate of the standardized population divided by the index death rate gives standardization factor ▪ Then standardizing factor is multiplied by the crude death to obtain standardized death rate

Significance
- Standardized death rate is the gold standard for comparison of mortality rate (vital statistics) across various countries[Q] as it does away with disparity in age-sex composition of a country.

5. Indices of thermal comfort.

- Thermal comfort being a complex entity, numerous indices have been put forward to express it.

Indices of Thermal Comfort

a. Air temperature
   - Was used as an indicator of thermal comfort for a long time
   - Not an adequate indicator alone.

b. Air temperature and humidity
   - Better indicator but still unsatisfactory.

c. Air temperature, humidity and air movement (Cooling power[Q])
   - Air temperature, humidity and air movement together are called cooling power
   - Measured using Kata thermometer[Q]
   - A reading of ≥6 by dry Kata thermometer and ≥20 by wet Kata thermometer are considered indices of thermal comfort.

d. Effective temperature
   - An arbitrary index which combines into a single value, the effect of temperature, humidity and movements of internal air on sensation of warmth or cold felt by human body
   - However, it does not include effect of radiation from surrounding structures (as reading are taken from dry bulb thermometer)
   - Numerical value of effective temperature is that of temperature of still saturated air which would induce same sensation of warmth or cold as that experienced in the given condition
   - Two scales are available depending upon clothing of individual, one of which refers to men who are stripped to waist and other fully clad men
   - Effective temperature may be obtained from special charts by reference to the three variables.

e. Corrected effective temperature
   - An improvement over effective temperature index by incorporating readings of Globe thermometer which allows for radiant heat
   - Therefore, preferred whenever there is a source of radiation present
   - Readings can be obtained from prepared normogram by reference to globe thermometer temperature, wet bulb temperature and air speed.

   Merit
   - Considers all four factors, namely air temperature, humidity, air movements and radiant heat.

   Application
   - Corrected effective temperature is used to describe the comfort zones as follows:

Ranges of corrected effective temperature	*Comfort zones*
69°F	Pleasant and cool
69–76°F	Comfortable and cool
77–80°F	Comfortable
81–82°F	Hot and uncomfortable
83+ °F	Extremely hot
86 + °F	Intolerably hot

f. McArdle's maximum allowable sweat rate
   - Rate at which a person sweats in hot environment and is expressed for four hours
   - Recorded as predicted four hour sweat rate (P_4SR)
   - Is an indicator of heat stress.

   Applications
   - Used to describe comfort zones as follows:

Predicted four hour sweat rate	*Comfort zones*
1–3 liters	Comfort zone
3–4.5 liters	Just tolerable
4.5+ liters	Intolerable

6. Criteria for healthful housing.

- Housing includes not only the physical structure but also the immediate surroundings and related community services and facilities.

Criteria of Healthful Housing (WHO Expert Committee)

i. Healthful housing provides physical protection and shelter
ii. Healthful housing provides adequately for cooking, eating, washing and excretory functions
iii. Healthful housing is designed, constructed, maintained and used in a manner such as to prevent spread of communicable diseases
iv. Healthful housing provides for protection from hazards of exposure to noise and pollution
v. Healthful housing is free from unsafe physical arrangements due to construction or maintenance and from toxic or harmful materials
vi. Healthful housing encourages personal and community development, promotes social relationships reflects a regard for ecological principles and by these means promotes mental health.

Housing Standards (Environmental Hygiene Committee)

a. Site	▪ Elevated, not subject to flooding, away from vector breeding places and nuisance ▪ Soil should be dry and safe for founding the structure ▪ Subsoil water should be below 10 feet
b. Setback	▪ As open space around house with no obstruction to lighting and ventilation
c. Floor	▪ Pucca, impermeable, easily washable, smooth, free of cracks and crevices and damp-proof
d. Walls	▪ Reasonably strong, low heat capacity, not easily damaged and should not harbor rats or vermin
e. Roof	▪ Height not less than 10 feet with low heat transmittance coefficient
f. Rooms	▪ At least 2 with number increasing according to family size
g. Floor area	▪ Should be 100 sq. ft for one person and at least 120 sq ft for more than one person
h. Cubic space	▪ At least 500 cuft per capita; optimum is 1000 cuft
i. Windows	▪ At least 2 windows per living room if room is not provided mechanical ventilation and artificial lighting, placed at a height of not more than 3 feet above ground ▪ Window area should be 1/5th of floor area
j. Lighting	▪ Daylight factor exceeding 1% over half floor area
k. Kitchen	▪ Should be separate for every dwelling, protected against dust and smoke, provided with storage space, water supply, drainage and adequately lighted
l. Sanitary privy	▪ In every house and readily accessible
m. Garbage and refuse	▪ Should be removed daily and sanitarily disposed
n. Bathing and washing facilities	▪ Should be exclusive to house
o. Water supply	▪ Should be safe and adequate

Significance

- Housing has important effect on health because house protects an individual from numerous environmental risk factors.

7. Cross-over type of study design.

- Cross-over type of study design is a study design of controlled trials
- In this type of study, each study subject or patient serves as his own control.

Revised Scheme 2

Procedure

- Like in a clinical trial, patients are randomly assigned to study group and control group
- The study group receives treatment and control group receives alternate form of active treatment or placebo
- Both groups are observed over time and then patients in each group are taken off their medication or placebo to allow for elimination of medication from body and for possibility of any carry over effects
- After this period, two groups are switched, i.e. crossed over

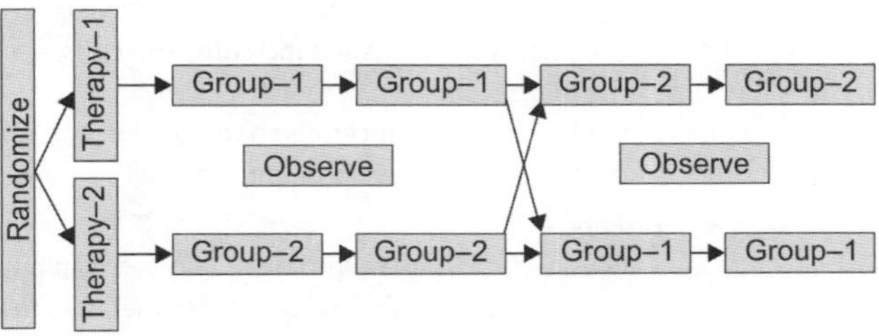

Fig. 3: Cross-over type of study design

Types

Planned cross-over	*Unplanned cross-over*
▪ Most common type ▪ After a certain period, patients are switched from treatment group to control group and vice versa	▪ In a study trial to assess effects of surgical and medical lines of treatment, if patients under surgical care decide to change line of treatment and similarly if condition of patient under medical care warrants surgery then such patients are crossed-over

Advantages	*Disadvantages*
▪ All patients are assured of new therapy sometime during course of investigation (Ethically better) ▪ Economical in terms of total number of patients required and time required ▪ All subjects serve as own controls and error variance is reduced ▪ Statistical tests assuming randomization can be used ▪ Blinding can be maintained	▪ Order in which treatments are administered may affect outcome ▪ Possibility of carry over effects ▪ Not suitable if treatment under study cures the disease or if treatment is effective only during a certain stage of disease ▪ Not suitable for the diseases which changes during the period of time required for the study. ▪ All subjects receive placebo or alternative treatment at some point ▪ Washout period lengthy or unknown ▪ Cannot be used for treatments with permanent effects ▪ Prolongs duration of trial

8. Occupational cancers.

- Occupational cancer (industrial cancers) is a serious problem in industry
- They differ from cancers in general population.

Characteristics

- Particular type of cancer is specific to a specific occupation
- Anatomical site of appearance of cancer is more or less fixed common to a particular occupational process and exposure
- They appear pretty long after exposure, may be 20–25 years
- They appear irrespective of continuation or cessation of exposure
- The age group affected is about a decade earlier compared to general population
- The early diagnosis through detection of precancerous lesions is possible and therefore are preventable
- Occupational carcinogens affect even population residing near industrial areas through air and water pollution
- Most commonly affected organs are skin, lungs, bladder and blood forming organs[Q].

OCCUPATIONAL CANCERS

a. Skin cancer	▪ Commonest[Q] of all occupational cancers (75%) ▪ Predominant type is squamous cell carcinoma[Q] ▪ Carcinogens incriminated include UV light, ionizing radiation, coal products, petroleum products, fuel oils, etc. ▪ Commonly occurs on exposed parts of body that have remained in direct contact with carcinogenic source ▪ Common sites are near hand cuffs, arm cuffs, neck, thigh above the knee, in between the thigh ▪ Workers with precancerous conditions like eczema, cracks and fissures on skin are more predisposed for development of cancer *Examples* ▪ Physical factors like exposure to sun and its ultraviolet rays over prolonged periods for long duration as in sailors and farmers can result in epitheliomas on exposed parts of skin ▪ Chemical agents in coal tar soot, asphalt, arsenic, benzene compounds, mineral oils are more likely to cause skin cancers in areas which are prone for being wet and friction in coal and gas worker, those using machine oil, spinning and oil, industry worker
b. Bladder cancer[Q]	▪ Increased incidence with rise in use of chemicals ▪ Carcinogens incriminated include aromatic amines such as aniline, naphthylamine[Q], benzidine, benzpyrene which are metabolised and excreted in urine ▪ Commonly seen in worker employed in rubber, shoe manufacturing, chemical, textile, gas, dyes, paints, plastics and synthetic polymer industries ▪ If manifests are sudden painless hematuria[Q] ▪ Most common type is transitional cell carcinoma (90%)[Q]
c. Lung cancer	▪ Respiratory passage from nose to alveoli may be affected by physical or chemical carcinogens in different industries ▪ In areas with high air pollution more prevalence of tobacco smoking and repeated attacks of respiratory infections the incidence is still higher ▪ Commonest type is squamous cell carcinoma of bronchus ▪ Industries using strong acids and alkalies have higher prevalence of sinus cancers ▪ In furniture workers nasal cancer is common ▪ Carcinoma bronchus in common in industries using or manufacturing chromium, nickel arsenic, aluminum, asbestos ▪ Lung cancer is also common industries mining hematite ore or uranium
d. Other cancers	▪ Leukemia and bone cancers are common with ionising radiations in mines, industrial and medical uses of radioactive energy, radium paints, benzene, vinyl chloride or rubber industry

Summery

Occupational cancer	*Occupation*	*Carcinogen*
a. Skin cancers[Q]	Gas work, oil refineries, tar distillation, road making, coke oven work	Anthracene, coal tar, soot, pitch, some oils, dyes, acids, UV rays, X-rays
b. Bladder cancer[Q]	Dye industry[Q], rubber/gas industry, electric cable making	B-naphthylamine, aniline dyes, aromatic amines, benzidine, auramine, magneta
c. Lung cancers[Q]	Asbestos factory, uranium mines, nickel-refineries, gas industry, tobacco industry	Arsenic, nickel[Q], asbestos, chromates, coal tar, tobacco, Radon[Q], Silica[Q]
d. Leukemia[Q]	Radiologists, radioactive mining, X-ray manufacture	Ionizing radiations, radioactive substances, X-ray, benzol

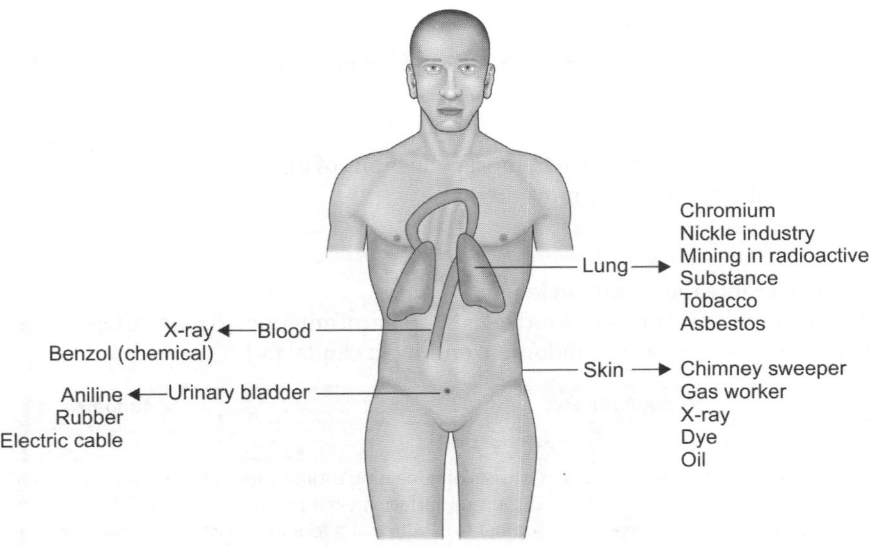

Fig. 4: Occupational cancers

PREVENTION AND CONTROL

a. Health Promotion	
i. Preplacement examination	▪ Consists of examination of individual for assessing his physical and psychological capacity, so as to place him in a suitable job (Ergonomics)
ii. Sanitation in working environment	▪ Good housekeeping, ventilation and cleanliness are mandatory in industries
iii. Health education	▪ To change their attitude towards cancer ▪ To know 'Danger signals' of cancers (Cancer education) ▪ To know hazards of smoking as an aggravating factor in dusty environment ▪ To maintain high standard of personal hygiene
iv. Control of dust in asbestos industry	
b. Specific Protection	
i. Primordial prevention	▪ Elimination or avoidance of carcinogens in industry ▪ Discouraging workers from adopting harmful lifestyle such as smoking
ii. Use of protective devices	▪ Masks in asbestos industry, lead apron, lead gloves and dark spectacles in radiology department ▪ Use of barrier creams in dyeing section of industry ▪ Worker safety by wearing 'Pocket dosimeter' for personal monitoring of radiation dose received ▪ Safety of machine by proper installation and maintenance of X-ray machine, use of efficient fitters so that unwarranted radiations are excluded. They are operated on high kilo-voltage with fast films, so that exposure is reduced to minimum dose
c. Early diagnosis and treatment	▪ Periodical examinations of at-risk group of industrial workers, especially in cancer clinics to detect lesions of early and curable stage ▪ Periodical examinations should be continued even after cessation of exposure to carcinogen ▪ Screening procedure consists of thorough physical examination followed by procedures like blood examination, urine examination, X-ray of chest, cytology, endoscopy and biopsy ▪ Treatment is given by chemotherapy, surgery, radiotherapy, hormonal therapy or immunotherapy depending upon type
d. Disability Limitation	▪ Consists of limiting the development of further disability by giving intensive treatment, when patients come in advanced stage
e. Rehabilitation	▪ Given for those who have become handicapped following major surgery such as amputation, lobectomy, etc. ▪ They are rehabilitated physically, socially, psychologically and vocationally

Significance

- Occupational cancers are very common constituting 5–10% of all cancers.

9. Cyclops.

- Cyclops or water flea is a crustacean present in most collections of fresh water
- It swims in water with characteristic jerky movements.

Morphology

- It is a tiny arthropod, not more than 1 mm in length
- It has a pear-shaped semitransparent body, a forked tail, 2 pairs of antennae, 5 pairs of legs and a small pigmented eye.
- It has broad cephalothorax and a narrow abdomen, ending in caudal fork.

Cephalothorax		***Abdomen***
Anterior part	***Posterior part***	
▪ Formed by fusion of head and first segment of thorax ▪ Anteriorly, there is a small, pigmented, single eye like that of giant of Greek mythology (thus the name) ▪ On either side of eye, are 2 pairs of antennae, first long is called antennules and second pair is short ▪ Antennules help in locomotion and seizing female during copualation ▪ On ventral surface, lie mouth, surrounded by two pairs of maxillae and one pair of mandible	▪ Consists of remaining thoracic segments ▪ On ventral surface are 6 thoracic segments of which first four bear each a pair of jointed feet with peddle like tips adapted for swimming in water, hence called swimming feet ▪ Fifth segment bears a pair of rudimentary feet ▪ Sixth and last thoracic segment bears genital aperture and is fused with first abdominal segment	▪ Composed of five distinct segments ▪ Fifth and last segment branches into two caudal forks and each fork terminates in a feathered filament or caudal hairs ▪ At junction of cephalothorax and abdomen in female cyclops, exists a bag like structure on either side called external ovisac or egg sac, in which eggs develop which is absent in male cyclops

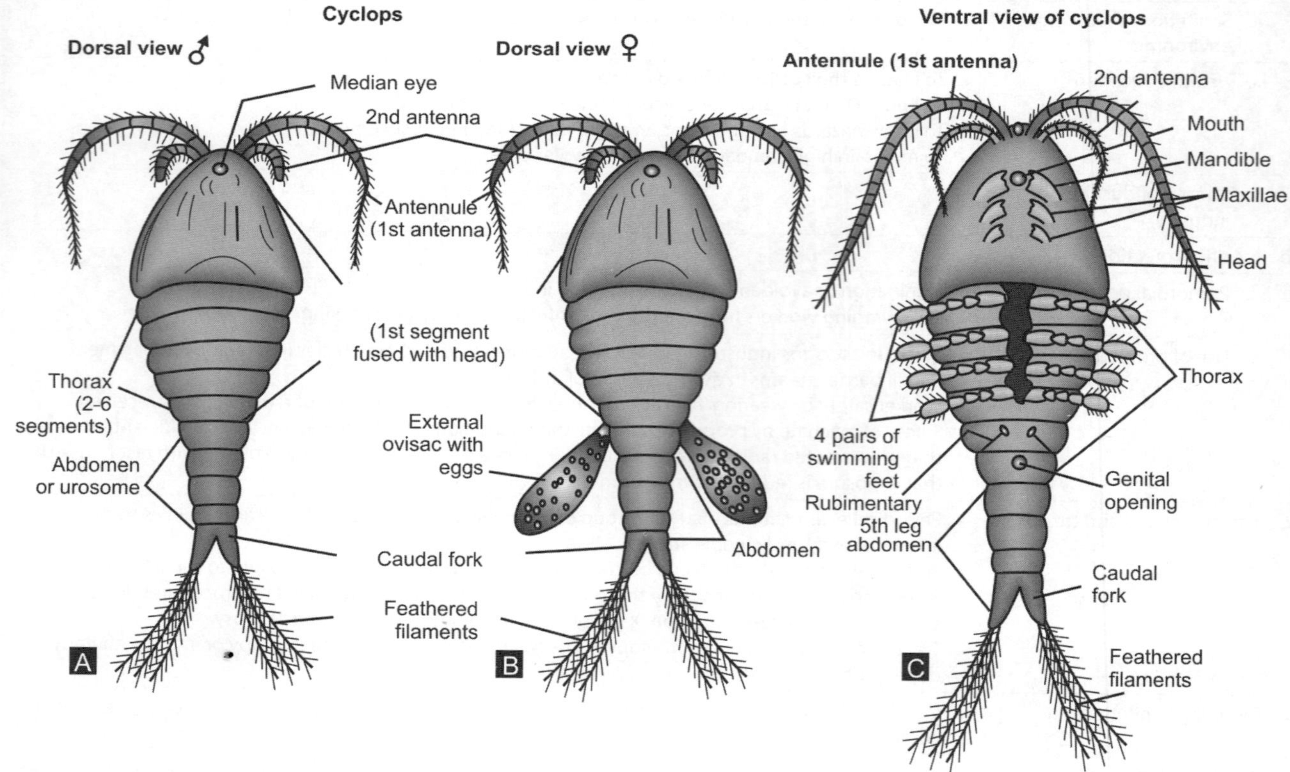

Fig. 5: Cyclops—morphology

Life Cycle

- Average life of a cyclops is about 3 months[Q]
- After copulation, eggs are fertilized in ovisac and sac gets detached from body of female cyclops
- Eggs come out of sac and are dispersed in water and hatch after 2–3 days releasing larvae
- Larva passes through two stages:

First stage	*Second stage*
▪ Called Nauplius, because of its resemblance to ships on sail ▪ Minute boat-shaped creature having a median eye and three pairs of legs ▪ Lasts for 5 days	▪ Called metanauplius ▪ Characterized by the addition of two more pairs of appendages and resembles adult ▪ Lasts for about 7 days

- Adult cyclops emerge from metanauplius and entire life cycle completes in 15 days, showing incomplete metamorphosis.

Control of Cyclops (Eradication of Guinea worm)

Physical (useful for individual prophylaxis)	*Chemical*	*Biological*	*Environmental*
▪ Filtration[Q] or straining through piece of fine cloth (double folded) ▪ Boiling at 60°C kills cyclops[Q]	▪ Chlorine[Q] (5 ppm of chlorine destroys cyclops and larvae of guinea worm) ▪ Lime (4 g of lime per gallon) ▪ Abate[Q] (an OP compound effective at a concentration of 1 mg/L)	▪ Fishes like barbell and gambusia feed on cyclops	▪ Abolish stepwells ▪ Provide piped water supply

Significance

- Cyclopes is intermediate host of dracunculus medinensis (guineaworm) and diphyllobothrium latum (fish tapeworm)
- Man acquires infection by drinking water with infected cyclops[Q]
- Control of cyclops was one of the important component of Guinea worm eradication program and its success.

10. Drug addiction

- Drug dependence is a state of psychic and sometimes also physical resulting from interaction between a living organism and a drug characterized by a behavioral and other responses that always include a compulsion to take the drug on a continuous or periodic basis in order to experience its psychic effects and sometimes to avoid discomfort of its absence (WHO).

Types

Psychological dependence	*Physical dependence*
▪ An overpowering desire to take the drug and obtain it by any means	▪ Withholding of drug causes withdrawal symptoms in form of irrational and violent behavior, nausea, vomiting, diarrhea, water of eye and nose, etc

Causes

Agent factors	*Host factors (Greatly responsible for drug dependence)*	*Social and environmental factors*
▪ Psychological dependence causing drugs do not disturb physiological activity and its withdrawal causes only apprehension or mental distress in user thus addiction liability is less and also easy to treat such persons ▪ Drugs causing psychological and physical dependence affects physiological activity of body on absence of drug thus addiction liability is more and hence such people are difficult to treat	▪ Physical and mental illness ▪ User's personality and mental make up ▪ Tolerance ▪ Threshold to different odds of life like failures or achievements ▪ Stress ▪ Emotional trends	▪ Family status ▪ Family environment ▪ Happenings in the family ▪ Family liability ▪ Attachment with family ▪ Social and mental status of friends and colleagues

Contd...

Contd...

Agent factors	***Host factors (Greatly responsible for drug dependence)***	***Social and environmental factors***
▪ Drugs causing dependence ▪ Alcohol ▪ Opioids ▪ Cannbinoids ▪ Sedative and hypnotics (Barbiturates) ▪ Cocaine ▪ Stimulants including caffeine ▪ Hallucinogens ▪ Tobacco ▪ Volatile solvents	▪ Habits and likingness ▪ Compulsive psychoeducational status ▪ Working engagements	▪ Capacity to meet social bindings and obligations ▪ Sense of responsibility towards family and society ▪ Residential and working environment

Predisposing Factors

- Therapeutic use of some drugs like morphine, pethidine may lead to addiction
- Once a drug is taken often even for recreational use, the user finds it difficult to do without it
- Repeated use to get relief from physical and mental exhaustion
- Use with desire to be freed from mental worry or distress
- Social structure and culture and influence of social environment
- Working conditions and influence of coworkers
- Economic factors
- Family structure, cohesion, environment, relation, culture, status
- Curiosity leading to repeated experimental use
- Status and influence of friends
- Environment in school, college or hostel
- Source and availability of the agent of the addiction
- Knowledge about immediate action of the drug
- Cost of the drug
- Handling drug as a peddler.

Manifestations

- Loss of interest in sports and daily routine
- Loss of appetite and body weight
- Unsteady gait, clumpsy movements, tremors
- Reddening and puffiness of eyes, unclear vision
- Slurring of speech
- Fresh, numerous injection marks on body and blood stains on clothes
- Nausea, vomiting and body pain
- Drowsiness or sleeplessness, lethargy and passivity
- Acute anxiety, depression, profuse sweating
- Changing mood, temper, tantrums
- Depersonalization and emotional detachment
- Impaired memory and concentration
- Presence of needles, syringes and strange packets at home.

Treatment

- Shift person to an institution to remove him from association with which addiction started
- Constant supervision
  - To assure nonuse of drug
  - To pay attention towards possible dangerous withdrawal symptoms
  - To prevent doing any harm to himself
  - To assure prevention of escape of the person

- Stop the supply of the drug of addiction
- Proper nursing care to improve general health
- Symptomatic treatment for ill health resulting from chronic use of drug
- Detoxification, i.e. reduction in dosage of drug over a period of 1–3 weeks
- Treatment of withdrawal symptoms, arising from the addiction
- Antidotes for prevention of use of the drug
- Administration of sedatives, benezidrine hyoscine
- Maintenance of adequate food intake, vitamins, electrolytes, etc.
- Mind diversion by engaging him physically and mentally in some occupation
- Giving proper education
- Psychotherapy to help develop personality, confidence and self respect
- Rehabilitation
  - Continuous process of weaning away the victims of drug dependency
  - Social rehabilitation and training for gainful employment are the most important components after weaning addicts away from drug dependence to prevent relapse.

Prevention and Control

Legal approach	*Education approach*	*Community approach*
▪ Legislation may be directed at controlling the manufacture, distribution, prescription, price, time of sale, or consumption of a substance ▪ Legislations to strong punishments for drug peddlers like "Narcotic Drugs and Psychotropic Substances Act"	▪ Education of target groups and the general public through TV, radio, leaflets and posters to create awareness	▪ Drug abuse can be prevented by provision of alternative activities that include establishment of groups or organizations interested in athletics, sports, music, public policy, religion, artistic activities of various kinds and improvement of environment through prevention of pollution ▪ NGOs play a crucial role in community approach

11. Chromosomal abnormalities.

- A chromosomal abnormality is an abnormality of chromosome number or structure
- Incidence of chromosomal abnormality is 5.6 per 1000 live births.[Q]

Cause	*Predisposing factors*
▪ Chromosome abnormalities usually occur when there is an error in cell division, i.e. mitosis and meiosis ▪ In both processes, correct number of chromosomes is supposed to end up in resulting cells ▪ However, errors in cell division can result in cells with too few or too many copies of a chromosome ▪ Errors can also occur when the chromosomes are being duplicated. ▪ Most commonly occur as an accident in egg or sperm; thus the abnormality is present in every cell of the body ▪ Some abnormalities, however, can happen after conception, resulting in mosaicism, where some cells have the abnormality and some do not ▪ Chromosome abnormalities can be inherited from a parent (such as a translocation) or be "de novo" (new to the individual)	▪ Advanced maternal age ▪ Women are born with all eggs they will ever have. Therefore, when a woman is 30 years old, so are her eggs ▪ Errors can crop up in eggs' genetic material as they age over time ▪ Therefore, older women are more at risk of giving birth to babies with chromosome abnormalities than younger women ▪ Since men produce new sperm throughout their life, paternal age does not increase risk of chromosome abnormalities ▪ Environment ▪ Although there is no conclusive evidence that specific environmental factors cause chromosome abnormalities, it is still a possibility that environment may play a role in occurrence of genetic errors

Types

a. Numerical abnormalities (non-dysjunction)
   - When an individual is missing either a chromosome from a pair (monosomy) or has more than two chromosomes of a pair (trisomy).

Examples
- Down syndrome (Trisomy 21)
- Turner syndrome (Monosomy X).

b. Structural abnormalities
- When chromosome's structure is altered

Type	Features
Deletions	A portion of chromosome is missing or deleted
Duplications	A portion of chromosome is duplicated, resulting in extra genetic material
Translocations	A portion of one chromosome is transferred to another chromosome Types: - Reciprocal translocation (segments from two different chromosomes have been exchanged) - Robertsonian translocation (an entire chromosome has attached to another at the centromere)
Inversions	A portion of chromosome has broken off, turned upside down and reattached, therefore genetic material is inverted
Rings	A portion of a chromosome has broken off and formed a circle or ring; with or without loss of genetic material.
Isochromosome	Formed by mirror image copy of a chromosome segment including the centromere

Ref:
http://www.genome.gov/11508982 - 6/18/2008
http://en.wikipedia.org/wiki/Chromosome_abnormalities - 6/18/2008

12. Cold chain equipment.

- Cold chain is a system of storage and transportation of vaccines at recommended, low temperature (+2° to +8°C) all along from the time and place of the manufacture to the time and place of its use.

Cold-chain System

- Cold-chain system consists of a series of transportation links with equipments and persons concerned from the manufacturer to the point of use
- Longer the chain, greater is the risk of cold-chain failure.

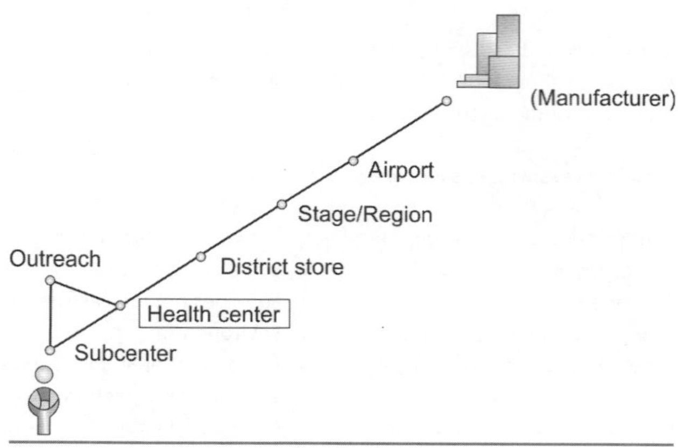

Fig. 6: Cold-chain system

Cold-chain Equipment

- Cold-chain equipment is so designed to keep cold air inside and to prevent warm air from entering, so when vaccines are placed inside these equipments, they are protected from heat and light.

Classification	*Equipment*	*Location*
a. Storage	Walk in coolers/Walk in freezer	At manufacturer
i. Electrical	Deep freezer	State and District HQ and Teaching Hospitals
	Refrigerators (Ice lined/conventional)	PHC, Urban Family Planning Centers, Postpartum Centers
ii. Solar	Refrigerators (battery drive/direct drive)	Subcenters
iii. Non-electrical	Vaccine carriers	Subcenter and Village level
	Cold box	For transportation
b. Transportation	Refrigerated/insulated vaccine van	Facility to facility transport
	Cold box/vaccine carrier/day carriers	In field

At Vaccine Institutes/Manufacturer

- Walk in coolers
  - Air conditioned cold rooms, maintaining temperature between +2° to +8°C.

  Applications
  - To store large bulk of vaccines

  Location
  - At manufacturer of vaccines i.e. Kasauli, Coonoor, Haffkine institute, etc.

At State and District Headquarters and Teaching Hospitals

- Deep Freezer
  - Top opening refrigerator, which maintains temperature at - 20° to - 40°C
  - Has electrical connections.

  Disadvantage
  - "T" series vaccines are never stored because they will be denatured
  - BCG vaccines are also not stored because ampoules may crack.

  Applications
  - To store only OPV and MV for long term use[Q]
  - To prepare ice-packs.

  Location
  - State and District headquarters and Teaching hospitals.

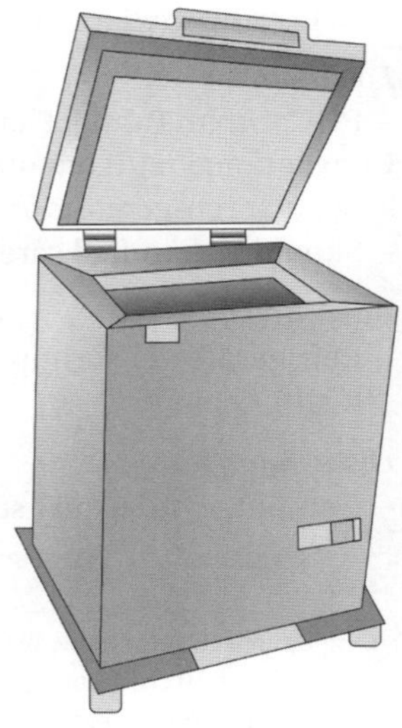

Fig. 7: Deep Freezer

At PHC, Urban Family Planning Centers, Postpartum Centers

- Ice-lined refrigerators
  - A top opening refrigerator.

  Types
  - Ice tubes lined (electrolux)
  - Ice packs lined (vest-frost).

  Features
  - Has single compartment for vaccine storage (0 to + 8°C) equipped with baskets and lined by preinstalled and water filled ice-lining ready for use
  - Works entirely as a cold-box with electrical connections
  - No freezer compartment in ILRs but electrolux type of ILR can also be used as deep freezer by changing the switch to appropriate position
  - Equipped with a "control panel" with:
    - Indicator- to indicate supply of electricity
    - Dial thermometer[Q]—to record temperature of compartment[Q]
    - Thermostat—to adjust inside temperature, from No. 1 to 8 signifying minimum to maximum cold
  - Bottom surface is the coldest place.

Do's
- Place vaccines in baskets because if kept directly on floor, they can freeze and get damaged
- Place water filled internal lids over the baskets
- Defrosting and cleaning once in 3 months for better performance because whenever it is opened, air enters and moisture settles on the inner cold surface and forms a layer of frost or ice
- Must be used only as a refrigerator for storing the vaccines.

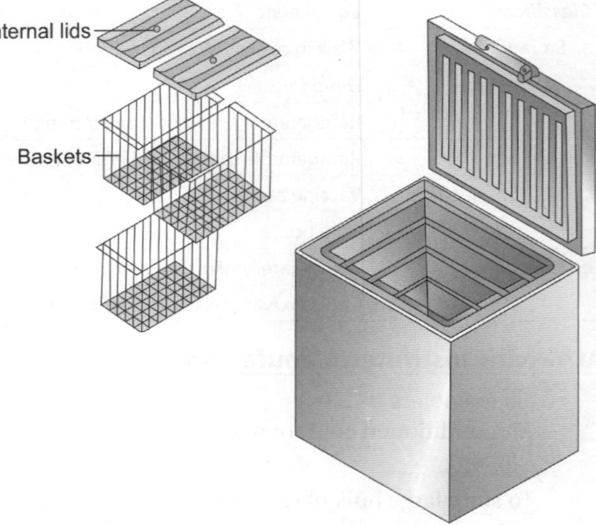

Fig. 8: Ice-lined refrigerators

Advantages
- Maintains cold life, during power failure, up to 18–20 hours/day
- Better than conventional refrigeration because risk of cold chain failure is far less, especially when there is periodic power failure
- Also the storage capacity is more.

Disadvantages
- Cannot be used to prepare ice-packs.

Location
- PHC, Urban Family Planning Centers, Postpartum Centers.

b. Conventional refrigerators
- Regular refrigerators found at every home
- Should be handled carefully so that temperature inside the cabinet does not rise above +8°C.

Advantages
- Refrigerator is so important in maintaining the cold chain that it is considered as one of the members of health team.

Disadvantages
- Gets out of order very soon only because of poor maintenance.

Do's	***Don'ts***
▪ Keep in a cool room away from direct sun light ▪ Should be 10 cm away from wall ▪ Level must be correct ▪ Plug must be properly and permanently fixed to the socket ▪ Voltage stabilizer to be used ▪ Vaccines should be placed in a definite order, neatly with space between the vials for free circulation of air ▪ If vaccines are stored in cartons, make sure there are holes in them for cold air circulation ▪ Should be opened only when necessary ▪ Ice-packs are placed in freezer compartment and water bottles in lowermost shelf, which act as buffer during power failure ▪ Defrosting is done periodically ▪ Temperature is recorded twice daily from a dial thermometer	▪ Do not open the door frequently and unnecessarily ▪ Do not keep the vaccines in the door ▪ Do not keep the food and drinks in the refrigerator ▪ Do not keep more than one month's requirements ▪ Do not keep "Date expired" vaccines

Location
- PHC, Urban Family Planning Centers, Postpartum Centers.

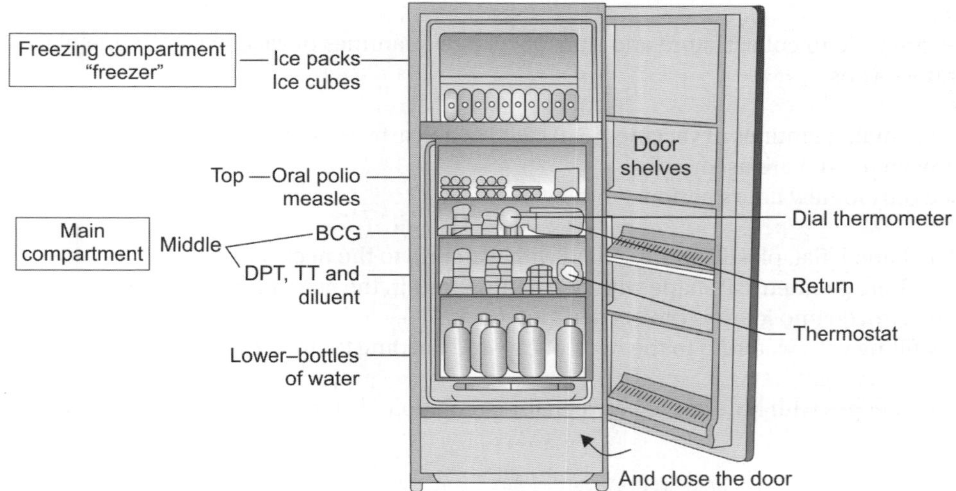

Fig. 9: Conventional refrigerators

At Subcenter and Village Level

- Vaccine carrier
  – A square shaped box, made up of a special insulated material, lined by 4 ice-packs, one on each side, which contains cold-life for 24 hours if not opened.

Do's	*Don'ts*
▪ Lid of the vaccine carrier should be secured tightly	▪ "T-series" of vaccines should not be in direct contact with ice packs, because they get frozen. Therefore, those vaccines are placed inside a polythene bag and closed with rubber band ▪ It should not be kept in the sun-light nor should be opened frequently and unnecessarily

Applications

– Used to carry small quantities of vaccines from primary health center or subcenter to the out-reach station (i.e. immunization camp), by the health worker.

Solar Cold Chain Equipment

a. Solar refrigerator battery drive
   – Similar to regular refrigerator except uses low voltage DC compressor which runs on battery charged by solar energy

   Features
   – Has good PUF insulation around storage compartments to maximize energy efficiency
   – Has two separate compartment, i.e.
     - Refrigerator (2–8°C) for storage of vaccines and does not have ON/OFF switch
     - Freezer (up to –7°C) for storing frozen icepacks and has ON/OFF switch (to allow defrosting).

b. Solar refrigerator direct drive
   – These refrigerators are directly connected to photovoltic generators thus directly use sun's energy to freeze water and use cooling from these frozen ice banks to cool the refrigerator during night and cloudy days.

For Transportation

a. Cold box
   – A big, rectangular box (90 cm × 60 cm) made up of an insulated material (bad conductor of heat), lined with 24 ice-packs, which act as buffers and maintain the cold life inside the box for about 5 days
   – Does not have electrical connections.

Applications
- Such boxes are used to collect, store and transport large quantities of vaccines from one place to another place by refrigerator—vans.

b. Day carriers
  - Used to carry small quantities of vaccines (6–8 vials) to a nearby session
  - Two fully frozen packed are used
  - Can be used only for few hours period.

c. Ice packs
  - Rectangular shaped, flat, plastic bottles, filled with water up to the neck
  - They have definite geometrical shape with two depressions in the center for finger grip
  - When water is frozen into ice, it is then called "Ice-pack"
  - Prepared by filling with water up to the neck of cap and keeping them in deep freezers and freezer compartment of refrigerator overnight
  - Placed on their edges with little space between for circulation of air and not flat on one another.

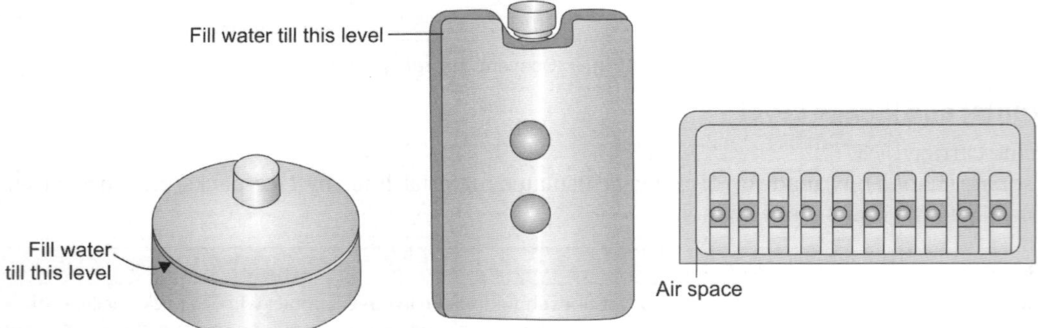

Fig. 10: Ice packs

Advantages
- Maintain cold-life for 5 days in cold box and for 1 day in vaccine carrier, if it is not opened.

Applications
- Used for lining walls of cold boxes and vaccine carriers, as buffers to maintain cold life inside the equipment.

Significance

- Cold chain system of maintaining cold-life for vaccines is necessary because vaccines are sensitive to heat and light, i.e. they lose their potency, when exposed to heat and light
- Once vaccine loses its potency, it cannot be restored and it becomes a waste.
- So care must be taken to see that the vaccines do not lose their potency, before the date of expiry, by maintaining Cold-chain
- All the vaccines retain their potency at temperatures between +2° and +8°[Q] and any fluctuation of temperature above or below this is considered cold chain failure
- The sensitivity of the vaccines in the descending order is as follows:

Vaccines sensitive to heat (in order)	***Vaccines sensitive to freezing***
▪ Can be stored at sub-zero temperature for long term use[Q]	
▪ BCG (after reconstitution) ▪ OPV ▪ Measles	▪ HepB ▪ DPT ▪ DT ▪ TT
Cannot be stored at sub-zero temperature	
▪ DPT ▪ BCG (before reconstitution)—cracks at sub-zero temperature ▪ DT ▪ Hep B ▪ JE ▪ TT (Least sensitive)	

- Risk of cold chain failure is greatest at subcenter and village level[Q] hence proper training should be provided to peripheral health workers.

SHORT ANSWERS

13. Human Genome Project.

- Human Genome Project (HGP) was an international scientific research project with a primary goal to determine the sequence of chemical base pairs which make up DNA[Q] and to identify the approximately 20,000–25,000 genes of the human genome[Q] from both a physical and functional standpoint.
- It began in 1990 initially headed by James D Watson
- A working draft of the genome was released in 2000 and a complete one in April 2003[Q], with further analysis still being published
- Preliminary count indicates about 20,000–23,000 genes in human genome.

Objective

- To understand the genetic makeup of the human species and complete map of all findings.

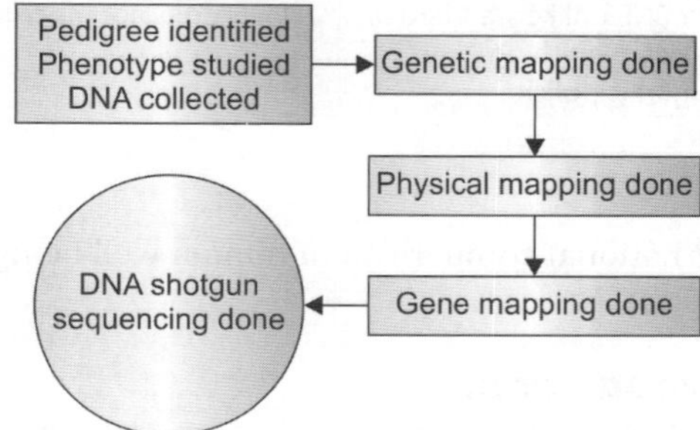

Fig. 11: Steps of Human Genome Project

Applications in Medicine

- Study of individual gene and its function
- Can show predisposition to a variety of illnesses, including breast cancer, cystic fibrosis, liver diseases and many others
- Deeper understanding of the disease processes at the level of molecular biology may determine new therapeutic procedures
- Help understand Genetic migration, genetic drift and genetic selection.

Ref: http://en.wikipedia.org/wiki/Human_Genome_Project dated 16th Nov. 2008

14. Effects of air pollution.

Refer Question No. 5 December 2014 (RS2) Paper I.

15. Hazards of immunization (adverse events following immunization).

Refer Question No. 2 December 2016 (RS2) Paper I.

16. Physical quality of life index.

- Physical quality of life index[Q] (PQLI) is a composite index which attempts to measure something which is difficult to measure quality of life
- It measures living standard of people[Q]
- It consolidates three different indicators which measure results rather than inputs.

Components[Q]

- Infant mortality rate[Q]

- Life expectancy at age one[Q]
- Literacy.[Q]

Calculation

- For each of component, performance of individual countries is placed on scale of 0 to 100, where 0 represents an absolutely worst performance, 100 represent an absolutely defined best performance and 50 represents average performance
- Composite index is calculated by averaging the three indicators, giving equal weightage to each of them
- The resulting PQLI thus is also scaled on 0 to 100.
  i. IMR weightage is on the scale of 0 to 100. IMR of 220/1000 live births is 0 and IMR of 7/1000 live births is 100. This is referred as A.
  ii. The weightage of life expectancy at age 1 is on the scale of 1 to 100. At 38 years it is 0 and at 77 years it is 100. This is referred as B.
  iii. Actual literacy rate is considered and is referred as C.
- Thus PQLI = A + B + C/3

Merits	*Demerits*
▪ PQLI does not depend upon per capita GNP unlike standard of living thereby showing that "money is not everything". ▪ PQLI measures result of social and economic policies	▪ PQLI does not measure economic growth

Significance

- PQLI is used for national and international comparison of human well being and ultimate objective is to achieve PQLI of 100.

17. Screening for diseases in blood bank.

- As per WHO guidelines regulating blood banks, any donor blood should be screened for following diseases to prevent their transmission to the patient:
  - ELISA test for HIV type 1 and 2 viruses
  - ELISA test for Hepatitis B and C viruses
  - VDRL test for syphilis
  - Peripheral smear for malarial parasites
  - Tests for Chagas disease and brucellosis.

18. Advantages and limitations of animal experiments.

- Animal experiments have contributed to our medical knowledge immensely
- However, like other studies they too have their advantages and limitations.

Advantages	*Limitations*
▪ Experimental animals can be breed in laboratories ▪ They can be manipulated easily as per the wishes of the investigators ▪ They multiply rapidly and enable the investigators to carry out certain experiments like genetic experiments which may take several years involving several generations in humans	▪ Not all human diseases can be reproduced in animals ▪ All conclusions derived from the animal experiments may not be strictly applicable to human beings

19. Tools of measurement of disease magnitude.

Refer Question No. 3 December 2015 (RS2) Paper I.

20. Give some examples of screening tests.

Refer Question No. 1 December 2010 (RS2) Paper I.

21. Relationship between incidence and prevalence.

Refer Question No. 3 June 2014 (RS2) Paper I.

22. Rodenticides.

- Rodenticides are chemical substances which are lethal to rats.

Types

Single dose (acute)	*Multiple dose (cumulative)*
▪ Lethal to rats after a single feeding ▪ Example: Zinc phosphide, barium carbonate	▪ Require repeated feedings over a period of 3 more days ▪ Example: Warfarin, courmfuryl

Classification (Examples)

Require ordinary care	*Require maximal precaution*	*Too dangerous for use*
▪ Red squill ▪ Norbromide ▪ Zinc phosphide	▪ Sodium fluorocetate ▪ Fluoroacetamide ▪ Strychnine	▪ Arsenic trioxide ▪ Phosphorus ▪ Thallium sulfate ▪ ANTU ▪ Gophacide

Commonly Used Rodenticides

	Barium carbonate	*Zinc phosphide*[Q]	*Warfarin, diphacinone, coumafuryl and pindone*
▪ Properties	▪ A white tasteless powder ▪ Baits are made by mixing it with wheat or rice flour in ratio of 1 part to 4 parts of flour and moistened with water and made into small round marbles ▪ Baits are placed near rat burrows and in dark, secluded places ▪ Fatal time is 2–24 hours	▪ When moist, zinc phosphide slowly gives off phosphine whose garlic odour is repellent to man and domestic animals, but seems to have no adverse effect on rats ▪ Used in ratio of 1 part to 10 parts of wheat or rice flour and mixed with a few drops of edible oil in order to render it more attractive to rats ▪ Fatal time is 3 hours	▪ Multiple dose poisons ▪ Cause internal haemorrhage and slow death (anticoagulant action) ▪ Fatal time is 4-10 days
▪ Advantages	▪ Cheap	▪ Good safety record ▪ Low cost ▪ Reasonably high effectiveness	
▪ Disadvantages	▪ Weak rodenticide of uneven performance ▪ Probably easily detected by rats in many baits	▪ Highly poisonous—requires use of rubber gloves for handling	▪ Appearance of resistance due to continued use

MBBS PHASE III EXAMINATION

DECEMBER 2007

(Revised Scheme 2)

PAPER II

LONG ESSAYS

1. What are the common causes of under 5 mortality in India? Describe the measures taken to ensure child survival in India.

- Under five mortality is the annual number of deaths of children under 5 years, expressed as a rate per 1000 live births.

$$\text{Child mortality rate} = \frac{\text{Number of deaths of children less than 5 years of age in a given year}}{\text{Numner of live births in the same year}} \times 1000$$

Current Statistics (India)

- 43 per 1000 live births (SRS 2015).

Common Causes of under 5 Mortality

a. Neonatal causes (37%)
   - Preterm birth (28%)
   - Severe infections (26%)
   - Birth asphyxia (23%)
   - Congenital anomalies (8%)
   - Neonatal tetanus (7%)

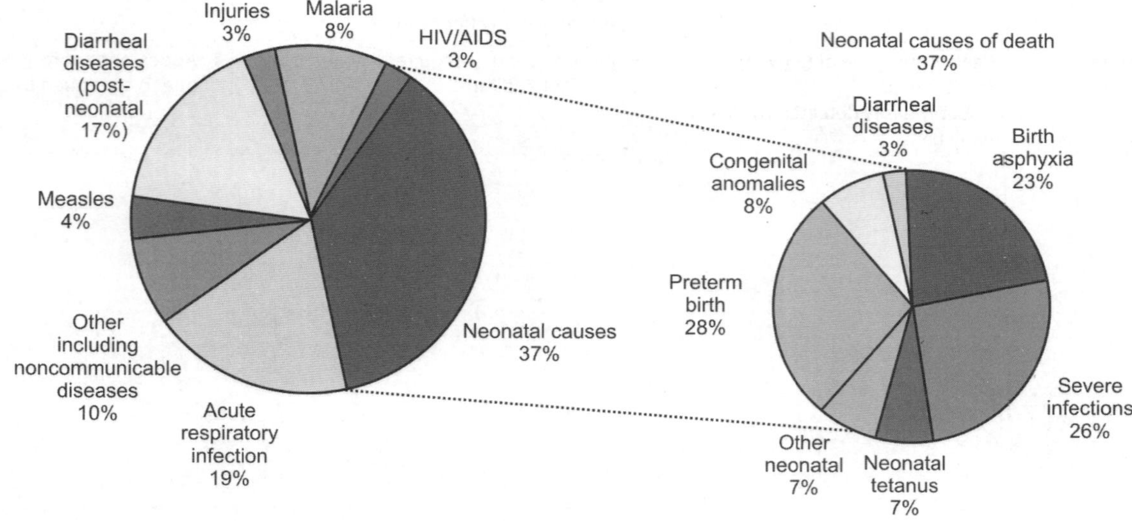

Fig. 1: Under 5 mortality—causes

 - Other causes (7%)
 - Diarrhea (3%).

b. Acute lower respiratory infections[Q] (19%)—Pneumonia (single most common cause)
c. Diarrhea—post-neonatal (17%)
d. Others including non-communicable (10%)
e. Malaria (8%)
f. Measles (4%)
g. Injuries (3%)
h. HIV/AIDS (3%).

Measures to Ensure Child Survival in India

a. Expanded program on immunization
 - Expanded program on immunization provides wide range of vaccination protecting child from major vaccine preventable diseases like tuberculosis, measles, polio, diphtheria, pertussis, tetanus
 - More recently pentavalent vaccine (DPT, Hep B and Hib), rotavirus vaccine, IPV have been added to the program
 - There is also launch of immunization strengthening project
 - This one measure alone has increased the child survival significantly.

b. Oral rehydration therapy
 - Widespread introduction of cheap and effective oral rehydration therapy has contributed largely to reducing the number of death from diarrhea
 - This has made management of diarrhea easy and possible at home by mothers.

c. ARI control program
 - With control in deaths due to vaccine preventable diseases and diarrhea, pneumonia turned out to be forerunner in the under 5 mortality cause
 - With introduction of acute respiratory infection control program, which simplified diagnostic and treatment technique, the deaths due to pneumonia are also brought under control.

d. Breastfeeding promotion
 - Breastfeeding especially during neonatal period offers many advantages and improves child survival
 - Antibodies in mother's milk protect the infant from numerous infectious diseases
 - Breastfeeding in infancy also protects child from malnutrition in childhood
 - Govt. of India is considering a policy for exclusive breastfeeding up to 6 months of age.

e. RCH program
 - This program has an exclusive component of child care to improve child survival
 - Under the program there is provision for organizing of RCH camps, health melas and RCH outreach scheme to reach disadvantageous segments of population.

f. Newborn care
 - New born care facilities are operationalised in identified weak districts
 - Operations research by ICMR for provision of home-based neonatal care through community level providers.

g. Safe delivery practices
 - Preparation and approval of concept note on development of community based midwives
 - Implementation of Dai training to provide key message for newborn health in 166 districts.

h. Integrated management of childhood illness
 - This is the recent program which addresses the principal cause of child mortality, i.e. diarrheal diseases, acute respiratory infection, measles, malaria and underlying malnutrition.
 - It combines effective interventions for preventing death and for improving healthy growth and development like oral rehydration therapy for diarrhea, antibiotics for sepsis, pneumonia and ear infections, antimalarials and insecticide treated bed nets, vitamin A, treatment of anemia, promotion of breastfeeding and complementary feeding for healthy nutrition and for recovery of illness and immunization.

Significance

- Under five mortality and child survival index is some of the best indicator of social development and well being rather than GNP per capita as they reflects income, nutrition, healthcare and basic education
- UNICEF considers under 5 mortality as single best indicator of socioeconomic development and well being[Q].

2. What is a "community health center"? Describe how healthcare is delivered to a population covered by a community development block.

- Community health center is an upgraded primary health center, one for each community development block, covering a population of 80,000–1,20,000 distributed over 100 villages[Q] covering area of 770 sq Km spread over radial distance of 15.6 Km.
- Also called first referral unit[Q] (FRU)
- One out of four PHCs is upgraded to CHC
- It acts as referral center for 4 PHCs.[Q]

Facilities

- 30 beds for in-patients[Q]
- Specialist services like surgery, medicine, obstetrics and gynecology and pediatrics[Q]
- X-ray facility
- Laboratory facility
- Blood bank.

Staffing Pattern (Total = 30-31[Q])

Existing clinical manpower (4[Q])

• General surgeon	1
• Physician	1
• Obstetrician/Gynecologist	1
• Pediatrician	1
Proposed clinical manpower (Under NHRM[Q])	
• Anesthetist (essential for utilization of surgical facilities)	1
• Eye surgeon (for every 5 lakh population as per Vision 2020 program)	1
Existing Non-clinical manpower	
• Community health officer (for strengthening preventive and promotive aspect of heath care)	1
Proposed Non-clinical manpower (Under NHRM[Q])	
• Public health program manager or Block Surveillance officer (for surveillance, coordination of national health programs, ASHA training, etc.)	1
Existing support manpower	
• Nurse—midwife	7 + 2
• Dresser	1
• Pharmacist	1
• Laboratory technician	1
• Radiographer	1
• Ophthalmic assistant	0-1
• Ward boy	2
• Sweepers	3
• Chowkidar	
• OPD attendant	
• Statistical assistant/Data entry operator	5
• OT attendant	
• Registration clerk	

Functions (Healthcare Delivery)

a. Care of routine and emergency case in surgery
   - This includes incision and drainage and surgery for hernia, hydrocele, appendicitis, hemorrhoids, fistula, etc
   - Handing of emergencies like intestinal obstruction, hemorrhage, etc.
b. Care of routine and emergency cases in medicine
c. 24 hours delivery services, including normal and assisted deliveries
d. Essential and emergency obstetric care including surgical interventions like cesarean sections and other medical interventions
e. Full range of family planning services including laparoscopic services
f. Safe abortion services
g. Newborn care
h. Routine and emergency care of sick children
i. Other management, including nasal packing, tracheostomy, foreign body removal etc
j. Delivery of all the national health programs and integration of existing programs to provide comprehensive services
   i. RNTCP
      - Provide diagnostic services through microscopy centers and treatment services as per the technical and operational guidelines
   ii. HIV/AIDS Control Program
      - Services under this program are also provided
   iii. National Vector Borne Disease Control Program
      - Provide diagnostic and treatment facilities for routine and complicated cases of malaria, filaria, dengue, Japanese encephalitis and kala azar in the respective endemic zones.
   iv. National Leprosy Eradication Program
      - Provide minimum services like diagnosis and treatment of cases and reactions of leprosy along with advice to patient on prevention of deformity
   v. National Program for Control of Blindness
      - Eye care services like diagnosis and treatment of common diseases, refraction services and surgical services including cataract surgery by IOL implantation at selected community health centers should be available.
   vi. Integrated disease surveillance project
      - Services for diagnosis for malaria, tuberculosis, typhoid and tests for detection of fecal contamination of water and chlorination level should be made available at community health centers
      - It will function as peripheral surveillance unit and collate, analyze and report information to district surveillance unit
      - It should initiate appropriate action in outbreak situation.
k. Others
   - Blood storage facility
   - Essential laboratory services
   - Referral or transport services.

Funding

- Community health centers are maintained by the state government under minimum needs program or basic minimum services program.

SHORT ESSAYS

3. What control measures would you recommend for control of chikungunya outbreak?

- Chikungunya is a viral fever caused by chikungunya virus, a group A virus
- It is transmitted by *Aedes, Culex* and *Mansonia* mosquitoes.

Control of Outbreak

Primary prevention	
a. Vector control (*Aedes aegypti* is the main target vector)	
i. Reduction of breeding places	▪ Keeping water storage containers free of mosquitoes and eliminating the breeding places of mosquitoes like stagnant water in and around houses
ii. Antilarval measures (useful to prevent epidemics)	▪ Using Abate, an organophosphorus insecticide which prevents breeding up to 3 months when applied on sand granules
iii. Antiadult measures (useful during an epidemic)	▪ Malathion or sumithion as aerosol spray of ultra low volume (250 mL/hectare) interrupts transmission and stops epidemics ▪ Tiny droplets of aerosol kills mosquitoes in the air as well as on water
iv. Personal protective measures	▪ Reducing exposure to mosquitoes by using mosquito nets and mats ▪ Use of repellents like DEET
b. Vaccination	▪ No vaccine is available
Secondary prevention	▪ Treatment of disease when it occurs ▪ Anti-inflammatory drugs for arthralgia ▪ Adequate bed rest and passive movements of joints to prevent stiffness ▪ Symptomatic treatment
Tertiary prevention	▪ Treatment of complications if any

4. Briefly discuss "National Program for Prevention of Blindness".

Refer Question No. 2 Dec. 2015 (RS2) Paper II.

5. Contribution of cultural, social and ecological factors to PEM in the community.

Refer Question No. 1 Dec. 2008 (RS2) Paper I.

6. How would you do counseling for a newly married couple for family planning?

- Counseling is a key component of family planning services
- Family planning counseling is an essential component of protection and supporting every person's right to make voluntary, informed decisions about sexuality and reproduction
- Proper and methodological counseling can help ensure correct use of and satisfaction with a chosen contraceptive method.

Services Offered During Family Planning Counseling

- Information: To understand the advantages and availability of family planning
- Access: To be able to obtain services, regardless of race, creed, social status or lifestyle
- Choice: To make decisions freely regarding family planning and contraceptive methods
- Safety: To practice safe and effective family planning
- Privacy: Access to a private space for receiving counseling and services
- Confidentiality: To be certain that any personal information will be kept confidential
- Dignity: To be treated with courtesy, consideration and complete attention
- Comfort: To feel comfortable when receiving services
- Continuity: To receive family planning services and supplies at the times when they are necessary
- Opinion: To express points of view regarding the services being offered.

Strategy

A family planning counselor should:

- Create a comfortable atmosphere for family planning users
- Have respect for the values and attitudes of users
- Present information clearly

- Encourage the formulation of questions
- Listen and observe attentively
- Be impartial or neutral
- Ask questions in a manner that encourages clients to share information and feelings
- Facilitate effective counselor-user interaction
- Speak the language of the client.

Topics to be Covered During Counseling in Regards to Individual Contraceptive Method

Intrauterine devices (IUDs)	*Barrier methods*	*Hormonal contraceptives*
▪ Characteristics of IUDs ▪ Current and possible future risk of contracting sexually transmitted infections (STIs) ▪ Mechanism of action and effectiveness of IUDs ▪ Procedures for inserting and extracting IUDs ▪ Instructions for use and follow-up visits ▪ Signs of possible complications ▪ Common side effects of IUDs	▪ How to use the method correctly ▪ Importance of regular/systematic use ▪ Ways to incorporate methods into intercourse (where appropriate) ▪ Common problems (and their solutions) associated with use ▪ Where to obtain additional supplies	▪ Possible changes in menstrual cycle, particularly prolonged or excessive bleeding, or amenorrhea ▪ Significance of amenorrhea ▪ Delays in return to fertility ▪ Need for regular and timely injections ▪ Lack of protection against STDs/HIV ▪ Other side effects ▪ Need to speak with providers about any particular concerns and need to return to clinic should any problems arise

Significance

- Family planning counseling helps the newly wed to make informed choices about your reproductive options and contraceptive methods and they learn about using a chosen method safely and effectively.

Ref:

Family Planning Counseling: A curriculum prototype; participant's handbook, AVSC International, New York, 1995. Contraceptive Technology Update (CTU) series, Family Health International, Research Triangle Park, NC.

7. What are the salient features of the National Population Policy?

- National Population Policy refers to policies intended to decrease the birth rate or growth rate
- Their common objective was improving quality of lives, enhancing the well being of the people and to provide them opportunities to become productive assets in society
- The National Population Policy 2000 is to be largely implemented at panchayat or nagar palika level with co-ordination of the state and union territory administration.

Objectives of National Population Policy

Immediate objectives	*Medium term objectives*	*Long term objectives*
▪ To provide integrated service delivery for basic reproductive and child healthcare ▪ To address unmet needs for contraception, healthcare infrastructure and health personal	▪ To bring total fertility rate to replacement levels (TFR = 2.1) by 2010[Q], through vigorous implementation of intersectoral operational strategies	▪ To achieve a stable population by 2045[Q], at a level consistent with requirement of sustainable social and economic growth

National Sociodemographic Goals to be Achieved by 2010

- Address unmet needs for basic reproductive and child health services, supplies and infrastructure
- Making school education up to age 14 free and compulsory and measures to reduce drop out rate below 20% for boys and girls
- Reduction of crude birth rate to 21 per 1000 population[Q]
- Reduction of infant mortality rate to below 30 per 1000 live births[Q]
- Reduction of maternal mortality rate to below 100 per 100,000 live births[Q]
- 100% immunization coverage against all vaccine preventable diseases
- Promote delayed marriage for girls not earlier than 18 years of age, preferably after 20 years of age[Q]
- Achieve 80% institutional deliveries and 100% by traditional birth attendants[Q]

- Achieve 100% registration of births, deaths, marriages and pregnancies[Q]
- Contain the spread of AIDS, management of reproductive tract infections, RTI and STDs
- Prevention and control of communicable diseases
- Integrate Indian system of medicine in the provision of RCH services and in reaching out to households
- Promote vigorously the small family norm[Q]
- Achieve universal access to IEC activities for fertility regulation and contraception
- Address the unmet needs for basic RCH services, supplies and infrastructure.

Strategic Themes

- Decentralizing planning and program implementation
- Convergence of service delivery at village level
- Empowering women for improved health and nutrition
- Child health and survival
- Meeting the unmet needs for family welfare services
- Underserved population groups:
  - Urban slums
  - Tribal communities, migrant population
  - Adolescents
  - Increased participation of men in planned parenthood
- Diverse healthcare providers
- Collaboration with NGOs and private sectors with commitment
- Mainstreaming Indian system of medicine and homeopathy
- Contraceptive technology and research on RCH
- Providing for geriatric population
- IEC activities—information, education and communication.

Promotion of Small Family Norms Through Promotional and Motivational Measures

- Panchayat and Zilla parishads will be rewarded for exemplary performance in universalizing small family norm and achieving reduced infant mortality rate, crude birth rate, promoting literacy
- Balika Samridhi Yojana providing cash incentive of ₹ 500 for birth of girl child at 1st and 2nd delivery
- Maternity Benefit Scheme providing cash incentive of ₹ 500 for mothers delivering their 1st and 2nd child above the age of 19 years[Q]
- Health Insurance Plan not exceeding ₹ 5000 for entire family for couple below poverty line upon sterilization after 1 or 2 child
- Rewards for couples below poverty line who marry after legal age of marriage, register their marriage, delivers after the age of 21 years, accepts small family norms and adopts terminal method after the birth of 2nd child
- Revolving fund for income generating activities by village level self-help groups
- Mother and child care centers in rural, urban slums to help women to participate in employment
- Strengthening of facilities of safe abortion
- Provision of ambulance services
- Availability of wider and affordable choices of contraceptives
- Innovative social marketing schemes for making products and services affordable
- Increased vocational training schemes for girls leading to self employment
- Soft loans at village levels
- Strict enforcement of Child Marriage Restraint Act, 1976
- Strict enforcement of Prenatal Diagnostic Technique Act, 1994.

Importance

- The National Population Policy 2000 drawn up by the Department of Family Welfare
  - Provides reliable and relevant policy framework for improving quality and coverage
  - Measures and monitors the delivery of family welfare program so as to enable increasingly literate and aware families to achieve their reproductive goals and the country to achieve rapid population stabilization

- Simultaneously aims at promoting synergy with the ongoing educational, infotechnology and socioeconomic transition so that India can achieve not only rapid population stabilization but also sustainable development, improvement in economic, social and human development in the new millennium.

8. Screening of school children under school health program.

Refer Question No. 4 Dec. 2013 (RS2) Paper II.

9. Vaccination for international travelers.

- International travelers may be at risk from a variety of potentially severe and life-threatening infections
- Some of these diseases are preventable, and vaccination remains a cornerstone of travel medicine.

Objectives

i. For the traveler, to prevent the risk of contracting an endemic disease during his stay abroad
ii. For the community to prevent the risk of importing an infectious agent yet unknown in the country (Exotic infection)

- To protect travelers from illnesses present in other parts of the world and to prevent importation of infectious diseases across international borders various international agencies have suggested vaccination for international travelers
- Which vaccinations you need depends on a number of factors including your destination, whether you will be spending time in rural areas, season of the year you are traveling, your age, health status, and previous immunizations

Categories

Routine vaccinations	*Recommended vaccinations*	*Required vaccination*
▪ Vaccinations against infections still common in most parts of the world ▪ If person is immunized with these vaccines then he should take booster doses to maintain protection	▪ Country specific vaccinations, i.e. certain countries require special vaccination before entering those countries	▪ These vaccines are must for international travel and should be accompanied by certificate of vaccination ▪ Only vaccine required by International Health Regulations is yellow fever vaccination for travel to certain countries in sub-Saharan Africa and tropical South America ▪ Meningococcal vaccination is required by government of Saudi Arabia for annual travel during the Haj

Status in India

- In India, Yellow fever vaccination certificate is must if the traveler is traveling from an endemic zone and also required for travelers arriving from or transiting from
  - **Africa:** Angola, Benin, Burkina Faso, Burundi, Cameroon, Central African Republic, Chad, Congo, Côte d'Ivoire, Democratic Republic of Congo, Equatorial Guinea, Ethiopia, Gabon, Gambia, Ghana, Guinea, Guinea- Bissau, Kenya, Liberia, Mali, Niger, Nigeria, Rwanda, São Tomé and Principe, Senegal, Sierra Leone, Somalia, Sudan, Togo, Uganda, Tanzania, and Zambia
  - **America:** Bolivia, Brazil, Colombia, Ecuador, French Guiana, Guyana, Panama, Peru, Suriname, and Venezuela
  - **Caribbean:** Trinidad and Tobago
- Any person (except infants ≤6 months) arriving without a certificate within 6 days of departure from or transit through an endemic area will be isolated for up to 6 days.

Ref:
http://wwwn.cdc.gov/travel/contentVaccinations.aspx - 6/18/2008
Marchou B, Picot N, Massip P.; Vaccinations of the traveler (Article in French); Ann Med Interne (Paris). 1998 Oct;149(6):332-9.
Kirkpatrick BD, Alston WK.; Current immunizations for travel; Curr Opin Infect Dis. 2003 Oct;16(5):369-74.

10. Job description of multipurpose health worker (female).

- Female multipurpose health worker is an auxiliary nurse midwife
- She is the front line staff and key person to deliver MCH services in the rural areas
- She is posted to sub-center to cover a population of about 5000 in areas in plains and 3000 in hilly or tribal areas
- Their salary is paid by the Central Govt.

Job Description

a. Record keeping (maintain following registers)
   - Antenatal register: Registers names of all pregnant mothers of her area, from 12th week of amenorrhea onwards and enters details of antenatal care provided
   - Postnatal register: Registers names of all postnatal mothers and details of postnatal check up
   - Under five children register: Registers names of all under five children in her area and enters details of the services provided, mainly immunization
   - Clinic attendance register
   - Eligible couple register: Registers names of all married women, in reproductive age group
   - Home visiting register
   - Birth and death registers[Q]
   - Family planning register: Registers about distribution of OC pills, condoms, tubectomies and vasctomies conducted and IUD fitted.

b. Antenatal care (at home and at subcenter)

   Care at home
   - She visits expectant mother's house at least 4–5 times and more often if mother is at high risk and gives advice on nutrition, exercise, rest, personal hygiene, cleanliness and sensitizes on family planning and breastfeeding

   Care at clinic
   - She distributes iron and folic acid tables to pregnant and nursing mothers
   - She immunize pregnant mothers with tetanus toxoid[Q].

c. Intranatal care
   - She conducts 50% of total deliveries in her area[Q]
   - She supervises deliveries conducted by dais and wherever called in
   - She recognizes danger signals during labor[Q] and refers all such cases to nearest primary health center.

d. Postnatal care
   - She pays at least 3–5 visits to newly delivered mother at home
   - She gives advice on early ambulation, nutrition, breastfeeding, personal hygiene and also motivates the mother for family planning.

e. Family planning services
   - She distributes conventional contraceptives and oral pills to newly married couples[Q]
   - She identifies eligible couples and motivates women for IUD insertion
   - She identifies target couples and motivates them for sterilization
   - She provides follow-up services to family planning adopters, identifies side effects, gives treatment on spot for side effects or minor complications and refers cases requiring specialized attention to the nearest PHC
   - She indentifies cases requiring help for medical termination of pregnancy[Q], provides information on the availability of services and refer them to the nearest approved MTP center
   - She will set up women depot holders for distribution of conventional contraceptives.

f. Care of children
   - She identifies infants of her area and assesses their growth and development, by plotting their weight on Road to Health card
   - She arranges for primary immunization with BCG, DPT, Polio and Measles vaccines
   - She distributes vitamin A solution of children.

g. Birth and deaths registration
   - She keeps a record of births and deaths occurring in her area and submits the registers to local Birth and Death Registrar and also to her supervisor.

h. Notification
   - She notifies notifiable diseases or outbreaks to medical officer incharge of the area.

i. Training
   - She gives training to Dais about observation of 5Cs while conducting deliveries[Q]
   - She also gives training to village health guides
   - She will indentify woman leaders and participate in the training of women leaders.

j. Health education
   - She gives health education to all the expectant mothers and lactating mothers, family planning acceptors and others coming to subcenter individually or in groups.

k. Healthcare
   - She conducts antenatal once a week when medical officer visits subcenter to conduct MCH and FP clinics
   - She assists MO and health assistant in conducting the clinic
   - She does routine examination of the urine and Hb%[Q]
   - She provides treatment for all minor ailments, distributes ORS packets to children with diarrhea and provides first aid in cases of emergencies
   - She refers cases beyond her competence to the nearest primary health center.

l. Miscellaneous
   - She maintains cleanliness of the subcenter.
   - She attends monthly meetings at PHC and submits her report.
   - She involves dais and village health guides of her area in promoting family welfare work[Q].
   - She participates in Pulse Polio Immunization.
   - She assists Medical officer and Health assistant Female in their works
   - She co-ordinates her activities with Anganwadi workers, Mahilamandals and others
   - Participate in Mahila Mandal meetings and utilize such gathering for educating women in family welfare program.
   - Utilize satisfied customers, village leaders, dais and others for promoting family welfare program
   - Prepare and maintain all registers and records and maps, charts for her area in subcenter and submit the prescribed reports in time to health assistant as per standing orders or instructions.

Significance

- Multipurpose Health worker is the face of healthcare delivery in rural areas at primary care level and this cadre has been created on recommendations of Shrivastav Committee.

11. Prevention of Food Adulteration Act.

- Prevention of Food Adulteration Act (PFA-Act) was enacted by the Indian parliament in 1954 and subsequently amended in 1964, 1976 and 1986 making it more stringent
- There is provision of implementation of the act by the state and local governments[Q] and the central Govt plays a role in proper coordination, monitoring and surveillance.

Objectives

- Ensuring pure and wholesome quality food to the consumers and to protect their health from fraudulent and deceptive trade practices and to encourage fair trade practices.

Provisions

- Act provides protection against adulteration or contamination of food that may have deleterious effects on consumer's health
- Act regulates use of chemicals, pesticides, flavors and other additives in food preparations
- There is also provision for enrichment and fortification of foods under the Act.

Adulterated Food

- Adulterant is a material which is employed for purpose of adulteration and an article is deemed to be adulterated:
  - If it is sold by a vendor and is not of the nature demanded by the purchaser and is not of the quality which it purports to be
  - If the articles contains any other substance so as to affect injuriously the nature or quality thereof
  - If it is substituted wholly or partially by an inferior substance
  - If the constituent of the article is abstracted partially or wholly as to affect its quality
  - If the article has been prepared, packed or kept under insanitary conditions and has become contaminated as to cause injury to the health

- If the article consists of filthy, rotten, putrid or decomposed substance and is unfit for consumption
- If the article is obtained from a diseased animal
- If the article contains any poisonous substance
- If the article contains prohibited preservative or coloring agent in excess of prescribed limits
- If the quality of the article falls below the prescribed limits.

Inspecting Authorities

- Powers are given to the State Government to appoint Public Analyst and Food Inspectors who control the food supply, storage and marketing of foods.
- There is also provision for in service training of the different functionaries like food inspectors, analysts and senior officers concerned with implementation of this act.
- There was a provision of establishment of chain of food laboratories (82 in number) and four regional appellant central food laboratories at Kolkata, Mysore, Ghaziabad and Pune whose report would be considered final
- A 1986 amendment empowers consumers and voluntary organizations to take the samples of food.

Revision of Rules

- Rules are subjected to revision from time to time by the "Central Committee for Food Standard" constituted by the central government
- According to rules, any food that does not conform to the minimum standards is said to adultered.

Punishment

- For proven cases of adulteration the minimum imprisonment of 6 months with a minimum fine of ₹ 1000
- For cases of adulteration rendering the food injurious to case death or such harm which may amount to grievous hurt (S. 320 IPC) is punishable with life imprisonment and fine which shall not be less than ₹ 5000.

Significance

- Food adulteration is a social evil and unless general public rises up against it, this evil cannot be curbed.

12. Primordial prevention of cancer.

- Primordial prevention is a new concept which is mainly applicable to chronic diseases
- It means prevention of emergence or development of risk factors in population in which they have not appeared
- Actually, it is primary prevention in its pure sense where the efforts are directed towards discouraging population from adopting harmful lifestyles.

Primordial Prevention of Cancer

- Control of tobacco consumption
- Immunization with hepatitis B vaccine
- Improvement of personal hygiene
- Food hygiene—preventing use of food colors, preventing growth of fungus
- Control of air pollution by containment, dilution, replacement, legislation
- Control of occupational cancers by health education, replacement, legislation
- Treatment precancerous lesions like warts, cervical tear, chronic cervicitis, chronic gastritis, intestinal polyps, adenoma, etc.
- Control of alcohol consumption prevents chances of developing Carcinoma liver[Q].

Strategies

- This can be done through health education (individual approach, mass approach, group approach, etc.) or legislation.

a. Health education
   - Main aim of cancer education is prevent people from adopting harmful lifestyles and making them aware of early signs of cancerous growth so they can seek timely help
   - People can be educated about harmful effects of smoking, alcohol consumption through means of mass media, street plays, lectures, etc

– They should be made aware about the available treatment facilities for cancer
– They should also be explained to notice warning (danger) signs of cancer

Warning (Danger) signals of Cancer

– Warning signals are certain changes in the body which if noticed should arouse suspicion of a cancer and should exhort people to seek medical advice.

Danger signals of cancer are (CAUTION)

i. **C**hange in bowel or bladder habits
ii. **A** wound or sore that does not heal
iii. **U**nusual bleeding or discharge (at menses or from any natural orifice)/**U**nexplained loss of weight
iv. **T**hickening or lump in the breast or elsewhere
v. **I**ndigestion or difficulty in swallowing
vi. **O**blivious change in a wart or mole
vii. **N**agging cough or hoarseness of voice.

Significance

– Danger signals of cancer forms an important part of health education on cancer
– With detection of these danger signals, numerous cancers can be diagnosed at stage where they can be effectively treated.

b. Prevention of emergence of risk factors
– Discouraging tobacco and alcohol consumption (prevents lung cancer, bowel cancer)
– Improvements in personal hygiene (prevents cancer cervix, skin cancer)
– Wearing protective gears in people exposed to radiations
– Occupational cancer can be prevented by health education of factory workers regarding exposure to industrial carcinogens and their effects at the time of employment
– Hepatocellular carcinoma can be prevented by immunization against hepatitis B virus
– Control of air pollution is another preventive measure.

c. Legislations
– Legislations like banning smoking in public places are being made and are welcome
– Factories Act and other occupational legislations reduce occupational risk of cancers
– Strict enforcement of motor vehicle act for pollution level can also be beneficial.

SHORT ANSWERS

13. Healthcare needs of the elderly.

Refer Question No. 2 June 2009 (RS2) Paper II.

14. Sentinel surveillance for HIV in India.

- Sentinel surveillance is a surveillance method to identify the missing cases and thereby supplementing diagnosed cases
- Data obtained is extrapolated to entire population to estimate the disease prevalence in total population

HIV Sentinel Surveillance

- HIV sentinel surveillance is a one of the surveillance method for prevalence of HIV infection in population.

Objectives

- To identify missing HIV cases and thereby supplementing diagnosed cases and estimate prevalence of HIV in adult population.

Strategy

- Annual cross sectional survey of risk group in same place over few years by unlinked anonymous serological testing procedures by two ERS i.e. HIV testing is carried out without identification of name of samples collected for other purposes like VDRL in STD clinics, Hb% estimation in Antenatal clinics, etc.
- Number of samples to be screened must represent risk group under study and determine sample size accordingly.

Analysis

- Data collected is compiled and analyzed by NACO and based on HIV prevalence rates in adult population, divides the states into three groups.

Groups	*Prevalence of HIV infection*		*States*
	In high risk groups	*In antenatal women*	
Group I (High prevalence[Q])	>5%	≥1%	Maharashtra, Tamil Nadu, Karnataka, Andhra Pradesh, Manipur, Nagaland[Q]
Group II (Moderate prevalence[Q])	>5%	<1%	Gujarat, Goa, Pondicherry[Q]
Group III (Low prevalence)	<5%	<1%	Remaining states

Advantage

- Minimization of selection bias and participation bias.

Significance

- HIV sentinel surveillance has provided an effective tool in estimating prevalence of HIV in an area thus help focus preventive measures in high prevalence areas.

15. Population explosion.

Refer Question No. 1 June 2011 (RS2) Paper II.

16. Management by objectives.

Refer Question No. 6 Dec. 2011 (RS2) Paper II.

17. Universal barrier precautions.

- Universal barrier precautions are a simple set of effective practices designed to protect health workers and patients from infection with a range of pathogens including blood-borne viruses.

Components

i. Hand washing after any direct contact with patients
ii. Safe collection and disposal of needles (hypodermic and suture) and sharps (scalpel blades, lancets, razors, scissors), with required puncture- and liquid-proof safety boxes in each patient care area
iii. Wearing gloves for contact with body fluids, non-intact skin and mucous membranes
iv. Wearing a mask, eye protection and a gown (and sometimes a plastic apron) if blood or other body fluids might splash
v. Covering all cuts and abrasions with a waterproof dressing
vi. Promptly and carefully cleaning up spills of blood and other body fluids
vii. Using a safe system for hospital waste management and disposal
viii. Do not recap the needle or recap with one hand only before disposal
ix. Resuscitator bags should be used preferably to mouth-to-mouth breathing
x. Do not mouth-pipette; always use pipette with rubber bulb
xi. Process all laboratory specimens as potentially infectious.

Significance

- These practices are used when caring for all patients regardless of diagnosis
- They are applied universally
- It is not feasible, effective or cost-effective to test all patients for all pathogens prior to giving care in order to identify those who are infected and take precautions only with them
- Knowing a patient is infected does not prevent occupational exposure to blood
- Thus, decisions regarding the level of precautions to use are based on the nature of the procedure and not on the actual or assumed serological status of the patient

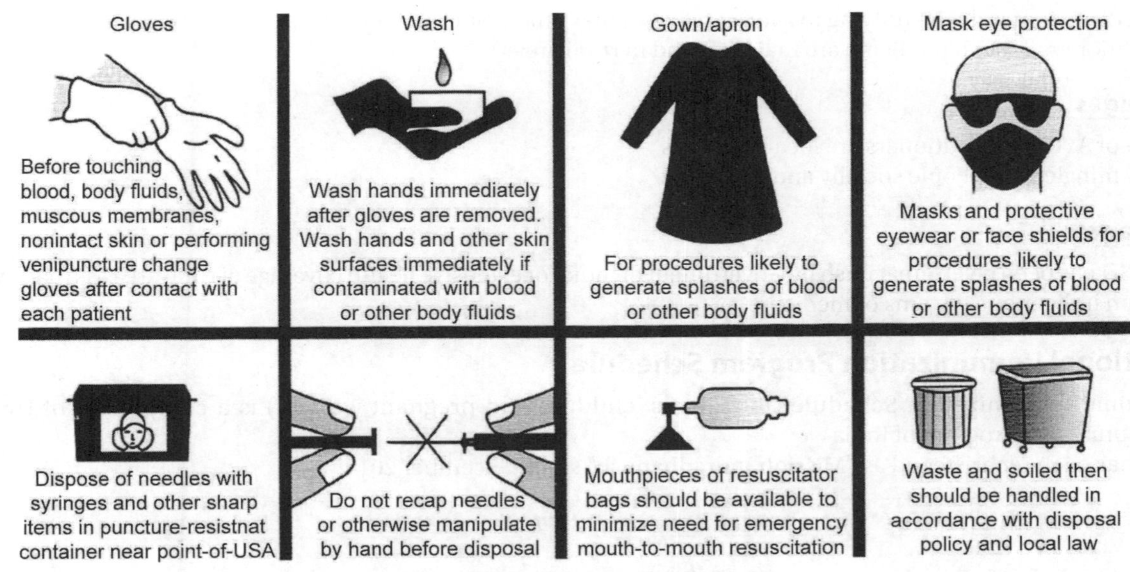

Fig. 2: Universal precautions

- It is not safe to take precautions only with those from so-called risk groups for infection with bloodborne pathogens as many people belonging to risk groups are not infected and many infected people do not belong to risk groups.

18. International quarantine.

- Quarantine is limitation of freedom of movements of such well person or domestic animals exposed to communicable diseases for period of time not longer than longest usual incubation period of the disease, in such manner as to prevent effective contact with those not so exposed
- International quarantine is quarantine of an international travelers for the diseases made notifiable by WHO, i.e. yellow fever[Q], small pox, cholera[Q] and plague[Q]
- Done at internal airports or seaports
- For most of the recorded history, nations acted alone, using quarantine for self survival
- First International Quarantine Rules were adopted in 1852 and are presently promulgated under auspices of WHO[#].

Objective

- Prevent international spread of a disease.

Procedure

- All travelers including infants exposed to risk of disease or passing through endemic zones must possess a valid International certificate of vaccination before they are allowed to enter receptive areas
- If traveler does not possess International vaccination certificate then he is placed under quarantine in a mosquito proof ward for 6 days for observation from date of leaving an infected area
- If travelers possesses the certificate and arrives before certificate becomes valid, he is isolated till certificate becomes valid.

Ref. # Larry Ogalthorpe Gostin; Public Health Law; Pg. 106

Significance

- Strict enforcement of International aerial and maritime traffic regulations in regards to quarantine is very important to prevent International spread of disease.

19. Indigenous system of medicine.

- Indigenous system of medicine constitutes Ayurveda, Unani, Siddha and Homeopathy
- This is termed as AYUSH (AYurveda, Unani, Siddha, Homeopathy)

- Government of India is studying to avail services of these medicines for effective and total health coverage
- Practitioners of such medicine are mainly found in rural areas.

Advantages

- Most of AYUSH practitioners are local residents
- They mingle with people socially and culturally.

Significance

- AYUSH has been given great push by Government of India for extensive health coverage of rural areas as many villages rely on indigenous systems of medicine.

20. National Immunization Program Schedule.

- National Immunization Schedule (for infants, children and pregnant women) is a component of Universal Immunization Program of India
- UIP has been rechristened as "Mission Indradhanush" since December 2014.

Age	Vaccine	Dosage	Route	Remarks
Infants^Q				
At birth	BCG^Q	0.05 mL	ID	Should be given as early as possible till 1 year of age
	OPV_0^Q	2 drops	Oral	Should be given as early as possible within first 15 days
	Hepatitis B_0	0.5 mL	IM	Should be given as early as possible within 24 hours
6 weeks	BCG^Q	0.1 mL	ID	If not given at birth
	OPV_1^Q	2 drops	Oral	
	$fIPV_1$ (inactivated polio vaccine)	0.1 mL	ID	Introduced in Odisha, Andhra Pradesh, Telangana, Tamil Nadu, Kerala, Karnataka, Maharashtra and Puducherry
	Pentavalent $vaccine_1$ (DPT + Hep B + Hib)		IM	Introduced in states of Kerala, Tamil Nadu, Goa, Delhi, Puducherry, Haryana, Gujarat, Karnataka and Jammu & Kashmir
	RVV_1 (Rotavirus vaccine)	5 drops (2 mL)	Oral	Introduced in Andhra Pradesh, Odisha, Himachal Pradesh, Haryana
	PCV_1 (Pneumococcal conjugate vaccine)	0.5 mL	IM	Introduced in Himachal Pradesh, Uttar Pradesh and Bihar
10 weeks	OPV_2^Q	2 drops	Oral	
	Pentavalent vaccine2			
	RVV_2	5 drops (2 mL)	Oral	
14 weeks	OPV_3^Q	2 drops	Oral	
	$fIPV_2$	0.1 mL	ID	
	Pentavalent $vaccine_3$ (DPT + Hep B + Hib)			
	RVV_3	5 drops (2 mL)	Oral	
	PCV_2	0.5 mL	IM	
9 months	$Measles_1$ or MR_1	0.5 mL	SC	MR (Measles—rubella vaccine) introduced in Karnataka, Tamil Nadu, Puducherry, Goa, Kerala, Andhra Pradesh, Lakshadweep
	JE_1	0.5 mL	SC	In select 110 endemic districts of Uttar Pradesh, West Bengal, Karnataka and Assam
	PCV (Booster)	0.5 mL	IM	
	Vitamin A^Q	100,000 IU (1 mL)	Orally	
	Vitamin A^Q	100,000 IU (1 mL)	Orally	

Contd...

Contd...

Age	Vaccine	Dosage	Route	Remarks
Preschool children				
16–24 months	DPT_{B1} booster1	0.5 mL	IM	
	OPV_B booster	2 drops	Oral	
	$Measles_2$ or MR_2	0.5 mL	SC	
	JE2 (SA14-14-2 vaccine)	0.5 mL	SC	In select 110 endemic districts of Uttar Pradesh, West Bengal, Karnataka and Assam
18 months	Vitamin A	200,000 IU (2 mL)	Orally	
24 months	Vitamin A	200,000 IU (2 mL)	Orally	
30 months	Vitamin A	200,000 IU (2 mL)	Orally	
36 months	Vitamin A	200,000 IU (2 mL)	Orally	
42 months	Vitamin A	200,000 IU (2 mL)	Orally	
48 months	Vitamin A	200,000 IU (2 mL)	Orally	
54 months	Vitamin A	200,000 IU (2 mL)	Orally	
60 months	Vitamin A	200,000 IU (2 mL)	Orally	
School children				
5–6 years	DT booster	0.5 mL	IM	Second dose given at an interval of 1 month if there is no clear history or documented evidence of previous immunization with DPT, DT or TT
10 years	TT booster	0.5 mL	IM	
16 years	TT booster	0.5 mL	IM	
Pregnant women				
Early in pregnancy	TT_1	0.5 mL	IM	Given at first contact
After 4 weeks	TT_2	0.5 mL	IM	Give TT-2 or booster doses before 36 weeks of pregnancy; however, give even if more than 36 weeks have passed Give TT to a woman in labor, if she has not previously received TT
	TT booster	0.5 mL	IM	If received 2 TT doses in a pregnancy within the last 3 years

* BCG is given intradermally on left upper arm
* PCV, DPT and hepatitis B vaccine is given intramuscularly on anterolateral side of mid-thigh
* Measles vaccine is given subcutaneously on right upper arm
* JE vaccine is given on left upper arm
* DPT booster and TT is given on upper arm
# On 25th April 2016, there was a switch from tOPV to bOPV all over the country

Rule of 2

1. Two vaccines are administered in the left upper arm: BCG and JE
2. Two vaccines are administered in the right upper arm: Measles/MR and IPV
3. Two vaccines are administered intradermally: BCG and IPV
4. Two vaccines are orally: OPV and rotavirus
5. Two vaccines are administered subcutaneously: Measles/MR and JE
6. Two injectable vaccines do not have a dose of 0.5 mL
   – BCG: 0.1 mL (0.05 mL up to 1 month of age)
   – IPV: 0.1 mL

Significance

- National Immunization Schedule besides covering the vaccine preventable diseases of children as per WHO EPI schedule, in addition also includes immunization for pregnant mothers
- UIP is inferior to recommendation of immunization schedule of Indian Academy of Paediatrics (IAP) as many vaccines are not included in UIP because of financial constraints.

21. Primary prevention of rheumatic heart disease.

Refer Question No. 11 Dec. 2016 (RS2) Paper II.

22. Essential newborn care.

Refer Question No. 1 Dec. 2008 (RS2) Paper II.

MBBS PHASE III EXAMINATION

JUNE 2008

(Revised Scheme 2)

PAPER I

LONG ESSAYS

1. How will you compare the health situation in two communities? What are the other uses of "indicators of health"?

- According to WHO, health status of a community can be measured and compared by comparing various health indicators[Q]
- However, there is no single indicator which can help compare health status amongst two communities because health is multidimensional, and each dimension is influenced by numerous factors, some known and many unknown therefore health must be measured multidimensionally
- Thus health must be conceived in terms of a profile, employing many indicators, which may be classified as:
  - Mortality indicators
  - Morbidity indicators
  - Disability rates
  - Nutritional status indicators
  - Healthcare delivery indicators
  - Utilization rates
  - Indicators of social and mental health
  - Environmental indicators
  - Socioeconomic indicators
  - Health policy indicators
  - Indicators of quality of life
  - Other indicators.

a. Mortality indicators

i. Crude death rate
- Crude death rate is number of deaths per 1000 population per year in a given community
- Indicates rate at which people are dying
- Considered a fair indicator of the comparative health of the people.

Disadvantage
- Health should not be measured by number of deaths that occur in a community, but in many countries, crude death rate is the only available indicator of health
- Usefulness of crude death rate is restricted for international comparison because it is influenced by the age-sex composition of the population.

Significance
- Although not a perfect measure of health status, a decrease in death rate provides a good tool for assessing the overall health improvement in a population.

ii. Expectation of life[Q]
- Life expectancy at birth is "the average number of years that will be lived by those born alive into a population if the current age-specific mortality rates persist"

- Life expectancy at the age of 1 excludes influence of infant mortality, and life expectancy at the age of 5 excludes influence of child mortality
- Life expectancy at birth is used most frequently and estimated for both sexes separately
- An increase in expectation of life is regarded, inferentially, as an improvement in health status

Disadvantage
- Life expectancy at birth is highly influenced by the infant mortality rate where that is high.

Significance
- Life expectancy is a good indicator of socioeconomic development in general
- As an indicator of long-term survival, it can be considered as a positive health indicator
- It has been adopted as a global health indicator.

iii. Infant mortality rate
- Infant mortality rate is ratio of deaths under 1 year of age in a given year to the total number of live births in the same year; usually expressed as a rate per 1000 live births.

Significance
- Infant mortality rate is a very comprehensive indicator, a sensitive indicator and a most important and universally accepted indicator of health status not only of infants, but also of whole population and of the socioeconomic conditions under which they live[Q]
- In addition, the infant mortality rate is a sensitive indicator of the availability, utilization and effectiveness of health care, particularly perinatal care.

iv. Child mortality rate
- It is defined as the number of deaths at ages 1–4 years in a given year, per 1000 children in that age group at the midpoint of the year concerned
- It excludes infant mortality.

Significance
- Apart from its correlation with inadequate MCH services, it is also related to insufficient nutrition, low coverage by immunization and adverse environmental exposure and other exogenous agents
- Indicates the magnitude of the gap and the room for improvement.

v. Under-5 proportionate mortality rate
- It is the proportion of total deaths occurring in the under-5 age group
- This rate can be used to reflect both infant and child mortality rates
- High rate reflects high birth rates, high child mortality rates and shorter life expectancy.

vi. Maternal mortality rate
- It is the ratio of death of women in the puerperal period in a given year to the total number of live births in the same year, usually expressed as a rate per 100000 live births.

Significance
- Maternal mortality also indicates the quality of services provided to mothers of reproductive age group, i.e. antenatal, natal and postnatal services.

vii. Disease-specific mortality
- It is the mortality rate computed for a specific disease.

viii. Proportional mortality rate
- It is the simplest measures of estimating the burden of a disease in the community[Q]
- It is the proportion of all deaths currently attributed to it.

Significance
- Proportional mortality rate from communicable diseases has been suggested as a useful health status indicator; it indicates the magnitude of preventable mortality.

Significance
- Mortality indicators represent the traditional measures of health status
- Even today they are probably the most often used indirect indicators of health
- With control of infectious diseases, mortality rates have declined to very low levels in many countries resulting in lesser sensitivity of mortality indicators as health indicators in developed countries.
- However, they continue to be used as the starting point in health status evaluation.

b. Morbidity indicators[Q] (assess ill health in community)

i. Incidence and prevalence
ii. Notification rates
iii. Attendance rates at out-patient departments, health centers, etc.
iv. Admission, readmission and discharge rates
v. Duration of stay in hospital
vi. Spells of sickness or absence from work or school

Disadvantage

– Morbidity indicators tend to overlook a large number of conditions which are subclinical or inapparent, that is, the hidden part of the iceberg of disease.

Significance

– Morbidity indicators supplement the mortality indicators to describe the health status of a community as they reveal the burden of illhealth in a community.

c. Disability rates[Q]

– Disability rates are based on premise or notion that health implies a full range of daily activities

Event-type indicators	*Person-type indicators*
▪ Number of days of restricted activity ▪ Bed disability days ▪ Work-loss days (or school loss days) within a specified period	▪ Limitation of mobility (confined to bed, confined to the house, special aid in getting around either inside or outside the house) ▪ Limitation of activity (limitation to perform the basic activities of daily living and limitation in major activity)

i. Sullivan's index[Q]

– Sullivan's index represents expectation of life free of disability[Q]
– Computed by subtracting from the life expectancy, the probable duration of bed disability and inability to perform major activities, according to cross-sectional data from the population surveys.

Significance

– Sullivan's index is considered one of the most advanced indicators currently available.

ii. HALE (Health-Adjusted Life Expectancy)

– Measures life expectancy at birth but includes an adjustment for time spent in poor health.
– Most easily understood as the equivalent number of years in full health that a newborn can expect to live based on current rates of ill-health and mortality.

iii. DALY (Disability-Adjusted Life Year) [Q]

– Measure of the burden of disease[Q] in a defined population and the effectiveness of interventions[Q]
– DALYs express years or life lost to premature death and years lived with disability adjusted for the severity of the disability
– One DALY is "one lost year of healthy life"
– DALYs are advocated as an alternative to QALYs and claimed to be a valid indicator of health
– DALY = YLL (years of lost life) + YLD (years lost to disability)
– Expressed as number of years lost due to ill health, disability or early death.

Disadvantage

– Use of DALY is limited because necessary data are not available or do not exist
– Moreover, the concept postulates a continuum from disease to disability to death that is not universally accepted, particularly by the community of persons with disabilities.

Significance

– Disability rates related to illness and injury are used to supplement mortality and morbidity indicators because death rates have not changed markedly in recent years, despite massive health expenditures.

d. Nutritional status indicators (positive health indicator)

i. Anthropometric measurements of preschool children, e.g. weight and height, midarm circumference
ii. Heights and weights of children at school entry
iii. Prevalence of low birth weight (less than 2.5 kg).

e. Health-care delivery indicators

i. Doctor-population ratio
ii. Doctor-nurse ratio
iii. Population-bed ratio
iv. Population per health/subcenter
v. Population per traditional birth attendant.

Significance

- These indicators reflect the equity of distribution of health resources in different parts of the country, and thus of the provision of health care.

f. Utilization rates

- Utilization of services—or actual coverage—is expressed as proportion of people in need of a service who actually receive it in a given period, usually a year
- Based on fact that there exists a relationship between utilization of health-care services and health needs and status.

Examples

i. Proportion of infants who are "fully immunized" against the 6 EPI diseases
ii. Proportion of pregnant women who receive antenatal care, or have their deliveries supervised by a trained birth attendant.
iii. Percentage of the population using the various methods of family planning.
iv. Bed-occupancy rate[Q] (i.e. average daily in-patient census/average number of beds).
v. Average length of stay[Q] (i.e. days of care rendered/discharges)
vi. Bed turn-over ratio[Q] (i.e. discharges/average beds).

Disadvantage

- Health-care utilization is also affected by factors such as availability and accessibility of health services and attitude of an individual towards his health and the health care system.

Significance

- Utilization rates give some indication of the care needed by a population, and therefore, the health status of the population
- These indicators direct attention away from the biological aspects of disease in a population towards the discharge of social responsibility for the organization in delivery of health care services

g. Indicators of social and mental health

- These include suicide, homicide, other acts of violence and other crime; road traffic accidents, juvenile delinquency; alcohol and drug abuse; smoking; consumption of tranquillizers; obesity, etc
- To these may be added family violence, battered-baby and battered-wife syndromes and neglected and abandoned youth in the neighborhood.

Significance

- These social indicators provide a guide to social action for improving the health of the people.

h. Environmental indicators

- Reflect quality of physical and biological environment in which diseases occur and in which the people live
- Include indicators relating to pollution of air and water, radiation, solid wastes, noise, exposure to toxic substances in food or drink.
- Most useful environmental indicators are those measuring the proportion of population having access to safe water and sanitation facilities.

i. Socioeconomic indicators[Q]

- These indicators do not directly measure health; nevertheless, they are of great importance in interpretation of healthcare indicators.

Examples

i. Rate of population increase
ii. Per capita GNP
iii. Level of unemployment
iv. Dependency ratio

v. Literacy rates[Q], especially female literacy rates
vi. Family size[Q]
vii. Housing[Q]: The number of persons per room
viii. Per capita "calorie" availability

j. Health policy indicators

– Single most important indicator of political commitment is "allocation of adequate resources".

Examples

i. Proportion of GNP spent on health services
ii. Proportion of GNP spent on health-related activities (including water supply and sanitation, housing and nutrition, community development)
iii. Proportion of total health resources devoted to primary health care

k. Indicators of quality of life

– Previous emphasis on using increased life expectancy as an indicator of health is no longer considered adequate, especially in developed countries, and attention has shifted more toward concern about the quality of life enjoyed by individuals and communities
– Physical quality of life index is one such composite index which consolidates three indicators, viz. infant mortality, life expectancy at age one, and literacy.

l. Other indicators

i. Social indicators
– Social indicators, as defined by United Nations Statistical Office, have been divided into 12 categories—population; family formation, families and households; learning and educational services; earning activities; distribution of income, consumption, and accumulation; social security and welfare services; health services and nutrition; housing and its environment; public order and safety; time use; leisure and culture; social stratification and mobility

ii. Basic needs indicators
– Basic needs indicators are used by ILO and include calorie consumption; access to water; life expectancy; deaths due to disease; illiteracy, doctors and nurses per population; rooms per person; GNP per capita.

iii. Health for All indicators
– For monitoring progress towards the goal of Health for All by 2000 AD, WHO has listed following four categories of indicators.

Health policy indicators	▪ Political commitment to Health for All ▪ Resource allocation ▪ Degree of equality of distribution of health services ▪ Community involvement ▪ Organizational framework
Social and economic indicators related to health	▪ Rate of population increase ▪ GNP or GDP ▪ Income distribution ▪ Work conditions ▪ Adult literacy rate ▪ Housing ▪ Food availability
Indicators for provision of health care	▪ Availability ▪ Accessibility ▪ Utilization ▪ Quality of care
Health status indicators	▪ Low birth weight ▪ Nutritional status and psychosocial development of children ▪ Infant mortality rate ▪ Child mortality rate (1–4 years) ▪ Life expectancy at birth ▪ Maternal mortality rate ▪ Disease specific mortality ▪ Morbidity—incidence and prevalence ▪ Disability prevalence

iv. Millennium development goal indicators
   – Millennium development goal indicators were adopted by United Nations in the year 2000 to improve global health
   – It has set forward certain goals and enumerates various indicators to evaluate attainment of the goal.

Goal	*Indicator*
Eradication of poverty and hunger	▪ Prevalence of underweight children under 5 years of age ▪ Proportion of population below minimum level of dietery energy consumption
Reduce child mortality	▪ Under five mortality rate ▪ Infant mortality rate ▪ Proportion of 1year old children immunized against measles
Improve maternal health	▪ Maternal mortality rate ▪ Proportion of births attended by skilled health personnel
Combat HIV/AIDS, malaria and other diseases	▪ HIV prevalence among young people aged 15–24 years ▪ Condom use rate of the contraceptive prevalence rate ▪ Number of children orphaned by HIV/AIDS ▪ Prevalence and death rates associated with malaria ▪ Proportion of population in malaria risk areas using effective malaria prevention and treatment measures ▪ Prevalence and death rates associated with tuberculosis ▪ Proportion of tuberculosis cases detected and cured under DOTS
Ensure environmental sustainability	▪ Proportion of population using solid fuel ▪ Proportion of population with sustainable access to an improved water source, urban and rural ▪ Proportion of urban population with access to improved sanitation
Develop a global partnership for development	▪ Proportion of population with access to affordable essential drugs on a sustainable basis

Significance

- To compare the health status of two communities, various health indicators are available but there is no single comprehensive indicator of a community's health
- An ideal index which combines the effect of a number of components measured independently is yet to be developed
- Currently the important health indicators proposed to measure the health status of a community and compare with others are:

Indicator	*Developed countries*	*Developing countries*	*Least developed countries*
Life expectancy at birth (years)	79	65	52
IMR (per 1000 live births)	5	52	98
Under 5 mortality rate (per 1000 live births)	6	87	155
MMR (per 100000 live births)	13	440	890
Doctor-population ratio (per 10000 population)	25.2	8.4	1.4
Nurse-population ratio (per 10000 population)	74.2	9.6	2.2
GNI per capita ($)	32232	1524	345
Per capita public expenditure on health (US $ in % of GDP)	14	4	5
Adult literacy rate (%)	97	77	54
Per capita calorie	3371	2663	2099
Access to safe water (% of population)	100	79	58
Access to adequate sanitation (% of population)	100	49	35

Uses/Applications of Indicators of Health

- To measure the health status of a country[Q]
- To describe the health of a community

- To compare the health status of one country with that another country or of one state with anther state in same country
- To assess the health-care needs and identification of priorities[Q]
- To plan and implement health care services and allocation of resources
- To evaluate health-care services
- To measure success of health services.

2. What are the health hazards of workers in coal mines? What steps you would take to reduce the hazards?

- India has numerous coal mines especially in the Chota Nagpur plateau and people working in these coal mines suffer from various occupational health hazards.

Health Hazards of Coal Mine Workers

a. Anthrocosis (coal worker's pneumoconiosis)
   - Anthrocosis is also called coal workers pneumoconiosis or Miner's black lung.

   Etiology
   - Inhalation of coal dust over a long period of time
   - Tuberculosis, smoking, nonspecific respiratory infections and autoimmunity predisposes.

   Pathology
   - Coal dust particles accumulate just before the bronchioles open into the alveoli
   - This aggregation of coal dust is known as coal maculae which look like nodular opacities or reticulation in the chest X-ray.

   Pathogenesis (2 phases)

Simple pneumoconiosis (first phase)	*Progressive massive fibrosis (second phase)*
▪ Characterized by little ventilatory impairment ▪ Requires about 10–12 years of exposure for its development[Q] ▪ Atrophy of bronchial smooth muscles and dilatation of bronchioles, give rise to focal emphysema	▪ Seen following simple pneumoconiosis even without further exposure ▪ Massive fibrosis of lungs leads to pulmonary hypertension and cor pulmonale ▪ There is severe respiratory disability followed by congestive cardiac failure and premature death

   Diagnosis
   - Chest X-ray shows multiple, nodular densities or reticulation (Black lung).

   Significance
   - Anthrocosis is notifiable under Indian Mines Act and compensable under Workmen's Compensation Act

b. Beat elbow or Beat knee
   - Produced as a result of the peculiar posture of coal mine workers
   - This is followed by bursitis which subsequently becomes the seat of septic cellulitis.

c. Miner's nystagmus
   - Caused due to poor lighting conditions in the mines.

For steps to prevent coal workers health hazards

Refer Question No. 2 June 2016 (RS2) Paper I.

SHORT ESSAYS

3. Benefits of forming self-help groups of mothers in villages.

- The term self-help group is used to describe a small group of 10 to 20 poor women who come together on voluntary basis to accumulate savings through thrift and self management, in order to prove their credit worthiness to financial institutions
- Establishment of the groups was envisaged under the women development and empowerment component Community Development Program
- The concept builds on mutual trust and help, shared ownership, peer pressure, emphasizing group solidarity and togetherness.

Self-help Groups in Karnataka

- A recent intervention is the Karnataka Government's Stree Shakthi (women power) program launched in 2000
- The Government of Karnataka realized that, despite implementing many programs which aimed at social, economic and overall development of rural women, it could not empower women or build up their confidence
- The Stree Shakthi program led to the formation of 100,000 SHGs, covering 2 million women.

Objective

- Poverty alleviation
- Women empowerment.

Benefits for Women

a. Economic benefits
   i. Increased entrepreneurial skills
      - This has allowed women to change from being wage workers to being self employed
      - Women also have gained the option to pursue two or three petty businesses, change from one type of business to another, combine wage employment with small business.
   ii. Increased access to credit
      - The micro credit facility of the SHG has encouraged women to save
      - They are at ease in their minds as they can avail money when they need, without having to pay any collateral.
   iii. Establishment of businesses
      - Many women see advantages in owning a petty enterprise as it allows flexibility in working hours and helps balance house keeping and child rearing along with earning for family
   iv. Changes in consumption patterns
      - Food items were purchased once a week or once a month, as and when wages were received was done
      - This saved not only the time spent but also saved on amounts as bulk/wholesale purchases are priced lower than retail purchases and ensure better quality
      - There is a noticeable change in the consumption pattern and better household nutrition
      - The financial mobility has led to an improvement in the quality of life
      - Overall, families were able to address their basic needs better than before.

b. Social benefits
   i. Increased mobility
      - This means a lot to poor women and to those who have been restricted by religious taboo
      - It has made women more bold and confident
      - Earlier, women were more confined to the four walls of the kitchen and some to the work place but now they are be able to meet each other, and discuss problems.
   ii. Increased exposure
      - This comes from more interactions with other women
      - It makes them more enthusiastic and positive about their lives
      - Interaction with other women has resulted in building congenial relationships and has ensured fewer conflicts.
   iii. Increased awareness
      - Awareness on health-related issues—personal hygiene, communicable diseases, effects of malnutrition and sanitation—has increased as a result of training programs
      - More importantly, awareness of the rights of women—as prescribed by the constitution and as prescribed by the religious doctrines—has also increased
      - Many women have come out of boundaries defined by their male companions or relatives.
   iv. Changes in decision-making
      - Women are more involved in decisions that affect their lives and that of their family/household
      - They have more freedom to decide how much time they could spend without having to seek permission from the men and worry about the conflicts that might ensue at home as a consequence
      - Women also felt they have more say in the education of the children, such as which school children were to be sent to

  - Men involved women in decision-making processes which were purely in the male domain before, such as house repairs and the purchase of a site.
- v. Increase in social security
  - Some of the SHGs have been successful in availing facilities like widow pensions, old age pensions, health and life insurance for its members
  - This has resulted in the women feeling more secure about themselves and their future
  - Women abuse is said to have reduced and deserted wives have witnessed the husband return home
  - The unequal power relation between men and women, with the increasing economic power and social mobility of women, is changing
  - However, many more changes are to be achieved, like achieving the rights of women to property, the reproductive rights and many more.

Significance

- Self-help groups are instrumental in providing women with collective access to services of different governmental programs and schemes that were hitherto usually denied them as individuals
- They are used to launch many of the awareness and skill training programs under Community Development Program
- They presented forums that were highly effective in reaching the overall communities.

Ref:
Shashikala Sitaram; Evaluation working paper, India: Promoting urban social development through self help groups in Karnataka Pg. 2, 14-16.

4. Describe briefly the various "tests of significance".

- Tests of significance are statistical test or mathematical methods employed to measure probability or chance of occurance of biological variation, in samples by standard error
- It defines limits of variation by chance and determines the probability of the factor playing the role
- They will measure the probability (p value) and p value less than 0.05 is significant and less than 0.001 is highly significant statistically[Q].

Types

i. Standard error of the mean
ii. Standard error of the difference between two means
iii. Standard error of proportion
iv. Standard error of difference between two proportions
v. 't' test
vi. Chi-square test

Choice of Tests of Significance

Sample size/Type of data	*Qualitative data*	*Quantitative data*
Sample size >30	▪ Standard error of proportion ▪ Standard error of difference between two proportions	▪ Standard error of mean ▪ Standard error of difference between two means
Sample size <30	▪ Chi-square test	▪ Paired 't' test ▪ Unpaired 't' test

a. Standard error of the mean
   - Standard error of mean is a parameter used to measure variation among the sample means
   - Simply denoted as SE $\overline{x}$
   - It is not an error, but it's the standard deviation of sample means from the population mean
   - Helps to measure the chance variation or biological variation.

   Calculations
   - Calculate the sample deviation by squaring summation of the difference between sample mean and population mean using the formula

$^{Q}SD = \sqrt{\frac{\sum(m - M)^2}{n}}$

- Calculate the standard error of the mean by the formula[Q]

$= \frac{SD}{\sqrt{n}}$

Example
- Mean and SD for height of 50 boys were 150 cm and 7 cm respectively. Find standard error of mean

Mean height = 150 cm
SD = 7 cm
n = 50 boys

$SE\bar{X} = \frac{SD}{\sqrt{n}} = \frac{7}{\sqrt{50}} = \frac{7}{7.07} = 0.98$

Applications
- To find confidence limits of population mean if standard deviation of the sample is known
- Population mean = Sample mean ± 2 SE of the mean
- To tell whether a particular sample is drawn from the known population or not, if the population mean is known. If the sample mean lies within the range of M ± 2 SE $\bar{x}$, it is considered as belonging to the known population because 95% of the sample lies within M + 2 SE $\bar{x}$.
- To find the SE of difference between two means to know if the observed difference between the means of two samples is real and statistical significant or it is apparent and insignificant due to chance.
- To calculate the size of the sample in order to have desired confidence limits, SD of population is known, by the formula SE

b. Standard error of difference between two means
- It measures chance difference between the means of two samples drawn from same population[Q]
- Denoted as SE $(\bar{x}_1 - \bar{x}_2)$
- In practice, it is not possible to find differences of large number of samples and then find SE of these differences
- Test is applied to one pair if standard deviation of two means are known
- If the observed difference between the two means is more than twice the SE of difference, it is significant at 95% confidence limits and if the observed difference between the two means is more than thrice the SE of difference, it is significant at 99% confidence limits
- SE of difference between two means is denoted as SE $(\bar{x}_1 - \bar{x}_2)$
- Mathematically it is the root of the sum of the squares of the standard error of two samples means.
- It is already seen that the SE of a sample mean is equal to $\frac{SD}{\sqrt{n}}$
- Therefore, SEDM denoted as $S\bar{d} = \sqrt{(SE_1)^2 + (SE_2)^2}$
- Substituting $SE = \frac{SD}{\sqrt{n}} = \frac{SD^2}{n}$

$$SEDM = \sqrt{\frac{(SD_1)^2}{n_1} + \frac{(SD_2)^2}{n_2}}$$

Calculations
- Calculate the two means $\bar{x}_1$ and $\bar{x}_2$, correspond to the two samples with sample sizes n_1 and n_2 respectively.
- Calculate the standard deviation of the two samples and their standard errors (SE_1) and (SE_2) respectively.
- Calculate the SEDM as $\sqrt{(SE_1)^2 + (SE_2)^2}$
- Calculate the equation $Z = \frac{\text{Difference between sample estimates}}{\text{SE of difference}}$
- Refer to normal distribution table and corresponding to this calculated value of Z, find the value of probability 'p'.
- If the p value is less than 0.05, then difference between two sample estimates is significant[Q]

Example

- In a study on growth of children, on group of 100 children had a mean height of 60 cms and SD of 2.5 cm, while another group of 150 children had a mean height of 62 cm and SD of 3 cm. Is the difference between the means statistically significant?

$$\text{SEDM} = \sqrt{(SE_1)^2 + (SE_2)^2}$$

$$= \sqrt{\frac{(SD_1)^2}{n_1} + \frac{(SD_2)^2}{n_2}}$$

$$= \sqrt{\frac{(2.5)^2}{100} + \frac{(3)^2}{150}}$$

$$= \sqrt{\frac{6.25}{100} + \frac{9}{100}}$$

$$= \sqrt{0.06 + 0.06}$$

$$= \sqrt{0.12}$$

$$= 0.35$$

$$Z = \frac{\bar{x}_1 - \bar{x}_2}{SE(\bar{x}_1 - \bar{x}_2)_2} = \frac{60 - 62}{0.35} = \frac{2}{0.35} = 5.71$$

- Since the observed difference is more than 3 times the SE, it is highly significant
- The growth is more in the second group than in the first

c. Standard error of the proportions
  - Standard error of proportions is a measure of variation occurring by chance between the sample proportion and the population proportion in a qualitative data.
  - It is the test of significance of variations in proportions of samples of qualitative data.
  - In qualitative data, the character remains the same while the frequency variations are dealt with.
  - Employed to find the efficacy of a drug or a vaccine or a surgical procedure.
  - If the sample consists of characters of two attributes only, it is a binomial distribution.
  - Proportion of individuals, having a specific character or attribute, in a binomial distribution, is expressed as "p", either as a fraction of 1 or percentage.

$$P = \frac{\text{No. of individuals having a specific character}}{\text{Total number in the sample}}$$

  - The remaining proportion of individuals having the other character is represented as "q"
  - Arithmetically "q" = 1 – p in terms of fractions of 1 or 100 – p in percentage.
  - Thus p is the probability of occurrence of a positive attribute and q is the probability of occurrence of the negative attribute.
  - To illustrate, proportion of 80 girls in a class of 200 strength and proportions of boys in same class is calculated as follows:

$$\text{Proportion of girls (p)} = \frac{80}{200} = 0.4 \text{ out of } 1$$

$$\text{Proportion of boys (q)} = \frac{200-80}{200} = \frac{120}{200} = 0.6 \text{ out of } 1$$

  - For statistical analysis, the proportion of girls (p) and boys (q) are expressed in percentage as below.

$$p = \frac{80 \times 100}{200} = 40\% \text{ girls}$$

$q = 100 - p = 100 - 40 = 60\%$ boys in the example

  - Sample proportions are symmetrically distributed around the population proportions, from which the samples are drawn, i.e. it gains the shape of a normal curve.
  - This distribution of the sample proportions is expressed arithmetically interms of standard error of proportions.
  - Binomial confidence limits are as follows"
    - 68% of sample proportions will lie within the range P ± 1SE of proportion
    - 95% value lies within the range of P ± 2 SE of proportions
    - 99% value lies within the range of P ± 3 SE of proportions.

Calculations

– Standard error of proportions is calculated using the formula:

$$SEP = \frac{p \times q}{n}$$

Where,
p = % of positive character (p)
q = % of negative character (100-p)
n = number of observations (sample size)

– Significance of difference is found by relative deviate (Z) test

$$Z = \frac{\text{Observed difference}}{\text{SEP}}$$

Example

- Proportion of blood group A among Indians is 30%. Find SEP and the 95% confidence limits. Could this sample be from an universe, in which the prevalence of blood group A is 40%
  P = 30; q = 100 – 30; n = 100

  $$SEP = \sqrt{\frac{p \times q}{n}} = \sqrt{\frac{30 \times 70}{100}} = \sqrt{21} = 4.58$$

95% confidence limit	= p ± 2 SE	
	= 30 + 2 X	= 30 – 2 X
	= 4.58	= 4.58
	= 30 + 9.16	= 30 – 9.1
	= 39.166	= 20.84

- Since the proportion 40 is outside the 95% confidence limits, we can say 95% confidence that the sample is not drawn from the universe having 40% prevalence of blood group A.

Applications

– SEP is used to find the confidence limits of population promotion if the sample proportion is given
– To tell whether the sample is drawn from the known population or not
– To find the standard errors of difference between two proportions, to know if the observed between proportions of two samples is real and statistically significant or due to chance and insignificant
– To find the sample size if SEP and the proportions are known.

d. Standard error of difference between two proportions

– Standard error of difference between two proportions measures the chance between the sample proportions of paired samples drawn from the same population or universe.
– If the observed difference between the two sample proportions is more than twice the standard error of difference, it is significant at 95% confidence limits and if more than 3, it is significant at 99% confidence limits.

Calculations

– SEDP is calculated by the formula:

$$SE\,(p_1 - p_2) = \sqrt{\frac{p_1 p_2}{n_1} + \frac{p_2 p_2}{n_2}}$$

Where,
p_1 and p_2 are the estimates of the proportions of the two samples
q_1 and q_2 = $(1-p_1)$ and $(1-p_2)$ respectively
n_1 and n_2 = number of observations in the two samples

– Significance of difference is found by relative deviate Z test

$$Z = \frac{\text{Observed difference between two sample proportions}}{\text{SE of difference between two proportions}}$$

Example

- In an epidemic of gastroenteritis in an area, the number of cases reported in two populations consuming water from two different sources were as follows:

Source of water	*No. of people consuming water from source*	*No. of cases*
Tap water	800	35
Hand pump	2400	120
Total	**3200**	**155**

Find out whether the difference in the proportion of cases in the two groups significant.

i. Calculate SE of first sample

p_1 = proportions of cases among tap water consumers = 0.044

$q_1 = 1 - p_1 = 1 - 0.044 = 0.956$

n1 = No. of water consumers = 800

Standard Error of proportion p_1 (SE_1)

$$= \sqrt{\frac{p_1 q_1}{n_1}} = \sqrt{\frac{0.044 \times 0.956}{800}}$$

$$= \sqrt{0.00005225}$$

$$= 0.0072$$

ii. Calculate SE of second sample

p_1 = proportions of cases among handpump water consumers = 0.05

$q_1 = 1 - p_1 = 1 - 0.05 = 0.95$

n1 = No. of water consumers = 2400

Standard error of proportion p_2 (SE_2)

$$= \sqrt{\frac{p_2 q_2}{n_2}} = \sqrt{\frac{0.05 \times 0.95}{2400}}$$

$$= \sqrt{0.0000197}$$

$$= 0.006$$

iii. Calculate difference between two proportions

$= p_1 - p_2$

$= 0.044 - 0.05$

$= 0.006$

iv. Calculate the standard error of difference

$$= \sqrt{(SE_1)^2 + (SE_2)^2}$$

$$= \sqrt{0.0000525 + 0.0000197}$$

$$= \sqrt{0.0000722}$$

$$= 0.0085$$

v. Calculate the significance of difference

$$Z = \frac{\text{Difference between the proportions}}{\text{Standard error of difference}}$$

$$= \frac{0.006}{0.0085}$$

$$= 0.706$$

- From the normal distribution table, p corresponding to this value is more than 0.48 thus the difference is insignificant

e. "t" test

- "t" test is a method of determining the significance of difference between standard errors for qualitative data in sample size less than 30
- It obtains a "t" value from which the probability of occurrence is determined by referring to "t" table
- The "t" value is calculated as a ratio of difference between two means or proportions to the standard error of the difference.

i.e., $t = \frac{\bar{x}_1 - \bar{x}_2}{SE} = \frac{\text{Mean difference}}{\text{SE of mean difference}}$

- Like confidence limits, "t" test has degrees of freedom which are expressed in percentage.
- If the numerical value exceeds 5%, then the difference is statistically significant.

Types

	Paired "t" test	*Unpaired "t" test*
Definition	▪ If the observations are made on a single sample and the values of a certain characterstic is noted before and after treatment with a particular drug, such comparison of values of observations is known as paired "t" test[Q]	▪ If the observations are made on two independent groups like control group and experimental group and their means are compared for significant difference, it is known as unpaired "t" test[Q]
Examples	▪ Mean BP before and after an interventional trial for significance (effect) of drug	▪ To study association between maternal uptake of iron supplements and birth weight of new born babies
Calculations	$t = \frac{\bar{d}}{SE\ of\ d}$	$t = \frac{\bar{x}_1 - \bar{x}_2}{\text{SE of difference between means}}$ $= \frac{\bar{x}_1 - \bar{x}_2}{SE(\bar{x}_1 - \bar{x}_2)}$

Where,
d = difference in the two values for each pair
$\bar{d}$ = mean of the n values for d

It may be remembered here that SE of $d = \frac{\text{SE of d}}{\sqrt{n}}$

f. Chi-square test (χ^2 test)
- Chi-square test involves the calculation of a quantity called χ^2 in a qualitative data.
- It is a non parametric test of significance[Q].

Calculations

- First a contingency table or association table (a two way table) is prepared out of the qualitative data where the actually observed frequencies of 2 sets of events are entered.
- Null hypothesis is set up stating there is no association between the events[Q]
- Then expected frequency for each cell is calculated on the assumption of no association using the formula

$$E = \frac{\text{Row total} \times \text{column total}}{\text{Grand total}}$$

- Then the difference between the observed and the expected frequencies for each cell is found.
- χ^2 value for each cell is calculated by using the formula $\chi^2 = \frac{(O-E)^2}{E}$
- Then the total of x^2 for all the four cells is calculated by the formula (Summation of all 4 cell x^2 – value)

$$\text{Total } \chi^2 = \sum \frac{(O-E^2)}{E}$$

Alternate formula for $\chi^2 = \frac{(ad-bc)^2 \times G}{(a+b)(c+d)(a+c)}$

Where a, b, c and d are observed frequencies of 4 cells and G is the grand total.
- Next the degree of freedom is calculated by suing the formula
Degree of freedom = (No. of columns – 1) (No. of rows – 1)
- Lastly to know whether the calculated $\chi 2$ value is significant or not, refer the Fisher's $\chi 2$ table for a particular degree of freedom, for a probability of 0.05, 0.01, etc.
- If the calculated value is higher than the table value, it is concluded that the association is significant.

Example

- Apply χ^2 test to find efficacy of a drug from the given data.

Group	*Result (Efficacy of drug)*		*Total*
	Died	Survived	
Control	(O) 10 (a) (E) (5.25)	(O) 25 (b) (E) (29.75)	35 (a + b)
Experimental	(O) 05 (c) (E) (9.75)	(O) 60 (d) (E) (55.25)	65 (c + d)
Total	**15 (a + c)**	**85 (b + d)**	**(G) 100**

i. Calculate the (E) value for each cell is calculated as follows:
   Expected number and χ^2 – value of "died" in the control group

$$E_a = \frac{\text{Row total} \times \text{Column total}}{\text{Grand total}}$$

$$= \frac{35 \times 16}{100} = 5.25$$

$$\chi^2 = \frac{(O-E)^2}{E} = \frac{(10-5.25)^2}{5.25}$$

$$= \frac{(4.75)^2}{5.25} = \frac{22.5226}{5.25} = 4.29$$

Expected number and χ^2 – value of "survived" in the control group.

$$E_b = \frac{85 \times 35}{100} = 29.75$$

$$\chi^2 = \frac{(O-E)^2}{E}$$

$$= \frac{(25-29.75)^2}{29.75} = \frac{(-4.75)^2}{29.75}$$

$$= \frac{22.56}{29.75} = 0.76$$

Expected number and χ^2 – value of "died" in the experimental group

$$E_c = \frac{15 \times 65}{100} = \frac{39}{4} = 9.75$$

$$\chi^2 = \frac{(O-E)^2}{E}$$

$$= \frac{(05-09.75)^2}{29.75} = \frac{(-4.75)^2}{29.75}$$

$$= \frac{22.56}{9.75} = 2.31$$

Expected number and χ^2 – value of "survived" in the experimental group

$$E_d = \frac{85 \times 65}{100} = 85 \times 0.65 = 9.75$$

$$\chi^2 = \frac{(O-E)^2}{E}$$

$$= \frac{(60-55.25)^2}{55.25} = \frac{(5.25)^2}{55.25}$$

$$= \frac{22.56}{55.25} = 0.408$$

ii. Calculate the sum total of 4 cells

$$\Sigma\chi^2 = \text{Total } \chi^2 \text{ value of all 4 cells}$$

$$= 4.29 + 0.76 + 2.31 + 0.41$$

$$= 7.77$$

iii. Calculate the degree of freedom
Degree of freedom = (c – 1) (r – 1) = (2 – 1) (2 – 1) = (1 X 1) = 1

iv. Find out the probability
- On referring the Fisher's χ^2 table with 1 degree of freedom, the tabulated χ^2 value, corresponding to probability of 0.05 is 3.84[Q]
- Since the calculated value is more than the table value, there exists a significant relationship between the two significant

Yate's correction

- Yate's correction or Correction for continuity is a correction suggested when the expected frequency in any cell of the fourfold table is less than 5.
- In such cases, $\chi 2$ value is obtained by following formulae:

$$\chi^2 = \frac{[(\bar{O} - E) - 1/2]^2}{E}$$

$$\text{Alternate formula } \chi^2 = \frac{[(ad - bc) - G/2]^2 \times G}{(a+b)(c+d)(a+c)(b+d)}$$

Applications

- It is an alternate method of testing the significance of the difference between two proportions
- As a test of goodness of fit, i.e. the $\chi 2$ test determines whether the observed frequency distribution table differs from the theoretical distribution by chance or the sample drawn from a different population.
- To find any association between two attributes is real or by chance[Q].

Significance

- Tests of significance play an important role in analysis of any epidemiological study by helping to determine association between two variables like smoking and lung cancer, etc.

5. Sensitivity and specificity of a screening test.

Refer Question No. 1 December 2010 (RS2) Paper I.

6. Methods for disinfection for control of communicable diseases.

Refer Question No. 2 December 2010 (RS2) Paper I.

7. Methods for control of "reservoir of infection".

Refer Question No. 1 June 2009 (RS2) Paper I.

8. Provisions under Factories Act.

Refer Question No. 1 December 2011 (RS2) Paper I.

9. Effective methods of communication to youths.

- Youth is a delicate age because of important changes in physique, secondary sexual characteristics and behavior.
- Considering this in mind, health education of such age group is very important.

Effective Communications to Youth

- Effective communication is central to working with youth
- Involves listening, questioning, understanding and responding to what is being communicated by them
- It is important to be able to communicate both on a one-on-one basis and in a group context
- Communication is not just about the words you use, but also your manner of speaking, body language and, above all, the effectiveness with which you listen
- To communicate effectively it is important to take account of culture and context, for example where English is an additional language

- Effective engagement requires the involvement of the audience in the design and delivery of services and decisions that affect them
- It is important to consult with them and consider their opinions and perspectives from the outset
- A key part of effective communication and engagement is trust, both between the communicator and the audience.
- To build a rapport with youth, it is important to demonstrate understanding, respect and honesty
- Continuity in relationships promotes engagement and the improvement of lives.

Components

a. Skills
   i. Listening and building empathy
      - Establish rapport and respectful, trusting relationships with the youths.
      - Develop and use effective communication systems appropriate to the audience.
      - Communicate effectively with them.
      - Be aware that some people do not communicate verbally and that you need to adapt your style of communication to their needs and abilities.
      - Understand the effects of nonverbal communication such as body language, and appreciate that different cultures use and interpret body language in different ways.
      - Build rapport and develop relationships using the appropriate form of communication (for example, spoken language, play, body and sign language).
      - Build open and honest relationships by respecting them and making them feel valued as partners.
      - Hold conversations at the appropriate time and place, understanding the value of day to day contact.
      - Actively listen in a calm, open, non-threatening manner and use questions to check understanding and acknowledge that you have heard what is being said.
   ii. Summarizing and explaining
      - Summarize situations in the appropriate way for the individual (taking into account factors such as background, age and personality).
      - Understand how to present genuine choices to young people and how to obtain consent to sharing information.
      - Explain to the audience what kind of information you may have to share with others.
      - Explain what has happened or will happen next and check their understanding and where appropriate, their consent to the process.
   iii. Consultation and negotiation
      - Consult them from the beginning of the process.
      - Inform, involve and help the youths to assess different courses of action, understand the consequences of each and, where appropriate, agree next steps.
      - Understand the key role and value of parents; know when to refer them to further sources of information, advice or support.
      - Identify what each party hopes to achieve in order to reach the best possible and fair conclusion for the youth.
      - Share reasons for action with the audience and those caring for them.
      - Provide support and encouragement to them.
      - Know when and how to hand over control of a situation to others.

b. Knowledge
   i. How communication works
      - Know that communication is a two-way process.
      - Know how to listen to people, make them feel valued and involved, and know when it is important to focus on the individual rather than the group.
      - Be aware of different ways of communicating, including electronic channels, and understand barriers to communication.
      - Be aware that the audience may not have understood what is being communicated.
      - Know how to report and record information formally and informally in the appropriate way for the audience concerned, including how the use of the Common Assessment Framework for youths (CAF) helps communication between practitioners.

ii. Confidentiality and ethics
   - Remember and understand the procedures and legislation relating to confidentiality issues that apply to your job role.
   - Understand the limits of confidentiality that apply to your job role and that sometimes it is necessary to go against a young person's expressed wishes in their best interests and, where this is the case, ensure that the young person understands what is happening and why.

iii. Sources of support
   - Know where education and support services for parents are available locally.
   - Know when and how to refer to sources of information, advice or support from different agencies or professionals.

iv. Importance of respect
   - Be self-aware: know how to demonstrate a commitment to treating all people fairly; be respectful by using active listening and avoiding assumptions.

Significance

- Youth form the majority of population of India and a fact effectively communicated to them would have far greater impact on the health of the community in the long run.

10. Nutritional anemia.

- Nutritional anemia is a condition in which the hemoglobin content of blood is lower than normal as a result of a deficiency of one or more essential nutrients, regardless of the cause of such deficiency (WHO).

Hemoglobin Cutoff Criteria for Anemia by WHO (of venous blood)

i. Adult male	13 g/dL[Q]
ii. Adult female	12 g/dL[Q]
iii. Pregnant woman[Q]	11 g/dL
iv. Child above 6 years	12 g/dL
v. Child below 6 years	11 g/dL[Q]

Causes

Iron deficiency anemia (due to deficiency of iron)	*Megaloblastic anemia (due to deficiency of vitamin B_{12} or folic acid)*
i. Decreased intake – Cereal and pulse based diet poor in iron – Inability to eat animal food due to poverty and strict vegetarianism – Seasonal non-availability of green leafy vegetables – Milk based diet ii. Increased demand for iron – Pregnancy – Infections iii. Excessive loss of iron due to hemorrhages – Menstruation, childbirth (physiological) – Anlyostomiasis, peptic ulcers, bleeding hemorrhoids, ulcerative colitis, etc. (pathological) iv. Other causes – Repeated pregnancies – Chronic infections – Presence of absorption interfering factors like phytates of wheat, phosphates of egg yolk, tannin of tea, oxalates of vegetables, etc.	i. Nutritional – Strict vegetarian diet[Q] ii. Increased demand – Pregnancy iii. Pathological – Tape worm infestation which absorbs vitamin B_{12} – Malabsorption syndrome

Detrimental Effects (Early warning signs of impeding anemia which becomes evident later)

a. Pregnancy	▪ Anemia during pregnancy will result in abortions, premature babies, low birth weight, still birth, excessive postpartum hemorrhage thus resulting in increased risk of infant mortality and maternal mortality
b. Infections	▪ Iron deficiency lower immunity by impairing cellular responses and immune functions thus increases the susceptibility to infections
c. Work capacity	▪ Anemia causes easy fatiguability, exhaustion and tiredness which results in decreased efficiency, decreased production and increased accidents affecting the economy of the country ▪ More severe the anemia, greater the reduction in work capacity
d. Child growth	▪ Anemia causes failure of growth in children, interferes with their learning and education process ▪ Decreased motor development results in decreased physical activity ▪ It also increases their susceptibility to infection

Clinical Features

- General appearance — Pale, plumpy, poor built and nourishment and easy fatiguability
- Head — Headache, giddiness
- Face — Pale and puffy
- Eye — Pale conjunctiva
- Hairs — Dry, lusterless
- Tongue — Pale, smooth with atrophied papillae
- Feet — Edematous
- Nails — Brittle, spoon shaped (koilonychia)
- Respiratory system — Exertional breathlessness
- Cardiovascular system — Rapid and weak pulse, lower BP, soft systolic murmur
- Abdomen — Anorexia, acidity, ascites, dysphagia

Prevention and Control

a. Health promotion
   - Adequate nutrition
   - Nutrition education to improve dietary habits
   - Heath education especially to pregnant mothers about hazards of anemia and its prevention
   - Periodical deworming especially amongst children and atleast once during second trimester of pregnancy
   - Nutritional supplementation under ICDS scheme.

b. Specific protection
   i. Food fortification
      - Consumption of salt fortified with ferric orthophosphate or ferrous sulfate with sodium bisulfate over a period of 12–18 months improves the hemoglobin content of the blood and thus results in prevalence of nutritional anemia significantly.
      - Govt. of India has accepted this as public health approach for prevention of nutritional anemia.

   ii. National nutritional anemia prophylaxis program
      - National nutritional anemia prophylaxis program was launced by the Govt. of India during fifth five year plan in 1970 to prevent nutritional anemia in mothers and children

Objective	*Beneficiaries*	*Eligibility criteria*
▪ To prevent and control nutritional anemia among mothers and children aged between 1–12 years	▪ Pregnant mothers ▪ Lactating mothers ▪ Children aged between 1–12 years	▪ Hb level between 10–12 g/dL ▪ Hb level below 10 g/dL referred to medical officer for treatment

Strategy

- Under the progam, all the beneficiaries who are eligible are distributed iron and folic acid tablets free of cost.
- These iron and folic acid tablets contain 100 mg of elemental iron[Q] (300 mg of ferrous sulfate) and 0.5 mg of folic acid[Q] for adults and 20 mg of elemental iron and 0.1 mg of folic acid for children[Q].
- These tablets are distributed through Govt. hospitals, CHCs, PHCs, Anganwadi, Female Health workers, etc.

Dosage

Group	*Dosage*	*Duration*
Pregnant mother with no visible signs of anemia	1 tablet	Last 100 days of pregnancy
Pregnant mother with visible signs of anemia	2 tablets	Daily until 2–3 months after hemoglobin level returned to normal[Q] so that iron stores are replenished
Pregnant mother with severe anemia	Admitted to hospital for treatment	
Anemic children between 1–12 years	1 tablet (pediatric)	Daily

Significance

- National nutritional anemia prophylaxis program has significantly reduced the prevalence of nutritional anemia in India and thus has contributed in reduction of infant mortality and maternal mortality rate.
- This program is now part of RCH program.

c. Early diagnosis and treatment
- By history of headache, giddiness, fatigue, loss of appetite
- By clinical signs
- By laboratory investigations like Hb%, peripheral smear, stool examination for ova or cysts of parasites
- Treatment of underlying etiology like parasitic infestation, bleeding piles, peptic ulcers, etc.
- Nutritional anemia is treated as follows:

Grade (WHO)	*Degree of anemia*	*Treatment*
11–14 g/dL	Nomal	No treatment
9–11 g/dL	Mild	Oral iron therapy
7–9 g/dL	Moderate	Parental iron therapy
<7 g/dL	Severe	Blood transfusion

d. Disability limitation
- This consists of treatment of cardiac failure associated with anemia with packed cell transfusion under the umbrella of digoxin, lasix and potassium salts.

Significance

- Nutritional anemia is a very important and very prevalent nutritional problem faced by India and needs to be addressed.

11. Main features of the ICDS program.

Refer Question No. 2 June 2010 (RS2) Paper II

12. Types of carriers.

Refer Question No. 1 June 2009 (RS2) Paper I.

SHORT ANSWERS

13. Stratified sampling.

Refer Question No. 1 June 2016 (RS2) Paper I.

14. Epidemiological case sheet for investigation of an epidemic.

Refer Question No. 2 December 2015 (RS2) Paper I.

15. Indicators of air pollution.

Refer Question No. 5 December 2014 (RS2) Paper I.

16. Soakage pit.

- Soakage pit is a cheap, simple and sanitary method of disposing sullage water in rural setup

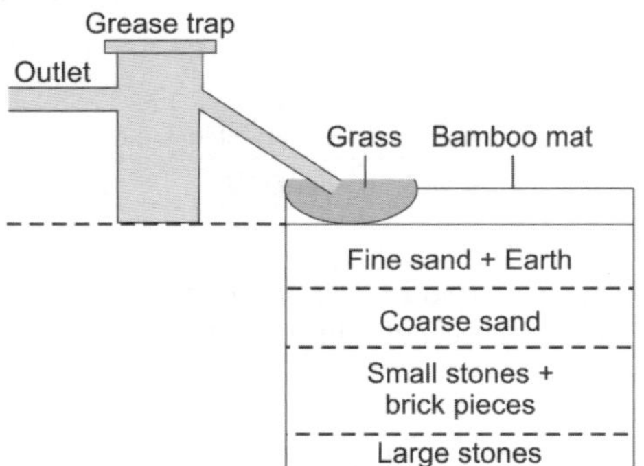

Fig. 1: Soakage pit

Steps of Constructing a Soakage pit

- Choose a proper site which should be at least 10 m distant from house wall and any well. Moreover, at the chosen site the water level should be more than 3–4 m below the ground level
- Dig a pit about 1 m long, broad and deep with a 15 cm slope at bottom directed away from house
- Divide the depth of pit into roughly 4 equal parts. Fill lower most part with stones or bricks the size of a coconut. Fill the second part with stones or bricks the size of a big apple. Fill the third part with tones of the size of an average lemon. The fourth or upper most part is for the inlet chamber.
- Construct the inlet chamber as follows:
  - Lay the foundation of the chamber at center in with 4 bricks leaving a central space of 12.5 × 12.5 cm
  - Lay on these bricks another layer bricks without leaving any space between the joints
  - If needed lay 3rd or 4th layer similarly depending upon the slope of the drain from the source outlet of waste water to the inlet chamber
- Cover the stone layer of the pit with 1 m^2 gunny cloth with a hole in the center about the size of inlet chamber
- Cover the gunny cloth with a similar sized polythene sheet having a hole in the center
- Cover the polythene sheet with soil and fill the pit. Compact the soil properly.
- Make a pucca drain of 7 cm wide and 10cm deep from the water outlet to the soak pit inlet with slope of 8 cm per meter. Cover the drain with bricks or flat stones to check entry of solid waste and rain water.
- A trap of 35 cm (length) × 25 cm (breadth) × 25 cm (height) is provided near the middle of the drain to check the entry of suspended solids from entering the pit.
- Cover the trap and the inlet chamber of the pit with a flat stone cover the top surface of the soak pit with soil so as to raise it 5 cm above the surrounding ground level.

Advantages

- Soakage pit is a cheap, simple and sanitary method of sullage disposal
- It can be built at home by the users themselves
- It also acts as a device for recharging of ground water.

17. Preplacement examination.

Refer Question No. 2 June 2016 (RS2) Paper I.

18. Nuclear family.

Refer Question No. 12 June 2013 (RS2) Paper I.

19. Lathyrism.

Refer Question No. 12 December 2009 (RS2) Paper I.

20. Sanitation barrier.

- Sanitation barrier is method of segregating the faeces and arranging for its proper disposal so that the disease agent cannot reach the new host, directly or indirectly.

Method of Ensuring Sanitation Barrier

- Sanitation barrier can be effectively provided by construction and use of sanitary latrines.

Advantage

- Sanitation barrier prevents access of pathogens from feces (F) through 6 Fs to the mouth of susceptible persons. The 6 Fs are:
  - **F**luid (water and milk)
  - **F**ood
  - **F**ruits and vegetables
  - **F**omites (soil, utensils)
  - **F**lies (vectors)
  - **F**ingers.

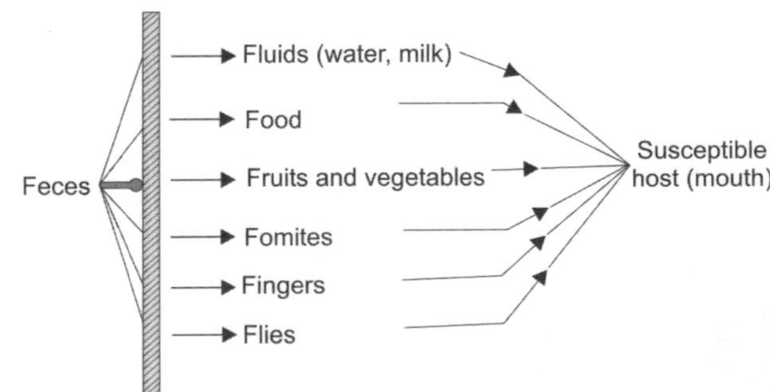

Fig. 2: Sanitation barrier

Significance

- Sanitation barrier breaks the disease cycle of fecal borne disease at the most vulnerable point, i.e. from feces to mouth of the host.

21. Social medicine.

- Social medicine is the study of man as a social being in his total environment comprising physical, biological and social environment.
- It is an expression of humanitarian tradition in medicine and people read into it any interpretation consistent with their own aspirations and interests.
- It is concerned with a body of knowledge embodied in epidemiology and the study of medical needs or medical care of the society.
- Concept first introduced by Neumann and Virchow[Q]
- Term was coined by Jules Guerin[Q]

Components	*Applications*
▪ Social anatomy ▪ Social physiology ▪ Social pathology ▪ Social therapy	▪ Development of epidemiological methods and their application to the investigations of disease

Advantages	*Limitations*
▪ Social medicine focuses on the health of the community as a whole ▪ It emphasizes the strong relationship between medicine and social science	▪ It is virtually isolated from the service world and confined mostly to academic study of health services and chronic diseases

Significance

- Social medicine is not a branch of medicine but rather new orientation of the medicine to the changing needs of man and society
- It is the precursor of preventive and social medicine which was formed by merger of preventive medicine and social medicine.

22. Integrated disease surveillance system.

Refer Question No. 12 June 2016 (RS2) Paper II.

MBBS PHASE III EXAMINATION

JUNE 2008

(Revised Scheme 2)

PAPER II

LONG ESSAYS

1. Discuss polio eradication in the light of epidemiological factors influencing poliomyelitis.

- Poliomyelitis is said to be eradicated from a country, when zero incidence is maintained for 3 continuous years with the absence of circulating wild polio virus in the environment and the people are free from the fear of getting the disease without immunization
- India has been certified polio free on 27th March 2014.

Epidemiological Basis for Polio Eradication

- Human beings are the only reservoir of infection[Q]
- There is no animal reservoir state
- There is no chronic carrier state[Q]
- Half life of excreted wild polio virus in sewage, is very short, i.e. 48 hours and the spread of infection through sewage can occur only during this period
- Available vaccine is a live vaccine, stabilized, highly potent, cheap, can easily be administered orally and highly safe
- As the live vaccine is administered orally, it mimics the natural route of infection
- There are no contraindications, under national program
- Oral polio vaccine helps in the indirect immunization of susceptible children in the community
- Simultaneous administration of vaccine within a short period of time by mass immunization campaigns like pulse polio immunization, vaccine helps in the replacement of the wild virus from the entire nature, by inducing the gut immunity and circulation of the vaccine progeny virus
- Correct and complete dosage schedule offers life long immunity.

Epidemiology of Poliomyelitis

- Poliomyelitis is an acute, highly infectious disease of children caused by a RNA virus[Q]

Agent factors	
a. Causative agent	▪ Poliovirus, the causative agent is a RNA virus belonging to the group of picarnovirus and family enterovirus ▪ It is 25 nm in size ▪ There are three of polioviruses, type 1 accounting for 80–90% of cases[Q], type 2 (rare) and type 3 (less frequent) ▪ The virus can survive outside the human body for fairly long period, however, the half life of excreted virus in sewer is only 48 hours and spread of infection occurs only during this period ▪ Virus can multiply only in human gut of unimmunized individual ▪ It selectively affects the motor neurons of the CNS resulting in flaccid paralysis[Q] ▪ There is no development of cross immunity

Contd...

Contd...

b. Reservoir of infection	▪ Humans are the only known host and reservoir of infection ▪ There is no animal reservoir ▪ The human reservoir may be an active clinical case or a carrier ▪ Even the carrier state in polio is temporary and there is no chronic carrier state
c. Infective material	▪ Throat secretions and feces of the diseased individual in early stage and only feces in later stages
d. Period of infectivity	▪ 1 week before and 3 weeks after the onset of signs and symptoms
Agent factors	
a. Age	▪ All age groups are susceptible but maximum incidence in age group of 6 months to 3 years[Q]
b. Sex	▪ Male : Female ratio 3 : 1
c. Risk factors (provocative poliomyelitis)	▪ Several risk factors or provocative factors favor precipitation of attack of paralytic poliomyelitis in susceptible individuals with latent virus ▪ These factors are: – Painful intramuscular injections especially of alum based DPT vaccine – Fatigue, trauma, exercise – Head and neck region surgeries like tonsillectomies, adenoidectomies, tooth extraction
d. Immunity	▪ After first 6 months of life the maternal antibodies gradually disappear ▪ Infection offers life long immunity ▪ However, there is no cross immunity[Q], i.e. infection with one poliovirus type does not offer immunity against the other types
Environmental factors	
a. Season	▪ Majority of cases seen in June to September and lowest transmission in November to March
b. Other factors	▪ Overcrowding, poor sanitation and contamination of food and water favor transmission of virus

Significance

- After successful eradication of smallpox, the WHO has targeted poliomyelitis for global eradication considering the epidemiological factors favoring its eradication and India is doing its bit for polio eradication through National Polio Eradication Program
- A country is certified for polio eradication if there is no viriologically confirmed diagnosed case of polio for last 5 years[Q]
- There is interruption of wild polio virus circulation in India
- Last case was reported on 13/01/2011 at Howrah, West Bengal.

2. Describe the natural history of stroke. What measures can be taken at the community level to control it?

- Stroke is an acute, focal or global disturbance of cerebral function, lasting for more than 24 hours or leading to death with no apparent cause other than vascular origin (WHO)
- 24 hours threshold excludes transient ischemic attach
- Also called apoplexy.

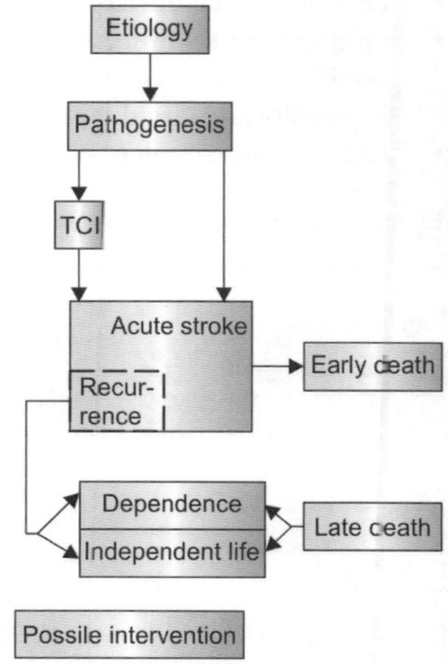

Fig. 1: Natural history of stroke

Natural History

Prepathogenic Phase (Epidemiology)

a. Agent factors (risk factors)—associated with >75% cases
   i. Hypertension
      - Main risk factor for cerebral thrombosis and cerebral hemorrhage.
   ii. Serum cholesterol
      - There exists a relationship between levels of serum cholesterol and incidence of cerebral hemorrhage or cerebral infarction.
   iii. Diabetes
      - Risk factor for cerebral thrombosis in cortical artery region.

iv. Others
   - Cardiac abnormality (left ventricular hypertrophy, cardiac dilatation), obesity, smoking, glucose intolerance, blood clotting and viscosity, oral contraceptive, etc.

v. Transient ischemic attack
   - Episodes of focal, reversible neurological deficit of sudden onset lasting for less than 24 hours
   - Caused due to microemboli and show tendency to recurrence
   - Occur in fair proportion of stroke cases and are a warning signs of stroke.

b. Host factors

i. Age
   - Can occur at any age but incidence rises steeply with age specially after 40 years of age.

ii. Sex
   - Twice as common in men as in women.

iii. Personal history
   - 1/3rd of patients have preexisting diseases mostly of cardiovascular system or diabetes.

Pathogenesis Phase

- Stroke is considered a number of syndromes which includes:
  - Transient cerebral ischemia (of more than 24 hours)
  - Subarachnoid hemorrhage
  - Cerebral hemorrhage
  - Cerebral thrombosis/embolism
  - Occlusion of precerebral arteries
  - Ill-defined cardiovascular disease
- In many instance, transient cerebral ischemia precedes the stroke
- In cerebral embolism, onset is almost instantaneous and signs tend to appear in steps
- Headache and other signs of raised intracranial pressure precedes intracranial hemorrhage
- Characteristic onset of focal neurological signs and sequence of events, a group of symptoms and signs make the diagnosis and localization possible.

Measures at Community Level to Prevent Stroke

- Under stroke control program, following measures are taken at community level to prevent stroke.

a. Control of arterial hypertension	▪ As arterial hypertension is the major cause of stroke, its preventions is first priority of stroke prevention ▪ This is achieved through health education, relief of stress, weight reduction, diet control, promotion of regular exercise, lifestyle modifications, self care, etc.
b. Early detection and treatment of TIA	▪ Association of transient ischemic attack with stroke makes its early detection and treatment important aspect of stroke prevention
c. Control of diabetes	▪ Early detection and treatment of diabetes is very essential
d. Elimination of smoking	▪ This could be achieved through health education and legislation
e. Management of other risk factors	▪ Management of other risk factors like hyperlipidemia, blood viscosity are very important
f. Improvement in health-care services for elderly	▪ Facilities for long-term follow-up of patients is essential ▪ There should also be facilities for treatment of complications
g. Community education	▪ Education and training of the public forms the integral part of community level prevention of stroke

Significance

- Stroke is an important noncommunicable disease in geriatric population rendering them incapable of self care and dignified death and thus requires sincere effort to bring it under control.

SHORT ESSAYS

3. Which are the factors influencing fertility in a community?

- Fertility means actual bearing of children.

Factors Influencing Fertility

- Fertility depends upon several factors
- In India, the fertility is very high evident from the fact that an average Indian woman gives birth to an average of 6–7 children if her married life is uninterrupted.

Factors enhancing fertility	
a. Universality of marriage	▪ In India, it is customary to get married at suitable age ▪ This is usually done to continue progeny
b. Lower age at marriage	▪ Age at which a female marries and enters the reproductive period of life has great impact on her fertility ▪ Women who marry before the legal age of marriage, i.e. 18 years give birth to more children than those marry after 18 years ▪ Woman married early have longer married life and more chances of conception ▪ Early marriage is a long established custom in India, the average age being 13 years ▪ This practice though reduced is still prevalent in parts of Madhya Pradesh, Rajasthan and Uttar Pradesh in name of Tradition where young brides are married on certain auspious occasions like Akha Teej ▪ Median age at marriage in India is 17.2 for females
c. Early menarche	▪ Early menarche increases the fertility by increasing the chances of conception and such women are married off at early age
d. Delayed menopause	▪ More delayed the menopause, longer the reproductive span and thus higher the fertility
e. Longer duration of married life	▪ Influence of duration of marriage on fertility is evident from the fact that 10–25% of all births occur within 1–5 years of married life and 50–55% within 5–15 yesrs of married life ▪ Thus longer the duration of marriage, more the number of babies born or higher the fertility
f. Spacing of children	▪ In India, concept of spacing is not widely popular and a woman conceives soon after delivery of previous child thus increasing the fertility
g. Age of population	▪ Younger the population more will be the fertility due to higher fecundity and more women in reproductive age group
h. Illiteracy	▪ Fertility is inversely related the education status of an individual ▪ Total fertility rate of illiterate women is 1.5 children higher than those educated up to high school
i. Poor economic status	▪ Economic status bears an inverse relation with fertility ▪ This is due to that family with poor economic conditions prefer to have more children who would work to earn bread and butter for family
j. Caste and religion	▪ Certain religious groups like Muslims have higher fertility ▪ Similarly lower castes in a religion have higher fertility
k. Poor nutrition	▪ High fertility in poorly fed societies shows the relationship between nutrition status and fertility ▪ However, this effect is indirect and mostly through economic condition
l. Family planning refusal	▪ Couples that do not opt for family planning methods have higher fertility
m. Other factors	▪ Higher fertility is also associated with other factors like degraded place of woman in society, important value of children in society, widow remarriage, customs and beliefs like that children are God's gifts, etc. good health conditions, opportunities for women and local community involvement
Factors decreasing fertility	
a. Higher age at marriage	▪ Age at which a female marries and enters the reproductive period of life has great impact on her fertility ▪ Women who marry before the legal age of marriage, i.e. 18 years give birth to more children than those marry after 18 years ▪ Woman married late has shorter married life and lesser chances of conception[Q] ▪ With legislation like Child Marriage Restrain Act, the legal age for marriage has been fixed at 18 years for females and 21 years for males ▪ This has declined the fertility in India
b. Early menopause	▪ More early the menopause, shorter the reproductive span and thus lower the fertility

Contd...

Contd...

c. Shorter duration of married life	▪ Influence of duration of marriage on fertility is evident from the fact that 10–25% of all births occur within 1–5 years of married life and 50–55% within 5–15 years of married life ▪ Thus shorter the duration of marriage, less the number of babies born or lower the fertility ▪ With advancing westernization, the system of divorce has taken root in India and thus decreasing the fertility
d. Spacing of children[Q]	▪ When all births are postponed by one year in each group, there is total decline in fertility[Q] ▪ It follows that spacing of children may have significant impact on the general reduction in fertility rates
e. Age of population	▪ Older the population less will be the fertility due to lower fecundity and less women in reproductive age group
f. Literary	▪ Fertility is inversely related to the education status of an individual[Q] ▪ Educated woman prefer methods of contraception early in marriage
g. Good economic status	▪ Economic status bears an inverse relation with fertility ▪ Good economic status provides for better health care thus ensuring child survival, good nutrition, better acceptance of family planning services
h. Caste and religion	▪ Certain religious groups like Christians have lower fertility and Hindus have medium fertility ▪ Similarly upper castes in a religion have lower fertility
i. Good nutrition	▪ Low fertility in well fed societies shows the relationship between nutrition status and fertility ▪ However, this effect is indirect and mostly through economic condition
j. Family planning	▪ Couples that opt for family planning methods early in marriage have lower fertility
k. Other factors	▪ Lower fertility is also associated with other factors like poor health delivery system, breastfeeding, industrialization and urbanization, opportunities for women and local community involvement

4. What are the main activities and benefits of an "under 5 clinic"?

Refer Question No. 2 December 2010 (RS2) Paper II.

5. Mid-day meals scheme.

- Mid-day Meal Scheme is a centrally sponsored scheme launched in 15th August 1995 (revised in 2004)
- Also known as Program of Nutritional Support to Primary Education
- It has undergone major revamp and covered by National Food Security Act, 2013.

Objective

- Universalization primary education by increasing enrolment, attendance and retention
- Impacting nutritional status of children in primary classes.

Beneficiary

- All school children in primary (Class I to V) and upper primary (Class classes studying in):
  - Government and government-aided schools
  - Education guarantee scheme and alternative and innovative education centers
  - Madarsa and Maqtabs supported under Sarva Shiksha Abhiyan and National Child Labor Project schools run by ministry of labor.

Nutrient Guidelines

- Meals provided should be hot and cooked locally.

	Primary class students	*Upper primary class students*
Calories	450	700
Proteins (in grams)	12	20
Rice/wheat (in grams)	100	150
Dal (in grams)	20	30
Vegetables (in grams)	50	75
Oil and fat (in grams)	5	7.5

Features

- Central and state governments share the cost of Mid-day Meal Scheme, with the center providing 60% and the states 40%
- Central assistance is provided by direct free supply of food grain to district administration from nearest Food Corporation of India godown at the rate of 100 g per student per day and subsidy for transport of food grain
- Costs for facilities, transportation and labor is shared by the Central and State Governments.

Significance

- Mid-day Meal Scheme is largest such program in the world
- Since 2017, the GOI as a monitoring tool, has mandated use of AADHAR for availing benefits under mid-day meal scheme.

6. What are the main health problems of urban slum dwellers and factors contributing to it?

Refer Question No. 9 December 2012 (RS2) Paper I.

7. Measures to prevent entry of yellow fever into India.

- Yellow fever is a zoonotic disease caused by an arbovirus[Q]
- It is an exotic disease as per India is concerned
- However, India is a yellow fever receptive area, i.e. an area in which yellow fever does not exist but where conditions would permit its development if introduced because:
  - Population is unvaccinated and susceptible
  - Vectors (*Aedes aegypti*) is found in abundance
  - onkey species found in India (*Macacus rhesus* and *Macacus sinicus*) are also susceptible
  - Climatic conditions are favorable in most parts of India for its transmission
- But still the disease does not exist because the missing link in chain of transmission is the yellow fever virus is not present in India[Q].

Measures to Prevent Entry of Yellow Fever in India

- The virus of yellow fever can gain entry into India through:
  - Infected travelers (clinical and subclinical cases)
  - Infected mosquitoes
- To prevent the entry of yellow fever virus, the Govt. of India adheres to International Health Regulations of WHO which are implemented through stringent aerial and maritime traffic regulations.

Travelers	*Mosquitoes*
▪ All travelers including infants exposed to the risk of yellow fever or passing through endemic zones of yellow fever must possess a valid international certificate of vaccination (validity 10 days to 10 years) against yellow fever before they are allowed to enter yellow fever receptive areas ▪ If the traveler does not possess the certificate then he is placed under quarantine in a mosquito proof ward for 6 days for observation from the date of leaving an infected area[Q] ▪ If the travelers possesses the certificate and arrives before the certificate becomes valid, he is isolated till the certificate becomes valid	▪ The aircrafts and ships arriving from endemic zones are subjected disinfection with aerosol spraying of prescribed insecticides on arrival for destruction of insect vectors ▪ The ships are moored about 400 meters from seaport and disinfected ▪ Further airports and seaports are kept free from the breeding of insect vectors over an area extending at least 400 meters around their perimeter[Q] ▪ The *Aedes aegypti* index is kept below 1[Q] (according to International Health Regulation)

Significance

- Strict implementation of aerial and maritime traffic regulations is very important to prevent entry of yellow fever in India as it is a receptive area for yellow fever.

8. Steps in the planning cycle.

- Planning is a process of "analyzing a system; defining a problem, assessing the extent to which the problem exists as a need, formulating goals and objectives to alleviate or ameliorate those identified needs, examining and choosing from among alternative intervention strategies, initiating the necessary action for its implementation and monitoring the system to ensure proper implementation of the plan and evaluating the results of intervention in the light of stated objectives

- Thus planning involves a succession of steps which are collectively called as planning cycle.

Planning Cycle

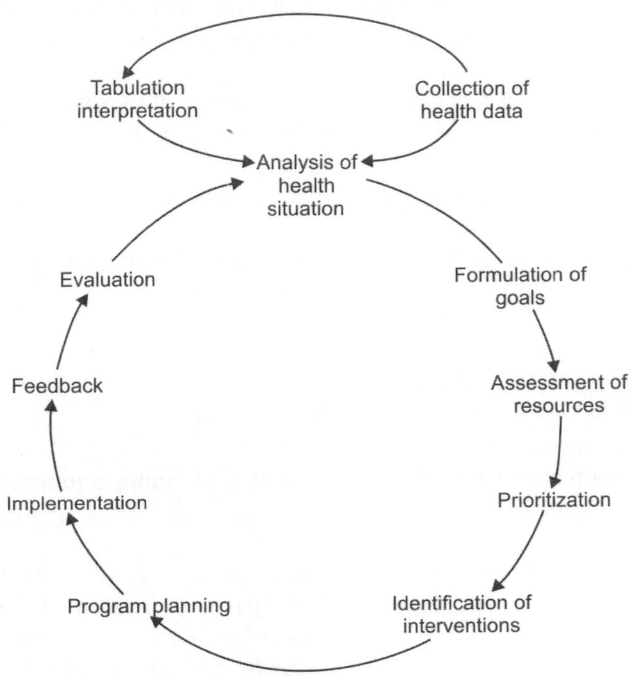

Fig. 2: Planning cycle

a. Analysis of the health situation[Q]
   - First step in planning cycle involves providing cycle involves providing a clear picture of health situation by collecting assessing and interpreting the information such as:
     i. Population its age and sex structure
     ii. Statistics of morbidity and mortality
     iii. Epidemiology and geographical distribution of different diseases
     iv. Medical care facilities like hospitals health centers and other health agencies
     v. Technical manpower of various categories
     vi. Availability of training facility
     vii. Attitudes and beliefs of the population towards disease, its cure and prevention.
     viii. Forementioned data is minimum essential requirement to bring about the health needs and health demands of the population.

b. Establishment of objectives and goals
   - After determining the health need and health demands of the population the objectives and goals of the program to address these needs has to be so that the efforts are guided in right direction
   - These objectives should be at all the level of organization down up to the smallest functional unit. Taking into consideration the time and resources at disposal
   - Objectives tend to be general at upper level but as the levels successively lower, they become more specified and detailed
   - Objectives guide the efforts and also serve as a Yard stick to measure the work done by means of cost benefit analysis and input–output study of health services
   - They are also important to prevent haphazard activity, uneconomical use of funds and poor performance.

c. Assessment of resources[Q]
   - Resources are the manpower, money, materials, skills, knowledge and technique needed or available for implementation of a health program
   - Availability of resources is important to formulate the objectives of the program
d. Fixing the priorities[Q]
   - Amongst all the health needs and demands, the priorities should be established in order of importance or magnitude
   - While fixing the priorities, attention should be paid to financial constraints mortality and morbidity data, diseases which can be prevented at lesser costs, saving lives of younger people and also political and community interests and pressure
   - Fixing of priorities is an important aspect of planning as resources always fall short of total requirement
   - Once priorities have been established, alternate plans for achieving them also formulated and assessed for their practibility and feasibility
   - Plan with greater effectiveness project is chosen and complete in all respects for execution.
e. Write up formulated plan
   - After a plan has been it should be prepared in detail containing following information:
     - Resources required
     - Results expected
     - Definition and cost of each stage
     - Time required for each stage to be implemented
     - Working guidance to all the people responsible for its execution
     - An in-built system of evaluation.
   - Any modification in a detailed plan can be done by the central planning authority and the government according to the resources available at hand.
f. Programming and implementation
   - Programming and implementation of the plan begin once a health plan is selected
   - Execution of the plan depends upon the existence of effective organization for which the plan must incorporate well define procedure to be followed sufficient delegation of authority to and fixation of responsibility of different workers for achieving the predetermined objective during the period prescribed.
   - Main considerations of this stage are:
     - Definition of roles and tasks
     - Selection, training, motivation and supervision of the manpower involved
     - Organization and communication
     - Efficiency of individual institutions such as PHCs hospitals.
g. Monitoring
   - Monitoring is a continuous day-to-day process of observing, recording and reporting of activities of or project curing stage of implementation to ensure that they are proceeding as planned and are on schedule
   - It thus identifies any deviations from the plan and helps to takes corrective measures if excessive deviations occur.
h. Evaluation[Q]
   - Evaluation assesses the achievement of the stated objectives of a program its adequacy, its efficiency and its acceptance by all the parties involved
   - It is concerned with the final outcome and with factors associated with it
   - A good plan has an in-built evaluation mechanism to measure the performance and effectiveness and for feedback to correct deficiencies or fill up gaps discovered during stage of implementation
   - Evaluation measures the degree to which objectives and targets are fulfilled and the quality of the result obtained. It measures the productivity of available resources in achieving clearly defined objectives it measures how much output or cost effectiveness is achieved. It makes possible the reallocation of priorities and of resources on the basis of changing health needs.

Significance

- Importance of planning can be summerized by the statement that "A work well planned is half done".

9. Activities of UNICEF in India.

Refer Question No. 8 June 2010 (RS2) Paper II.

10. Integrated management of a sick child.

- Integrated management of childhood illness (IMCI) is an international strategy developed by WHO and UNICEF for an integrated approach to the management of childhood illness as it is important for child health program to look beyond the treatment of a single disease
- Strategy combines improved management of childhood illness with aspects of nutrition, immunization and other important disease prevention and health promotion elements
- Indian version of IMCI has been renamed as Integrated Management of Neonatal and Childhood Illness (IMNCI).
- It has been started in four selected districts each in 9 states (Uttaranchal, Madhya Pradesh, Odisha, Rajasthan, Maharashtra, Gujarat, Delhi, Haryana and Tamil Nadu).

Difference in IMNCI from IMCI (Highlights of IMNCI[Q])

- Inclusion of 0–7 days age in program (hence the word Neonatal)
- Incorporating national guidelines on malaria, anemia, vitamin A supplementation and immunization schedule[Q]
- Training of the health personnel begins with sick young infants up to 2 months
- Proportion of training time devoted to sick young infant and sick child is almost equal
- Is skill based

Objectives	*Components*	
	Curative component[Q] includes management of	*Health promotive and preventive component*
▪ To reduce deaths in children. ▪ To reduce frequency and severity of illness and disability ▪ To contribute to improved growth and development of child	▪ Diarrhoea ▪ Measles ▪ Acute respiratory infections (pneumonia) ▪ Malaria ▪ Severe malnutrition and nutritional counseling	▪ Breastfeeding ▪ Nutritional counseling ▪ Vitamin A and iron supplementation ▪ Immunization ▪ Treatment of helminthic infestations

Strategy

a. Syndromic approach
   - Children mostly suffer from a constellation of symptoms and need to be treated as a whole
   - Syndromic approach gives advantage of not missing out on coexisting conditions while presenting with a particular condition.

b. Holistic approach
   - Taking care of all the factors that determine the health of the child
   - Like, while treating for diarrhea, the immunization and nutritional factors are also addressed.

c. Triage
   - Management is planned after triage of the patient into those needing emergent, early treatment, referral or care at home.

d. Standardized case management
   - Based on the classification/severity of illness.

e. Primary health-care model
   - Based on primary health-care model and referral to a facility when required.

f. Community participation
   - IMNCI approach gives due importance to role of the mother in the whole process of prevention, early diagnosis and management of the case at home by providing counseling to the caretaker.

Case Management Process[Q] (*ACT—Assess, Classify and Treat*)

a. Assessment
   – Assess a child by checking first for danger signs, asking questions about common conditions, examination the child and checking nutrition and immunization status and also checking the child for other health problems.

b. Classification
   – Classify a child's illness using a color-coded triage system as follows:
     - Red: Urgent prereferral treatment and referral
     - Yellow: Specific medical treatment and advice
     - Green: Simple advice on home management.

c. Identification of specific treatment
   – If the child requires referral, give essential treatment before referring the patient
   – If the child needs treatment at home, develop an integrated treatment plan and give the first dose in the clinic
   – If the child needs immunization, immunize the child.

d. Treatment instructions
   – Provide practical treatment instructions, including teaching the caretaker how to give oral drugs, how to feed and give fluids during illness and how to treat local infections at home
   – Ask caretaker to return for follow-up on a specific date
   – Teach then how to recognize danger signs to seek immediate medial attention.

e. Counseling
   – Assess feeding, including assessment of breastfeeding practices and counsel to solve any feeding problems found
   – Then counsel mother about her own health.

f. Give follow-up care
   – Instruct the parents when to return for follow-up and provide follow-up care when the child is brought back
   – Reassess the child for new problem if necessary.

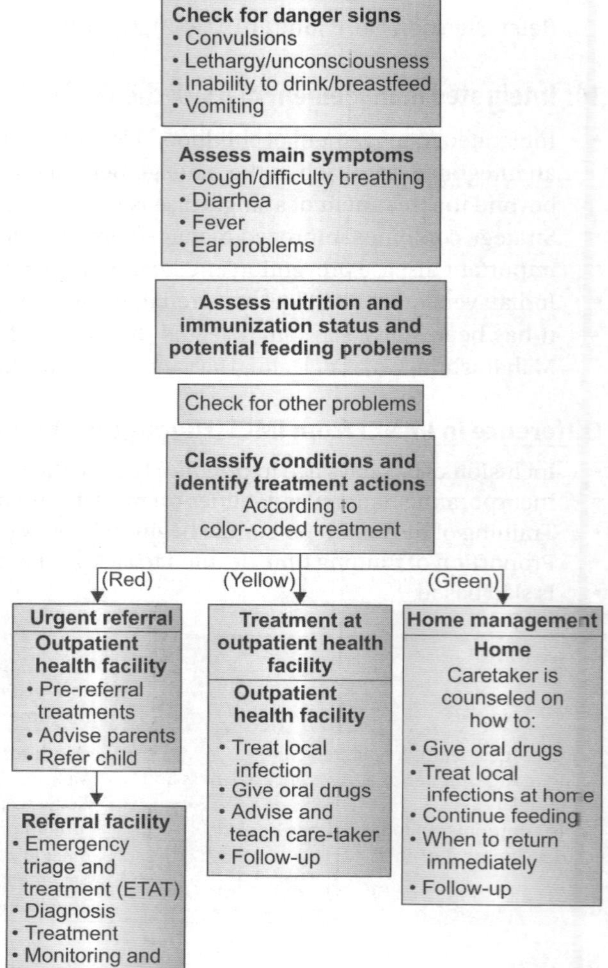

Fig. 3: Integrated management of childhood illness

Advantages	*Disadvantages*
▪ The program promote evidence-based assessment and management, using a syndromic approach that supports the rational, effective and affordable use of drugs ▪ The program besides management of sick child also includes health education to parents regarding child care ▪ It is cost effective	▪ The program does not address the management of trauma or other acute emergencies due to accidents or injuries ▪ It does not address AIDS specifically

Significance

IMNCI is the only child health strategy that emphasizes on prevention of disease and promotion of child health and development besides provision of standard case management of childhood illness.

11. Primary care services for the aged.

Refer Question No. 2 June 2009 (RS2) Paper II.

12. Essential obstetric care for ensuring safe motherhood.

Refer Question No. 1 December 2008 (RS2) Paper II.

SHORT ANSWERS

13. "Rule of Halves" in hypertension control.

Refer Question No. 12 December 2008 (RS2) Paper II.

14. Voluntary counseling testing center.

Refer Question No. 2 June 2015 (RS2) Paper II.

15. Demographic gap.

- The difference between the birth rate and the death rate marked in a graph is called demographic gap[Q].

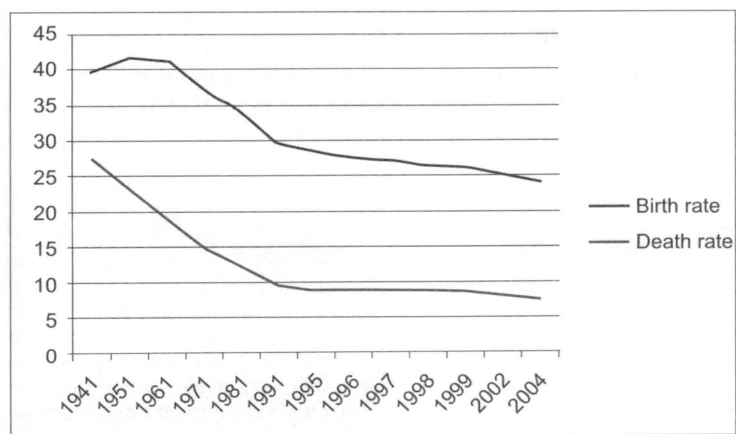

Fig. 4: Demographic gap

Significance

- Demographic gap can be used to compare the health status among various communities or countries
- It also serves an indicator for noting health progress of a community.

16. Pre-disaster phase of disaster management.

Refer Question No. 8 December 2012 (RS2) Paper II.

17. AYUSH in health-care services for the community.

Refer Question No. 19 December 2007 (RS2) Paper II.

18. Objectives of school health.

Refer Question No. 4 December 2013 (RS2) Paper II.

19. Social marketing of condoms.

- Social marketing of condoms is a component of condom programming/promotion by NACO.

Objectives	*Strategy*
▪ Increasing the acceptability and availability of condoms	▪ Social advertisement ▪ Phasing out unlubricated condom NIRODH and production of condoms adhering to WHO prescribed quality control specifications ▪ Providing easy access to condoms ▪ Improved sustainability in condom provision

Advantages	Disadvantages
▪ Condoms are the most cost effective method of controlling sexually transmitted infections including HIV/AIDS if used correctly and consistently ▪ It also prevents unwanted pregnancy thus alleviating the fear and enhancing the pleasure associated with sex	▪ Market research is required as the target groups for condom promotion for disease protection and for family planning are different

Significance

- Social marketing has been accepted as the most effective strategy for condom promotion.

20. DOTS strategy under RNTCP.

Refer Question No. 2 December 2012 (RS2) Paper II.

21. Measures for control of Urban malaria.

- Urban malaria poses a significant problem for malaria eradication prorgram.
- Hence to control the urban malaria, Urban Malaria Scheme was launched in 1971.
- Major vector for urban malaria is Anopheles stephensi.[Q]

Urban Malaria Scheme

Objectives	Area selection criteria	Control strategies
▪ To control malaria by controlling the vector population through antilarval measures	▪ Population >50,000 ▪ Slide positivity rate >5 ▪ API >1 ▪ Fever cases >30%	▪ Early diagnosis and treatment of malaria cases ▪ Bioenvironmental management of source reduction measures such as emptying water containers including overhead tanks, ponds, etc. once a week and observing weekly dry day ▪ Controlling larvae by weekly application of larvicidal oil, temephos, fenthion or by use of larvivorous fish

Significance

- Control of urban malaria primarily lies in implementation of civic by-laws to prevent mosquito breeding in domestic and peridomestic areas.

22. Five-year plans.

- Five-year plans are the component of the development strategy of Govt. of India.
- It is formulated by the National Planning Commission consisting of a chairman, a deputy chairman and 5 members
- First five-year plan was developed in 1951[Q] and currently 12th five-year plan (2012–2017) is being implemented.

Objectives

- To rebuild the rural India
- To lay foundation of industrial progress
- To secure the balanced development of all parts of the country
- Improve the health for better utilization of manpower and uplifting economic condition of the country by:
  - Control or eradication of major communicable diseases
  - Strengthening the basic health services through the establishment of primary health centers and subcenters
  - Population control
  - Development of health manpower resources.

Twelfth Five-Year Plan—2012–2017 (from Public Health Perspective)

Objective

- To improve the health status of the population by optimizing coverage and quality of care by indentifying and rectifying the critical gaps in infrastructure, manpower, equipment, essential diagnostic reagents and drugs.

Strategy

- Improve access to and enhance the quality of primary health care in urban and rural areas by providing an optimally functioning primary health-care system as a part of basic minimum services
- Improve the efficiency of existing health care infrastructure at primary, secondary and tertiary care settings through appropriate institutional strengthening and improvement in referral linkages.

Targets

Parameter	*Goal*
▪ Infant mortality rate	25 per 1000 live births
▪ Maternal mortality rate	100 per 100,000 live births
▪ Total fertility rate	2.1
▪ Under 3 year-old malnutrition	Reduction by 50%
▪ Anemia in 15–49 years old women	28%
▪ 0–6 years child sex ratio	950
▪ Poor household's out of pocket expenditure	Reduction
▪ Non-communicable disease burden	Reduction
▪ Communication disease burden	
– Tuberculosis	Reduce incidence and mortality by 50%
– Leprosy	▪ Prevalence <1/10,000 ▪ Incidence Zero in all districts
– Malaria	Incidence <1/1,000
– Filariasis	Microfilaria prevalence <1% in all districts
– Dengue	Case fatality rate <1%
– Chikungunya fever	Containment of outbreaks
– Japanese encephalitis	Mortality reduction by 30%
– Kala-azar	Elimination by 2015 (<1/10,000 in all blocks)
– HIV/AIDS	▪ Zero new infections ▪ Care and support ▪ ART to all PLHA

MBBS PHASE III EXAMINATION

DECEMBER 2008

(Revised Scheme 2)

PAPER I

LONG ESSAYS

1. What are the sociocultural factors contributing to PEM in India? What measures Government of India is taking to control malnutrition?

- Protein energy malnutrition (PEM) is a major health and nutrition problem[Q] occurring particularly in weakling and children in the first year of life.

Socioeconomic and Cultural Factors Contributing to PEM

- Socioeconomic and cultural factors related to nutrition are many in a country like ours
- Cultural beliefs traditions and practices influence the food behavior particularly at family level
- Influence of these factors in child nutrition starts in his embryonic days itself where mother is not allowed to eat more especially food of animals origin thinking that the babies to be delivered would be bigger and labor would be difficult
- Similarly because of poor economic status, a pregnant mother does not get enough nutrition to deliver a healthy baby thus predisposing the newborn to malnourishment in future
- A newborn child is denied colostrum because many people consider it equivalent to pus and blood
- In some communities it is a customary practice to feed the infant honey or sugar water during first 48 hours which is harmful to infant
- Rural India does not recognize the importance of weaning and the child is exclusively breastfed for a year and sometimes up to two thus depriving the child of supplemental nutrition when required the most
- There numerous false beliefs regarding the some of the nutrition food like eggs and meat are through to produce jaundice and edema and considered unsuitable for delicate stomach of child and citrus fruit, butter milk curd are also for bidden for fear of cold and dals for fear of diarrhea
- A girl at menarche is fed only sweet things and salt is restricted in diet commonly consisting of jaggary, fat and sesame oil mixed with raw egg
- Certain foods which are considered cold like milk, and milk products, citrus fruits, ragi, melon, etc. are avoided during winter season
- In rainy season, many people eat pulp of date palm
- There is even belief that drinks like toddy and arrack are suppose to increase the potency in adolescent boys
- Religion also plays an important role in child nutrition as Hindus and Jains do not eat protein rich eggs and meat and have to rely on pulses for their protein requirement
- Children as known to exhibit food fads that is a personal like and dislike towards particular foods which may lead to nutritional deficiencies
- Harmful cooking practices like draining away the rice water at the end of cooking, prolonged boiling in open pans, peeling of vegetables, etc. alter the nutritious value of food
- In modern society, many mothers prefer bottle feeding their infants considering their figure which is harmful
- Excessive reliance on commercially available baby food products is also harmful
- A child suffering from diarrhea is kept hungry with belief that if nothing is fed nothing would be defecated thus stopping diarrhea which relay a dangerous practice, as it is the time that child requires additional nutritional to make up for the loss

- Similarly if child is severely ill and unable to demand food, some mothers consider it as their children do not need food
- Belief of dangerous food combinations like spinach and tomato, fish and milk also deprives nutrition to children
- Nutrition of children living in poor sanitary conditions is also affected due to higher incidence of feco-oral diseases and parasitic infestations in them
- Poverty force children into child labor and even their nutrition is compromised at the cost of the head of family or other adults
- Ignorance regarding importance of child nutrition is also contributory to the malnutrition
- Even in large family, the child nutrition is compromised at the cost of adults
- Hence socioeconomic and cultural factors play an important role in child's nutrition.

Measures by Government of India to Control Malnutrition

- Government of India has initiated numerous measures at various levels to prevent malnutrition.

Measures at family level	*Measures at community level*	*Measures at national level*
▪ Malnutrition at the family level is combated through nutrition education of both the husband and wife on selection of right kind of local foods and planning of nutritionally adequate diets within the limits of their purchasing power ▪ Harmful food taboos and dietary prejudices are identified and corrected ▪ Improvement of breastfeeding and improvement in infant and child feeding practices is achieved through health education ▪ Misleading commercial baby food advertising is regulated ▪ Encouragement is provided to plan kitchen garden or rear poultry to meet shortage of protective food	▪ Malnutrition at community level is managed by supplementary feeding programs, midday school meals, vitamin A prophylaxis program ▪ Availability of food is increased in terms of both quality and quantity and is made accessible to the malnourished population ▪ Various types of protective foods are produced by the community for community under Applied Nutrition Program ▪ Supplementary nutrition is provided to vulnerable age groups, i.e. children under 6 years of age, adolescent girls and pregnant and lactating mothers through ICDS program	▪ Rural development is attempted to increase the food production, raising the standard of living and improving the purchasing power of the poor ▪ Agriculture production is increased by application of modern farming practices, expansion of cultivated areas, use of fertilizers and better seeds, etc. ▪ The food is supplied to the needy and poor through public distribution system or fair price shops ▪ Numerous nutritional intervention programs have been initiated like prevention and control of endemic goiter through iodized salt, distribution of iron and folic acid tablets to prevent nutritional anemia, fortification of food, supplementary feeding programs for preschool children

Significance

- Measures to prevent malnutrition require coordinated approach many disciplines like nutrition, food technology, health administration, health education, marketing, etc.

2. You are in-charge of a primary health centre. How will you make a community diagnosis of the health situation in order to formulate intervention measures?

- Community diagnosis is the pattern of disease in a community described in terms of the important factors which influence this pattern
- It is defined as the study of pattern of mortality and morbidity in the community and factors which influence this pattern
- It is made by the epidemiologist and is concerned with defined population involving both sick and healthy people.

Objectives	*Strategy*
▪ Identification of basic health needs and health problems of the community	▪ Community diagnosis is based on collection and interpretation of relevant data such as: – Age and sex distribution of a population – Social distribution of the population – Vital statistics rates such as birth rate, death rate – Incidence and prevalence of important diseases of the area

Significance

- Community diagnosis helps to prioritize the health problems and implement control measures.

Community diagnosis at Primary Health Center

- Community medicine is based on collection, analysis and interpretation of following data.

Age and sex distribution of population	*Social distribution of population*	*Vital statistics*	*Incidence and prevalence of diseases in the area*
▪ It is collected from census reports of the area ▪ It helps to understand the structure of community	▪ It involves study of social relationships, social groups and socioeconomic status of the community to determine functioning of community	▪ Vital statistics like crude birth rate, crude death rate, age specific death rate, disease specific death rate, etc. are indicators of the health and morbidity of the community ▪ For community diagnosis, morbidity data is preferred but mortality data is widely used because of its easy availability ▪ These are considered the signs and symptoms for community diagnosis	▪ It involves study of disease pattern in the community, risk groups for various illnesses, characteristics of diseased people, nutritional status of the community, environmental sanitation of the community, etc.

- Analysis and interpretation of the above data, helps in diagnosing the health need of the community
- Based on the community diagnosis, the proper intervention measures are adopted to control and cater the health needs of the community.

Application

- Community diagnosis diagnoses national and local health problems and the changing pattern of disease in the community
- It identifies the risk groups in the community
- It helps to compare the health status of a community with another.

SHORT ESSAYS

3. Steps in conducting a "Cohort study".

Refer Question No. 1 December 2016 (RS2) Paper I.

4. Effects of noise on health.

- Noise is an unwanted sound, causing disturbance or annoyance to the hearer
- Human ear is sensitive to sound frequency of 20–20,000 Hz[Q]
- Daily maximum tolerable sound level to human ear (without sustained damage to hearing) is 85–90 dB[Q]
- Hazards of noise pollution are seen above acceptable noise level of 85 dB[Q].

Effect of Noise on Health (Hazards of Noise Pollution)

Auditory hazards	*Non – auditory hazards*
a. Auditory fatigue[Q] – Appears in region of 90 dB[Q] and greatest at 4,000 Hz[Q] – May be associated with side effects such as whistling and buzzing in the ear b. Deafness – Most serious hazard and may be temporary or permanent – Person is generally loss results from a specific exposure to noise and disappears after a period of time up to 24 hours following the noise exposure – Usually occurs in the frequency range of 4,000–6,000 Hz – Permanent hearing loss may occur due to repeated or continuous exposure to noise around 100 dB[Q] – Changes may be as minor as changes in hair cell endings or major as complete destruction of organ of Corti – Sometimes even rupture of tympanic membrane due to noise above 160 dB[Q] may also lead to permanent hearing loss	a. Interference with speech – Sound frequencies in range of 300–500 Hz (commonly produced due to road and air traffic) may cause interference speech communication b. Annoyance – Primarily a psychological response which is evident from the observation that people working in noisy environment are more likely to be short tempered, often irritated and impatient – Neurotic people are more sensitive than balanced people c. Efficiency – Noise level is inversely proportional to work efficiency – Low noise levels are desired where mental concentration is to be undertaken d. Physiological changes – Numerous physiological changes occur in body as a direct result of noise exposure such as: o Rise in blood pressure o Rise in intracranial pressure o Increased heart rate and breathing o Increased sweating. – Noise interferes with sleep, causes visual disturbances due to narrowing of pupils, affection of color perception and reduction of night vision – May also general symptoms such as giddiness, nausea and fatigue e. Economic loss – Noise is a significant factor in economic losses

Control and Prevention	
a. Control at source	• Planned maintenance of the machines • Modification of the speed of the machines • Used of resilient materials • Enclosure of machines • Sound proofing of walls • Replacement of equipment, insertion of silencer
b. Increasing the distance from source of noise	• Possible in open field • In closed space achieved by sound proof lining of the walls
c. Reduction of exposure time	• By job rotation
d. Acoustic barrier	• Around the source: insulation, damping • Around the receiver: ear muffs, ear plugs
e. Miscellaneous	
i. Careful planning of cities	• Division of cities into residential zones, industrial zones, transportation zone, etc. • Separation of residential areas from the main roads by means of wide green belts of about 15 meters with thick trees and bushes • Widening of main roads to reduce level of noise penetration into dwellings
ii. Control of vehicles	• Avoiding routing of heavy vehicles into narrow lanes • Reduction in vehicular traffic in residential areas • Prohibition of indiscriminate use of horn
iii. Improving acoustic insulation of building	• Construction of detached building • Prohibition of noise producing installations
iv. Legislation	• Supreme Court has prohibited use of loudspeakers after 11 PM in residential areas
v. Education	• Through all media, general public should be educated such as avoiding honking near hospitals, schools, offices, etc. using horns free from shrills, enforcement of speed limits, restriction on loudspeakers, etc.

5. Disability indicators.

Refer Question No. 1 June 2008 (RS2) Paper I.

6. Qualities of a good screening test.

Refer Question No. 1 December 2010 (RS2) Paper I.

7. Natural history of a disease.

Refer Question No. 1 December 2007 (RS2) Paper I.

8. Diseases of poverty.

- Poverty has long been associated with health inequities and poverty and ill-health are interlinked
- Association between poverty and ill-health reflects causality running in both directions
- Ill-health is often associated with substantial health care costs but poverty and low income also cause ill-health
- Thus poor people are thus caught in a vicious circle—poverty breeds ill health, ill-health maintains poverty.

Role of Poverty on Health

- Poverty has indirect influence on health at almost every stage of life, right from conception till death
- Poverty predisposes people to greater risk of unhealthy conditions at home and at work
- Poor live in slums surrounded by filth and vector breeding places which pose a great health hazard
- Poor are forced into occupations that are injurious to their health
- Poverty is the reason for nonimmunization, poor access to clean water and sanitation and unavailability of curative drugs and other treatments
- It is one of the causative factors for low life expectancy, low birth weight babies, higher maternal mortality, handicap, disability, mental illness, stress, suicide, family disintegration and substance abuse
- Poverty is a major component of the vicious cycle of malnutrition and has an important role to play in causation of malnutrition by poor nutrition, increased risk of infections, delayed recovery, etc.
- Moreover, even the ill health of forces the family to eat less and work harder to cope up with temporary financial loss.

Significance

- More than 19% of world population lives under poverty line and thus is exposed its deleterious effects
- Most of the poor are involved in production industry and hence vital for growth of an economy
- Thus investments in health care of the poor and social insurance would always be a better bet.

9. Housing standards for rural areas.

- In rural areas, the housing standards are lower than the urban areas.

Minimum Housing Standards for Rural Areas

- Site — Should be located on high elevation, firm ground
- Set back and layout — Provision for ample verandah space
- Built up area — Built up area should not exceed 1/3rd of total area[Q]
- Floor — Must be impermeable, smooth, dry and washable
- Walls — Must be strong, heat resistant, rat proof and smooth
- Roof — Should be at least 3.5 meters and made up of low heat transmitting substances
- Rooms — Should have at least 2 living rooms with 4–5 m^2 per person
- Kitchen — Should have a separate kitchen with a paved sink or platform for washing utensils
- Window — Window area must be at least 10% of floor area
- Doors — Door area must be at least 10% of floor area
- Lightening — Day light factor of +1% on floor
- Water supply — Sanitary well or tube well should be within a distance of quarter of a mile with provision of 40–50 liters/person/day
- Cattle shed — Cattle shed must be at least 25 feet away and should be open on all sides with provision of about 8 × 4 feet space for each cattle head
- Excreta disposal — Provided with sanitary latrine
- Waste disposal — Adequate arrangement for disposal of waste water, refuse and garbage

Significance

- Though rural housing standards are a bit compromised but at least minimum standard should be adhered to, so as to promote healthy living.

10. Measures for safe disposal of sullage.

- Sullage is the waste water coming from kitchen[Q] and bathroom
- It is liquid waste without excreta[Q].

Disposal of Sullage

Pervious pits like soakage pit	*Impervious pits or non-soakage pits like septic tank*	*Surface irrigation like kitchen garden*	*Underground drainage or sewerage system*
▪ Soakage pits are rectangular shaped pits filled with large stones, brick bats and gravel to dispose sullage in rural areas and small towns	▪ These are rectangular concrete tanks employed to dispose sullage in urban areas along with night soil	▪ It done by digging small pits in front of individual homes to collect sullage and is conveyed through proper drains to water trees, kitchen gardens, agriculture fields or natural streams	▪ These are big underground pipes laid in concrete bed which collect sullage from several houses and is carried to ultimate place of disposal ▪ To ensure self-cleansing velocity, these pipes are laid with sufficient gradient

Significance

- Sullage is most abundant liquid waste generated by humans and its proper systemic drainage is must so as avoid nuisance and disease prevention.

11. Types of carriers.

Refer Question No. 1 June 2009 (RS2) Paper I.

12. Principles of health education.

Refer Question No. 2 December 2011 (RS2) Paper I.

SHORT ANSWERS

13. Dietary needs of pregnant women.

- Pregnancy increases the calorie requirement of the woman by 350 kcal[Q] and protein requirement by 23 g per day throughout the pregnancy (New Guidelines, 2011)
- This additional calorie is provided through addition to balanced diet.

	Nonpregnant women	*Additional allowances*	*Additional calories*
Cereals	440 g	35 g	118 kcal
Pulses	45 g	15 g	52 kcal
Leafy vegetables	100 g	—	
Other vegetables	40 g	—	
Roots and tubers	50 g	—	
Milk	150 g	100 g	83 kcal
Oils and fats	25 g	—	
Sugar or jaggery	20 g	10 g	40 kcal
		Total	**293 kcal**

- This calorie requirement should be provided through all the nutritive as follows:

Net energy	*2525 kcal*
Protein	65 g
Fat	30 g
Calcium[Q]	1200 mg
Iron[Q]	35 mg
Retinol[Q]	800 mg
Thiamine	1.3 mg
Riboflavin	1.5 mg
Nicotinic acid	16 mg
Pyridoxine	2.5 mg
Ascorbic acid[Q]	40 mg
Folic acid	400 μg
Vitamin B_{12}[Q]	1 μg

Significance

- This additional energy is required during pregnancy is must for proper growth and development of the child and prevention of maternal mortality.

14. Dark green leafy vegetable.

- Dark green leafy vegetables are the indigenous leafy vegetables consumed by the people
- Darker the green leaves, greater their nutritive value.

Examples
- Spinach, amaranth, cabbage, fenugreek, coriander, etc.

Recommended dietary allowance
- 40 g for an adult man and 100 g for adult woman.

Dietary benefits	*Disadvantages*
▪ Sources of important nutrients ▪ Rich source of carotene, calcium, iron and vitamin C ▪ Good source of riboflavin, folic acid and others micronutrients ▪ Leaf proteins are good source of lysine ▪ They are high in water content and dietary fiber	▪ They are poor source of vitamin $B_{12,}$ proteins and carbohydrates ▪ Leaf proteins are deficient in sulfur containing amino acids ▪ Because of high oxalate content, the bioavailability of calcium and iron from greens is poor ▪ They are bulky and their calorific value is less (25–50 kcal/g)

Significance

- Green leafy vegetables are cheap, easily available source of essential nutrients
- Besides an essential component of balanced diet, they are recommended for obese people and diabetics to cut down their calorie intake and increase dietary fiber in their diet and also to treat constipation.

15. Environmental antilarval measures.

Refer Question No. 11 June 2010 (RS2) Paper I.

16. Asbestosis control.

Refer Question No. 14 June 2013 (RS2) Paper I.

17. Bar diagram.

Refer Question No. 8 June 2017 (RS2) Paper I.

18. Warning signs of poor mental health.

Refer Question No. 6 June 2009 (RS2) Paper I.

19. Modified Prasad's classification.

- Dr BG Prasad's method of social stratification employs per capita family monthly income as an indicator and classifies status in 5 classes
- It is used for rural families and based on per capita monthly income
- When BG Prasad proposed this method in 1961, he had considered the per capita family income in those days for classification but with economic growth, a need was felt to apply a correction factor.
- This correction factor is obtained from multiplying the All India Consumer Price Index (AICPI) of rupee with 4.93% as suggested by Kumar (1991) and has been used ever since
- Thus we have

$$\text{Per capita family monthly income} = \frac{\text{Total monthly come of the family}}{\text{Total members of the family}} \times \text{AICPI} \times \frac{4.93}{100}$$

Classification (Based on Per Capita Family Monthly Income)

Socioeconomic status	*Prasad's classification (1961)*	*Modification proposed by Kumar (1991)*	*Modification Prasad's classification (April 2012) Consumer price Index = 949*
I	₹ 100 and above	₹ 1000 and above	₹ 4700 and above
II	₹ 50–99	₹ 500–999	₹ 2350–4699
III	₹ 30–49	₹ 300–499	₹ 1410–2349
IV	₹ 15–29	₹ 150–299	₹ 705–1409
V	Less than ₹ 15	Less than ₹ 150	Less than ₹ 704

Significance

The BG Prasad classification considers the per capita monthly income of the family not the individuals but overlooks other important factors which play important role in rural society.

20. Normal curve.

Refer Question No. 6 December 2014 (RS2) Paper I.

21. International quarantine.

Refer Question No. 18 December 2007 (RS2) Paper II.

22. Crude death rate.

Refer Question No. 4 December 2007 (RS2) Paper I.

MBBS PHASE III EXAMINATION

DECEMBER 2008

(Revised Scheme 2)

PAPER II

LONG ESSAYS

1. Describe the components and strategies under reproductive and child health (RCH) program.

- RCH program is example of old wine in new bottle as it replaced the National Child Survival and Safe Motherhood program in 1994
- The first phase of the program was launched in 1996 and the second phase of the program was launched in 2005

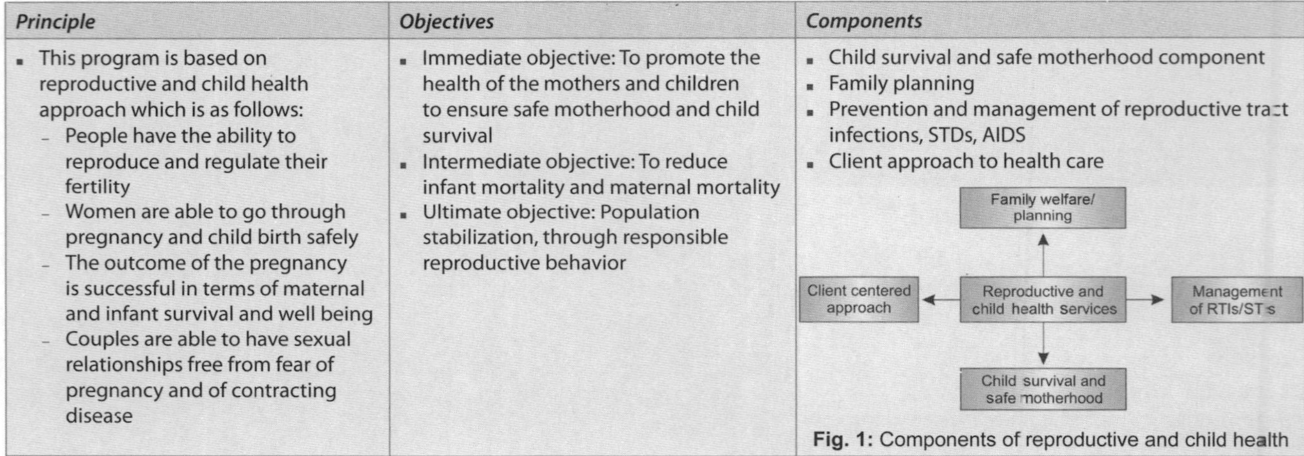

Principle	*Objectives*	*Components*
▪ This program is based on reproductive and child health approach which is as follows: – People have the ability to reproduce and regulate their fertility – Women are able to go through pregnancy and child birth safely – The outcome of the pregnancy is successful in terms of maternal and infant survival and well being – Couples are able to have sexual relationships free from fear of pregnancy and of contracting disease	▪ Immediate objective: To promote the health of the mothers and children to ensure safe motherhood and child survival ▪ Intermediate objective: To reduce infant mortality and maternal mortality ▪ Ultimate objective: Population stabilization, through responsible reproductive behavior	▪ Child survival and safe motherhood component ▪ Family planning ▪ Prevention and management of reproductive tract infections, STDs, AIDS ▪ Client approach to health care

Fig. 1: Components of reproductive and child health

Goals (RCH-II)

- Reduction of decadal rate of population growth between 2001–2011 to 16.2%
- Reduction of IMR to 45 per 1000 live births by 2007 and <30 per 1,000 live births by 2010
- Reduction of total fertility rate to 2.2 by 2010
- Reduction of MMR to 1.5 per 1000 live births
- Increased couple protection rate to 65% by 2010
- To improve coverage of full antenatal care in the rural areas to 89% by 2010
- To improve the coverage of rural institutional deliveries to 80% by 2010
- To improve quality, coverage and effectiveness of the existing family welfare and essential RCH services with special focus on empowered action groups
- To improve management performance
- To develop the human resource intensively
- To expand the essential RCH services to the tribal areas also.

Operational Profile (Strategy)

A. Maternal health (Safe motherhood)

a. Essential obstetric care

Objectives[Q]

- Provision of basis maternity services to all pregnant women[Q]
- Ensuring safe motherhood[Q]

Services provided

Phase I	*Phase II*
▪ Registration of all expectant mothers after 12 weeks of amenorrhea ▪ Provision of minimum three antenatal check ups (20, 32, 36 weeks) by ANM or medical officer to monitor progress of the pregnancy and to detect risk/complication so that appropriate care including referral could be taken in time ▪ Two doses of tetanus toxoid injections ▪ Prophylaxis of nutritional anemia during pregnancy by distribution of 100 tablets of iron folic acids[Q] ▪ Provision of safe delivery at home by observing five cleans or in an institution ▪ Provision of postpartum check ups to monitor the postnatal recovery and to detect complications	▪ Institutional delivery ▪ 50% of the PHCs and all the CHCs would operate as 24 hours delivery centers providing basic emergency obstetric care and essential newborn care and basic newborn resuscitation services round the clock ▪ Skilled attendance at delivery ▪ Provision of skilled attendance at every birth and its linkage with appropriate referral services ensures safe motherhood ▪ Formulation and dissemination of guidelines for normal delivery and management of obstetric complications at PHC/CHC for medical officers and for ANC and skilled attendance at birth for ANM/LHVs ▪ Policy decisions ▪ ANMs/LHVs/SNs have been permitted to use drugs in specific emergency situations to ensure safe motherhood ▪ They have also been permitted to carry out certain emergency interventions when the life of the mother is at stake

b. Emergency obstetric care

Objectives

- Operationalization of first referral units for providing emergency and essential obstetric care.

First referral units

Facilities	*Services provided*
▪ Minimum bed strength of 20–30 (10–12 in North East and under served areas) ▪ Fully functional operation theater ▪ Fully functional labor room ▪ An area embarked and equipped for newborn care in labor room and in the ward ▪ A functional laboratory ▪ Blood storage facility ▪ 24 hours water supply and electricity supply ▪ Arrangements of disposal of waste ▪ Ambulance facility	▪ 24 hours delivery services included normal and assisted deliveries[Q] ▪ Emergency obstetric care including surgical interventions like cesarean sections[Q] ▪ Newborn care ▪ Emergency care of sick children ▪ Full range of family planning services including laproscopic services ▪ Safe abortion services ▪ Treatment of STI/RTI ▪ Blood storage facilities[Q] ▪ Essential laboratory facilities ▪ Referral services

c. 24 hours delivery services at PHCs and CHCs

- To promote institutional deliveries, provision is made to give additional honorarium to the staff to encourage round the clock delivery facilities at the health centers.

d. Strengthening referral system

- Involvement of Panchayats (RCH I) and local self-help groups, NGOs and women groups (RCH II) to provide assistance to poor in case of obstetric emergencies.

e. Infection control measures

- Women are advised to maintain genital hygiene during menstruation to prevent RTI
- They are educated to keep their parts clean by frequent washing and by using sanitary towels and to avoid using dirty linen

- They are advised to prevent STDs by using condoms
- Early pregnant mother is immunized against tetanus with two doses of tetanus toxoid
- Traditional birth attendant is trained to observe 5 cleans while conducting delivery.

f. Nutrition promotion
- All mothers are given nutrition education
- They are explained that pregnancy drains out their nutrient stores and unless substantial improvement is made in their diet, they would develop malnutrition which can impair their health and adversely affect the future pregnancies
- They are instructed to consume food rich in iron content
- They are also additionally motivated to consume one large IFA tablet daily during the last trimester to prevent anemia

g. New initiatives
- Training of MBBS doctors in life-saving anesthetic skills for emergency obstetric care in numbers who are required for functioning of FRU and CHC and shall be limited to the requirement of tacking emergency obstetric situations only
- Setting up blood storage centers at FRU
- Janani Suraksha Yojana under Rural Health Mission
- Vandemataram Scheme for provision of safe motherhood services through private practioners.

B. Child health (Childhood survival)

a. Essential newborn care

Objectives	*Components*	*Strategy*
▪ To reduce perinatal and neonatal mortality	▪ Resuscitation of newborn with asphyxia ▪ Prevention of hypothermia ▪ Prevention of infection ▪ Exclusive breastfeeding ▪ Referral of sick newborn	▪ Train medical and other health personnel in essential newborn care ▪ Provide basic facilities for care of low birth weight and sick newborns in first referral units and district hospitals, etc.

b. Infection control measures
- Starting from observing 5 cleans while conducting delivery
- Early initiation of breast feeding while avoiding prelactal feeds
- By adopting warm chain with the mother
- By minimum handling and handling by barely minimum number of persons
- By keeping the room clean, dust free and warm
- By giving bath about one week after birth
- By getting primary immunization during infancy
- By educating the mother about ORS therapy of the child with the onset of diarrhea
- By early recognition and giving home remedy to treating upper respiratory infections of child with ginger syrup and/or pediatric cotrimoxazole tablets.

c. Nutrition promotion
- By promotion of breastfeeding of the child
- By proper complimentary feeding after 6 months of exclusive breastfeeding
- By 5 mega doses of vitamin A syrup between 9 months to 3 years with interval of 6 months.

C. Reproductive health

a. Fertility control
- Distribution of conventional contraceptive and oral pills for newly married couples
- Condoms and IUDs for spacing after one child
- Sterilization for either of the partners after two children, including services of laproscopic surgery
- Monitory compensation of ₹ 200/- for female sterilization and ₹ 180/- for male sterilization
- Meeting expenditure incurred by state governments on sterilization services such as transportation, drugs, dressing, diet, etc.
- Offering facilities for post-vasectomy semen testing.

b. MTP services

Objective	*Strategy*
▪ To reduce maternal deaths from unsafe abortions for unwanted pregnancies	▪ Provision of MTP services at district and taluka hospitals, CHCs and PHCs ▪ Involvement of adequately equipped and trained doctors of private hospitals ▪ Supportive assistance in form of training in MTP techniques, supply of MTP equipments, assistance of trained doctors to PHC on fixed weekdays

c. Adolescent counseling

Objectives	*Strategy*
▪ Dispelling misgivings, misconceptions and misapprehensions from the adolescent minds	▪ Counseling on problems related to sex and sexuality including various forms of sexual dysfunction, sexual aberrations, sexual abuse, impotence, etc. ▪ Education of adolescent girls on menstruation and menstrual hygiene ▪ Warnings about effects of unprotected sex such as transmissions of STIs including hepatitis B, HIV besides resulting in pregnancy ▪ Advise on adequate nutrition for proper growth and development

d. Prevention and management of sexually transmitted diseases and reproductive tract infections
  - These services are currently available only at district hospitals and teaching hospitals but their provision in CHCs, PHCs and FRUs is being considered.

Significance

- RCH program is a paradigm shift from rigid, target based, centralized, coercive system to non-rigid, target free, decentralized, participatory, demand driven, client-based approach system aimed at satisfaction of individual clients with a range of quality services.

2. Describe the epidemiology of rabies and its prevention and control in India.

- Rabies is an acute, highly fatal and highly infectious viral disease of the central nervous system
- It is a zoonotic disease^{Q}, primarily affecting carnivorous animals, dogs especially
- Also called as hydrophobia^{Q} (Pathognomic feature)
- It is a dead end infection in man^{Q}.

Epidemiology

▪ Agent factors	
i. Causative agent	▪ Causative agent is the rabies virus^{Q} (Lyssavirus type 1^{Q}), a RNA virus belonging to Rhabdoviridae family ▪ It is a bullet shaped, single stranded, nonsegmented virus measuring 120 mm × 80 mm ▪ The virus particle contains two distinct virus antigens ▪ G protein, a glycoprotein from the virus membrane ▪ Nucleoprotein antigen from the virus interior
ii. Reservoir of infection	▪ Principle reservoir of rabies in India are the rabid, wild carnivorous animals like tigers, wolves, foxes, etc. and the rabid stray dogs or domestic dogs in urban and rural areas
iii. Source of infection	▪ Among the rabid animals the infectious material are body fluids like saliva, serum, urine and milk ▪ But virus is mainly excreted in saliva which remains the most infectious material for source of infection ▪ In humans though virus is present in body fluids like saliva, sweat, semen and tears, they are not considered infectious because of lack of viruses in optimum number, however, cornea an constitute infective material
iv. Period of infectivity	▪ Rabid animal is infectious during the last 3–5 days of incubation period, i.e. before appearance of clinical features and also during the entire period of illness, i.e. 8–10 days
v. Incubation period	▪ 3–8 weeks (average)

Contd...

Contd...

<table>
<tr><td>▪ Host factors</td><td></td></tr>
<tr><td>i. Susceptibility</td><td>▪ All warm blooded animals including man are susceptible
▪ In humans, rabies is a dead end infection
▪ Most of victims belong to age group of 1–24 years and certain occupations like laboratory staff handling rabies virus, veterinarians, dog handlers, hunters, etc. are at greater risk
▪ However, not all persons bitten by rabid animals get the disease because the virus is shed intermittently in the saliva of the rabid animals</td></tr>
<tr><td>▪ Route of entry</td><td>▪ Percutaneous route</td></tr>
<tr><td>▪ Modes of transmission</td><td><table><tr><th>Animal bites</th><th>Licks</th><th>Aerosols</th><th>Person to person</th></tr><tr><td>Bite by rabid animal—MC mode of transmission in India (dogs, cats, monkey, cow, goat, sheep, buffalo, horses except rat bite and human bite[Q])</td><td>Licking of abraded skin or mucosa by the rabid dog can transmit the disease</td><td>It is observed in laboratories and in nature in certain caves harboring rabid bats[Q]</td><td>Though rare, can be possible by human bites or organ transplantation especially cornea</td></tr></table></td></tr>
<tr><td>▪ Incubation period</td><td>▪ Quite variable from 15 days to 1 year but is usually 3 weeks to 3 months depending upon:
i. Site of bite: Nearer the site to CNS, shorter the incubation period
ii. Severity of bite: More severe the bite, shorter the incubation period
iii. Species of biting animal: Bite of wild animals have shorter incubation period
iv. Richness of nerve supply: Bites over highly innervated areas like perineum, palms and fingers have shorter incubation period
v. Amount of saliva deposited: More the quantity of saliva deposited, shorter the incubation period
vi. Protection through clothes: Bites over bare skin have shorter incubation period
vii. Partial treatment: Incomplete treatment with antirabies vaccine prolongs incubation period</td></tr>
</table>

Prevention and Control

Prophylaxis for rabies (depending upon exposure to dog bite)

a. Pre-exposure prophylaxis
  - Employed before exposure to rabies in person belonging to high-risk groups

High-risk group (indicated in)	*Vaccines used*	*Regimen*	*Boosters*
▪ Laboratory staff handling virus and infected material ▪ Veterinarians ▪ Animal handlers and catchers ▪ Wildlife officers and naturalists ▪ Taxidermist and quarantine officers	▪ Tissue culture vaccine	▪ 3 injection in doses of 1 mL IM or 0.1 mL ID on days 0, 7 and 28 in deltoid region or anterolateral area of thigh in children (0 indicating day of first injection[Q])	▪ Serum samples are drawn one month after 3rd injection and if titres are less than 0.5 10/mL booster doses are administered in dose of 1 mL IM or 0.1 mL ID till the antibodies becomes demonstrable ▪ Further booster injections should be administered at interval of 2 years an long as exposed person remains at risk

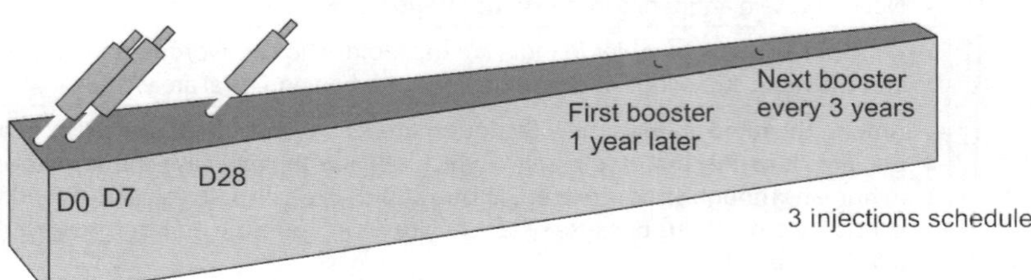

Fig. 2: Pre-exposure prophylaxis of rabies—regimen

b. Post-exposure prophylaxis
  - Employed after exposure to the infection therefore it is called antirabic treatment.

  Indications
  - When a person has been bitten, scratched or licked by an animal apprehended.

Components

i. Local treatment
   - Animal bite deposits the virus in the wounds therefore the wound should be immediately washed well with soap and water for at least 15 minutes under a running tap and then treated with quaternary ammonium compound, tincture iodine or 40–70% alcohol[Q].
   - In severe wounds, antirabic serum may be applied topically and infiltrated around the wound with prior sensitivity testing.
   - Suturing is not recommended but if necessary done in 24-48 hours later[Q]
   - Observe the animal for 10 days[Q].

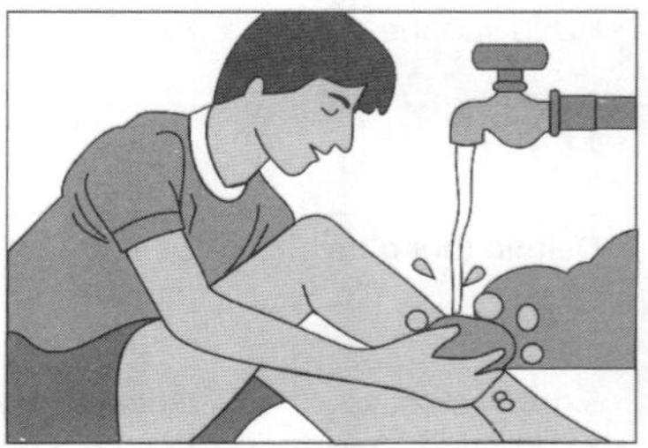

Wash the wound with plenty of water and soap

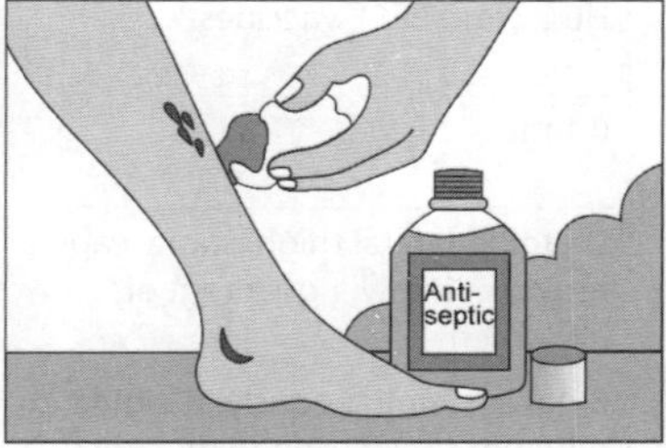

Apply an antiseptic or even alcohol

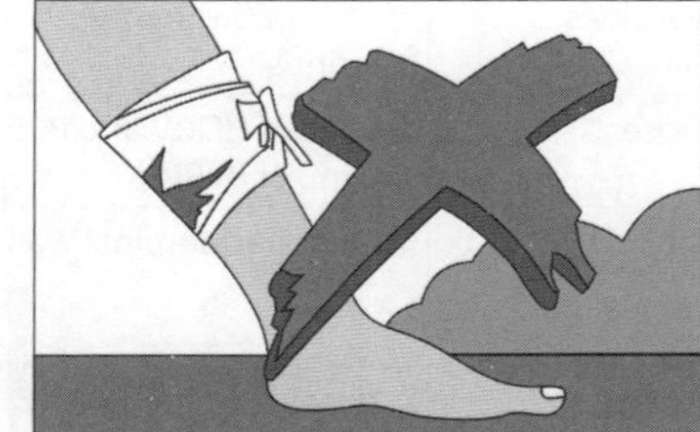

Do not cover the wound

Fig. 3: Rabies—local treatment

ii. Antirabic vaccines (active immunization)
   Classification of patients for risk (to determine dose of vaccine)

Class and risk	*Types of exposure*	*Recommended for PEP*
Class I (slight risk[Q])	▪ Licks on unbroken skin ▪ Licks on intact mucosa or conjunctiva ▪ Scratches without oozing of blood ▪ Consumption of unboiled milk suspected animal ▪ Handing raw flesh of suspected animals	▪ None (if history is reliable)
Class II (moderate risk)	▪ Licks on fresh cuts ▪ Scratches with oozing of blood ▪ All bites except on head, neck, face, palms, fingers ▪ Minor wounds <5	▪ Start vaccine immediately (may be discontinued if animal remains healthy after an observation period of 10 days or found –ve for rabies by diagnostic technique)
Class III (severe risk)	▪ All bites or scratches with oozing of blood on head, neck, face, palms, fingers ▪ All bites penetrating true skin and drawing blood with 5 teeth marks or more[Q] ▪ Lacerated wounds ▪ Multiple wounds >5 ▪ Bites from wild animals (jackal and wolves) ▪ Class II patient who has not received treatment within 14 days of exposure	▪ Start rabies immunoglobulin and vaccine immediately (may be discontinued if animal remains healthy after an observation period of 10 days or found –ve for rabies by diagnostic techniques)

Vaccination schedule/Regimen

Nerve tissue vaccine (BPL vaccine)

Class	*Pasteur Institute, Coonoor*		*Central Research Institute, Kasuali*		
	Adult	Children	Adult	Children	Booster (after completion of 10th injection)
Class I	2 mL x 7 days	1 mL x 7 days	2 mL x 7 days	2 mL x 7 days	Nil
Class II	3 mL x 10 days	3 mL x 10 days	5 mL x 10 days	2 mL x 10 days	1 after 3 weeks
Class III	5 mL x 10 days	3 mL x 10 days	5 mL x 10 days	2 mL x 10 days	2 on 7th and 21st day

- Vaccine is administered deep subcutaneously on the anterior abdominal wall. The immunity following vaccination lasts for 6 months only and any exposure later should receive fresh treatment
- Chief and dreaded complications of vaccine treatment is neuroparalysis (1 in 2,000).

Tissue vaccines (HDCS, PCEC, PVRV vaccines)

Route of administration	***Intradermal regime***		***Intramuscular regime***	
Regimen	2 site intradermal regimen (2-2-2-0-1-1)	8 site intradermal regimen (8-0-4-0-1-1)[Q]	WHO regime (Essen regimen) (1-1-1-1-1)	Zagreb abbreviatec multisite regime (2-1-1)
Vaccines	HDCV, PECE and PVRV vaccines	HDCV and PECE vaccines	HDCS vaccine	HDCS vaccine
Dose	0.2 mL of HDCV and PCEC 0.1 mL of PVRV	0.1 mL	1 mL	1 mL
Site	Anterior abdominal wall	Deltoids, lateral thigh, suprascapular region and lower quadrant of abdomen	Deltoid (not gluteal)	Deltoid (not gluteal)
Schedule	2 doses simultaneously on 2 sites on days 0, 3 and 7, no dose on day 14 and one dose each on day 28 and 90[Q]	8 doses simultaneously at eight different sites, i.e. deltoids, lateral thigh, suprascapular region and lower quadrant of abdomen on day 0, no dose on day 4, then 4 doses simultaneously at four sites, i.e. deltoid, thighs, no dose on day 14 and single dose each on day 28 and 30	5 doses on days 0, 3, 7, 14 and 30 with booster dose on day 90[Q]	2 doses, one each in right arm and left arm at day 0 followed by single dose on days 7 and 21

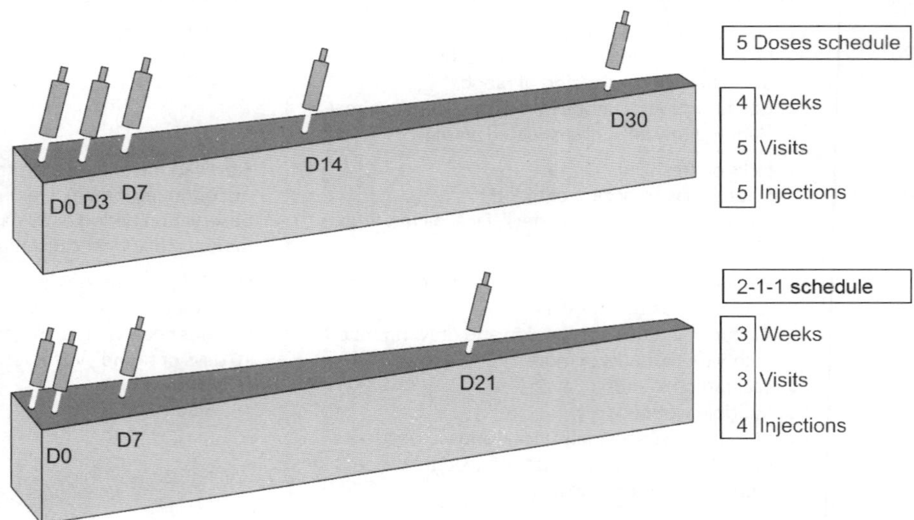

Fig. 4: Rabies—Essen and Zagreb regimen

iii. Antirabic serum (Passive immunization)
  - Human rabies immunoglobulin[Q] is safest antirabies antiserum

  Dosage
  - 20 IU/kg body weight.

  Procedure
  - Most of the antiserum is infiltrated locally and rest is administered intramuscularly at a site away from that of vaccine usually gluteal.

Other Measures[Q]

- Licensing of all domestic dogs
- Restraint of dogs in public places
- Vaccination of dogs
- Control of stray dogs.

Significance

- Rabies widely prevalent in India (Lakshadweep is rabies free zone[Q]) and gains a lot of importance from preventive medicine point of view because it has no treatment and prophylaxis is the only modality of reducing the mortality due to rabies
- Most logical and cost effective approach for control of urban rabies is elimination of stray dogs and swift mass immunization of at least 80% entire dog population of the area.

SHORT ESSAYS

3. Primary prevention of disabilities in handicaps.

- Handicap is reduction in a person's capacity to fulfill a social role as a consequence of an impairment, inadequate training for the role or other circumstances.

Primary Prevention of Disabilities

- These are the measure adopted before the occurrence of debilitating disease.

Health promotion	*Specific protection*
▪ These are general measures to prevent an individual from getting the disease *Examples* ▪ Good living conditions with safe environment ▪ Adequate nutrition ▪ Health education ▪ Personal hygiene ▪ Sex education ▪ Genetic counseling ▪ Efficient antenatal care	▪ These are specific measure to prevent certain diseases *Examples* ▪ Immunization with oral polio vaccine to prevent paralytic polio ▪ Vitamin A supplementation to prevent nutritional blindness ▪ Immunization of all potential mothers with rubella to prevent congenital rubella ▪ Immunization of Rh antibody to Rh -ve mothers to prevent erythroblastosis fetalis ▪ Provision of nutrition to mothers to prevent prematurity ▪ Prevention of exposure to radiation to pregnant mothers to prevent congenital anomalies

4. How will you identify 'at risk infants'.

- At risk infants are the babies at a very high risk of dying due to underlying risk factors.

Identification of 'at Risk Infants'

- Low birth weight, i.e. birth weight less than 2.5 kg[Q]
- Preterm babies, i.e. gestation less than 35 weeks[Q]
- Small for date (<3 percentile) or large for date (>97 percentile) babies
- Birth asphyxia
- Birth injury following instrumental delivery
- Loss of mother
- Loss mother's milk
- Artificial feeding[Q]
- Born within 2 years of previous birth
- Loss of previous sibling[Q]
- Twins
- Weight below 70% of the expected weight[Q], i.e. 2nd and 3rd degree malnutrition
- Failure to gain weight during three successive months[Q]

- Children with PEM, diarrhea
- Working mother[Q] or one parent
- Illegitimacy
- Birth order of 5 and above[Q]
- With congenital defect or disease
- With jaundice at birth
- Born to hypothyroid mother
- Born to unimmunized mother with tetanus toxoid during pregnancy
- Born to infected mother with hepatitis B, HIV, syphilis, tuberculosis, etc. (infected newborn)
- With APGAR score less than 5.

Significance

- At risk infants are the cases which contribute largely to perinatal, neonatal and infant mortality hence such cases should be identified and provide special care.

5. Multidrug therapy in leprosy.

- Under National Leprosy Eradication Program the treatment strategy for leprosy eradication is based on the multidrug therapy.

Principle	*Objectives*
▪ Prevent the development of not only resistance but also the relapse and the reactions ▪ To convert the infectious case into noninfectious as soon as possible to reduce reservoir of infection in community	▪ To interrupt transmission of the infection in the community by sterilizing infectious patients as rapidly as possible with bactericidal drugs ▪ To ensure early detection and treatment of cases to prevent deformities ▪ To prevent drug resistance ▪ Curtailing duration of treatment

Recommended Regimen of Chemotherapy (WHO)

Type of leprosy	*Drug*	*Adult dose*	*10–14 years child dose*	*Frequency of administration*	*Duration*	*Follow up*
Multibacillary	Rifampicin	600 mg	450 mg	Monthly under supervision	12 months[Q] extendable up to 18 months	Once a year for 5 years[Q]
	Dapsone	100 mg	50 mg	Daily self administered		
	Clofazimine	300 mg	150 mg	Once monthly supervised		
		50 mg	50 mg* (alternate days)	Daily self administered		
Paucibacillary[Q]	Rifampicin[Q]	600 mg	450 mg	Monthly under supervision[Q]	6 months[Q]	Once a year for 2 years[Q]
	Dapsone[Q]	100 mg	50 mg	Daily self administered[Q]		
Single skin lesion	Rifampicin	600 mg	450 mg	Single dose	Single dose treatment of ROM	
	Ofloxacin	400 mg	200 mg	Single dose		
	Minocycline	100 mg	50 mg	Single dose		

* Currently single skin lesion patients are treated at par with paucibacillary leprosy
Dose is adjusted appropriately for children under 10 years

Significance

- Multidrug treatment has curtailed the duration of treatment and thus has increased patient compliance, made it cost-effective and decreased workload on health delivery system.

6. Natural history of Japanese encephalitis.

- Japanese encephalitis is an acute, inflammatory disease of the brain, caused by an arbovirus called Japanese encephalitis virus
- It is a zoonotic disease[Q], transmitted accidently to humans by bite of infective female culex mosquito.[Q]

Natural History

Pre-pathogenesis phase (epidemiology)	
a. Agent factors	
i. Agent	▪ Causative agent is an arbovirus called Japanese encephalitis virus belonging to Castle's group B, family *Togaviridae* and genus *Flavi* virus ▪ It is a neurotropic RNA virus, filterable, ultramicroscopic (25–40 μm in diameter), enveloped by a lipid layer, showing varied morphology
ii. Animal hosts	▪ Pigs are natural hosts[Q] but even with viraemia they do not manifest any illness[Q] and remain infective to mosquitoes ▪ They acts as amplifier hosts[Q] by helping the virus multiplication
iii. Reservoir of infection	▪ Animals like cattle and horses are reservoir of infection and are next attractants for mosquitoes but only horses show manifestation of disease ▪ Among birds, ardeid birds, pond herons, poultry ducks and cattle egrets constitute reservoirs
iv. Immunity	▪ Repeated subclinical infection confers immunity
b. Host factors	
i. Age	▪ Occurs in any group but incidence is high amongst under five children[Q] (85%) especially rural children ▪ Infrequent in infancy[Q]
ii. Sex	▪ Minimally more among boys than girls because of outdoor activities
iii. Type of infection	▪ Man is incidental dead end host[Q] ▪ Man to man transmission is not seen
c. Environmental factors	
i. Climatic conditions	▪ Favorable climatic conditions are temperature of about 20°C and relative humidity of 70%
ii. Vectors (in India)	▪ Females Culex mosquitoes especially *Culex vishnui* and *Culex tritaeniorhyncus*[Q] ▪ Some anophelines are also acts as vectors ▪ These vectors mainly feed on animal blood, mainly pigs then cattle whereas man is only accidental victim[Q] ▪ They bite during night time ▪ Culex mosquito usually breeds in water collections with acquatic plants like water hyacinth ▪ In monsoons, paddy fields become best breeding place[Q] ▪ Extrinsic incubation period is about 10–12 days during which virus multiplies in vector to reach an optimum number to render it infective ▪ Once infected, the mosquito remains infective throughout its life
d. Risk factors	▪ High density of culex mosquito ▪ Presence of amplifying hosts like pig[Q] ▪ Paddy cultivation
e. Mode of transmission	▪ From animal to animal and birds and animal to man by bite of infected female culex mosquito ▪ No man to man transmission because of short period of viremia, low levels of circulating viruses and preference of vector for animal blood ▪ Not all humans bitten by mosquito develop disease ▪ JE overt disease to inapperent infection ratio is 1:300 to 1:1000[Q]
Pathogenesis phase ▪ After entering the body through the percutaneous route, the virus circulates in blood for a short period and lodge in the brain resulting in encephalitis	
a. Incubation period	▪ 5–15 days

Contd...

December 2008 (Paper II)

Contd...

b. Clinical features (3 stages)	*Prodromal stage*	*Acute encephalitic stage*	*Late stage and sequelae*
	▪ Characterized by sudden onset of fever with severe headache, vomiting, bodyache, anorexia and malaise ▪ Lasts 1–2 days[Q]	▪ Characterized by rise in fever, neck rigidity, vomiting, positive Kernig's sign, convulsions, altered sensorium, disorientation, state of confusion, stupor, coma and death ▪ Case fatality rate is 40% at this stage and child may die within 8–10 days	▪ Occur among those who recover ▪ Characterized by amnesia, abnormal movements, ataxia, personality changes, emotional instability, paralysis, etc.

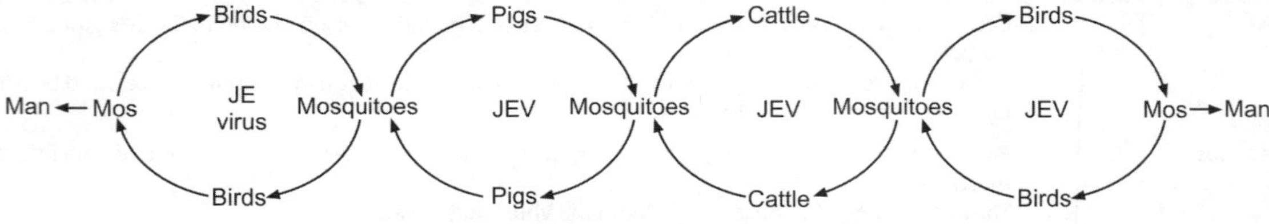

Fig. 5: Japanese encephalitis—natural history

Prevention and Control

A. Elimination of animal reservoirs
 – Pigs and cattle are eliminated by construction of pigsties and cattle shed at least 3 km away from human habitation (beyond flight range of vector)

B. Breaking channel of transmission
 – It consists of vector control (best method of control)
 a. Antilarval measures

Physical methods	*Chemical methods*	*Biological methods*	*Biocide method*
• Source reduction through improvement in sanitation by deweeding of ponds, removal of submerged grasses, using herbicides	• Larvicides like abate, temephos in concentration of 1 ppm in breeding places	• Larvivorous fish like Gambusia fish	• *Bacillus sphaericus* and *Bacillus thuringensis* which infect larvae and kill them

 b. Antiadult measures
 - Consists of indoor and outdoor spraying of insectides in all villages within radius of 3 km
 - It should cover vegetation around houses, breeding sites and animal shelters also
 i. Indoor spraying
 - 5% malathion is used sprayed in pigsties, cattle shed and inside house
 - It is done once every 15 days for 3 times
 ii. Outdoor sprays—ultra-low volume fogging (dry fogging)

Agent used	*5% malathion*
Principledes	• Insecticide is heated to vapor at high temperature in a special machine • Vapors coming out of machine when comes into contact with moisture of cooler air, form a fine fog or cloud of insecticide • When this fog comes into contact of mosquitoes, it kills them
Timing	• Early morning or late evening because air is cool and forms fine fog • Ideal temperature is about 20°C
Frequency	• Done on 1st, 3rd and 12th day
Methods	• Ground level application technique – Here special vaporizer TIFA is fitted onto an open jeep and jeep is driven slowly at speed of 5–6 km/hr • Aerial application technique – Here spraying is done by a special aircraft which flies about 40 meters above ground level

C. Protection of susceptible
 a. Immunization
 - Currently three types of vaccines are used for vaccination against JE

Vaccine	*Type*	*Strain*	*Used in*
• Mouse brain derived	Purified and inactivated	Nakayama or Beijing strain	Asian countries
• Cell culture derived	Inactived	Beijing P-3 strain	China
• Cell culture derived	Live attenuated	SA 14-14-2 strain	China and India

Contd...

Contd...

- Most commonly used vaccine in India is mouse brain derived JE vaccine (Produced at Kasuali)

Type	*Purified and inactivated*
Constitution	• Nakayama JE strain
Efficacy	• 50%
Route of administration	• Subcutaneously
Dosage	• Children <3 years: 0.5 mL • Children >3 years: 1.0 mL
Schedule (during interepidemic period)	• Primary immunization • 2 primary doses 4 weeks apart • Booster doses • 1st booster after 1 year and subsequently at 3 yearly interval until age of 10–15 years
Immunity	• Develops 1 month after 2nd primary dose
Indications	• All under five children living in endemic areas (most useful in interepidemic period) • Travellers to endemic areas
Contraindications	• Infants below 6 months (due to likely interference from maternal antibodies)
Disadvantages	• Limited duration of induced protection • Need for multiple doses • Relatively high price per dose

b. Health education
- People in endemic areas are educated about the reservoirs of disease and are encouraged to located their pigsties far away from house
- Use of mosquito nets is advocated.

Significance

- Japanese encephalitis is significant from public health perspective because of its high epidemic potential, high case fatality rate (20–40%), permanent sequel, no treatment and most importantly because it is preventable
- However, major problem for its elimination is presence of large number of inapperent cases[Q].

7. Anganwadi worker (AWW).

Refer Question No. 2 June 2010 (RS2) Paper II.

8. Millennium development goals.

Refer Question No. 2 December 2013 (RS2) Paper II.

9. Basic steps of planning cycle.

Refer Question No. 8 June 2008 (RS2) Paper II.

10. List out fertility related statistics.

- Fertility can be measured by a number of indicators collectively called fertility indices.

Fertility Indices

a. Birth rate[Q]
- It is number of live births per 1000 estimated mid year population in a given year

$$\text{Birth rate} = \frac{\text{No. of live births during a year}}{\text{Estimated mid year population}^{Q}} \times 1000$$

Current statistics (SRS September 2017)
- 20.4 per 1000 midyear population

Advantages	*Disadvantage*
▪ Unaffected by age distribution ▪ Excludes death rate	▪ Unsatisfactory measure of fertility as entire population is not exposed to child bearing

b. General fertility rate
   - It is the number of live births per 1,000 women in the reproductive age group (15–44 or 49 years) in a given year

$$\text{General fertility rate}^{Q} = \frac{\text{No. of live births during a year}}{\text{Estimated mid year population of women in 15–44 years age}} \times 1000$$

Current statistics (2015)
- 76.2

Advantage	*Disadvantage*
Better measure of fertility because denominator is restricted to number of women in the child-bearing age rather than entire population	Not all women in denominator exposed to the risk of childbirth

c. General marital fertility rate
   - It is the number of live births per 1,000 married women in the reproductive age group (15–44 or 49 years) in a given year

$$\text{General marital fertility rate}^{Q} = \frac{\text{No. of live births during a year}}{\text{Estimated mid year population of married women in 15–44 years age}} \times 1000$$

Current statistics (2015)
- 113.4

d. Age-specific fertility rate
   - It is the number of live births in a year to 1,000 women in any specified age group

$$\text{Age-specific fertility rate} = \frac{\text{No. of live births in particular age group during a year}}{\text{Estimated mid year population of women in same age group}} \times 1000$$

Advantages
- A more precise indicator
- Can provide fertility patterns
- Sensitive indicator of family planning achievement.

e. Age-specific marital fertility rate
   - It is the number of live births in a year to 1,000 married women in any specified age group

$$\text{Age-specific marital fertility rate} = \frac{\text{No. of live births in particular age group during a year}}{\text{Estimated mid year population of married women in same age group}} \times 1000$$

f. Total fertility rate
   - It represents the average number of children a woman would have if she were to pass through her reproductive years bearing children at the same rates as the women now in each age group[Q]
   - Also known as period total fertility rate
   - Is standardized index for fertility level
   - It helps in estimating total family size[Q]
   - It gives magnitude of approximately completed family size[Q]—No. of children in a family
   - It is obtained by summing single year age-specific rates at a given time[Q]
   - It is synthetic rate[Q], i.e. it is actually not counted as this would involve waiting until woman completes child bearing.

Current statistics (2015)
- 2.3 (Urban 1.8 and Rural 2.5).

g. Total marital fertility rate
   - It represents the average number of children that would be born to a married woman if she experiences the current fertility pattern throughout her reproductive span.

Current statistics (2015)
- 4.6.

h. Gross reproduction rate
   - It represents the average number of girls that would be born to a woman if she experiences the current fertility pattern throughout her reproductive span (15–44 or 49 years) assuming no mortality[Q].
   - Gross reproduction rate is same as net reproduction rate, except that like total fertility rate, it ignores life expectancy.

   Current statistics (2015)
   - 1.1.

i. Net reproduction rate
   - It is the number of daughters a newborn girl will bear during her lifetime assuming fixed age specific fertility and mortality rates[Q].

j. Child woman ratio[Q]
   - It is the number of children 0–4 years of age per 1000 women in child-bearing age (15–44 or 49 yesrs)[Q].

k. Pregnancy rate
   - It is the ratio of number of pregnancies (includes live births, still births, abortions and not yet terminated) in a year to married women in child-bearing age (15–44 or 49 years).

l. Abortion rate
   - It is the number of all types of abortions per 1,000 women of child-bearing age.

m. Abortion ratio[Q]
   - It is the ratio of number of abortions per year to the number of live births in a year[Q].

n. Marriage rate
   - It is the number of marriages in a year per 1,000 population.

11. Newer contraceptive pills.

- With population explosion emerging a global and serious problem for major world economies, research into contraceptive methods is on rise.

Newer Contraceptive Pills (Nonhormonal Long-acting Oral Pills)

- Its composition is methoxychroman hydrochloride which it differs from the hormonal pills in that it does not contain hormones, not to be taken daily and the side effects are minimal
- It is taken twice a week, starting on the first day of the menstrual cycle, for the first three months and subsequently once in a week, irrespective of the duration of the cycle, as long as contraception is required hence also called as once-a-week pill
- Each pill contains 30 mg of Centchroman[Q]
- It was developed by Central Drug Research Institute, Lucknow, India.

Commercial Preparation

- Saheli or Centron.

Mechanism of action

- It is a selective estrogen receptor modulator
- Works through unique combination of weak estrogenic and potent antiestrogenic action
- Exerts its contraceptive effect by interfering with nidation, which is an estrogen dependent post-ovulatory process
- Induces a mismatch between embryo transport and endometrial suitability.

Missed Dose

- Should be taken as soon as possible within 2 days of missing and normal schedule days adhered to
- If the dose is missed by 2 or more days, but less than 7 days, normal schedule is continued, preferably with condom, till the next period
- If the dose is missed for more than 7 days, adopt condom till the next cycle then the dosage regimen is reinitiated as a fresh one, i.e. biweekly for 3 months, followed by once a week schedule.

Failure rate	Contraindications	Merits	Demerits
▪ 1.83–2.84 per 100 WYE	▪ Lactation period, especially during the first 6 months ▪ Hypersensitivity ▪ Hepatic dysfunction (jaundice), chronic lung and renal disease ▪ Polycystic ovarian disease ▪ Cervical hyperplasia	▪ Does not affect hypothalamo-pituitary-ovarian axis ▪ Does not inhibit ovulation ▪ Once a week dosage hence convenient and increases client privacy ▪ Safe and economical ▪ No adverse effects	▪ Fertility returns about 6 months after cessation of therapy ▪ Sometimes menstruation is delayed (8%)

Noncontraceptive Benefits

- Treatment of dysfunctional uterine bleeding (DUB)^Q^.

Significance

- Centchroman is the only anti-implantation agent approved for clinical use globally.

12. "Rule of Halves".

- "Rules of Halves" is a representation of the ice-berg phenomenon^Q^ exhibited by the hypertension
- It was demonstrated in 1970s that only about ½ of the hypertensive subjects in the general population of most developed countries were aware of the conditions, only about ½ of those aware of the problem were being treated and only about ½ of those treated were considered adequately treated
- It can be illustrated by the following figure where circles within circles depict a specific section of population.

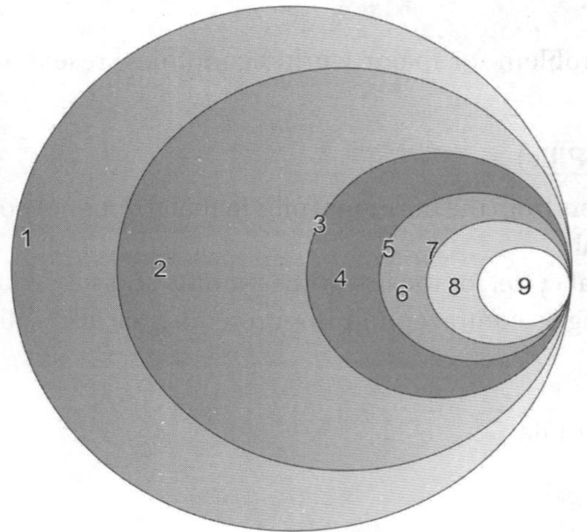

They are:
1. The whole community
2. Normotensive subjects
3. Hypertensive subjects
4. Undiagnosed hypertension
5. Diagnosed hypertension
6. Diagnosed but untreated
7. Diagnosed and treated
8. Inadequately treated
9. Adequately treated

Fig. 6: Rules of Halves in hypertension

Significance

- "Rules of Halves" is a represents the patient load of the hypertension which remain undiagnosed.

SHORT ANSWERS

13. Birth and death registration.

- Birth and death registration is the procedure mandated by Central Births and Deaths Registration Act, 1969 to register any birth and death in the family within 21 days^Q^
- This helps keep continuous check on the demographic changes.

Reasons for Under-registration

By the pubic	*Due to the system*
▪ Illiteracy ▪ Ignorance ▪ Lack of concern ▪ Lack of motivation	▪ Lack of uniformity in the collection, compilation and transmission of data between urban and rural areas ▪ Multiple registration agencies

Significance

- Registration of birth and deaths is very important as they serve as an important source of health information thus helping to formulate better and effective health-care programs.

14. Intrauterine contraceptive device.

Refer Question No. 6 June 2009 (RS2) Paper II.

15. Natural history of stroke.

Refer Question No. 2 June 2008 (RS2) Paper II.

16. Domestic accidents.

Refer Question No. 11 June 2014 (RS2) Paper I.

17. Vision 2020: The right to sight.

Refer Question No. 5 June 2013 (RS2) Paper II.

18. Age pyramid.

- Age pyramid or population pyramid is a graphical representation of the age-sex composition wherein the breakdown of the population is done in form of horizontal bar diagram, horizontal axis referring to the sex and vertical sex to the age
- It shows the age distribution of the population
- Also called as age-sex pyramid or age structure diagram[Q].

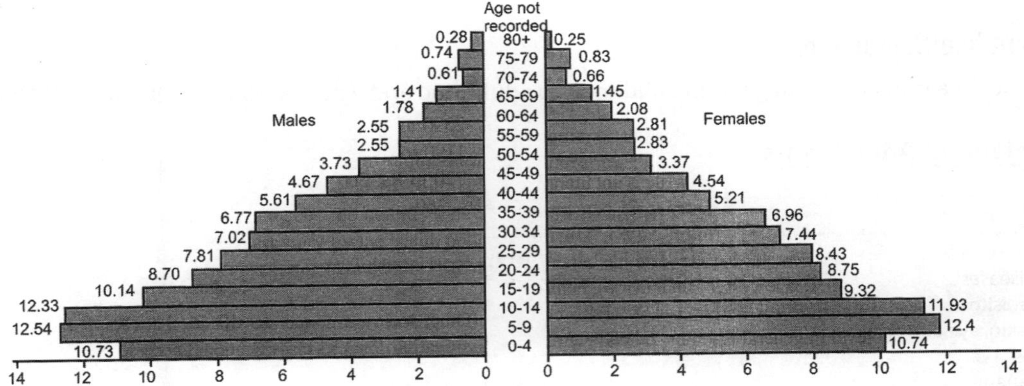

Fig. 7: Age pyramid of India (2001 census)

Features

- It is a double histogram[Q] placed back to back

- One of them showing male population (conventionally placed on left) and other showing female population (placed on right)
- Population is plotted on X-axis and age on Y-axis in 5 years age group interval.

Types

Stationary	*Expansive*[Q]	*Constrictive*
▪ A population pyramid showing an unchanging pattern of fertility and mortality	▪ A population pyramid showing broad base indicating a high proportion of children, a rapid rate of population growth and a low proportion of older people ▪ Indicates a population in which there is high birth rate and death rate and short life expectancy ▪ It is typical pattern of less economically developed countries including **India**	▪ A population pyramid which means the people are generally older

- The age pyramid of India is typical of under developed countries with a broad base (indicating high birth rate) and a tapering top (indicating less number of elderly people)
- In the developed countries as in UK the pyramid generally show a narrow base (low birth rate), and bulge in the middle.

Significance (Application)

- Age pyramid helps in calculations of:
  - Age-sex specific death rate
  - Age specific sex ratio
  - Standardization of death rate
- Shape of age pyramid helps determine

	Developing countries[Q]	*Developed countries*[Q]
▪ Population composition (based on shape)	▪ Broad base and narrow top (upright triangle) ▪ High proportion of younger population	▪ Bulge in middle (spindle shaped) ▪ High population of adults
▪ Life expectancy (based on height)	▪ Short (short pyramid)	▪ High (taller pyramid)
▪ Sex ratio (based on symmetry)	▪ Unfavorable (<1,000) (asymetrical pyramid)	▪ Ideal (symmetric pyramid)

19. Adolescent health problems.

- Adolescence is a transitional stage from childhood to adulthood and extends from 10–19 years[Q] (WHO).

Health Problems of Adolescents

Both boys and girls	*Girls*
▪ Malnutrition ▪ Infectious diseases ▪ Intestinal parasites ▪ Diseases of skin, eye and ear ▪ Dental caries ▪ Nutritional anemia ▪ Sexually transmitted diseases ▪ Addiction	▪ Irregular menstrual cycle ▪ Teenage pregnancy

Significance

- Adolescence is a formative period of life and crucial because major physical, psychological and behavioral changes take place.

20. Community need assessment approach.

- Community need assessment approach is a novel practice utilized in the delivery of family planning method adopted since 1995–1996
- As per this method, the earlier method of target-based achievement of family welfare program was retained only for state and national level and done away with for the district level
- Now it was up to the health worker to fix the performance norms for themselves which would be cumulatively calculated to obtain the target for the district.

Strategy

- Health workers would consult the families and local community at the beginning of the year in order to access their needs and preference and then work out the program and workload of the coming year for themselves
- This way requirement of each village would be workload for the auxillary nurse midwife for the year, total workload of different auxillary nurse midwife under one PHC would determine the workload of that PHC and similarly total orkload of all PHCs in a district would be the requirement of the district.

Advantages

- Reflects user preferences
- Improved quality of service.

Significance

- Community need assessment approach is really unique approach wherein the needs of the community is fulfilled as per their requirement.

21. Antenatal care.

Refer Question No. 9 December 2010 (RS2) Paper II.

22. Mid-upper arm circumference.

- Mid-upper arm circumference is an anthropometric measurement used to assess nutritional status of a child in age group of 1–5 years
- It gives information about the muscle mass because muscle wasting is a cardinal feature of PEM especially during early childhood
- In field, Shakir's tape[Q] is used to measure mid-arm circumference.

Mid-arm circumference	*Color zone*	*Interpretation*	*Management*
>13.5 cm[Q]	Green	Well nourished	—
12.5–13.5 cm	Yellow	Mild-to-moderate malnourishment	At home, through diet
<12.5 cm	Red	Severe malnutrition	Refer to institute

- For a quick nutrition survey, a bangle with an internal diameter of 4 cm can be used
- If it goes over the child's upper arm, it means the child is malnourished.

Disadvantage

- Child between 1 year and 4 years of age will have almost the constant measurement.

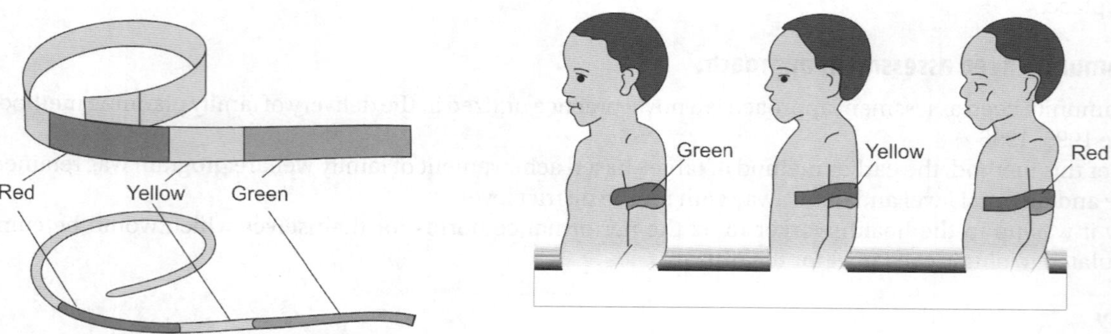

Fig. 8: Mid-arm circumference with Shakir's tape

Significance

- Mid-upper arm circumference is an easy to use and easy to understand and interpret tool for in field assessment of nutrition.

MBBS PHASE III EXAMINATION

JUNE 2009

(Revised Scheme 2)

PAPER I

LONG ESSAYS

1. What is chain of infection? What are the various modes of disease transmission?

Chain of Disease Transmission/Infection

- Chain of disease transmission method of transmission of communicable diseases from the reservoir or source of infection to susceptible host
- Basically there are three links in the chain of transmission, *viz.* the reservoir, modes of transmission and the susceptible host.

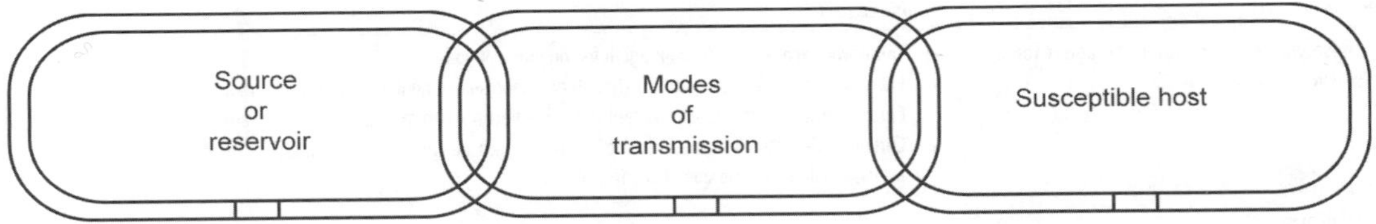

Fig. 1: Chain of disease transmission

A. Source or reservoir
   - It is the starting point for the occurrence of a communicable disease
   - A source of infection is the person, animal, object or substance from which an infectious agent passes or is disseminated to the host[Q] whereas a reservoir is any person, animal, arthropod, plant, soil or substance (or combination of these) in which an infectious agent lives and multiplies, on which it depends primarily for survival, and where it reproduces itself in such manner that it can be transmitted to a susceptible host
   - In short, the reservoir is the natural habitat in which the organism metabolizes and replicates[Q]
   - The terms reservoir and source are not always
   - Synonymous[Q] and the term source refers to the immediate source of infection and may or may not be a part of reservoir

   Types

   i. Human reservoir
   - A human case or carrier is the most important source or reservoir of infection for man.
     a. Cases
       - A case is a person in the population or study group identified as having the particular disease, health disorder or condition under investigation
       - The clinical illness may be mild or moderate, typical or atypical, severe or fatal depending upon the gradient of involvement
       - Epidemiologically, mild cases may be more important sources of infection than severe cases because they are ambulant and spread the infection wherever they go, whereas severe cases are usually confined to bed
       - The subclinical cases are variously referred to as inapparent, covert, missed or abortive cases and they are equally important as sources of infection because the disease agent may multiply in the host but does not manifest itself by signs and symptoms and it is eliminated[Q] and contaminates the environment in the same way as clinical cases
       - Persons who are thus sick contribute more than symptomatic patients to the transmission of infection to others and what is more, they do not appear in any of the statistics.
       - Subclinical cases play a dominant role in maintaining the chain of infection (endemicity) in the community
       - Subclinical infection can be detected only by laboratory tests, e.g. recovery of the organism, antibody response, biochemical and skin sensitivity tests
       - Barring a few (e.g. measles[Q]), subclinical infection occurs in most infectious diseases
       - Since subclinical infections occur frequently during a person's life time, they are responsible for the immunity shown by adult humans to a variety of disease-producing microbes
       - In latent infection, the host does not shed the infectious agent[Q] which lies dormant within the host without symptoms
       - In epidemiological terminology, the term primary case refers to the first case of a communicable disease introduced into the population unit being studied
       - The term index case refers to the first case to come to the attention of the investigator; it is not always the primary case
       - Secondary cases are those developing from contact with primary case
       - Whatever may be the gradient of infection, all infected persons, whether clinical or subclinical, are potential sources of infection, because the disease agent is leaving the body through frequent stools, vomiting, coughing, sneezing or other means and is potentially available for transfer to a new host

Contd...

Contd...

b. Carriers
- Carrier is an infected person or animal that harbors a specific infections agent in the absence of discernible clinical disease and serves as a potential source of infection for others.

Characteristics
- Presence in the body of the disease agent
- Absence of recognizable symptoms and signs of disease
- Shedding of the disease agent in the discharges or excretions[Q]
- Acts as a source of infection of others
- Number of carriers may outnumber the sick patients in community
- Carrier and his contacts do not know that he is infected hence neither takes precautions to avoid transmission of infection
- Carrier is apparently healthy and continues with his normal life

Types

Based on health status

Incubatory carriers	*Convalescent carriers*	*Healthy carriers*
• Those who shed the infectious agent during the incubation period of the disease, i.e. they are capable of infection others before the onset of illness • It usually occurs during the last few days of the incubation period • At the end of incubation period these carriers become case • Examples: Measles[Q], mumps[Q], polio[Q], pertussis[Q], influenza[Q], chickenpox[Q], diphtheria[Q] and hepatitis B[Q]	• Those who continue to shed the disease agent during the period of convalescence • This means the person is cured clinically but not bacteriologically • Examples: Typhoid fever, dysentery, cholera[Q], diphtheria[Q] and whooping cough[Q] • A convalescent carrier poses a serious threat to the unprotected household members and those in the immediate environment	• Healthy carriers are victims of subclinical infection who have developed carrier state without suffering from overt disease but are nevertheless shedding the disease agent • Example: Poliomyelitis[Q], cholera[Q], meningococcal meningitis, salmonellosis[Q] and diphtheria[Q]

By duration

Temporary carriers	*Chronic carriers*
• Those who shed the infection agent for short period of time	• Those who excrete the infections agent for indefinite periods • Example: Typhoid fever, hepatitis B, dysentery, cerebrospinal meningitis, malaria[Q], gonorrhea[Q] etc. • Chronic carriers are far more important source of infection than cases and longer the carrier state, greater the risk to the community • Chronic carriers can reintroduce disease into areas which are otherwise free of infection therefore their early detection and treatment are essential to limit the spread of infection

By portal of exist

Urinary carriers	*Intestinal carriers*	*Biliary carriers*	*Cutaneous carriers*	*Nasal carriers*	*Genital carriers*
Focus of organism is kidney as in typhoid[Q]	Focus of organism is intestine as in typhoid[Q], amoebiasis[Q], poliomyelitis[Q]	Focus of organism is gall-bladder as in typhoid[Q]	As in staphylococci	As in nasal diphtheria[Q]	As in gonorrhea[Q], AIDS

Significance
- Carriers are less infectious than cases but epidemiologically more dangerous than cases they escape recognition and continue to live a normal life among the population or community, they readily infect the susceptible individuals over a wider area and longer period of time under favorable conditions
- Carriers are responsible for endemicity of the disease in the community
- They may also spread infection to areas which are free of infection
- They correspond to the submerged portion of the iceberg phenomenon

ii. Animal reservoir
- Source of infection may sometimes be animals and birds and like the human sources of infection, may be cases or carriers
- Diseases and infections which are transmissible to man from vertebrates are called zoonoses
- Best known examples are rabies, yellow fever and influenza
- The migrations and movements of animals and birds may carry serious epizootiological and epidemiological risks
- Genetic recombination between animal and human viruses might produce new strains of viruses

iii. Reservoir in non-living
- Soil and inanimate matter can also act as reservoirs of infection
- For example, soil may harbor agents that cause tetanus, anthrax, coccidioidomycosis and mycetoma

B. Modes of transmission
- Communicable diseases may be transmitted from the reservoir or source of infection to a susceptible individual in many different ways, depending upon the infectious agent, portal of entry and the local ecological conditions
- Usually an infectious disease is transmitted by only one route, e.g. typhoid fever by vehicle transmission
- But some diseases may be transmitted by several routes, e.g. AIDS which enhance the survival of the infectious agent.

Classification

Direct transmission	*Indirect transmission*
▪ Direct contact ▪ Droplet infection ▪ Contact with soil ▪ Inoculation into skin or mucosa ▪ Transplacental (vertical)	▪ Vehicle-borne ▪ Vector-borne ▪ Mechanical ▪ Biological ▪ Air-borne ▪ Droplet nuclei ▪ Dust ▪ Fomite-borne ▪ Unclean hands and fingers

i. Direct transmission

a. Direct contact

- Infection may be transmitted by direct contact from skin to skin, mucosa to mucosa, or mucosa to skin of the same or another person
- This implies direct and essentially immediate transfer of infectious agents from the reservoir or source to a susceptible individual, without an intermediate agency, e.g. skin-to-skin contact as by touching, kissing or sexual intercourse or continued close contact
- It not only reduces the period for which the organism will have to survive outside the human host but also ensures a larger dose of infection.

Examples

- STD and AIDS, leprosy, leptospirosis, skin and eye infections.

b. Droplet infection

- This is direct projection of a spray of droplets of saliva and nasopharyngeal secretions during coughing, sneezing, or speaking and spitting, talking into the surrounding atmosphere
- Expelled droplets may impinge directly upon the conjunctiva, ororespiratory mucosa or skin of a close contact
- Particles of $\geq$10 μm in diameter are filtered off by nose and those $\leq$5 μm can penetrate deeply and reach the alveoli
- Droplet spread is usually, limited to a distance of 30–60 cm between source and host
- Potential for droplet spread is increased in conditions of close proximity, overcrowding and lack of ventilation
- In infectious diseases, these droplets, which may contain millions of bacteria and viruses can be a source of infection to others and when a healthy susceptible person comes within the range of these infected droplets he is likely to inhale some of them and acquire infection.

Examples

- Common cold, diphtheria, whooping cough, tuberculosis, meningococcal meningitis, etc.

c. Contact with soil

- Disease agent may be acquired by direct exposure of susceptible tissue to the disease agent in soil, compost or decaying vegetable matter in which it normally leads a saprophytic existence.

Examples

- Hookworm larvae, tetanus, mycosis, etc.

d. Inoculation into skin or mucosa

- Disease agent may be inoculated directly into the skin or mucosa.

Examples

- Rabies virus by dog bite, hepatitis B virus through contaminated needles and syringes, etc.

e. Transplacental (or vertical) transmission

- Disease agents can be transmitted transplacentally.[Q]

Examples

- TORCH[Q] agents (Toxoplasma gondii, rubella virus, cytomegalovirus and herpes virus), varicella virus, syphilis, hepatitis B, coxsackie B and AIDS.

ii. Indirect transmission
  – This embraces a variety of mechanisms including the traditional 5 F's—"flies, fingers, fomites, food and fluid".

Essential requirement	Factors determining external survivability of disease agent
Infectious agent must be capable of surviving outside the human host in the external environment and retain its basic properties of pathogenesis and virulence till it finds a new host	▪ Characteristics of the agent ▪ Inanimate object ▪ Influence of environmental factors like temperature and humidity ▪ Drug resistance

a. Vehicle-borne
  - Vehicle-borne transmission implies transmission of the infectious agent through the agency of water, food, ice, blood, serum, plasma or other biological products such as tissues and organs
  - Of these water and food are the most frequent vehicles of transmission, because they are used by everyone
  - The infectious agent may have multiplied or developed in the vehicle before being transmitted; or only passively transmitted in the vehicle.

Features
  - If the dose of contamination is heavy, the outbreak may be explosive
  - Cases are initially confined to those who are exposed to the contaminated vehicle
  - When secondary cases occur, the primary case may be obscured
  - Distance travelled by the infectious agent may be great
  - It is not always possible to isolate the infectious agent in the incriminated vehicle
  - When the vehicle is controlled or withdrawn, the epidemic subsides
  - Common source of infection is often traceable.

Examples
  - Diseases transmitted by water and food: Acute diarrheas, typhoid fever, cholera, polio, hepatitis A food poisoning and intestinal parasites
  - Disease transmitted by blood: Hepatitis B, malaria, syphilis, brucellosis, trypanasomes (Chaga's disease), infectious mononucleosis and cytomegalovirus infection
  - Disease transmitted by organ transplantation: Cytomegalovirus in association with kidney transplants.

b. Vector-borne
  - Vector is an arthropod or any living carrier (e. g. snail) that transports an infectious agent to a susceptible individual.

Epidemiological classification of vector-borne diseases

By vector	▪ Invertebrate type – Diptera—flies and mosquitoes – Siphonaptera—fleas – Orthoptera—cockroaches – Anoplura—sucking lice – Hemiptera—bugs, including kissing bugs – Acarina—ticks and mites – Copepoda—cyclops ▪ Vertebrate type—mice, rodents, bats
By transmission chain	▪ Man and a non-vertebrate host – Man-arthropod-man (malaria) – Man-snail-man (schistosomiasis) ▪ Man, another vertebrate host, and a non-vertebrate host – Mammal-arthropod-man (plague) – Bird-arthropod-man (encephalitis) ▪ Man and 2 intermediate hosts – Man-cyclops-fish-man (fish tape worm) – Man-snail-fish-man (*Clonorchis sinensis*) – Man-snail-crab-man (paragonimiasis)

Contd...

Contd...

By methods in which vectors transmit agent^Q	▪ Biting ▪ Regurgitation ▪ Scratching-in of infective feces ▪ Contamination of host with body fluids of vectors
By methods in which vectors are involved in transmission and propagation of parasites	▪ Mechanical transmission – Infectious agent is mechanically transported by a crawling or flying arthropod through soiling of its feet or proboscis; or by passage of organisms through its gastrointestinal tract and passively excreted – There is no development or multiplication of the infectious agent on or within the vector ▪ Biological transmission – Infectious agent undergoing replication or development or both in vector and requires an incubation period before vector can transmit *Types* ▪ Propagative^Q – Agent merely multiplies in vector, but no change in form *Examples* – Plague bacilli in rat fleas^Q, yellow fever in aedes^Q ▪ Cyclopropagative^Q – Agent changes in form and number *Example* – Malaria parasites in mosquito^Q ▪ Cyclodevelopmental^Q – Agent undergoes only development but no multiplication *Example* – Microfilaria in mosquito^Q, guineaworm in cyclops
By intervector transmission	▪ Transovarial transmission – When the infectious agent is transmitted vertically from the infected female to her progeny in the vector ▪ Trans-stadial transmission – Transmission of the disease agent from one stage of the life cycle to another

Factors influencing ability of vectors to transmit disease
- Host feeding preferences
- Infectivity (ability to transmit the disease agent)
- Susceptibility (ability to become infected)
- Survival rate of vectors in the environment
- Domesticity (degree of association with man)
- Suitable environmental factors.

c. Airborne

i. Droplet nuclei
- These are a type of tiny particles (1–10 μ) that represent the dried residue of droplets.

Formation
- By evaporation of droplets coughed or sneezed into the air
- By purposeful generation by a variety of atomising devices (aerosols)
- By accident in microbiological laboratories, in abattoirs, rendering plants or autopsy rooms.

Features
- The droplet nuclei may remain airborne for long periods of time, some retaining and others losing infectivity or virulence
- They not only keep floating in the air but may be disseminated by air currents from the point of their origin
- Particles in the 1–5 μ range are liable to be easily drawn into the alveoli of the lungs and may be retained there.

Examples
- Tuberculosis, influenza, chickenpox, measles, Q fever and many respiratory infections.

ii. Dust
- Some of the larger droplets which are expelled during talking, coughing or sneezing, settle down by their sheer weight on the floor, carpets, furniture, clothes, bedding, linen and other objects in the immediate environment and become part of the dust.
- A variety of infectious agents and skin squamae have been found in the dust and some of them may survive in the dust for considerable periods under optimum conditions of temperature and moisture
- During the act of sweeping, dusting and bed-making, the dust is released into the air and becomes once again airborne
- Dust particles may also be blown from the soil by wind; this may include fungal spores.

Examples
- Streptococcal and staphylococcal infection, pneumonia, tuberculosis, Q fever and psittacosis.

d. Fomite-borne
- Fomites are inanimate articles or substances other than water or food contaminated by the infectious discharges from a patient and capable of harboring and transferring the infectious agent to a healthy person
- It include soiled clothes, towels, linen, handkerchiefs, cups, spoons, pencils, books, toys, drinking glasses, door handles, taps, lavatory chains, syringes, instruments and surgical dressings
- They play an important role in indirect infection.

Examples
- Diphtheria, typhoid fever[Q], bacillary dysentery, hepatitis A, eye and skin infections.

e. Unclean hands and fingers
- Hands are the most common medium by which pathogenic agents are transferred to food from the skin, nose, bowel, etc. as well as from other foods
- The transmission takes place both directly (hand-to-mouth) and indirectly.

Examples
- Staphylococcal and streptococcal infections, typhoid fever, dysentery, hepatitis A and intestinal parasites.

C. Susceptible host
- Susceptible host is one who is likely or prone to develop the disease and shows the four stages of successful parasitism

Stages of successful parasitism

Portal of entry	*Site of selection*	*Portal of exit*	*Survive in external environment*
• Infectious agent must find a portal of entry by which it may enter the host • There are many portals of entry, e.g. respiratory tract, alimentary tract, genitourinary tract, skin, etc. • Some organisms may have more than one portal of entry, e.g. hepatitis B, Q fever, brucellosis	• On gaining entry into the host, the organisms must reach the appropriate tissue or site of election in the body of the host where it may find optimum conditions for its multiplication and survival	• Disease agent must find a way out of the body (portal of exit) in order that it may reach a new host and propagate its species • If there is no portal of exit, the infection becomes a dead-end infection as in rabies, bubonic plague, tetanus and trichinosis	• After leaving the human body, the organism must survive in the external environment for sufficient period till a new host is found • In addition, a successful disease agent should not cause the death of the host but produce only a low-grade immunity so that the host is vulnerable again and again to the same infection

Control Measures

A. Control of reservoir
- A reservoir of infection is any person, animal, arthropod, plant, soil or substance or combination of these in which an infectious agent lives and multiplies, on which it depends primarily for survival and where it reproduces itself in such manner that it can be transmitted to a susceptible host
- It is the first link in chain of causation and also the weakest
- Thus it is logically the most control measure of disease would be eliminating or controlling the reservoir of infection

Methods for control of reservoir

I. Elimination of environmental reservoir
- Elimination of environmental reservoirs such as air, water, soil, etc. is impossible and out of question

II. Elimination of animal reservoirs
- Achieved by keeping animals away from the human habitation

III. Elimination of human reservoirs

a. Early diagnosis
- Rapid identification of a disease is the first step in control of a communicable disease
- Earlier the disease is detected and earlier the treatment started, further transmission can be prevented
- Delay in disease diagnosis can result in further transmission of the disease
- Frequently, it should be aided by laboratory procedure to confirm the diagnosis

Contd...

Contd...

- Early diagnosis is need for:
  - The treatment of patients
  - For epidemiological studies, e.g. to trace the source of infection from the known or index case to the unknown or primary source of infection
  - To study the time, place and person distribution
  - For institution of prevention and control measures.

b. Notification
- Notification is compulsory reporting of a disease under legal provisions under certain times or at all times to the health authorities whose responsibility is to rush to the spot and implement control measures early in order to prevent further spread
- The notification is usually made by the attending physician or the head of family but any person including lay public can report, even on suspicion
- Certain diseases are statutorily notifiable and the list varies from country to country, however, cholera, plague and yellow fever are notifiable as per International Health Regulations prescribed by WHO

c. Epidemiological investigations
- Epidemiological investigations are done whenever there is a disease outbreak to:
  - Know the distribution of the disease with reference to time, place and person
  - Know the causative agent, source of infection, mode of transmission, factor influencing
  - Know the magnitude of problem by estimating the attack rate and case fatality rate.

d. Isolation
- Isolation is separation, for the period of communicability of infected persons or animals from others in such and under such conditions, as to prevent or limit direct or indirect transmission of the infectious agent form those infected to those who are susceptible or whom may spread the agent to others (physical isolation).

Objective
- To contain the disease, i.e. it remains confined to infected individual
- To protect community by preventing transfer of infection from the reservoir to the possible susceptible hosts.

Types

Depending upon mode of spread and severity of disease	*Depending upon place of isolation*	*Based on method*	*Special types*
• Standard isolation • Strict isolation • Protective isolation • High security isolation	• Hospital isolation • Home isolation	• Physical isolation • Isolating person from rest of community • Chemical isolation • Giving rapid domicilary treatment to render the patient noninfectious as quickly as possible	• Ring isolation[Q] • Encircling a infected person with a barrier of immune persons through whom the infection is unable to spread

Isolation in cases of various diseases
- Isolation has distinctive value in control of highly infectious diseases like diphtheria, cholera, plague[Q], etc.
- Even strict isolation is of no importance where large component of subclinical infection and carrier state like polio, hepatitis A, typhoid fever, etc.
- It futile in diseases which are highly infectious even before diagnosed like mumps
- Isolation fails in containing diseases like tuberculosis, leprosy, STD, etc.

Significance
- Isolation which is a barrier approach was once well established method of disease control
- However, with advancement in epidemiological and disease control technologies, isolation should be more judiciously applied and recommended when the risk of transmission of infection is exceptionally serious.

e. Disinfection

Concurrent disinfection	*Terminal disinfection*
• Disinfection of body discharges like sputum, urine and stool of the patient • Should be carried out as long the patient is in isolation ward	• Disinfection of the left over articles of the patient, after death or discharge

f. Treatment

Objectives
- To kill the infectious agent when it is still within the reservoir, i.e. before its dissemination so that the patient becomes non-infectious

Types

Individual treatment	*Mass treatment*	*Blanket treatment*
• Patient alone is treated • Example: Tuberculosis	• In high endemic zone, entire population is given treatment with drugs irrespective of whether they have the disease or not • Example: Malaria, filariasis	• Form of treatment in which the whole family is treated if one member of the family is suffering from a communicable disease • Example: In scabies benzoyl benzoate (25%) is given for the whole family member

Advantages	*Disadvantages*
• Reduces the communicability of disease • Cuts short the duration of illness • Prevents development of secondary cases	• If the treatment is inadequate or inappropriate, it may induce drug resistance in the infectious agent and may frustrate attempts to control the disease by chemotherapy

Contd...

Contd...

g. Quarantine
   - Quarantine (meaning 40 days) is the limitation of freedom of movements of such well person or domestic animals exposed to communicable diseases for period of time not longer than the longest usual incubation period of the disease[Q], in such manner as to prevent effective contact with those not so exposed
   - It applies to those who have exposed to a contagious disease but how may or may not become ill
   - Quarantine was first applied to plague[Q]

Types

Absolute quarantine	*Modified quarantine*	*Segregation*
• Limitation of freedom of movements to prevent effective contact with those not so exposed	• Selective partial limitation of the movement, such as exclusion of children from school during period of treatment as in scabies, diphtheria, chickenpox, etc	• Separation for special consideration, control of observation of some part of a group of person or domestic animals from the others to facilitate control of a communicable disease, such as removal of susceptible children to homes of immune persons

Significance

   - Quarantine has been currently replaced by active surveillance.

B. Interruption of transmission
- Breaking the chain of transmission or interruption of transmission means changing some components of man's environment to prevent the infective agent from a patient or carrier from entering the body of susceptible person.

Measures
- Water treatment will eliminate typhoid, dysentery, hepatitis A, cholera and gastroenteritis which are transmitted through water[Q]
- Clean practices such as handwashing, adequate cooking, prompt refrigeration of prepared foods and withdrawal of contaminated foods will prevent most foodborne illnesses
- When the disease is vector-borne, control measures should be directed primarily at the vector and its breeding places
- Vector control also includes destruction of stray dogs, control of cattle, pets and other animals to minimize spread of infection among them, and from them to man
- On the other hand, episodes of infection either by droplets or droplet nuclei are not usually controlled effectively by attempting to interrupt their mode of spread; reliance is placed on early diagnosis and treatment of patients, personal hygiene and proper handling of secretions and excretions.

Significance
- Blocking the routes of transmission imply an attack on environmental factors, i.e. to bring about an adjusted equilibrium between host and environment through encouraging some ecological influences and inhibiting others.

C. Susceptible host

a. Active immunization
   - One effective way of controlling the spread of infection is to strengthen the host defences which may be accomplished by active immunization
   - There are some infectious diseases whose control is solely based on active immunization like polio, tetanus, diphtheria and measles and vaccination against these diseases is given as a routine during infancy and early childhood, with periodic boosters to maintain adequate levels of immunity
   - Then there are immunizations against certain diseases which are offered to high-risk groups or restricted to definite geographic areas
   - Low grade fever, mild respiratory infections or diarrhea and other minor illnesses should not be considered as contraindications to immunization because these are the very children who are most in need of immunization and they are most likely to die should they acquire a vaccine preventable disease.

b. Passive immunization
   - Passive immunity can be provided by:
     - Normal human immunoglobulin
     - Specific (hyperimmune) human immunoglobulin
     - Antisera or antitoxins
   - Passive immunization is a short-term expedient useful only when exposure to infection has just occurred or is imminent within the next few days
   - The duration of immunity induced is short and variable (1–6 weeks)
   - Undesirable reactions may occur, especially if antiserum is of non-human origin
   - Passive immunization has a limited value in the mass control of disease
   - It is recommended for non-immune persons under special circumstances.

c. Combined
   - In some diseases (e.g. tetanus, diphtheria, rabies) passive immunization is often undertaken in conjunction with inactivated vaccine products, to provide both immediate (but temporary) passive immunity and slowly developing active immunity
   - However, the immunoglobulin should not be given within 3 weeks before, or until 2 weeks after administration of a live attenuated vaccine
   - If the injections are given at separate sites, the immune response to the active agent, may or may not be impaired by immunoglobulin .

d. Chemoprophylaxis
   - Chemoprophylaxis implies the protection from, or prevention of, disease.

Types

Causal prophylaxis	*Clinical prophylaxis*
• Implies complete prevention of infection by the early elimination of the invading or migrating causal agent	• Implies the prevention of clinical symptoms; it does not necessarily mean elimination of infection

e. Nonspecific measures
   - Most of the nonspecific measures to interrupt pathways of transmission are of general applicability
   - Improvements in the quality of life (e.g. better housing, water supply, sanitation, nutrition, education) fall into this category
   - It also includes legislative measures, wherever needed, to formulate integrated program and permit effective program implementation
   - Another important nonspecific measure is community involvement in disease surveillance, disease control and other public health activities.

Significance

- Knowledge about the chain of disease transmission and the methods to control a disease forms an essence of the community medicine.

2. What are the various methods used in health communication?

- Information, education and communication are important approaches to bring about changes in the knowledge, attitude and behavior of the people for betterment of their health and the health of the family and community in which they live.

Concept

Information	*Education*	*Communication*
▪ Consists of providing scientific knowledge to the people about the health problems and how to prevent them and promote and maintain good health ▪ Based on principle that it is right of the people to know the facts about health and disease ▪ It is a one way process and is also called as health propaganda ▪ It brings about awareness in the people	▪ Consists of educating or motivating the people to change their lifestyle or behavior for betterment of their health ▪ May be either one way or two way process	▪ It is a complex process in which a source of information gives the information through various channels to the audience and in turn gets the feedback to know the effect of the process ▪ It is a two way process ▪ It is the main weapon to change the behavior of the people ▪ Its final goal is to change the people's knowledge, attitude, behavior and practices

Components[Q]

Sender (source)
- Communicator or originator of the message and should know the audience, the message to be given and the methods or channels to communicate

↓

Message (content)
- Technical know how of the information being communicated to the audience
- It should be clear, understandable, interesting, meaningful, related to the objective, specific, precise and acceptable by the audience

↓

Media (channel)
- Channel which bridges between the sender and the receiver
- Types of media used are interpersonal communication, mass media and traditional or folk media

↓

Audience (receiver)
- May be a single person or a group of persons with common interest (controlled) or gathered out of curiosity (uncontrolled or free)

↓

Feedback (effect)
- Reverse flow of information or remarks made by the audience about the message to the sender so that the sender can make modification and improve the communication to make it more effective and acceptable to the audience.

Methods to Deliver IEC (Methods of Health Communication)

- IEC can be carried out at three main levels:
  - i. Individual and family health education
  - ii. Group health education
  - iii. Health education of the general public

a. Individual and family health education
- There are plenty of opportunities for individual health education
- It may be given in personal interviews in the consultation room of the doctor or in the health center or in the homes of the people
- When an individual comes to the doctor or health center because of illness, the opportunity is taken in educating him on matters of interest—diet, causation and nature of illness and its prevention, personal hygiene, environmental hygiene, etc.
- Topics for health counselling may be selected according to the relevance of the situation
- In working with individuals, the health educator must first create an atmosphere of friendship and allow the individual to talk as much as possible.

Objective
- Equipping the individual and the family to deal more effectively with the health problems.

Role of health personnel
- The responsibility of the attending physician in this regard, is very great because he has the confidence of the patient therefore the patient will listen more readily
- A hint from the doctor may have a more lasting effect
- The nursing staff has also ample opportunities for undertaking health education
- Similarly public health nurses, health visitors and health inspectors are visiting hundreds of homes and thus, have plenty of opportunities for individual health teaching.

Advantage	*Disadvantage*
▪ Provides ample opportunity to discuss, argue and persuade the individual to change his behavior ▪ Provides opportunities to ask questions in terms of specific interests	▪ Numbers reached is small, and health education is given only to those who come in contact with health personnel

b. Group education
- Educating a group of individuals is called group education
- It is an effective way of educating the community.

i. Lecture
- A lecture may be defined as carefully prepared presentation of facts, organized thoughts and ideas qualified person
- It has still a very important place in small group education
- Its effectiveness depends to a large extent on the speaker's ability to write legibly and draw with chalk on a black board.

Criteria for good lecture	*Criteria for good health educator*
▪ The talk should be on a topic of current interest or health needs of the group ▪ The group should not be more than 30[Q] ▪ The talk should not exceed 15 to 20 minutes[Q] because if the talk is too long people may become bored and restless ▪ Ideal time is morning and the subject matter should not deal with more than 6 points ▪ Divide the topic into various subheadings ▪ Summerize at the end	▪ Should be clear about the basic principles of the subject ▪ Should present the material clearly ▪ Should be clearly audible and legible ▪ Should maintain appropriate pace in lecture ▪ Should illustrate with practical applications ▪ Should stimulate the learner to think ▪ Should have good sense of humor, consider learner's view and invite their views ▪ Should be friendly and skilled ▪ Should appear confident and at ease ▪ Should not lose temper by the behavior of the group

Advantages[Q]	*Disadvantages*
▪ Continuity will be present ▪ Lectures can be taken anywhere and at any time ▪ Not many instruments required ▪ Most economical method ▪ Information transfer in a short time to a large group ▪ Less preparation and minimal resources	▪ Students are involved to a minimum extent[Q] ▪ Learning is passive, does not motivate ▪ Suitable only for small group ▪ Do not stimulate thinking or problem-solving capacity ▪ Comprehension of a lecture varies with the student ▪ Health behavior of the listeners is not necessarily affected ▪ Mainly depends on the skills of the educator

Aid for lecture delivery

Flipcharts	*Flannelgraph*	*Exhibits*	*Films and charts*
▪ Consist of a series of charts (or posters), about 25 by 30 cm or more, each with an illustration pertaining to talk to be given ▪ They are meant to be shown one after another ▪ Each chart is "flashed" or displayed before a group as talk is being given ▪ Message on charts must be brief and to the point ▪ These charts are primarily designed to hold attention of group and help the lecture to proceed	▪ A piece of rough flannel or khadi fixed over a wooden board provides an excellent background for displaying cut-out pictures, graphs, drawings and other illustrations ▪ The cut-out pictures and other illustrations are provided with a rough surface at the back by pasting pieces of sand paper, felt or rough cloth and they adhere at once when put on the flannel *Advantages* ▪ Pre-arranged sequence of pictures displayed one after another helps maintain continuity and adds much to the presentation ▪ Very cheap medium, easy to transport and promotes thought and criticism	▪ Objects, models, specimens, etc. convey a specific message to the viewer ▪ They are essentially mass media of communication, which can also be used in group teaching	▪ These are mass media of communication and if used with discrimination, they can be of value in educating small groups

ii. Demonstrations
- A demonstration is a carefully prepared presentation to show how to perform a skill or procedure[Q]
- Here a procedure is carried out step by step before an audience or the target group, the demonstrator ascertaining that the audience understands how to perform it
- Demonstration as a means of communication has been found to have a high educational value in programs like environmental sanitation, mother and child health and control of diseases
- The clinical teaching in hospitals is based on demonstrations.

Advantages	*Application*
▪ Involves the audience in discussion ▪ Dramatises by arousing interest ▪ Persuades the onlookers to adopt recommended practices ▪ Upholds the principles of "seeing is believing" and "learning by doing" ▪ Can bring desirable changes in the behavior pertaining to the use of new practice	▪ Environmental sanitation (use of sanitary latrine) ▪ MCH (ORS feeding) ▪ Control of diseases (scabies)

Significance
- This method has a high motivational value.

iii. Group discussion
- A group is an aggregation of people interacting in a face to face situation[Q]
- It is a two way method of communication
- It is considered a very effective method of health communication
- Where long-term compliance is involved (e.g. cessation of smoking, obesity reduction) group discussion is considered valuable.

Procedure
- For effective group discussion, the group should comprise not less than 6 and not more than 12 members[Q]
- The participants are seated in a circle, so that each is fully visible to all the others
- There should be a group leader who initiates the subject, helps the discussion in the proper manner, prevents side-conversations, encourages everyone to participate and sums up the discussion in the end
- If the discussion goes well, the group may arrive at decisions which no individual member would have been able to make alone
- It is also desirable to have a person to record whatever is discussed who is called recorder and he prepares a report on the issues discussed and agreements reached
- Group discussion is successful if the members know each other beforehand, when they can discuss freely

Rules[Q]	Advantages	Disadvantages
▪ Express ideas clearly and concisely ▪ Listen to what others say ▪ Do not interrupt when others are speaking ▪ Make only relevant remarks ▪ Accept criticism gracefully ▪ Help to reach conclusions	▪ Permits the individuals to learn by freely exchanging their knowledge, ideas and opinions ▪ Provides a wider interaction among members than is possible with other methods ▪ A very effective method ▪ Valuable to ensure long-term compliance	▪ Shy people may not take part in the discussions ▪ Some may dominate the discussion ▪ There may be unequal participation of members in a group discussion unless properly guided ▪ Some members may deviate from the subject and make the discussion irrelevant or unprofitable

Significance

- A well-conducted group discussion with adequate resources is very effective[Q] in reaching decisions, based on the ideas of all people
- The decision taken by the group tends to be adopted more readily than in situations where the decision is a solitary one
- Thus the group acceptance has a binding effect on the individual member to translate their acceptance into action
- A well-conducted group discussion is effective for changing attitudes and the health behavior of people.

iv. Panel discussion

- It is a setting where 4–8 qualified people[Q] talk about the topic, sit and discuss a given problem[Q], or the topic, in front of a large group or audience.

Procedure

- The panel comprises, a chairman or moderator and from 4 to 8 speakers
- The chairman opens the meeting[Q], welcomes the group and introduces the panel speakers
- He introduces the topic briefly and invites the panel speakers to present their points of view
- There is no specific agenda, no order of speaking and no set speeches
- After the main aspects of the subject are explored by the panel speakers, the audience is invited to take part
- The discussion should be spontaneous and natural
- The members on the panel may have a preliminary meeting, prepare the material on the subject[Q] and decide upon the method and plan of presentation if they are unacquainted with this method.

Advantages[Q]	Disadvantages
▪ Provides views from different speaker thus help to arrive at a solution which will be acceptable to all ▪ Audience is also involved actively ▪ Flexible, spontaneous ▪ Helps understand various perspectives	▪ Success of the panel depends upon the chairman as he has to keep the discussion going and develop the train of thought ▪ Needs a thorough planning and preparation in advance ▪ Panelist needs to be of sufficient experience ▪ Audience is usually passive

Significance

- Panel discussion can be an extremely effective method of education, provided it is properly planned and guided.

v. Symposium

- A symposium is a series of speeches on a selected subject[Q].

Procedure

- Each person or expert presents an aspect of the subject briefly
- There is no discussion among the symposium members[Q] like in panel discussion
- In the end, the audience may raise questions
- The chairman makes a comprehensive summary at the end of the entire session.

Advantages	Disadvantages
▪ Transfers concise information to audience at one time ▪ Audience remains alert ▪ Analysis of different aspects of a topic at one time ▪ Good tool for integrated teaching	▪ There is no discussion among the members of symposium ▪ It requires long-term preparation and time and hence cannot be conducted frequently

vi. Workshop

- The workshop is the name given to a novel experiment in education.

Procedure

- Workshop consists of a series of meetings, usually four or more[Q], with emphasis on individual work[Q], within the group[Q], with the help of consultants and resource personnel.
- The total workshop may be divided into small groups and each group will choose a chairman and a recorder.
- The individuals work, solve a part of the problem through their personal effort with the help of consultants, contribute to group work and group discussion and leave the workshop with a plan of action on the problem.

Advantages	*Disadvantages*
▪ Learning takes place in a friendly, happy and democratic atmosphere, under expert guidance ▪ It provides each participant opportunities to improve his effectiveness as a professional worker	▪ Needs a lot of baseline ground work[Q] ▪ Benefits a small number of people

vii. Role playing

- Role playing or socio-drama is based on the assumption that many values in a situation cannot be expressed in words, and the communication can be more effective if the situation is dramatised by the group[Q].

Procedure

- The size of the group is thought to be best at about 25[Q]
- The group members who take part in the socio-drama enact their roles as they have observed or experienced them
- The audience are supposed to pay sympathetic attention to what is going on, suggest alternative solutions at the request of the leader and if requested, come up and take an active part by demonstrating how they feel a particular role should be handled, or the like
- Role playing is followed by a discussion of the problem.

Advantage

- The audience is not passive but actively concerned with the drama.

Significance

- Role playing is a useful technique to use in providing discussion of problems of human relationship[Q]
- It is a particularly useful educational device for school children[Q].

viii. Conferences and seminars

- This category contains a large component of commercialized continuing education
- The programs are usually held on a regional, state or national level[Q] and range from once half-day to one week in length and may cover a single topic in depth or be broadly comprehensive
- They usually use a variety of formats to aid the learning process from self instruction to multimedia.

c. Mass approach (general public education)

- It is achieved through mass media of communications
- Mass media are a "one-way" communication.

i. Television

- Television has become the most popular[Q] of all effective in not only creating awareness, but also to an extent influencing public opinion and introducing new ways of life.

Advantages	*Disadvantages*
▪ It raises levels of understanding and helps people familiarise with things they have not seen before ▪ It has much potential for health communication ▪ It can reach illiterate population not accessible through printed words	▪ TV is a one-way channel, no much opportunity for feedback and discussion ▪ It can only be an aid to teaching ▪ It cannot cover all areas of learning

ii. Radio

- Radio is found in almost every house
- Doctors and health workers may speak out on radio
- Local health issues may be identified and discussed leading to increased general awareness.

Advantages	*Disadvantages*
▪ Radio is much cheaper than TV ▪ It is valuable aid in "putting across" useful health information in the form of straight talks, plays, questions and answers and quiz programs	▪ Radio is a purely didactic medium

June 2009 (Paper I)

iii. Internet
- It is new mean of computer-based communication system
- This is a fast growing communication media[Q] and holds very large potential to become a major health education tool
- It has opened vast capability of transfer of knowledge and has made it possible to get into direct and instant communication across the world by means of e-mail and even an online chat
- Already a fairly large number of persons in India are using this media, and the numbers are growing everyday
- Vast amount of health-related literature from WHO and other health agencies is available online
- The health-related information from the ministry of health and family welfare government of India is available on their websites.

iv. Newspapers
- Newspapers have been a media for health education since a century.

Advantages	*Disadvantages*
▪ Most widely disseminated of all forms of literature[Q] ▪ News in newspapers is newsworthy ▪ Provide more factual, detailed and even statistical material	▪ Health problems have little of value to newspapers ▪ Limitation of having low readership in rural areas because of illiteracy ▪ Reach only a limited group, i.e. the literates in the community

v. Printed material
- Magazines, pamphlets, booklets and hand-outs have long been in use for health communication

Advantages	*Disadvantages*
▪ They can convey detailed information ▪ They can be produced in bulk for very little cost, and can be shared by others in the family and community	▪ They are aimed at those who can read

vi. Direct mailing
- This is a new innovation in health communication in India
- The intention is to reach the remote areas of the country with printed word (e.g. folders and newsletters and booklets on family planning, immunization and nutrition, etc.)
- These are sent directly to village leaders, literate persons, panchayats and local bodies and others who are considered as opinion leaders
- It is possibly the most personal of mass communication.

vii. Posters, billboards and signs
- These are intended to catch the eye and create awareness; therefore, the message to be communicated must be simple, and artistic
- The message of the poster should be short, simple, direct and one that can be taken at a glance and easy to understand immediately, in places where the exposure time is short whereas the poster can present more information in places where people have some time to spend
- The right amount of matter should be put up in the right place and at the right time.

Advantages	*Disadvantages*
▪ Posters are not expensive when one considers they are seen by a large number of people ▪ Motives such as humor and fear are introduced into posters in order to hold the attention of the public	▪ Short life span and require frequent change ▪ Have much less effect in changing behavior ▪ Indiscriminate use of posters by pasting them on walls serves no other useful purpose than covering the wall

viii. Health museums and exhibitions
- If properly organized, health museums and exhibitions can attract large numbers of people
- By presenting a variety of ideas, they do increase knowledge and awareness
- Photographic panels attract more persons than graphic panels because photos give a humanized touch to the communication
- The three-dimensional models with lighted visuals are even more effective than photos
- In exhibitions, there is a big element of personal communication through workers who explain each item on the exhibit
- Printed literature explaining the exhibits is often freely distributed
- Health exhibitions and museums thus offer a package of both personal and impersonal methods of communication.

ix. Folk media
- Folk (or indigenous) media such as keerthan, katha, folk songs, dances and dramas and puppet shows which have roots in our culture are also modes of mass media.

Advantages of mass media	*Disadvantages of mass media*
▪ Mass media are useful in transmitting messages to people even in the remotest places ▪ The numbers of people who are reached are usually in millions ▪ Their effectiveness can give high returns for the time and money involved ▪ Reaches a relatively larger population in a shorter time than with other means ▪ More influential with average and below average education level ▪ Gets public attention	▪ Mass media alone are generally inadequate in changing human behavior and for effective health communication, they should be used in combination with other methods ▪ Impersonal ▪ One way communication, carry messages from center to periphery ▪ Feedback mechanism is poorly organized

Significance
- The mass media are only instruments to disseminate the information but what is important is the content of the message and the target audience.

SHORT ESSAYS

3. Describe the concept of disability with an example.

- Disability is any restriction or lack of ability to perform an activity in the manner or within the range considered normal of a human being (WHO)
- It results from an impairment due to a disease and results in handicap
- Thus pathogenesis and outcome of disability can be represented as follows:
  Disease → Impairment → DISABILITY → Handicap

Examples

- To illustrate examples for disability, we have:

		Example 1	*Example 2*	*Example 3*
Intrinsic pathology	Disease	Accident	Vitamin A deficiency	Leprosy
⇓	⇓	⇓	⇓	⇓
Anatomical and functional abnormality	Impairment	Loss of foot	Corneal xerosis	Involvement of nerves
⇓	⇓	⇓	⇓	⇓
Activity restrictions	Disability	Cannot walk	Blurring of vision/ blindness	Claw hand
⇓	⇓	⇓	⇓	⇓
Psychological disadvantage	Handicap	Loss of job	Unemployment	Loss of job

Causes

- Communicable diseases
- Malnutrition
- Low quality of perinatal care
- Accidents.

Prevention

Primary prevention	*Secondary prevention*	*Tertiary prevention*
▪ Reducing occurrence of impairment ▪ For example, immunization against polio	▪ Disability limitation by appropriate treatment	▪ Prevention of transition of disability into handicap

Significance

- Disability has mostly social and environmental components associated with it but interventions in disability also includes medical component besides social and environmental and primary prevention is the most effective way of dealing with it.

4. Classification of carriers.

Refer Question No. 7 December 2011 (RS2) Paper I.

5. Occupational hazards of agricultural workers.

- Occupation hazards of agricultural workers are:

Zoonotic diseases	*Accidents*	*Toxic hazards*	*Physical hazards*	*Respiratory diseases*
▪ Close contact of agricultural worker with animals or their products increases the likelihood of zoonoses ▪ Example: Brucellosis, anthrax, leptospirosis, tetanus, bovine tuberculosis and Q fever	▪ Common due to increasing use of machinery in agriculture ▪ Even snake and insect bites are also grouped under accidents which are very common	▪ Chemicals like insecticides or pesticides, fertilizers, may cause poisoning due to chronic exposure ▪ Susceptibility to poisoning is increased by associated factors such as malnutrition and parasitic infestations	▪ Extreme climatic conditions such as temperature, humidity solar radiation are part of the job due to its outdoor environment ▪ Other physical hazards such as excessive noise and vibrations, inadequate ventilation and uncomfortable working position may also add to stress	▪ Exposure to dusts of grains, rice husks, coconut fibers, tea, tobacco, cotton, hay and wood may lead either to byssinosis, bagassosis, farmer's lung and occupational asthma

Significance

- Agricultural worker has magnitude occupational health hazards but they are not given importance because in the today's industrial society occupational diseases denote diseases of workers working in factories or industries not agriculture workers.

6. Warning signals of poor mental health.

- Warning signals of poor mental health are set of questions designed by Dr William C Menninger, President, Menninger Foundation, Topeka, Kansas, USA

Warning Signals of Poor Mental Health

i. Are you always worrying?
ii. Are you unable to concentrate because of unrecognized reasons?
iii. Are you continually unhappy without justified cause?
iv. Do you lose your temper easily and often?
v. Are you troubled by regular insomnia?
vi. Do you have wide fluctuation in your moods from depression to elation, back to depression which incapacitate you?
vii. Do you continually dislike to be with people?
viii. Are you upset if the routine of our life is disturbed?
ix. Do your children consistently get on your nerves?
x. Are you browned off and constantly bitter?
xi. Are you afraid without real cause?
xii. Are you always right and other person always wrong?
xiii. Do you have numerous aches and pains for which no doctor can find a physical cause?

Significance

- Each of these 13 questions characterize major psychiatric conditions and help is required if answer to any of these question is yes.

7. Comparison of growth monitoring and nutritional surveillance.

- Growth monitoring and nutritional surveillance are two similar but confusing phrases which are different from one another.

Points of comparison	*Growth monitoring*	*Nutritional surveillance*
Strategy	Preservation and promotion of normal growth	Detection of malnutrition
Approach[Q]	Educational and motivational	Diagnostic[Q] and interventional
Subjects	All infants	Representative sample
Orientation	To individual child	To group of individuals
Age	Starts before 6 months	Representative age
Periodicity	Done monthly	Done periodically
Sample size	Small, preferably 10–20	Any size, 50–100
Recorder[Q]	Mother guided by worker	Trained worker[Q]
Weight card[Q]	Simple	Precise[Q]
Focus on	Growth	Nutritional status
Response	Early home intervention based on local knowledge	Nutritional rehabilitation often with nutritional supplement
Interventions	Primary health care, oral rehydration therapy, immunization, vitamin A supplementation, deworming, contraception, chloroquine, other treatment, etc.	Nutritional supplement of community through food subsidy
Response time	Brief, till resumption of normal growth	Long, till regain of good community nutrition
Referral	Health system for check up and possible brief food supplementation	Malnutrition rehabilitation in special centers

Significance

- Growth monitoring and nutritional surveillance are two approaches to prevent malnutrition and promote growth in children.

8. Concept of "lead time".

- Lead time is the period between diagnosis by early detection and diagnosis by other means[Q]
- It is the advantage gained by screening

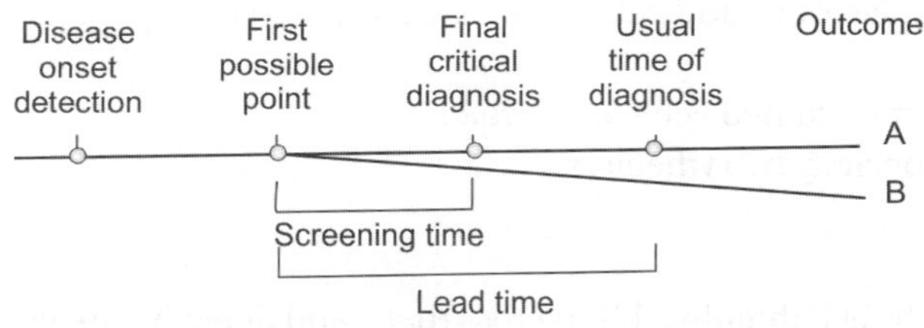

Fig. 2: Concept of lead time

Advantages	*Disadvantages*
▪ Can help in altering the outcome of disease by early detection and diagnosis	▪ Can only be applied the diseases with considerable time lag between disease onset and the usual time of positive diagnostic tests

Significance

- It helps to determine whether detection strategy should be applied to a disease or not.

9. Propagated epidemic.

Refer Question No. 4 December 2016 (RS2) Paper I.

10. Spectrum of iodine deficiency disorders.

Refer Question No. 1 June 2013 (RS2) Paper I.

11. Anthropometry.

Refer Question No. 2 June 2010 (RS2) Paper I.

12. Pasteurization of milk.

Refer Question No. 6 December 2009 (RS2) Paper I.

SHORT ANSWERS

13. Amplifier host in zoonoses.

- Amplifier hosts are the hosts which help in multiplication of the disease agent and help to continue the natural history of the disease.

Examples

Amplifier host	*Disease*
• Pigs[Q]	Japanese encephalitis[Q]
• Monkey	Kyasanur forest disease

Significance

- Amplifier hosts increases the weight of infection to which man is exposed.

14. Risk factors for road traffic accidents.

- Road traffic accidents accounts for most number of mortality[Q] from accidents besides causing innumerable morbidity.

Risk Factors for Road Traffic Accidents

- No segregation of road for pedestrians and vehicular traffic and also no segregation between fast moving and slow moving traffic
- Large number of old, poorly maintained vehicles on road
- Large number of vehicles especially two wheelers
- Overloading of vehicles
- Low driving standards
- Poor road conditions, poor street lightening, blind cross roads and defective speed breakers
- Widespread disregard for traffic rules
- Over speeding
- Indulgence in drug and alcohol by drivers
- Diversion of attention of drivers by road side advertisements, etc.

Significance

- Fatalities due to road traffic accidents can be easily prevented with a change in attitude of the community and little planning by the government.

15. Definitions of control, elimination and eradication.

	Disease control	*Disease elimination*	*Disease eradication*
Definition	Permitting the disease agent to persist in the community at a level where it ceases to be a public health problem according to the local population[Q] (Keeping the frequency of disease within acceptable limits[Q])	Interruption of disease transmission from large geographical areas, with prevalence of disease reduced to very low levels[Q] but organism persists in the environment	Termination of disease transmission by extermination of disease agent[q] (tearing out by roots of disease[Q])
Disease transmission	At minimal but not interrupted	Interrupted	Terminated.
Disease prevalence	In all areas but under control	In some areas or geographical areas	Disease ceases to exist
Prevalence rate	<1/1000	<1/100000	0
Examples	Malaria, leprosy	MeaslesQ, polio[Q], diphtheria, drancunculosis[Q], yaws	Smallpox (only disease that is eradicated worldwide)[Q] – 8th May 1980[Q]
Remarks	Aimed at reducing incidence of disease, financial burden to community and disease duration[Q]	Disease elimination is a geographical term, i.e. can be used only for a country or a region	Exhibits all or none phenomenon[Q] Is a global term, i.e. can be used for enter planet

16. Record linkage.

Refer Question No. 12 June 2014 (RS2) Paper I.

17. Spurious association.

Refer Question No. 12 December 2017 (RS2) Paper I.

18. Contingency table.

- A contingency table is a statistical table that shows the observed frequencies of data elements classified according to two variables, with the rows indicating one variable and the columns indicating the other variable
- It is a display of data in columns and rows, arranged to facilitate the discovery of any relationship that may exist between different sets of data
- The term was first used by Karl Pearson in 1904.

Features

- It is table displaying the frequencies for each combination of two or more variables which either categorical or numerical for which the possible outcomes have been arranged in groups
- Each location in a table is called a cell, and the corresponding frequency is the cell frequency
- Simplest type of contingency table displays two sets of data, one each in the columns and rows and is a fourfold, or 2 × 2, table
- More complex contingency tables can be constructed with a further subclassification of data in the columns or rows, or in both columns and rows
- Many varieties of data exist that can be arranged in this sort of table.

Example

- A random sample of 100 to demonstrate dietary habits in major religions may be represented as follows:

	Vegetarian	*Mixed*	*Total*
Hindu	43	9	52
Muslim	4	44	48
Total	**47**	**53**	**100**

- The figures in the right-hand column and the bottom row are called marginal totals and the figure in the bottom right-hand corner is the grand total.

Application

- Contingency tables are used to record and analyze the relationship between two or more variables, most usually categorical variables.

19. Effects of atmospheric pressure on health.

- Atmospheric pressure is the pressure exerted by the air
- Atmospheric pressure at sea level is 760 mm Hg which is called "One atmosphere of pressure" and it falls as altitude increases and rises as altitude decreases.

Effects of Atmospheric Pressure on Health

- Man is physiologically adopted to live at 760mm Hg or around it and any change in this has adverse effect on health

Effects of diminished atmospheric pressure at high altitude	*Effects of increased atmospheric pressure or low altitudes*
▪ At high altitude, air becomes thinner, low in temperature and partial pressure of oxygen also becomes less and man cannot survive at an altitude of 25,000 feet without breathing equipment i. Acclimatization – Long period of exposure to high altitude forces human body to acclimatize to high altitude of about 15–20 thousand feet without ill effects bringing about - Increase in rate and depth of respiration - Increase in Hb concentration of blood - Increase in cardiac output ii. Acute mountain sickness ▪ Results due to sudden exposure to high altitude of above 10,000 feet. Clinical features – Headache, mental fatigue – Irritability, irrational behavior – Loss of muscular coordination, impaired vision – Insomnia – Nausea, vomiting – Breathlessness – Bleeding from nose, ringing in ears, palpitation and collapse in severe cases Treatment – Bringing the person to lower altitude as soon as possible iii. High altitude pulmonary edema – Serious complication of acute mountain sickness occurring around 3rd day at high altitude Clinical features – Cough – Irregular or Cheyne–Stokes breathing – Oliguria – Mental confusion, hallucination – Stupor, seizures and coma Treatment – Bringing the person to lower altitude as soon as possible	▪ Seen at low altitudes like in mines and under sea and amongst miners, sea divers, etc. i. Dissolution of blood gases – At high atmospheric pressure, blood gases dissolve into blood and tissue proportionately to their partial pressure which causes various manifestations Clinical features – Loss of mental function and consciousness due to narcotic action of nitrogen which is facilitated by carbon dioxide – Convulsions and death due to excess oxygen ii. Decompression sickness or Caisson's disease – As the person rises to high altitude, the dissolved gases are liberated causing bubbles in the tissue and blood Clinical features – Euphoria, sensation of increased strength – Deeper and quicker respiration – Stronger and slower heart – Nasal voice, disturbances in hearing, changing in smell or taste – Hemorrhages from mouth, tympanic cavity and lung – Severe pain in muscles and joints by the gas bubbles (Bends or screws) – Death due to gas emboli in blood Treatment – Recompression followed by gradual decompression

Significance

- Any drastic change in altitude either low or high is hazardous therefore one should give enough time to the body to acclimatize to avoid these serious and sometimes fatal events.

20. Assessment of dietary intake.

Refer Question No. 2 June 2010 (RS2) Paper I.

21. Exotic diseases with examples.

- Exotic diseases are the diseases imported into a country in they do not occur otherwise[Q].

Examples

- Yellow fever in India
- Rabies in UK

Significance

- Exotic diseases pose a challenge to health-care delivery system of any country because being exotic, they are seldom diagnosed early and their treatment also becomes difficult because of paucity of available remedial measures.

22. Histogram.

- Histogram is a graphical representation of frequency distribution table for continuous data in which the vertical axis represents the frequency and the horizontal axis the class interval
- It consists of a series of blocks adjoining each other, the length of each block or rectangle is proportional to the frequency and the width of each block to the class interval.

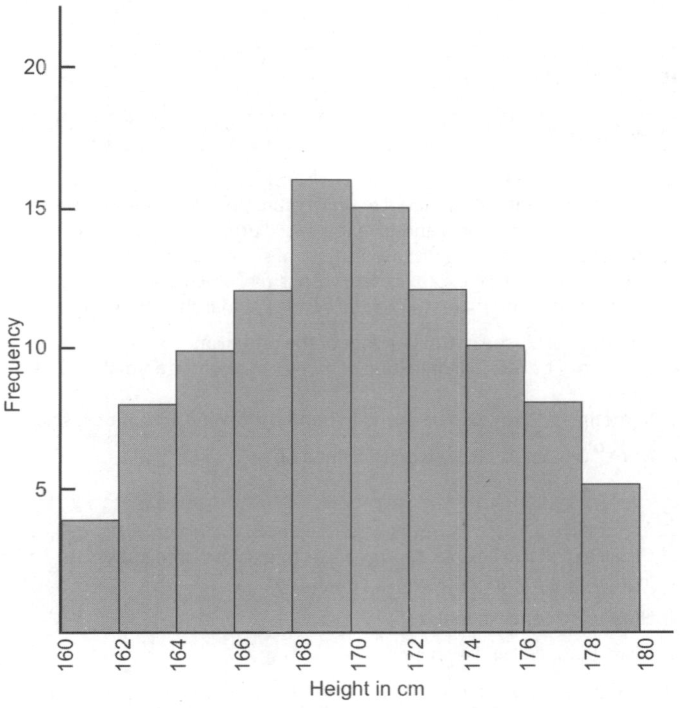

Fig. 3: Histogram

Concept

- Area under each rectangle represents the proportion of the total area of all the rectangles considering as one.

Advantages	*Disadvantages*	*Application*
▪ Histogram provides a better understanding of quantitative data of continuous type than frequency distribution tables[Q]	▪ Only one histogram can be placed clearly on one set of axis ▪ More time consuming to construct than a frequency polygon ▪ Applicable only for continuous data	▪ Ideally suited to represent distribution of anthropometric values like height[Q], weight[Q], midarm circumference, etc. ▪ Can also represent other types of continuous data series such as blood pressure, pulse rate, hemoglobin level, etc.

MBBS PHASE III EXAMINATION

JUNE 2009

(Revised Scheme 2)

PAPER II

LONG ESSAYS

1. Describe the natural history of tetanus and outline the strategies adopted for its prevention.

- Tetanus is an acute infectious disease caused by *Clostridium tetani*, characterized by muscular rigidity with persists throughout the illness.

Natural History of Tetanus

Pre-pathogenesis phase (epidemiology)	
a. Agent factors	
i. Agent	▪ Causative agent is *Clostridium tetani*, a gram positive, anerobic, spore-bearing bacilli ▪ The spores are terminal and give the bacilli drumstick appearance ▪ Spores are highly resistant to a number of sterilization methods and germinate under anerobic conditions to produce a potent exotoxin, tetanospasmin which brings about the pathogenesis of the bacilli by acting on the motor end plates in skeletal system, spinal cord, brain and sympathetic nervous system
ii. Reservoir of infection	▪ Soil and dust is the natural habitat of the organism ▪ Bacilli may be found in intestine of many herbivorous animals like cattle, sheep and is excreted in their feces ▪ Sometimes it may also be found in human intestine without causing any ill effect
iii. Period of communicability	▪ None[Q] (no person-to-person transmission)
b. Host factors	
i. Age	▪ Disease of active age, i.e. 5–40 years as this period predisposes to all kinds of trauma ▪ In infants, it occurs as tetanus neonatorum
ii. Sex	▪ Higher incidence in males
iii. Occupation	▪ More in agricultural workers
iv. Rural-urban difference	▪ Incidence is more in rural areas compared to urban areas
v. Immunity	▪ No age is immune unless protected by immunization ▪ Herd immunity does not protect
c. Environmental factors	▪ Unhygienic customs and habits ▪ Unhygienic delivery practices ▪ Ignorance of infection ▪ Lack of primary health-care services
d. Mode of transmission	▪ Spores of the bacilli are the infective forms which inter the body through wounds including microscopic injuries and cut end of umbilical cord of the newborn ▪ The vehicle of transmission is dust, soil, contaminated dressing or instruments ▪ Pathogen never spreads from person to person

Contd...

Contd...

Pathogenesis phase	
a. Pathogenesis and pathology	▪ After percutaneous entry into the body, the spores germinate into vegetative form under favorable conditions like pus and anerobic conditions and start multiplying ▪ On autolysis, they produce an enterotoxin called tetanospasmin (2nd most lethal toxin) ▪ Lethal dose for 70 kg man 0.1 mg[Q] ▪ Sensitivity to toxin is more in males ▪ The enterotoxin enters the circulation and gets fixed into the anterior horn cells of spinal cord[Q] and blocks the inhibition of spinal reflexes[Q] thus making the patient highly sensitive to sensory stimuli like touch, pain, heat, cold, etc.
b. Incubation period	▪ Varies from 3 days to 30 days with average of 6–10 days[Q]
c. Clinical features	▪ Sudden onset of fever which increase gradually ▪ Headache, bodyache, anorexia and malaise ▪ Low jaw or trismus, i.e. difficulty in opening of mouth due to painful spasm of masseter muscle ▪ Rigidity of muscles of neck, back and extremities making entire body stiff ▪ Opisthotonus position, i.e. hyperextension of neck, vertebral column and extremities ▪ Sensitivity to sensory stimuli like touch, pain, cold breeze manifesting as severe, painful and exhaustive convulsions ▪ Partial contraction of muscles persists between convulsions ▪ Clear mental faculties and pain consciousness persists throughout the illness ▪ Death due to continuous, painful exhaustive convulsions, asphyxia or aspiration pneumonia

Prevention and Control

A. Health promotion
   - Health education of the people about mode of transmission of tetanus and its complications
   - Educated people about wound care and wound hygiene
   - Motivate high-risk people and expectant mothers for immunization
   - Conduct all hospital procedures under strict aseptic conditions with meticulous care and caution
   - All home deliveries to be conducted by trained dais and following 5 cleans of safe delivery.

B. Specific protection
   a. Prevention before injury
      i. Active immunization
         - Aim is to vaccinate entire community
         - To ensure protection level of antitoxin ~0.01 IU/mL of serum throughout life
         - Primary immunization as per National Immunization Schedule
            - 3 doses of DPT of 0.5 mL each IM in children below 2 years at 6, 10 and 14 weeks
            - 2 booster doses of DT of 0.5 mL each IM at 18th months of age and 5–6 years of age
            - 1 booster dose of TT of 0.5 mL IM at 10 years of age

      ii. Passive immunization

Human tetanus hyperimmunoglobulin	*Equine antitetanus serum*
▪ Best for prophylactic use ▪ 250–500 IU is used IM ▪ Gives immunity for 30 days	▪ 1500 IU injected subcutaneously after sensitivity testing ▪ Carries the risk of hypersensitivity reaction ▪ Immunity is also short lasting for about 7–10 days

      iii. Active and passive immunization[Q]
         - Preferred in nonimmune persons who have sustained injury to provide immediate immunity by antitoxin and long-lasting immunity by vaccine

- Patient is given 1500 IU of ATS or 250–500 units of human immunoglobulin in one arm and 0.5 mL of TT into the other arm or gluteal region
- TT vaccine is repeated at 6 week and 1 year.

b. Prevention of tetanus after injury
   - For steps of prevention of tetanus following injury, the injury or wound is classified into two types and the injured into four types depending upon the immunity status
   - Active immunization with tetanus toxoid is best prevention.

Classification of wound

i. Clean, minor wound — Wound less than 6 hours old, clean, nonpenetrating wound with negligible tissue damage

ii. Other wound — Wound contaminated with dirt, feces and soil, puncture wound, burns, crush injury, bites and frost bite

Classification of individuals based on immunity status

i. Category A — Has had a complete course of toxoid or a booster dose within past 5 years[Q]

ii. Category B — Has had a complete course of toxoid or a booster dose more than 5 years ago and less than 10 years ago

iii. Category C[Q] — Has had a complete course of toxoid or a booster dose more than 10 years ago[Q]

iv. Category D — Has not had a complete course of toxoid or with unknown immunity status

Procedure

- Thorough cleaning of the wound with removal of foreign substance if any to abolish the anaerobic conditions which favor germination of tetanus spores
- Categorize the patient based on wound and immunity status and administer treatment as follows:

	Clean, minor wound	*Other wound*
Category A[Q]	Nothing[Q]	Nothing
Category B	Tetanus toxoid 1 dose	Tetanus toxoid 1 dose
Category C[Q]	Tetanus toxoid 1 dose[Q]	Tetanus toxoid 1 dose + Human tetanus Ig[Q]
Category D	Tetanus toxoid compete course	Tetanus toxoid complete dose + Human tetanus Ig

- 1 dose of TT comprises 0.5 mL intramuscularly
- Complete course of TT comprise 0.5 mL of TT at O, 6 weeks and 1 year later
- Human tetanus hyperimmunoglobulin is given in dose of 250–500 IU.

Significance

- Tetanus is a rapidly fatal but preventable disease thus every effort should be made to prevent it.

2. What are health problems of the aged and how will you control them?

- Science dealing with the study of diseases and their treatment peculiar to old age is called geriatrics.
- Geriatric age group in India is above 60 years[Q] and about 8.1% of population of India is aged[Q]

Revised Scheme 2

Health Problems of the Aged

Physiological (normally occurring due to aging process resulting in disabilities)	*Pathological*	*Psychological*	*Social*
▪ Senile cataract (MC health disorder[Q]) ▪ Glaucoma ▪ Nerve deafness ▪ Bony changes like osteoporosis ▪ Emphysema ▪ Special sense failure ▪ Changes in mental outlook ▪ Changes in physical outlook like wrinkling of skin	i. Diseases of CVS (MC–COD[Q]) – Atherosclerosis – Hypertension ii. Cancers – Cancer prostate – Cervical cancer iii. Accidents – At home – Outside home iv. Fractures of bones – Very common due to fragility of bone especially neck of femur v. Diabetes vi. Diseases of bones and joints – Spondylosis – Myositis – Fibrositis – Osteoarthritis – Gout – Rheumatoid arthritis vii. Respiratory diseases – Chronic bronchitis – Bronchial asthma – Emphysema viii. Genitourinary system – Enlargement of prostate – Prolapse of uterus – Incontinence of urine – Dysuria, nocturia – Fecal incontinence	▪ Mental changes ▪ Loss of memory (senile dementia) associated with impaired comprehension and impaired intellectual performance ▪ Decline in sexual performance resulting in physical and emotional disturbances ▪ Isolation due to death of kith and kin, lack of care by younger generation, social maladjustment, etc. ▪ Depression and even suicide because of isolation, poverty, illness, suffering, emotional disturbances, lack of happiness, etc.	▪ Poverty (due to retirement, loss of income, more expenditure due to illness) ▪ Isolation (due to death of friends, colleagues and family members, etc.) ▪ Maladjustment with younger generation ▪ Unhealthy life style like smoking, alcoholism ▪ Idleness and boredom

Primary Care of the Aged (Remedial Measures)

A. Pre-geriatric care (Primordial prevention)

Objectives

– To take health promotive measures in childhood and adolescence to prevent geriatric problems

Measures

– Maintenance of optimum body weight and prevention of obesity with correct food habits
– Regular moderate physical activity
– Abstain from nicotine and alcohol
– Avoidance of drug abuse and self medication
– Cultivation of interest in reading, writing, listening to music, hobbies, social work, pet keeping or other diversional activities to keep them busy post-retirement
– They should plan for future financial, housing and disease security
– They should build a large circle of friends and well wishers by selfless behavior, kindness and social service.

B. Geriatric care proper

Objectives

– To reduce disability and improve the quality of life

Primary prevention	*Secondary prevention*	*Tertiary prevention*
i. Health promotion (heath education on topics such as): – Self care – Abandoning smoking, alcoholism, over eating and sedentary life style – Use and upkeeping of hearing aids, ear moulds, prostheses and such other devices used by them – Instructed on various self-help mechanism such as avoiding fall and fracture, burns, accidents, etc. – Maintenance of optimum body weight – Personal hygiene – Exercise, yoga and meditation ii. Specific protection – Immunization against influenza, pneumococcal pneumonia, tetanus, hepatitis B, diphtheria, varicella – Selective immunization against hepatitis A, meninogococcal meningitis, Japanese encephalitis, typhoid and rabies	i. Early diagnosis and treatment – Most old age diseases are predictive and progressive and can be identified by periodic screening for health – Timely detection and intervention can preserve quality of life in old age – Old age people must be educated about the warning signals of the cancer – Women must be educated about self examination of breast for early detection of breast cancer and they should be advised to undertake Pap smear on routine basis for early detection of cervical cancer	i. Disability limitation – Intensive treatment of a disease can help reduce disability in old age ii. Rehabilitation Objective – To make the old people self caring by building up self confidence and self reliance Measures – Cataract surgery, provision of spectacles – Hearing aids – Artificial limbs – Provision of prostheses – Physiotherapy, vocational therapy, psychotherapy and social therapy – De-addiction counseling in addicts – Old age homes for needy

Significance

- Besides an important part of health care, care of old age people is very important because they give their present for our future and thus it is our obligation to take care of their present.

SHORT ESSAYS

3. List out the basic steps involved in evaluation.

- Evaluation is the process of collecting and analyzing information at regular intervals about the effectiveness and impact of a program[Q]
- Evaluation measures the degree to which the objectives and targets are fulfilled and the quality results obtained[Q] (WHO).

General Steps of Evaluation

a. Determine what is to be evaluated (three types of evaluation)

Evaluation of structure	*Evaluation of process*	*Evaluation of outcome*
▪ Evaluation of whether facilities, equipment, manpower and organization meet a standard accepted by experts as good	▪ Process (includes the problems of recognition, diagnostic procedures, treatment and clinical management, care and prevention) is evaluated by comparing with a predetermined standard ▪ Medical/nursing audit: An objective and systematic way of evaluating the performance of a physician (or nurse)	▪ Concerned with the end results either positive (improved survival/ reduced disability or negative ("5 Ds", i.e. disease, discomfort, dissatisfaction, disability and death)

b. Establishment of standards and criteria
   – Prerequisite to determine how well the desired objectives have been attained
   – Developed in accordance with the focus of evaluation

   Examples

Structural criteria	*Process criteria*	*Outcome criteria*
▪ Physical facilities and equipment	▪ Every prenatal mother must receive 6 check-ups ▪ Every laboratory technician must examine 100 blood smears	▪ Alterations in patient health status (cured, death, disability) ▪ Behavior resulting from health care (satisfaction, dissatisfaction) ▪ Educational process (e.g. cessation of smoking, acceptance of a small family norm)

c. Planning the methodology
   - Desired information is gathered in a preformed format keeping in purpose of evaluation
   - Standards and criteria must be included at the planning stage.
d. Gathering information
   - Evaluation requires collection of data or information which may include political, cultural, economic, environmental and administrative factors influencing the health situation as well as mortality and morbidity statistics
   - Amount of data required depends on the purpose and use of the evaluation.
e. Analysis of results
   - Once information is gathered, data should be analyzed and interpreted within the shortest time feasible. Feedback should be sent to all individuals concerned and evaluation results should be discussed.
f. Taking action
   - For evaluation to be truly productive, emphasis should be placed on actions—actions designed to support, strengthen or otherwise modify the services involved
   - This may also call for shifting priorities, revising objectives, or development of new programs or services to meet previously unidentified needs.
g. Re-evaluation
   - Evaluation is an on-going process aimed mainly at rendering health activities more relevant, more efficient and more effective.

Significance

- Evaluation though different from planning, they both must be viewed as a continuous interactive process, to continually modify both the objectives and the plan
- For successful evaluation, means of evaluation should be built into the design of the program before implementing it.

4. Functions of multipurpose health assistant (female).

- Female multipurpose health assistant is also called as Lady Health Visitor
- She is link between the Medical Officer and the Multipurpose Health Worker
- She is posted at PHC to cover a population of about 30,000 in areas in plains and 20,000 in hilly or tribal areas
- Their salary is paid by the Central Government.

Job Description

a. Supervision and guidance of multipurpose health worker (female)
   - Female Health Assistant is in-charge of 6 subcenters and responsible for 6 multipurpose health workers (female) manning these subcenters
   - They visit each subcenter at least once a week on a fixed day to supervise and guide/help them as follows:
     - In delivery of health-care services to the community
     - Strengthen their knowledge and skills
     - Improving their skills in working in the community
     - Planning and organizing her program of activities
     - Periodically assess their progress of work and submit an assessment report to the medical officer
     - Carrying out supervisory home visits in their area.
b. Team work
   - Help health worker (female) to work as part of the health team and coordinate their activities with those of health assistant (male) and other health personnel including the dais
   - Conduct regular staff meetings with the health workers in coordination with the health assistant (male)
   - Attend staff meetings at the primary health center
   - Assist the medical officers in organization of different health services in the area
   - Participate as a member of the health team in mass camps and campaigns in health programs
c. Supplies, equipment and maintenance of subcenter
   - At regular intervals, check the subcenter stores and help in procurement of supplies and equipment in collaboration with the health assistant (male)

- Check proper storage of drugs and maintenance of equipments at subcenter
- Ensure proper maintenance of general and midwifery kit by the health worker (female)
- Ensure cleanliness and proper maintenance of subcenter

d. Records and reports
- Scrutinize maintenance of records by the health worker (female) and guide them in their proper maintenance
- Maintain the prescribed records and prepare the necessary reports
- Review reports of health workers (female), consolidate them and submit periodical reports to the medical officer.

e. Role in control of communicable diseases (in endemic areas of kala-azar, lymphatic filariasis, Japanese encephalitis)
- Along with health assistant (Male)
- Check minimum of 10% of house in a village to verify visits by the health worker (female)
- Responsible for ensuring complete treatment
- Ensure more than 80% compliance of drug during mass drug administration
- Maintain proper record forms, diary and guidelines for identifying suspected cases
- Ensure complete coverage during the spray activities and search operation.

f. Acute respiratory infection (ARI)
- Ensure early diagnosis of pneumonia cases
- Provide suitable treatment to mild/moderate cases of ARI
- Ensure early referral in doubtful/severe cases

g. Maternal and child health
- Conduct weekly MCH clinics at each subcenter with the assistance of the health worker (female)
- Respond to calls from the health worker (female) and trained dais, and from the health worker (male) and render necessary help
- Conduct deliveries when required at PHC level and provide domiciliary and midwifery services.

h. Family welfare and MTP
- Conduct weekly family welfare clinics (along with MCH clinics) at each subcenter with the assistance of the health worker (female)
- Personally motivate resistant cases for family planning
- Provide information on the availability of services for MTP and refer suitable cases to the approved institutions
- Guide the health worker (female) in establishing female depot holders for the distribution of conventional contraceptives and train the depot holders with the assistance of the health worker (female)
- Ensure that health worker (female) maintains up-to-date eligible couple register
- Provide IUD services and their follow-up
- Assist medical officer in organizing family planning camps.

i. Nutrition
- Identify cases of malnutrition among infants and under five children and give them the necessary treatment and advice and refer serious cases to PHC
- Ensure distribution of iron and folic acid tablets and vitamin A solution to the beneficiaries
- Educate the expectant mother regarding breastfeeding.

j. Immunization
- Supervise immunization of all pregnant women and under five children
- Guide the health worker (female) to procure supplies, organize immunization camps, provide guidance for maintaining cold chain, storage of vaccine and health education about immunization.

k. School health
- Help medical officer in school health services.

l. Primary medical care
- Provide treatment for minor ailments, provide first aid for accidents and emergencies
- Attend to cases referred by the health workers
- She must refer cases beyond her competence to the PHC or nearest hospital.

m. Training
- Organize and conduct training for dais/ASHA with the assistance of the health worker (female).

n. Health education
   - Undertake health education activities particularly through interpersonal communication, arrange group meetings with leaders and organizing and conducting training of community leaders with the assistance of health team
   - Carry out educational activities for MCH, family planning, nutrition and immunization with the assistance of the health worker (female)
   - Organize and conduct training of woman leaders with the assistance of health worker (female)
   - Organize and utilize mahila mandals, teachers and other women in the community in the family welfare programs.

Significance

- Concept of health assistants were first proposed by Bhore Committee in their recommendations about primary health care
- They serve as an important link between the qualified medical practitioners (MO) and the multipurpose workers, thus forming an effective team to deliver health care, family welfare and nutritional services to the people.

5. World Health Organization.

- World Health Organization (WHO) is a specialized nonpolitical health agency established under agesis of United Nations with its headquarters at Geneva^{Q}.
- It came into existence on 7th April 1948^{Q}, hence 7th April is celebrated every year as World Health Day^{Q}.

Objective

- Attainment of highest level of health by all the people of the World^{Q}.

Constitution

- WHO is an autonomous body with its own constitution, own governing bodies, own membership and own budget
- The constitution of WHO is a master piece in medical literature and was drafted by Dr Rene Sand of Brussels in 1947^{Q}
- The preamble of constitution:
  - Defines the health as a "state of complete physical, mental and social well being and merely the absence of disease or infirmity"
  - Declares that the attainment of highest level of health in one of the fundamental rights of every human being without distinction of race, religion, political belief, economic and social condition
  - Recognizes that the health of all people is fundamental to the attainment of peace and security and to the abolition of wars
  - Fixes the responsibility on the governments of the countries to provide adequate health and social welfare measures for the benefit of the their citizens
  - Recognizes that understanding and active cooperation of the people is of utmost importance in the improvement of health of the people
  - Affirms that the health of one country is of benefit to all other countries
  - Suggest that healthy development of a child is of basic importance and ability to live harmoniously in a changing total environment is essential to such development
  - Suggest that health education of all the people is essential to the fullest attainment of health.

Membership

- Membership is open to all the countries and countries not maintaining international relations are admitted as associated members
- WHO has 190 member countries and 2 associate members by 1996
- The member countries contribute yearly to the budget and are entitled to the services of WHO.

Organizational Profile

a. World Health Assembly
   - It is the supreme governing body of WHO^{Q} and is like a health parliament where all member countries are represented by up to 3 delegates
   - It meets once a year usually in month of May at its headquarters.

Activities
- Lays down international health policy and program
- Reviews the yearly progress
- Approves the yearly budget
- Elects members of Executive Board
- Appoints the Director General, nominated by the Executive Board.

b. Executive Board
- It is body of 30 technically qualified experts from medical field designated by member countries but they do not represent their countries
- One third of membership is renewed every year
- It meets twice in a year, usually in January and in May after the meeting of health assembly.

Activities
- Implementation of policy decisions of assembly
- Take actions independently to tackle emergencies like epidemics, floods, earthquakes, etc.

c. Secretariat
- It is the administrative wing of WHO, headed by the Director General, the chief technical and administrative officer of the organization[Q]
- He has five Assistant Director General subordinate to him.

Activities
- Looks after routine official work
- Extend technical and administrative support to the member countries in planning, programming and implementing their National Health Programs

d. Regional Offices
- There are 6 regional offices headed by a Regional Director and is assisted by the technical and administrative officers and members of the secretariat
- It has a regional committee composed of representative of member countries of that region which also functions similar to World Health Assembly

Region	*Headquarter*
i. South East Asia[Q]	New Delhi (India)
ii. Africa	Brazzaville (Congo)
iii. Americas	Washington, DC (USA)
iv. Europe	Copenhagen (Denmark)
v. Eastern Mediterranean	Alexandria (Egypt)
vi. Western Pacific	Manila (Philippines)

Functions (Activities of WHO)

- Acting as directing and coordinating authority on all International health work[Q] is the first constitutional function of WHO
- The broad area of WHO activities are:

a. Prevention and control of specific diseases:[Q]
- WHO helps its members states in prevention and control of specific diseases of public health importance through:
  - Epidemiological surveillance of the diseases
  - Collection and dissemination of epidemiological information on diseases subject to International Health Regulations and occasionally other communicable diseases of international importance through Automatic Telex Reply Service (ATRS) and the Weekly Epidemiological Record (WER) containing complete detail and brief reviews of communicable disease of international importance
  - Offering use of "WHO Emergency Scheme for Epidemics" to the member states
  - International Health Regulations regarding immunization and quarantine of travelers to prevent international spread of disease without affecting world traffic
  - Emphasis on Extended Immunization Program to target six killer diseases of childhood.

- Prevention and control of diseases covers communicable diseases like smallpox (eradicated) malaria, filariasis, tuberculosis, leprosy, diarrheal diseases, AIDS, etc. and also noncommunicable diseases like cancer, cardiovascular diseases, genetic disorders, mental disorders, drug addiction and dental diseases
- These activities now even comprise vector biology and control, immunology, quality control of drugs and biological products, drug evaluation and monitoring and health laboratory technology.

b. Development of comprehensive health services
  - WHO helps its member states to strengthen their health services through:
    - Organizing health systems based on primary health care
    - Development of health manpower and utilization
    - Building long-term national capability particularly in health infrastructure and managerial capabilities and health service research
    - Encouraging self sufficiency in solving health problems through Appropriate Technology for Health Program
    - Provision of drugs and equipments.

c. Family health
  - WHO is trying to improve the quality of life of the family as a unit
  - Its main components are maternal and child health, human reproduction, nutrition and health education.

d. Environmental health
  - WHO is promoting environmental health by:
    - Advising its member states on problems like quality of air, water and food, health conditions of work, radiation, identification of new hazards, etc.
    - Monitoring the environment through 'WHO Environmental Health Monitoring Program".
    - Establishing the criteria for environmental health in 'Environmental Criteria for Health Programs"
    - Extending technical and financial help to member states on specific issues.

e. Health statistics
  - WHO has contributed greatly to health statistics by:
    - Laying down uniform procedure for reporting, registering and collecting health and vital statistics
    - Collection and publication of various health and vital statistics in weekly epidemiological report, world health statistics quarterly and world health statistics annual
    - Bringing uniformity in statistics through International Classification of Diseases, Injuries and Causes of Death.

f. Biomedical research
  - WHO stimulates and coordinates research work by:
    - Establishing a worldwide network of WHO collaborating centers
    - Providing fellowship and grants to research workers and institutions involved with research
    - Deciding priority areas through its regional advisory committees
    - Promoting training of workers.

g. Health literature and information
  - WHO acts as a clearing house for information on health problems which are disseminated through
    - Its publications like:
      - ❖ WHO Bulletin
      - ❖ WHO Chronicle
      - ❖ Weekly Epidemiological Report
      - ❖ World Health Statistics (quarterly and annual)
      - ❖ World Health (monthly)
      - ❖ WHO Technical Report
      - ❖ WHO Monograph
      - ❖ International Digest of Health Legislations
      - ❖ World Health Forum
    - MEDLARS, i.e. Medical Literature Analysis and Retrieval System, the one and only fully computerized indexing system covering the whole of medicine on an international basis
    - Its website www.who.int
    - Its headquarter and regional headquarters.

h. Cooperation with other organization
   - WHO promotes health by working in close liaison with UN and other specialized agencies like UNICEF, FAO, ILO, CARE, USAID, etc.

6. Advantages and contraindications for intrauterine device (IUD).

- An intrauterine device is a small, stiff but flexible, nontoxic, polyethylene plastic frame, incorporated with barium sulfate, to make it radiopaque and prevents conception by acting as a foreign body when inserted into the uterus of the woman, through vagina
- The IUD has two strings, made up of nylon, which hang through the opening of the cervix into the vagina, to check by the user to know whether it is in-situ and also to remove it by pulling when pregnancy is desired.

Types

a. First generation IUDs

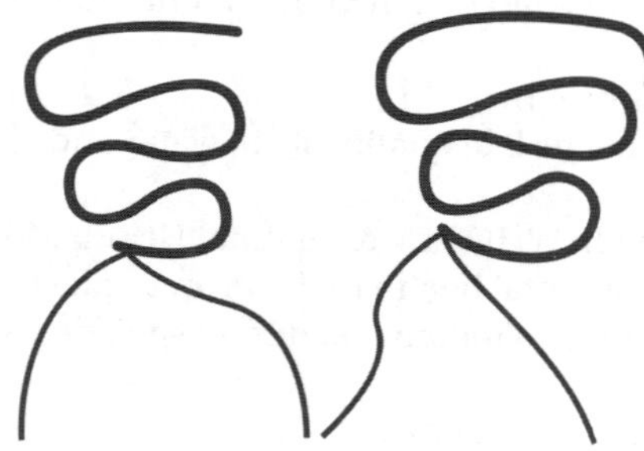

Fig. 1: First generation IUDs

- These are inert[Q], nonmedicated devices
  i. Lippe's loop
     - It is a double S shaped, serpentine device, made up of polyethylene, nontoxic, nontissue reactive material, incorporated with barium sulfate
     - It has 2 nylon transcervical threads, attached to lower end of the loop
     - It is available in 4 sizes, A, B, C and D, latter being the largest, recommended for multiparous women.

     Failure rate
     - 19 pregnancy per 100 WYE

     Demerit
     - Side effects
     - More expulsion rates
  ii. Grafanberg's ring[Q]
     - It is a flexible ring of silver wire used as birth control device as precursor to IUD.

b. Second generation IUDs

Earlier devices	*Newer devices*	*Multiload (mL) devices containing copper[Q]*
T Cu 200, T Cu 200 B, Copper 7, Shangai-V-Cu-200	T Cu-220 c, T Cu-380 A, T Cu 380 S (Slim line), CuNova- T 200, Cu Nova T 380	mL - Cu - 250, mL - Cu – 375

- Number in name of the device indicates the surface area of copper in square mm[Q]
- Nova T and Copper T 380 Ag are distinguished by a silver core[Q] over which copper wire is wrapped
- All copper T and multiload devices are effective for at least 3 years[Q], except TCu 380 A, which is much more effective for prevention of pregnancy up to 10 years[Q].

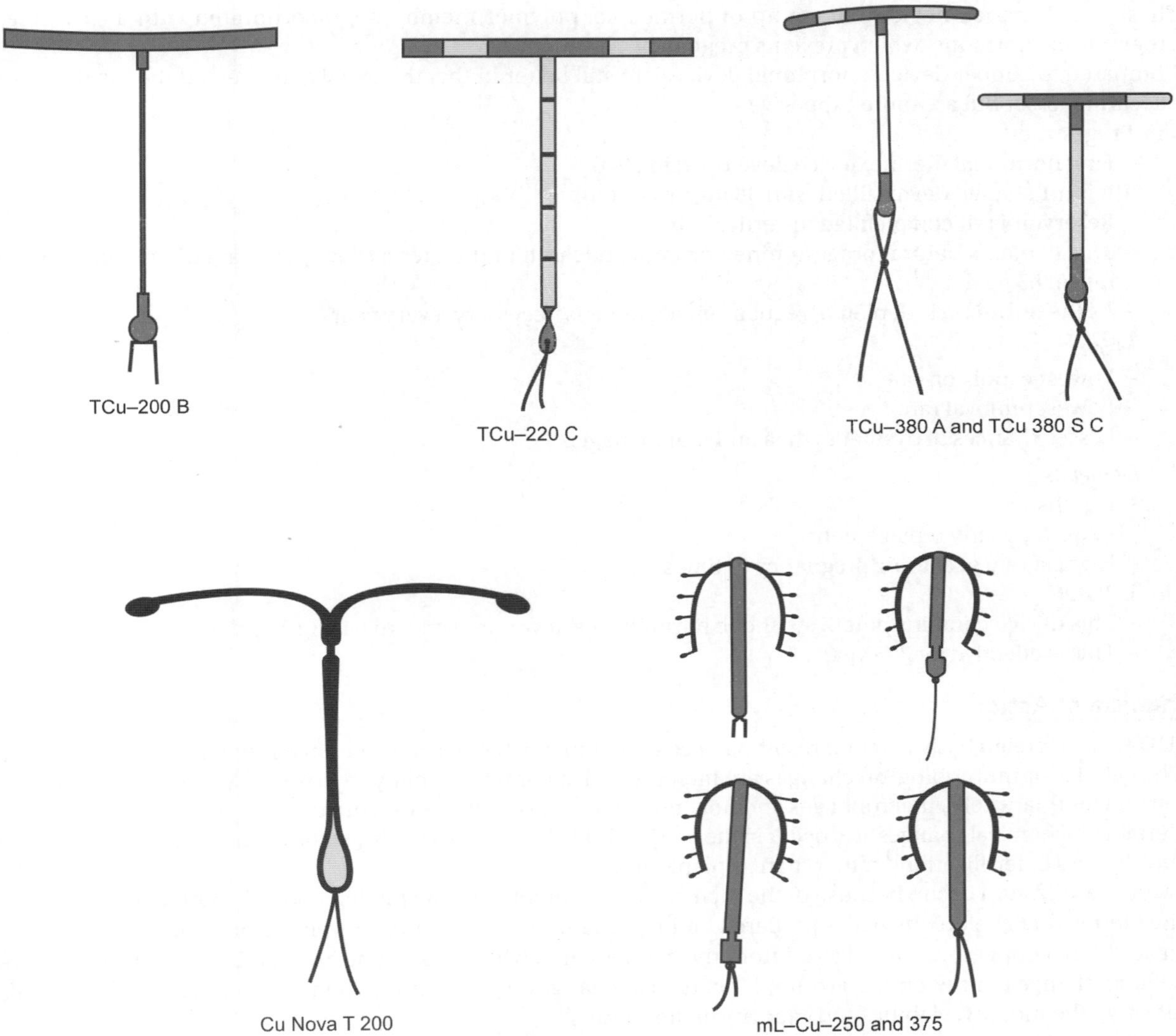

TCu–200 B

TCu–220 C

TCu–380 A and TCu 380 S C

Cu Nova T 200

mL–Cu–250 and 375

Fig. 2: Second generation IUDs

c. Third generation IUDs (Medicated IUDs/Bioactive IUDs[Q])

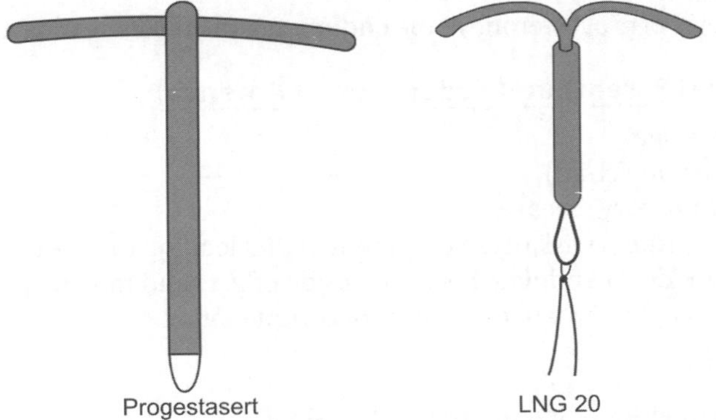

Fig. 3: Third generation IUDs

- These are T shaped devices, made up of permeable, polymer membrane, incorporated with a slow releasing progesterone hormone, which prevents pregnancy
- Compared to copper devices, hormonal devices are still better in that the expulsion rate and the incidence of side effects are lesser but are more expensive:
  i. Progestasert
    - First hormonal uterine device developed in 1976
    - It is a T shaped device filled with 38 mg progesterone[Q]
    - Reservoir is silicon oil filled in vertical stem
    - This contains natural progesterone hormone, released in the uterus slowly over a period of one year, at the rate of 65 μg daily[Q]
    - As the hormone is depleted, regular replacement is necessary, every year[Q].

    Merits
    - Lowest expulsion rate
    - Lowest removal rate
    - Lesser chances of dysmenorrhea and menorrhagia.

    Demerits
    - Expensive
    - Requires yearly replacement
    - Highest rate of ectopic pregnancy (9 times).
  ii. LNG-20
    - This device contains potent synthetic hormone, i.e. levonorgestrel, releasing 20 g daily
    - This is effective for 3–5 years.

Mechanism of Action

- IUDs cause foreign body reaction resulting in cellular and biochemical changes in endometrium/uterine fluid
- The cellular or morphological changes are increased vascular permeability (hyperemia), edema and infiltration of leukocytes (giant cells, macrophages and polymorphs) in the endometrium of uterus
- Certain biochemical changes also occur in the uterine fluid, thereby the viability of the ovum is impaired, thus reducing the chances of fertilization[Q] rather than implantation
- Even if fertilization occur, because of the increased tubal motility by the foreign body, the fertilized ovum moves to the uterus much before the bed is prepared for implantation and dies, thus preventing pregnancy
- In addition, copper ions are released from the copper IUDs, which has strong antifertility effect, by enhancing the cellular changes in the endometrium, biochemical changes in the uterine fluid and cervical mucus and also by affecting the motility, viability and capacity of the sperms[Q]
- Further, Cu-T also causes the release of prostaglandin which increases the contractility of uterus and makes it uncongenial for the nidation of zygote
- The hormone releasing devices release the progesterone hormone, which increases the viscosity of cervical mucus and prevent the sperms from entering the cervix
- They also maintain a high level of progesterone in the endometrium, making it unfavorable for implantation of zygote.

Ideal IUD Candidate (Planned Parenthood Federation of America)

- A woman in the reproductive age
- Given birth to a child (at least one child)
- Not having any pelvic inflammatory disease
- Not having multiple sexual partners (risk of development of PID leading to infertility)
- Nulliparous woman is not an ideal candidate because of side effects and more expulsions but IUD can be preferred in her if she cannot use or accept alternative methods of contraception
- Has normal menstrual cycle
- Is willing to check IUD tail
- Has access to followup and treatment of potential problems.

Procedure of IUD Insertion

- The placement of IUD is done by using a plastic syringe called IUD inserter, which is presterilized by gamma radiation
- The device is thus made available in a presterilized packet
- Hands to be washed, sterile gloves to be worn, thorough pelvic examination to be done to exclude any pathology, the genitalia (vagina and cervix) is cleaned with iodine, working slowly and gently, the provider inserts the IUD by opening the new, presterilized packet
- After insertion, if the woman fells dizzy, she should lie down quietly for 5–10 minutes.

Timing of Insertion

Ideal Time

- After the 5th day and before 10th day of menstrual period[Q] (intermenstrual insertion)
- Because cervical canal diameter is greatest, lesser expulsion and least risk of pregnancy
- However, IUD can be inserted at any time during the menstrual cycle, if it is reasonable sure that she is not pregnant.

Other Timings

i. Postplacental insertion
   - Insertion of IUD immediately following delivery of the placenta, at any time between 10 minutes to 48 hours after childbirth (immediate postpartum insertion)
   - High expulsion rate and high risk of infection and perforation of uterus.

ii. Postpartum insertion
   - Insertion of IUD about 6–8 weeks after delivery[Q] (postpuerperal insertion)
   - Can be combined with follow-up visit of mother and child
   - Expulsion rate is almost half of postplacental insertion.

iii. Postabortum insertion
   - Insertion of IUD about 12 weeks after an abortion
   - Not recommended for 2nd trimester abortion
   - However, following spontaneous abortion, IUD can be inserted after the first menstrual period.

iv. Postcesarean section insertion
   - Insertion of IUD, about 6–8 weeks after cesarean section
   - Risk of infection is high.

v. Postcoital insertion
   - Insertion of IUD within 3–5 days of unprotected or forced intercourse, to provide postcoital contraception (emergency contraception).

Precautions

- She must feel for the filaments in the vagina, every month
- She must report if it is not felt or expelled out or if it causes any problem
- In the absence of any complaints, she must report for the examination 1 year and 2 years after insertion
- Depending upon the types of IUD, it has to be removed after its life span is over
- In case she becomes pregnant and if she desires that pregnancy, it is better to remove the IUD to avoid infection and spontaneous abortion.

IUD Removal

- Using aseptic precautions, the IUD strings are pulled slowly and gently with forceps
- Indications for removal
  - Development of side effects such as severe pain and heavy bleeding
  - Occurrence of pregnancy
  - Development of pelvic inflammatory disease (PID)

- Perforation of uterus
- Partial expulsion of IUD
- When the life span of IUD has passed
- When the woman reaches menopause.

Contraindications

Absolute[Q]	*Relative*
▪ Pregnancy[Q] ▪ STDs[Q] ▪ Previous ectopic pregnancy[Q] ▪ Pelvic pathology such as infections, tumors, bleeding disorder[Q] ▪ Congenital defects in the uterus[Q] ▪ Cancer of cervix, uterus or adnexa[Q] ▪ Vaginal bleeding of undiagnosed etiology	▪ Multiple sexual partners ▪ Anemia ▪ Wilson's disease for copper IUDs only ▪ Menorrhagia ▪ History of PID since last pregnancy ▪ Purulent cervical discharge ▪ Unmotivated person ▪ Distortion of uterine cavity

Failure Rate

- Average: 2–3 per 100 WYE
- Nonmedicated devices: 6–13 per 100 WYE
- Copper devices 1–8 per 100 WYE.

Restoration of Fertility after Removal

- Fertility is not impaired after removal of IUD, provided there is no episode of PID and 70% of IUD users conceive within one year of removal.

Merits (Advantages)

- Simple to insert, safe to use
- Visit to the clinic is only once
- Effective to the tune of 97% (i.e. High success rate), thus reliable
- High continuation rate (stays in place for several years)
- Reversible contraceptive method (IUD can be removed easily)
- Free from systemic, metabolic side effects, unlike oral pills
- Does not interfere with sexual intercourse (so increased sexual enjoyment)
- Does not interfere with lactation (ideal contraceptive for lactating woman[Q] as it has no effect on quality and composition of breast milk)
- Collateral benefit is thorough pelvic examination of the woman, before IUD insertion
- Effective as "postcoital emergency contraceptives", if inserted within 3 to 5 days of unprotected intercourse
- Less risk of ectopic pregnancy.

Noncontraceptive Benefits of IUDs[Q]

- Synechiolysis in Asherman's syndrome[Q]
- Reduction of risk of endometrial cancer
- Treatment of anemia
- Treatment of nemorrhagia (LNG IUD)
- Hormone replacement therapy (LNG IUD)
- Adjuvant therapy to tamoxifen (LNG IUD).

Demerits (Side Effects and Complications)

a. Menstrual changes (bleeding) [Q]—ost common[Q]
   - Common during the first three months[Q] and can occur in form of spotting between the periods, longer and heavier menstrual periods (menorrhagia), more cramps or pain (dysmenorrhea) during periods

- Removal of IUD restores the normal pattern of the cycle
- Usually disappears by 1–2 months
- Leads to 10–20% of IUD removals
- Greater bleeding with nonmedicated IUDs
- Managed by reassuring the woman (do not remove IUD[Q]), ferrous sulfate 200 mg TDS for 1–2 months or remove IUD if bleeding is heavy or persistant.

b. Pain—most common cause of removal[Q]
- 2nd most common side effect
- Occurs in nearly 30–40% of the users
- Pain is experienced as low backache, abdominal cramps or pain down the thighs
- Usually pain disappears by third month
- More common in nullipara and those who have not had child for many years
- Mild pain is managed by analgesics
- If it is intolerable, IUD has to be removed
- Leads to 15–40% of all IUD removal (most common)
- If pain is severe during insertion, it indicates that either the IUD is large, incorrectly placed inside the uterus, uterine perforation or uterine infection

c. Pelvic infection or PID (pelvic inflammatory disease)
- PID is a collective term including acute, subacute or chronic inflammatory conditions of pelvic organs such as ovaries, fallopian tubes, uterus, the related connective tissues and the pelvic peritoneum
- It can occur if aseptic precautions are not adopted, while placing the IUD
- IUD increases risk of PID by 2–8 times
- PID is clinically characterized by fever, intermenstrual bleeding, leukorrhea, dysuria, pelvic pain and tenderness and palpable painful adnexal swelling
- One or two such episodes can result in blocking of fallopian tubes and infertility
- Thus PID is a threat to woman's fertility therefore when PID is diagnosed, IUD has to be removed
- PID can be prevented by proper selection of cases, thorough examination of pelvis before IUD insertion and by following aseptic precautions while inserting IUD and by avoiding multiple sexual partners
- Managed by prompt broad-spectrum antibiotics or removal of IUD if no response to antibiotics in 24–48 hours

d. Uterine perforation
- It is rare but potentially a serious complication following IUD insertion
- It used to be more with Lippe's loop than with copper IUDs
- It is more common following postplacental insertion[Q] than postpartum insertion (within 48 hours to 6 weeks postpartum)
- It is also more when inserted by an untrained person
- Perforation of uterus results in migration of the device into the peritoneal cavity causing obstruction of bowel, and peritoneal adhesions, it could be asymptomatic also
- Uterine perforation is suspected when a search is made for a missing IUD and diagnosis is made by pelvic X-ray or ultrasound examination
- IUD is removed by laprotomy.

e. Expulsions
- Nonmedicated devices like Lippe's loop have higher expulsion rates than copper devices
- Higher expulsion is seen in younger women, mulliparous, inert IUDs and postpartum insertion
- Among the parous women, it is more among lactating mother than nonlactating mothers
- Most expulsions take place within 3 months of IUD insertion and frequently occur during menstruation
- About 20% of the expulsions go un-noticed and may lead to unwanted pregnancy.

f. Ectopic pregnancy
- Pregnancy itself is rare among IUD users but when pregnancy occurs, 3% cases it is ectopic
- Highest in 1st year[Q]
- It is life threatening and requires immediate treatment
- Ectopic pregnancy is characterized by history of amenorrhea, lower abdominal pain and tenderness, scantly or dark vaginal bleeding, anemia and fainting and is confirmed by pelvic ultrasonography

- It may result in rupture of fallopian tubes
- Treatment is lapratomy and removal of trophoblast, fetal parts and tubes
- History of previous ectopic pregnancy is associated with an increased risk of ectopic pregnancy; therefore, such women should not use IUD.

g. Mortality
- Very low (~1 death per 100,000 years of case)
- Safer than OC pills.

7. National Cancer Control Program.

- National Cancer Control Program was initiated by the Government of India in 1975–1976[Q] has been revised since then in 1984 and then again in 2004
- During 2010, the program was integrated with National Program on Prevention and Control of Diabetes, Cardiovascular Disease and Stroke (NPCDCS).

Objectives

- Primary prevention of cancer by health education
- Secondary prevention by early detection and diagnosis of common cancers like cancers of cervix, mouth, breast and tobacco-related cancers by screening or self-examination method
- Tertiary prevention by strengthening of the existing institutions of comprehensive therapy including palliative care.

Strategy

a. Regional cancer center scheme
- Regional cancer centers are strengthened by providing one time assistance of 3 crores rupees for them to act as referral centers for complicated and difficult cases at tertiary levels.

b. Oncology wing development scheme[Q]
- To fill the geographical gap in availability of cancer treatment, a grant of 3 crores rupees per institution is provided to state governments or health institutes to purchase equipment[Q] including cobalt therapy unit, brachytherapy unit, linear accelerator, etc. and civil works to develop an oncology wing in existing health infrastructure.

c. District cancer control program
- Another central-state partnership project wherein a total of 90 lakh rupees is provided by the central government over 5 years (22 lakh in first year and 17 lakh in subsequent 4 years) for the district cancer institutes selected by the state government to provide health education, prevention, early detection and pain relief measures.

d. Decentralized NGO scheme
- Nodal agencies and NGOs (recommended by State Government) are given financial assistance of 5 lakh rupees for undertaking health education and early detection activities of cancer preferably in rural areas and urban slums.

e. IEC activities at central level
- These activities include widespread publicity about the rules formulated for implementation of antitobacco legislation and ill effects of consumption of tobacco and tobacco-related products to discourage consumption of cigarettes and other tobacco-related products
- It also includes celebration of National Cancer Awareness Day on 7th November every year.

f. Research and training
- It includes conducting training programs and monitoring and research activities
- Many training manuals have also been developed for cancer control at district levels:
  - Manual for health professional
  - Manual for cytology
  - Manual for palliative care
  - Manual for tobacco cessation.

g. Legislation
- Central Government passed "The Cigarettes and other Tobacco Products (Prohibition of Advertisement and Regulation of Trade and Commerce, Production, Supply and Distribution) Act, 2003" to reduce the tobacco consumption in the society

– Its important provisions are:
  - Prohibition of smoking in public places
  - Prohibition of direct or indirect advertisement of cigarette and other products
  - Prohibition of sale of cigarette and other tobacco products to a person below the age of 18 years
  - Prohibition of sale of tobacco products near educational institutions
  - Mandatory depiction of statutory warning including pictorial warning on tobacco or tobacco product packs
  - Mandatory depiction of tar and nicotine contents along with maximum permissible limits on tobacco products.

Targets Achieved (As of 2004)

Tertiary Cancer Centers (2012)	45
Districts selected (Under NPCDCS)	100
NGOs selected (1994)	33
Total number of radiotherapy centers	217
No. of brachytherapy centers	136
Equipment purchased	
No. of telecobalt units	262
No. of telecobalt—Cs-137 units	9
No. of linacs	77
No. of remote HDR units	83
No. of remote LDR units	36
Manual intracavitary	75
Manual intrastitial	29

Significance

- National Cancer Control Program is based on Central-State partnership wherein the financial assistance is provided by the central government and the state government provides the manpower and health-care infrastructure for implementation of the program.

8. Maternal mortality rate.

Refer Question No. 2 June 2012 (RS2) Paper II.

9. Health hazards of health-care waste.

- Health-care waste means any waste generated during the diagnosis, treatment or immunization of human beings or animals or in research activities pertaining thereto or in the production or testing of biological.

Health Hazards of Health-care Waste

- Health-care waste poses a great threat of disease or injury to those exposed because:
  – It contains infectious agents
  – It contains toxic or hazardous chemicals or pharmaceuticals
  – It contains sharps and needles
  – It is genotoxic
  – It is radioactive.

"At Risk" Groups

- Medical professionals including doctors, nurses, auxiliaries and hospital maintenance staff
- Patients and their visitors in hospitals
- Workers of allied services of hospitals like house keeping, waste handling, transportation, etc.
- Workers involved with waste disposal
- Scavengers or rag pickers.

Health Hazards

From infectious waste and sharps	*From chemical and pharmaceutical waste*	*From genotoxic waste*	*From radioactive waste*	*Public sensitivity*
Pathogens like HIV, hepatitis viruses, antibiotic resistant bacteria present in health-care waste may gain access to humans directly though puncture wounds, abrasions or cuts on the skin, mucous membranes or by inhalation or ingestion	Though present in small quantities, they are toxic, genotoxic, corrosive, inflammable, reactive or explosive and cause intoxication by acute or chronic exposure and injuries including burns	May cause toxicity by inhalation, inhalation or absorption through skin and severity depends upon the toxicity of the substance, extent and duration of exposure	Toxicity ranges from headache, dizziness and vomiting to much more severe form depending upon the type and extent of exposure	Health-care waste particularly anatomical waste may offend public sensitivity

Significance

- Health-care waste unlike regular household waste is very toxic and harmful posing various hazards to community besides the health professionals and need to be disposed off safely and meticulously.

10. List out the principles of health education.

Refer Question No. 2 December 2011 (RS2) Paper I.

11. Intensified pulse polio program.

- Intensified Pulse Polio Program was started in 1999 by Government of India because of inspite of all efforts, there occurred focal outbreaks of acute flaccid paralysis.

Objective

- Reduction of number and size of high-risk areas for poliomyelitis by not missing any child for OPV and achieving 100% immunization.

Strategy

- Increase the involvement of health-care officials especially peripheral health officers in the planning process and make them accountable
- Maintain high level of AFP surveillance and promote use of AFP surveillance information in planning immunization activities
- Focus on better conversion of X house (house with unimmunized target child) to P house (house with immunized target child)
- Consistently vaccinate the children
- Effectively improve the microplans so as not miss any house
- Improve IEC activities and social mobilization
- Improve program management and monitoring
- Sustain and maintain high level of routine immunization in high-risk areas
- Carry out supplementary immunization activities (SIA) if necessary.

Activities

- Original program was intensified by making it a 3-day program to detect and immunize missed and eligible children who were not immunized on National Immunization Day

Day 1 (National Immunisation Day)	*Day 2 (house-to-house visits)*	*Day 3*
▪ Administer OPV to all children visiting immunization booths and mark their finger with Gentian violet for later identification	▪ Conduct house to house visits in the area and look for immunization status of the target children (Gentian violet mark on finger) ▪ Mark the houses as "X" for houses which are not cooperative, or locked or target child is not immunized or else mark the houses as "P" if the target children are immunized or target children are not available	▪ Visit the houses marked "X" and immunize the target children and remark the house as "P"

Targets Achieved

- Even with intensification there were lots of setbacks for the program as the polio transmission increased, reporting as much as 383 cases in 2006 mostly from Western UP and Bihar
- This was due to:
  - High density of population
  - Poor quality of health-care services
  - Very poor sanitation
  - Interference by nonpolio enteric viruses in the development of immunity with OPV
  - Malpractices like false marking of children without immunization or unimmunized houses as "P" or under immunization, etc.
  - Weak performance by vaccination team such as non-identification of eligible children or wrong marking of houses.

Significance

- With intensification of pulse polio program, the polio-free day does not seems very far provided there is commitment and cooperation, both by the health-care providers and public.

12. Mass chemotherapy in filariasis control.

Refer Question No. 11 June 2011 (RS2) Paper II.

SHORT ANSWERS

13. Accredited social health activist.

Refer Question No. 2 June 2014 (RS2) Paper II.

14. What are the risk factors for coronary heart diseases?

Refer Question No. 11 June 2015 (RS2) Paper II.

15. Brief out the indigenous systems of medicine in India

Refer Question No. 19 December 2007 (RS2) Paper II.

16. Rockefeller foundation.

- Rockefeller foundation is a non-governmental philanthropic agency[Q] established in USA in 1913 by Mr John D Rockefeller
- It started its activities in India from 1920.

Objectives	*Activities*
▪ Promote the well being of mankind all over the world	▪ Public health and medical education in early days ▪ Advancement of life sciences, social sciences, humanities and agricultural sciences were included subsequently

Activities in India

- It started its activities in India with scheme for control of hookworm disease in then Madras Presidency
- It has helped establishment of:
  - All India Institute of Hygiene and Public Health, Kolkata
  - All India Institute of Medical Sciences, New Delhi
  - King George's Medical College, Lucknow
  - Christian Medical College, Vellore
  - Christian Medical College, Ludhiana
  - SGS Medical College, Mumbai

- Field Demonstration Project, Ballabhgarh
- National Institute of Viriology, Pune

- It sponsors educational visits for advanced training of health professionals of India to other countries through fellowship and travel grants
- It sponsors the visits of specialists from USA
- It provides grants in aid to selected institutions for carrying out researches, libraries and medical education
- Currently it gives active support for improvement of agriculture, family planning and rural development besides medical education.

17. Input-output analysis.

Refer Question No. 6 December 2011 (RS2) Paper II.

18. Shrivastav committee, 1975.

Refer Question No. 6 June 2010 (RS2) Paper II.

19. Vaccine for meningococcal meningitis.

- Internationally licensed vaccine for meningococcal meningitis are either bivalent, i.e. prepared from group A and C[Q] or tetravalent, i.e. prepared from groups A, C, Y and W-135[Q]
- However, they may be monovalent, i.e. prepared from either A, C, Y or W-135 groups
- Meningococcal vaccine is not available for group B meningococcus[Q] because group B polysaccharide is not immunogenic.

Nature	▪ It is purified, heat stable, lyophilized capsular polysaccharides from meningococci (cellular fractions) ▪ Each dose contains 50 μg of each of the individual polysaccharides
Dose	▪ 0.5 mL
Route	▪ Subcutaneously in middle 1/3rd of anterolateral thigh
Schedule	▪ 1st dose at 11–12 years followed by booster dose at 16 years of age
Immunity	▪ Starts within 10 days and lasts for 3 years and booster required after 3 years
Indications	▪ Active immunization of high-risk groups against meningococcal meningitis Routinely – All adolescents in age group of 11–12 years Others – Adolescents in group of 13–18 years – Young people 19–21 years – 2 years and above (splenectomised chronic diseases, laboratory workers and travelers to endemic areas) ▪ International travelers at high risk of infection
Contraindications[Q]	▪ Pregnancy [Q] ▪ Infants and children under 2 years of age (due to development of immunological tolerance)

20. Diarrheal disease control program.

- National Diarrheal Disease Control Program was started by Government of India in 1978 during 7th five year plan

Objectives	*Goal*	*Principle*
▪ Creation of awareness that most diarrhea cases can be managed at home using home-based solutions ▪ Education mothers on feeding children with diarrhea ▪ Promotion of oral rehydration therapy and making it widely available ▪ Reducing morbidity and mortality due to diarrheal diseases	▪ Reduction in under five mortality due to diarrheal diseases by 50% over 5 years	▪ 90% of all diarrheal diseases can be managed at home ▪ 9% develop some dehydration which can be managed with ORS packets ▪ 1% only develops severe dehydration requiring hospitalization

Revised Scheme 2

Strategy

- Education of mothers to use home available fluids with the onset of diarrhea among under five children[Q]
- Education of mothers to use ORS and to continue feeding
- Training of health workers, village health guides and Anganwadi workers in oral rehydration therapy
- Distribution of ORS packets and booklets on Home Treatment of Diarrhea, published in various regional languages to health workers and village health guides through Primary Health Centers
- Supplying every village health guide with 100 ORS packets and every health worker at subcenter with 200 ORS packets every year
- Establishing Diarrhea Training and Treatment Units in all medical colleges to serve as demonstration centers of Oral Rehydration Therapy for medical students, nurses and health workers besides treating diarrhea with dehydration cases.

Status

- Currently the program component of supply of ORS packets and home management of diarrhea is integrated with RCH program.

Significance

- Diarrheal diseases which claim many lives in under five age group can easily be managed at home and thus save lots of human lives if detected early and properly treated[Q].

21. Baby friendly hospitals.

- Baby friendly hospital initiative is a concept jointly developed and promoted by WHO and UNICEF in 1992 in 12 countries which has now spread to 171 countries.

Aim	*Objectives*	*Benefits to hospital*
▪ To ensure that every newborn baby gets the best start in its life ▪ To encourage correct scientific practices in breastfeeding	▪ To protect, to promote and to support breastfeeding practices ▪ To reduce infant mortality rate	▪ Professional satisfaction of helping lactating mothers ▪ Reduction of infant mortality rate ▪ National and International recognition for hospital without any financial investment

Characteristics of Body friendly Hospital (10 Steps to Successful Breastfeeding)

- Baby friendly hospital initiative has set up for ten steps to be followed in a hospital to make it a "baby friendly hospital". (Mnemonic—SERENDIPITY)
  i. **S**how mothers how to breastfeed and how to maintain lactation even if they should be separated from their babies.
  ii. Foster the **E**stablishment of breastfeeding support groups and refer mother to them on discharge from hospital or clinic.
  iii. Practice "**R**OOMING IN", i.e. allow mother and infant to remain together 24 hours/day[Q].
  iv. Give **N**o artificial teats or pacifiers[Q] to breast feeding infant.
  v. Encourage breastfeeding on demand[Q] or "**D**emand feeding".
  vi. **I**nform all pregnant women about the benefits and management of breastfeeding.
  vii. Have a written breastfeeding **P**olicy that is routinely communicated to all health delivery staff.
  viii. Help mother **I**nitiate breastfeeding within half an hour of birth[Q].
  ix. **T**rain all health-care staff in skills necessary to implement this policy.
  x. Give newborn infants no food or drink other than breast milk[Q] unless medicall**Y** indicated.

Certification

- In India, the National Task Force at New Delhi provides policy guidelines and technical support
- The State Task Force is entrusted with responsibility of certification of baby friendly hospital wherein the professional assessor conducts an inspection and if satisfied, the hospital certified baby friendly hospital.

Significance

- The concept of baby friendly hospital Initiative came into practice because of malpractices in breastfeeding, which in turn, is due to ignorance and lack of knowledge and also because of hindrance in breastfeeding by marketers of infant milk substitutes and infant foods.

22. Street children.

- These are the children living and working on the streets
- They form a large proportion of children without family support in metropolitan cities.

Causes	*Exposed risks*	*Services offered for betterment*
▪ Physical and sexual abuse at home ▪ Poverty ▪ Rapid urbanization	i. Health risk – Malnutrition, tuberculosis, sexually transmitted diseases including HIV, parasites and worm infestations and skin diseases ii. Social risk – Drug abuse, prostitution and criminal exploitation	▪ Health and welfare services ▪ Housing ▪ Counseling centers ▪ Adoptions ▪ Educational opportunities ▪ Employment

MBBS PHASE III EXAMINATION

DECEMBER 2009

(Revised Scheme 2)

PAPER I

LONG ESSAYS

1. Describe the levels of prevention of disease. Apply each level of prevention to the prevention of coronary heart disease in a population.

Refer Question No. 1 December 2007 (RS2) Paper I.

2. What is social security? Describe the benefits under ESI scheme.

- Social security is the security that society furnishes through appropriate organizations, against certain risk to which its members are exposed
- It primarily refers to a social insurance program providing social protection or protection against socially recognized conditions including poverty, old age, disability, unemployment and others.

Risks Covered

- Sickness
- Invalidity
- Maternity
- Old age
- Death.

Components (Approaches)

Social insurance[Q]	*Social assistance*[Q]
▪ It provides income security in form of cash benefits ▪ It is a contributory benefit extended to individuals as a matter of right *Examples* i. For industrial workers[Q] – Workmen's Compensation Act, 1923 – Central Maternity Benefit Act, 1961 – Employees State Insurance Act, 1948 – The Family Pension Scheme, 1971 – Factories Act – Disablement Benefit Act – Personal Benefit Act ii. For civil servants – Pension, Gratuity and Provident fund – The Family Pension Scheme, 1971 iii. For general public – Life Insurance Corporation of India – Public Provident Fund	▪ It is not insurance, i.e. there is not contribution system but fund comes from general revenues ▪ It is non-contributory benefit extended to vulnerable groups *Beneficiaries* ▪ Unemployed ▪ Disabled ▪ Old widows ▪ Children ▪ Handicapped *Examples* ▪ National Rural Employment Guarantee Scheme ▪ Sanjay Gandhi Niradhar Yojna ▪ Savithri Phule Dattak Palak Yojna ▪ Indira Gandhi National Old Age Pension Scheme

Significance

- Social security is basis of social welfare and is essential because those who are not secured in this way, may cause social harm for fulfilling their own needs
- Social security was first introduced in Germany in 1883 by Bismark[Q] which become model for other European countries to emulate.

For benefits under ESI scheme

Refer Question No. 4 December 2012 (RS2) Paper I.

SHORT ESSAYS

3. What is human development index?

- Human development index (HDI) is defined as a composite index combining indicators representing three dimensions, i.e. longevity (life-expectancy at birth), knowledge (adult literacy rate and combined school enrollment ratio) and income (real GDP per capita in purchasing power parity in US dollars)
- The value of human development index varies between 0 to 1[Q] which allows International comparison
- It was created by Amrtya Sen (Indian Economist and Nobel Laureate) and Mahbub ul Haq (Pakistani Economist) in 1990.

Calculations

Reference Ranges

- To calculate the index, fixed minimum and maximum values have been established for each of the components.

Component[Q]	*Fixed maximum*	*Fixed minimum*
Life-expectancy at birth (longetivity)[Q]	85 years[Q]	25 years[Q]
Adult literary rate (knowledge)[Q]	100%	0%
Combined gross school enrollment ratio	100%	0%
Real GDP per capita (purchasing power/income)[Q]	$ 40000	$ 100

New Goalposts (2010 onwards)

Parameters	*Country*	*Maximum value*	*Minimum value*
Life-expectancy (in years)	Japan	83.4	20.0
Mean years of schooling (in years)	Czech republic	13.1	0
Expected years of schooling (in years)	Capped at	18.0	0
Combined education index	New Zealand	97.8%	0
Per capita income (in Dollors)	Qatar	$ 107,721	$ 100

Calculation

- The individual component index can be calculated using following general formula

$$\text{Index} = \frac{\text{Actual value} - \text{Minimum value}}{\text{Maximum value} - \text{Minimum value}}$$

- HDI is geometric mean of three dimensions
- Indices = $I_{Life}^{1/3} \times I_{Education}^{1/3} \times I_{Income}^{1/3}$
- Thus, human development index of India can be calculated as follows:
  a. Life-expectancy at birth (actual value of India is 62.8)

$$\text{Life-expectancy at birth} = \frac{62.8 - 25}{85 - 25} = \frac{37.8}{60} = 0.63$$

b. Adult literacy rate (Actual value of India is 53.5%)

$$\text{Adult literacy rate} = \frac{53.5-0}{100-0} = \frac{53.5}{100} = 0.535$$

c. Combined gross school enrollment ratio (Actual value of India is 55%)

$$\text{Combined gross school enrollment ratio} = \frac{55-0}{100-0} = \frac{55}{100} = 0.55$$

d. Real GDP per capita (Actual value of India is ₹ 1670/-)
 - Adjusted real GDP per capita would be

$$\text{Real GDP per capita index} = \frac{\log(1670) - \text{Log}(100)}{\log(40000) - \text{Log}(100)} = 0.47$$

- The human development index is simple average of above three indices as follows:

$$\text{Human development index} = \frac{0.63 + 0.54 + 0.47}{3} = \frac{1.64}{3} = 0.546$$

Interpretation

- Based on human development index, countries have been graded as follows:

Human development index	*Grading*	*Example*	*HDI*	*Rank (2012–13)*
> 0.8	High	Norway	0.955	1
0.79 – 0.50	Medium	India	0.554	136
< 0.5	Low	Niger	0.304	186

Advantage

- Human development index is a comprehensive indicator of development which does not only measure economic prosperity but other factors which are essential to maintain this economic prosperity thus the countries with same GDP differ in their HDI index.

Significance

- The human development index reflects achievements in the most basic human capabilities, i.e. leading a long life, being knowledgeable and enjoying a decent standard of living
- Human development index is used for international comparison of degree of development of a country and countries are awarded ranking as per their HDI
- India ranks 136 out of 186 countries (2012–13).

4. How is randomized controlled trial done?

Refer Question No. 1 December 2015 (RS2) Paper I.

5. Briefly discuss the various approaches to health education.

- Health education is a process aimed at encouraging people to want to be healthy, to know how to stay healthy, to do what they can individually and collectively to maintain health and to seek help when needed. (Declaration of Alma Ata).

For approaches and applications of health education

Refer Question No. 2 June 2009 (RS2) Paper I.

6. How is pasteurization of milk carried out? What are the tests done for checking the efficiency of pasteurization?

- Pasteurization is process of preservation of milk by the heating of milk to such temperature and for such periods of time as are required to destroy and pathogens that may be present while causing minimal changes in the composition, flavor and nutritive value. (WHO).

Methods

Holder method (Vat method[Q])	HTST method[Q] (flash method or High Temp & Short Time method)	UHT method (Ultra high temperature method)
▪ Milk is heated to 63–66°C[Q] and maintained at this temperature for 30 minutes followed by rapid cooling quickly to 5°C or lower ▪ Recommended for small and rural communities	▪ Milk is rapidly heated to 72°C and maintained at this temperature for not less than 15 seconds followed by rapid cooling quickly to 4°C or lower ▪ Recommended for urban areas and is the most widely used method as it very large quantities of milk can be pasteurized	▪ Milk is heated in two stages ▪ In 1st stage, heating is done under normal pressure to 88°C for few seconds, and in 2nd stage, it is heated to 125°C under pressure for few seconds only ▪ It is then rapidly cooled and bottled as quickly as possible

Tests for Pasteurization

a. Phosphatase test	▪ Most widely used test to access quality of pasteurization[Q] *Principle* ▪ Raw milk contains an enzyme, phosphatase which is completely destroyed on heating at temperature which corresponds closely with standard time and temperature required for pasteurization (at 60°C for 30 min) *Procedure* ▪ Add disodium phenyl phosphate buffer to sample of milk and incubate ▪ Add Felin's reagent to this milk *Observation* ▪ Observe for color change of milk to blue *Interpretation* ▪ If milk turns blue, indicates presence of phosphatase enzyme in milk which acts upon buffer to liberate phenol which is indicated by Felin's reagent ▪ Positive phosphatase indicates milk is not pasteurized or raw milk is added *Significance* ▪ Phosphatase test is most widely used test to check efficiency of pasteurization
b. Methylene blue reduction test	▪ Indirect method for detection of microorganism in milk[Q] ▪ Carried on out milk accepted for pasteurization *Principle* ▪ Detects destruction of bacilli *Procedure* ▪ Add 1 mL methylene blue to 10 mL of sample milk and incubate in water bath for 5 hours *Observation* ▪ Observe for any discoloration of milk *Inference* ▪ Discoloration of milk indicated presence of bacteria
c. Standard plate count	▪ Permissible limit is 30,000 bacteriae per mL of pasteurized milk
d. Coliform count	▪ Pasteurization completely destroys coliform organisms hence they should be zero or absent in 1 mL sample of milk ▪ Presence of coliforms indicates improper pasteurization or post-pasteurization contamination

Significance

- Pasteurization is the simplest, safest and cheapest and modern method of rendering the milk safe
- By these methods, all nonsporing pathogens such as mycobacteria, brucellae and salmonellae are destroyed but a relatively heat resistant bacteria *Coxiella burnetii* may survive the holder method.

7. What are the medical measures for prevention of occupational diseases?

Refer Question No. 2 June 2016 (RS2) Paper I.

8. What are the methods for determining the bacteriological quality of water?

Refer Question No. 5 June 2016 (RS2) Paper I.

9. Write short notes on residual insecticides.

- Residual insecticides are long acting insecticides used in form of residual spraying.

Characteristics of good residual insecticide
- Be toxic to target vector
- Have long-lasting effect on a given surface
- Be safe to human a domestic animals
- Be acceptable to house owners
- Be cost-effective
- Be stable during storage and transport
- Not be irritant or repellent to target insects to ensure that insects pick up a lethal dose
- Mix well with water and be harmless to spraying instrument.

Examples

	Dosage (g/m²)	*Duration of action*
a. Organochlorines		
– DDT[Q]	1–2[Q]	More than 6 months
– Lindane (BHC)	0.2–0.5	3 or more months
b. Organophosphorus		
– Malathion[Q]	1–2	1–3 months[Q]
– Fenitrothion	1–2	1–3 months
– Methyl pirimphos	1–2	2–3 months
c. Carbamates		
– Propoxus	1–2	2–3 months
– Bendiocarb	0.2–0.4	2–3 months
d. Pyrethroids		
– Permethrin	0.5	2–3 months
– Cypermethrin	0.5	4 or more months
– Deltamethrin	0.05	2–3 months

Application

- Residual insecticides are used for residual spraying wherein these insecticides are sprayed on walls[Q], ceiling and other surfaces where mosquitoes rest
- Spraying is also done in dark corners, under surface of furniture, cots and also in cattle sheds and stables using knapsack sprayers
- This method is especially suited for rural areas because of mud walls, which absorb insecticides and retain effect for long time.

10. How will you measure morbidity?

- Morbidity indicators are the direct indicators of health status of a country.[1]

Ref:

1. T. Bhaskara Rao TB. Textbook of Community Medicine, 2nd edition. Paras Medical Publisher, Hyderabad;2006.p.22.

Measures of Morbidity

a. Incidence rate
   – Incidence rate is the number of new cases occurring in a defined population during a specified period of time.

$$\text{Incidence rate} = \frac{\text{Number of new cases of specific disease during a given time period}}{\text{Population at risk during that period}} \times 1{,}000$$

- Incidence rate includes
  - Only new cases
  - During a specified period of time
  - In a specified population, i.e. population at risk
- Incidence rate also refers to new spells or episodes of disease arising in a given period of time per 1,000 population.
- Incidence rate is not influenced by the duration of the disease.
- Its use is generally restricted to acute conditions

b. Prevalence rate
- Prevalence rate is the number of persons having disease (both old and new cases) at a given point of time or over a period of time in a given population.

Point prevalence	*Period prevalence*
▪ Number of all current cases (old or new) of a disease at one point in time in relation to a defined population ▪ Point may consist of a day, several days or even a few weeks depending upon the time needed to examine the population $\frac{\text{Number of all current cases (old and new) of a specified disease existing at a given point in time}}{\text{Estimated population at the same point in time}} \times 100$	▪ Number of all current cases (old and new) of a disease during a defined period of time in relation to a defined population. ▪ Includes the cases arising but extending into or through the defined period as well as those arising during the defined period $\frac{\text{Number of existing cases (old and new) of a specified disease existing at a given point in time}}{\text{Estimated mid-interval population at risk}} \times 100$

Significance

- Morbidity indicator is direct indicators of health of a community and thus most widely used data for comparison and in planning and evaluation of health programs.

11. Food fortification.

- Food fortification is a public health measure whereby nutrients are added to food (in relatively small quantities) to maintain or improve the quality of the diet of a group a community or a population[Q]. (WHO)

Objective	*Criteria for food fortification*	*Examples*
▪ Reinforcing the usual dietary intake of nutrients with additional supplies to prevent/ control some nutritional disorder	▪ Vehicle to be fortified must be consumed regularly in diet by population ▪ Amount of nutrient added must not cause deficiency or toxicity in consumers ▪ On addition of nutrient, there should be no change in taste, odor, consistency or appearance ▪ Cost of fortification must be affordable by consumers	▪ Flouridation of water as a preventive of dental caries ▪ Iodization of salt for combating endemic goiter[Q] (first introduced in India[Q]) ▪ Food fortification (e.g. vanaspati, milk) with vitamin A and D[Q] ▪ Addition of iron to common salt to prevent nutritional anemia ▪ Addition of lysine to wheat flour[Q] while making bread ▪ Twin fortification of table salt with iodine and iron

Significance

- Food fortification has proved that it is a long-term measure for mitigating specific problems of malnutrition in the community
- Food fortification is an example of primary level of prevention.

12. What is lathyrism? How to prevent and control it?

- Neurolathyrism (Lathyrism) is a type of food toxicity, produced due to a toxin, Beta-oxalylamino-alanine (BOAA) which is found in the khesari dal[Q] (*L. sativus*)

- Neurolathyrism is prevalent in regions where khesari dal is eaten (diet containing more than 30% of khesari dal[Q] over a period of 2–6 months), i.e. Madhya Pradesh[Q], Uttar Pradesh[Q], Bihar[Q] and Odisha[Q]. It is also reported in Maharashtra, West Bengal, Rajasthan, Assam and Gujarat.

Toxin

- Beta-oxalylamino-alanine (BOAA[Q])
- Can be isolated in crystalline form and is water soluble
- Can cross the blood brain barrier and affect the nervous system.

Clinical Features

- Disease mainly affects young men between the age of 15–45 years and manifests as:

Latent stage	*No stick stage*	*One stick stage*	*Two stick stage*	*Crawler stage*
▪ Apparently healthy individual but exhibit ungainly gait when subjected to physical stress ▪ Characterstic physical signs on neurological examination ▪ Complete remission if diet is withdrawn at this stage	▪ Patient walks with short jerky steps without aid of a stick	▪ Patient walks with a stick to maintain balance and overcome muscular stiffness	▪ Patient needs two sticks (crutches) due to excessive bending of knees and crossed legs ▪ The gait is slow and clumpsy and walking for short distance tires the patient easily	▪ In final stages, knee cannot support the body weight thus making erect posture impossible ▪ Atrophy of thigh and leg muscles and patient is reduced to crawling by throwing his weight on hands

Prevention and Control

a. Vitamin C prophylaxis[Q]	▪ Daily administration of 500–1000 mg of ascorbic acid for a week or so can repair the damage in certain instances
b. Banning the crop or its consumption	▪ It is an extreme and unfeasible step
c. Removal of toxin[Q]	i. Steeping method – Toxin being water soluble can be removed by soaking the dal in hot water for 2 hours and washing the dal again with clean water and let to dry before consumption ii. Parboiling[Q] – Similar to parboiling of rice where large quantity of dal is soaked in lime water over night followed by boiling.
d. Education	▪ About the dangers of the consumption of dal and the need and methods of removal of toxins
e. Genetic approach	▪ Selective propagation and cultivation of strains of kesari dal which have very low levels of toxin
f. Socioeconomic changes	▪ Socioeconomic change or overall development can root out the problem

Significance

- Prevalence of lathyrism is very common in certain geographical regions in lower socioeconomic classes due to cost of the dal, however, with efforts of State Government in Health Education regarding removal of toxin, incidence is lowering.

SHORT ANSWERS

13. What is standardized death rate?

Refer Question No. 4 December 2007 (RS2) Paper I.

14. Orthotoludine test.

Refer Question No. 5 June 2011 (RS2) Paper I.

15. What are the maternity benefits under ESI Act?

Refer Question No. 4 December 2012 (RS2) Paper I.

16. Meaning of the term "Interquartile range".

- Interquartile range in a measure of statistical dispersion or variation
- Also called midspread or middle fifty
- It indicates 2 values of a variate in set which contains middle 50% observations when series is arranged in ascending or descending order of measurement.

Calculations	*Comparison to range*	*Applications*
▪ Interquartile range is calculated by arranging series in ascending or descending order followed by dividing series into 4 parts ▪ Each part is called quartile and it includes 25% of total observations ▪ Interquartile range equals difference between third and first quartiles ▪ Thus QR = Q3–Q1	25% 25% 25% 25% A B C D A = Lowest value in range B = Lower value in interquartile range C = Median D = Higher value in interquartile range E = Highest value in range **Fig. 1:** Interquartile range	▪ Used to build box plots, simple graphical representation of a probability distribution

Significance

- Unlike range, interquartile range is a robust statistic, having a breakdown point of 25% and is thus often preferred to range.

Ref:

1. http://en.wikipedia.org/wiki/Interquartile_range accessed on 2nd June 2011.

17. What are the warning signals of poor mental health?

Refer Question No. 6 June 2009 (RS2) Paper I.

18. Sampling errors.

- Sampling error is variation in result obtained from one sample to another taken from same population.

Factors Influencing Sampling Errors

Size of sample	*Natural variability of individual readings*	*Sampling methods*
▪ Sampling error decreases with increase in sample size	▪ Individual readings vary widely from one another resulting in variability from one sample to another	▪ Faulty sampling methods results in sampling errors

Significance

- Sampling errors can be minimized with proper sampling methods.

19. What are the types of epidemics?

Refer Question No. 4 December 2016 (RS2) Paper I.

20. What do you mean by breakpoint chlorination?

Refer Question No. 9 December 2016 (RS2) Paper I.

21. List three sources of health information in India.

Refer Question No. 10 December 2009 (RS2) Paper II.

22. List the Indian systems of medicine.

- Ayurveda and Siddha system of medicine are considered Indian system of Medicine in true sense
- Ayurveda is practised throughout India but Siddha is practised in Tamil speaking areas of south India
- Both these systems differ very little in their theory and practice.

Indian Systems of Medicine

Ayurveda system	*Siddha system*
▪ Ayurved means 'Science of life' ▪ Based on Tridosha theory of disease[Q] ▪ Diseases occur when there is disequilibrium in three doshas (humor), namely vata (wind), pitta (gall) and kapha (mucus)	▪ Siddha means 'Achievement' ▪ Based on notion that medical treatment has to take into account the patients environment, age, sex, race, physiological constitution, etc.

Significance

- Indian system of medicine is very much alive in India today and is being promoted by Government of India under AYUSH Scheme.

MBBS PHASE III EXAMINATION

DECEMBER 2009

(Revised Scheme 2)

PAPER II

LONG ESSAYS

1. Describe the epidemiology of tuberculosis and current strategy in the prevention and control of tuberculosis.

- Tuberculosis (TB) is a chronic infectious disease caused by *Mycobacterium tuberculosis* affecting lungs, bones, joints, meninges, intestines, lymph nodes, kidneys, etc.
- Also known as barometer of social welfare.

TB Statistics

- About 40% (2 out of every 5) of Indian population is infected with TB bacilli and 20,000 people become infected daily
- About 14 million people are suffering from the disease and more than 5000 develop disease daily[Q]
- About 4 million cases are sputum positive for sputum, i.e. infectious and 0.8 million become sputum positive every year[Q]
- About 1.8 million cases are added every year
- About 0.37 million cases die every year[Q], i.e. about 1,000 per day or 2 per minute
- It amount to loss of about 12,000 crores every year to the Government of India
- About 80 working days are lost per year per case
- Annual risk of becoming infected with TB is 1.5%[Q]
- Life time risk of disease among infected is 10%[Q]

Indian Scenario (2014)

- India is the country with highest TB burden in the world
- India accounts for 1/4th of worldwide TB cases (Mantoux positive[Q])
- Prevalence is 195 per lakh population
- Incidence is 167 per lakh population
- Tuberculosis mortality is 17 per lakh population
- About 2.4 lac cases die annually from TB[Q]
- About 124 per lac population new and relapse cases were notified.

Indices to Measure Tuberculosis (Epidemiological Indices)

a. Frequency of infection

Prevalence of infection (Tuberculin index)	*Incidence of infection (Annual infection rate or Tuberculin conversion index[Q] or Annual risk of infection)*
▪ Percentage of population infected with tuberculosis bacilli and shows positive reaction to tuberculin test ▪ About 40% in India[Q] ▪ Represents cumulative experience of population in recent as well as remote infection with TB[Q] ▪ Tuberculin test is the only way of estimating the prevalence of infection in a population[Q] ▪ Only limitation is false positive reaction by BCG vaccinated individuals	▪ Number of uninfected persons getting tuberculosis infection newly per 1,000 midyear population during a given year ▪ About 1–2% (~1.7%), i.e. 10–20 per 1,000 population ▪ Explains the attacking force of the disease and is the best and a sensitive indicator to evaluate the tuberculosis problem and its trend[Q] ▪ In developing countries, 1% ARI corresponds to 50 sputum smear +ve cases per 100,000 general population[Q] ▪ Most informative index of magnitude of problem of TB[Q]

b. Frequency of disease

Prevalence of disease (Case rate)	*Incidence of disease*
▪ Percentage of population suffering from tuberculosis (both old and new cases) and sputum is positive of tuberculosis bacilli on microscopic examination[Q] ▪ About 0.2% or 256 per 100,000 population (2011) ▪ Reflects the case load of tuberculosis in community ▪ Best available practical index to estimate case load in community[Q] ▪ Age specific prevalence is most relevant index	▪ Number of new cases of tuberculosis occurring in a given population during a given year per 1,000 midyear population ▪ About 1.7 per 1,000 population ▪ Reveals trend of problem including impact of control measures ▪ Is of utility only in countries where high proportion of new cases are detected and notification is reliable ▪ Sputum smear examination for AFB is a reliable method for estimation[Q]

d. Prevalence of drug resistant cases
   - It is the percentage of tuberculosis resistant to routine antituberculosis drugs
   - It is directly related to chemotherapy
e. Tuberculosis mortality rate
   - It is the number of deaths due to tuberculosis per 1,000 midyear population
   - It is about 26 per 1 lakh population every year in India
   - Was earlier used as an index of magnitude of TB problem.

Natural History of Tuberculosis

Pre-pathogenesis phase (Epidemiology)	
a. Agent factors	
i. Agent	▪ Tuberculosis is caused by Mycobacterial group of bacilli namely – *Mycobacterium* tuberculosis var hominis—affecting humans and accounts most cases – *Mycobacterium bovis*—affecting mainly cattle but also humans through milk – Atypical mycobacteria, namely photochromogens, scotochromogens, non-photochromogens and rapid growers—causing opportunistic infections ▪ Mycobacteria are both acid fast and alcohol fast and stain readily with Ziehl Neelsen (ZN) stain ▪ It is a facultative intracellular parasite, i.e. it is readily ingested by phagocytes and is resistant to intracellular killing ▪ Remains single, both extracellularly and intracellularly ▪ Infectivity of the bacilli is very high but pathogenicity is low
ii. Reservoir of infection	▪ Sputum positive case of tuberculosis acts as the reservoir of infection
iii. Infective material	▪ Sputum of tuberculosis patient is infective
iv. Period of infectivity	▪ Period of infectivity is determined by the sputum positivity of the tuberculosis cases
v. Period of communicability	▪ As long as not treated ▪ Every TB sputum positive case can infect up to 10–15 people per year[Q]
b. Host factors	
i. Age	▪ Occurs in all age groups but a shows small peak in early childhood, extensive peak in adolescence and a moderate peak in old age
ii. Sex	▪ More preponderance in males but death rate is more in females
iii. Heredity	▪ Not a hereditary disease but susceptibility is inherited in some families due to common environment
iv. Nutrition	▪ Malnutrition is a risk factor ▪ Degree of malnutrition is proportional to the severity of disease
v. Socioeconomic factors	▪ Poverty, illiteracy, ignorance, poor standard of living, over crowding, etc.
vi. Immunity	▪ No inherited immunity but can be acquired through active immunization with BCG vaccine or infection
c. Mode of transmission	▪ Infected droplet method (direct and major mode) ▪ Infected dust (Indirect) ▪ Drinking of unpasteurized raw milk of infected cattle—causes intestinal bovine tuberculosis ▪ Congenital transmission (possible but extremely rare)
Pathogenesis phase	
a. Incubation period	▪ Varies from several weeks to several months
b. Pathogenesis	
i. Primary complex	▪ After entering the body through the respiratory route, the bacilli traverse through small bronchioles to lodge in subpleural part of lower 2/3rd of the right lung (because of best ventilation and greatest exposure to contaminated inspired air) ▪ After multiplication, the bacilli reach regional (hilar and mediastinal) lymph nodes and multiply there too forming tubercles ▪ Meanwhile, cell-mediated immunity develops against the pathogen resulting in reduction in bacilli multiplication and caseous necrosis of the tubercles ▪ The disease is asymptomatic or minimally symptomatic ▪ The infection resolves by either or combination of resolution, fibrosis or calcification within 1–2 months

Contd...

Contd...

ii. Post-primary or disseminated tuberculosis	▪ In 1–5% cases with impaired immunity, the bacilli disseminate from the primary focus to the apical portion of right lung as it provides favorable environment for growth of bacterial like poor ventilation, rich oxygen concentration and poor blood supply (Pulmonary tuberculosis) ▪ It also spreads to other parts of the body such as meninges, bones, joints, intestines, kidney, etc. (Extra-pulmonary tuberculosis)
c. Clinical features	▪ Gradual onset of low grade fever, associated with evening rise of temperature and subsides at night with sweating ▪ Malaise, headache, loss of appetite, loss of weight ▪ Progressive cough associated with expectoration producing yellowish, copious, viscid and foul smelling sputum especially in morning ▪ Exertional and progressive breathlessness ▪ Hemoptysis in severe cases

Diagnosis

a. Sputum examination
   - Best criteria to diagnose tuberculosis according to WHO[Q]
     i. Direct smear microscopic examination for acid fast bacilli by ZN staining
       - Simple, cheap, easy, reliable, confirmative and practical diagnostic test
       - Helps to identify infectious cases[Q]
       - First line of investigation and considered gold standard test in adult tuberculosis[Q]
       - Sputum should contain 10^4 bacilli for detection[Q]
       - Method of choice as a case finding tool[Q]
     ii. Concentration method
       - Concentration of sputum by centrifusion and examination of sediment for acid fast bacilli by direct microscopy
       - Indicated in clinically suspected cases with negative smear in 2–3 slides
     iii. Culture test
       - Sputum can also culture for acid fast bacilli
       - Not done routinely because requires about 6 weeks for growth of mycobacteria
       - Instead of diagnosis, carried out for sensitivity testing and monitoring drug treatment
       - Offered as centralized service at district and regional chest clinic laboratories
       - Only meant for chest symptomatic who are smear negative

b. X-ray of the chest
   - Only a complimentary test, not done routinely because of:
     - Cost
     - Low yield
     - Compulsory sputum examination even in X-ray positive cases
     - Other disease resembling tuberculosis

c. Tuberculin test (Mantoux test or PPD test)
   - An intradermal, hypersensitivity test to know TB infection status of an individual
   - Discovered by Von Pirquet (1907)
   - It is a test of prognostic significance

   Principle
   - Detects the delayed hypersensitivity to tuberculin protein

   Test material
   - PPD-S (Purified protein derivative–standardized) which is purified and standardized tuberculin, a protein derived from RT-23 strain of tuberculosis bacilli (WHO)

   Test dose
   - 1 tuberculin unit (TU) of PPD-S containing 0.00002 mgm of tuberculin antigen (used in suspected cases of extreme hypersensitivity[Q])
   - 10 or 100 TU when 5 TU test is negative

Procedure

– 0.1 mL of 1TU of PPD is administered intradermally[Q] with help of tuberculin syringe on the flexor aspect of forearm to raise a wheal of 8 mm in diameter

Observation

– Results are read after 48–72 hours[Q] which consists of a hypersensitivity reaction characterized by an erythema and induration
– Induration is measured for interpretation[Q] and erythema is not considered[Q] while measuring
– Horizontal transverse diameter[Q] of induration is measured at its widest point

Interpretation

Diameter of induration	*Interpretation*	*Indicates*
▪ 10 mm or more	Positive	Infection either in past or present
▪ 5 mm or less[Q]	Negative	No infection with tuberculosis bacilli thus at a greater risk of infection[Q]
▪ 6–9 mm	Nonspecific or doubtful (equivocal)	Present or past infection with tubercle bacilli or atypical mycobacteria

– A positive tuberculin test indicates hypersensitivity to tuberculoprotein denoting infection with tubercle bacillus or BCG immunization, recent or past with or without clinical disease[Q]
– The test becomes positive 4–6 weeks after infection or immunization and gradually wanes and disappears by 4–5 years.
– Persons who had no contact with the bacilli are tuberculin negative.

False positive tests[Q]	*False negative tests*[Q] *(anergy)*	*Limitations*
▪ Infections with atypical mycobacteria[Q]. ▪ Faulty injection technique ▪ Using degraded tuberculin ▪ Too deep injection ▪ Repeated tuberculin testing ▪ Prior BCG vaccination[Q]	▪ Miliary tuberculosis ▪ Convalesce from some viral infections like measles ▪ Lymphoreticular malignancy ▪ Sarcoidosis ▪ Severe malnutrition ▪ Immunosuppressive therapy ▪ Impaired cell-mediated immunity ▪ Inactive PPD preparations ▪ Improper injection technique ▪ HIV/AIDS[Q] ▪ Whooping cough	▪ Significant only in children below 2 years ▪ Positive test among BCG vaccinated ▪ Negative in dissociative tuberculosis[Q] ▪ Limited validity due to lack of specificity

Significance

– Most appropriate test and only method to assess prevalence of tuberculosis in a community[Q]
– However, it lost its sensitivity as an indicator of true prevalence of infection in countries with high coverage of BCG[Q]

d. Erythrocyte sedimentation rate (ESR)
   – It is a nonspecific test and carries only prognostic importance.

Prevention and Control

• According to WHO tuberculosis is said to be under control when the prevalence of infection among children below 14 years is reduced to less than 1%

a. Elimination of reservoir
   i. Early diagnosis
      - If detected early tuberculosis cases can be easily treated and made noninfectious thus preventing further spread of disease
      - It done by clinical and microbiological diagnosis of the tuberculosis cases
      - Cardinal features of tuberculosis
        ❖ Productive cough for more than 3 weeks

Flowchart 1: Tuberculosis-diagnostic algorithm (RNTCP)

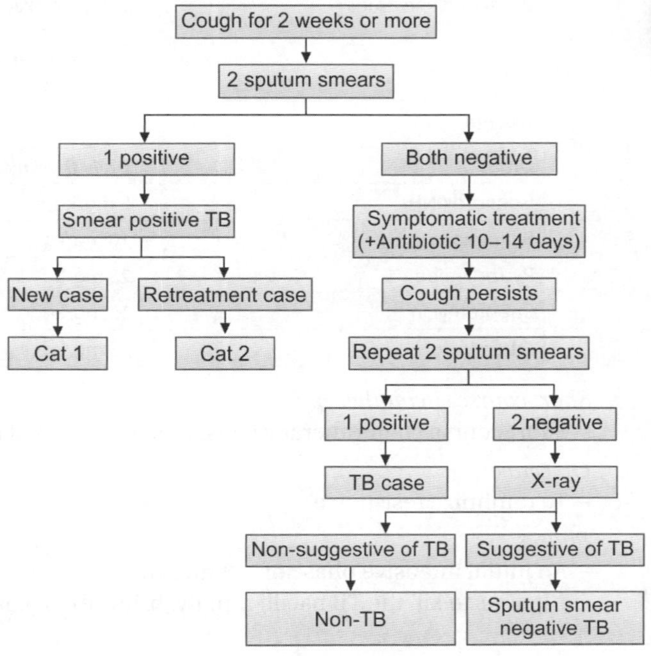

- Intermittent fever
- Loss of appetite
- Loss of weight
- Chest pain
- Hemoptysis
- Diagnostic confirmation
  - Direct sputum microscopy[Q]
  - Chest X-ray

ii. Treatment
- Achieved through multidrug short course chemotherapy and is the only effective means of tuberculos s in community

Objectives
- To make the infectious cases noninfectious rapidly[Q]
- To make lesions sterile quickly and completely
- To prevent development of complications like resistance[Q] and relapse[Q]
- To prevent further spread of disease in community
- To prevent death due to tuberculosis

Principles
- Choose drugs to which bacteria are susceptible
- Start the treatment with a combination of 3–4 drugs to simultaneously attack all groups of bacteria, i.e. persisters, intracellular, extracellular, rapid growers, slow multipliers, etc.
- Give complete and regular treatment
- Give all drugs before breakfast in single dose for better absorption
- Prefer single dose to ensure peak concentration for a longer period

Drugs used

	Bacteriocidal[Q]	*Bacteriostatic*[Q]
▪ First line drugs	▪ Isoniazide (INH) ▪ Rifampicin ▪ Pyrazinamide ▪ Streptomycin	▪ Ethambutol
▪ Second line drugs	▪ Ciprofloxacin ▪ Ofloxacin ▪ Kanamycin	▪ Thiacetazone ▪ Cycloserine ▪ Para-amino salicylate sodium ▪ Ethionamide

Dosage

Drugs	*Daily therapy*[Q]	*Thrice weekly therapy*[Q]
Isoniazid (INH)	5 mg/kg	10–15 mg/kg
Rifampicin	10 mg/kg	10 mg/kg
Pyrizinamide	25 mg/kg	35 mg/kg
Streptomycin	15 mg/kg	15 mg/kg
Ethambutol	15 mg/kg	30 mg/kg

Short course chemotherapy
– Short course chemotherapy consists of regimens of 6–9 months duration.

Objective
– To minimize resistance[Q]

Phases
– An initial intensive phase of 2–3 months.
  - It aims to kill the TB bacilli rapidly, bring about sputum conversion and afford symptomatic relief.

Revised Scheme 2

– A continuation phase of 4–6 months
  - It aims of eliminate all the remaining bacilli to prevent relapses.

Categories

– Treatment of tuberculosis is categorized into three categories by:

- Site of disease	Either pulmonary or extrapulmonary
- Severity of disease	Bacillary load and acute threat to life or permanent handicap
- Sputum smear positivity/negativity	Positive cases are infectious and have higher mortality
- History of previous treatment	Irregularly treated patients have risk of drug resistance

Flowchart 2: Tuberculosis—categorization of patients (RNTCP)

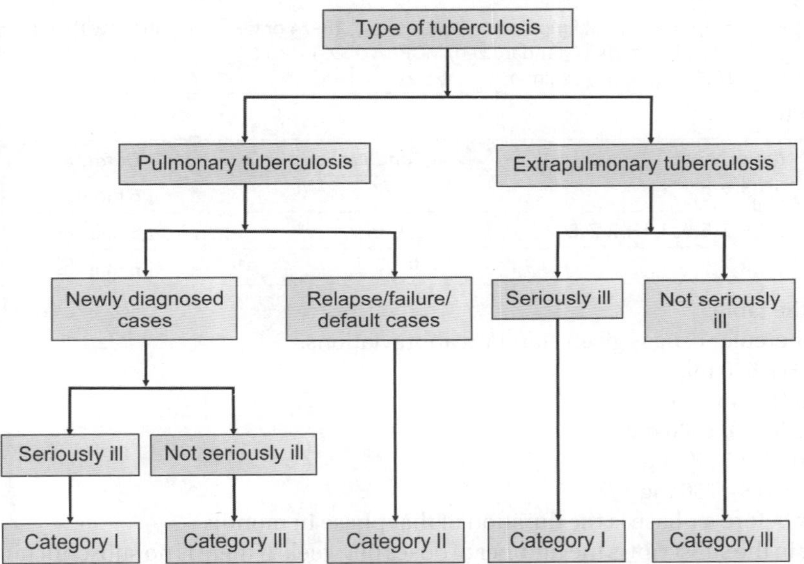

Categories	*Includes*
Category I	▪ New smear positive pulmonary tuberculosis ▪ Seriously ill smear negative pulmonary tuberculosis with extensive parenchymal involvement ▪ Seriously ill cases of extrapulmonary tuberculosis like meningitis, miliary, pericarditis, peritonitis, bilateral or extensive pleural effusion, spinal, intestinal, genitourinary tuberculosis[Q]
Category II	▪ Patients who remain or again become smear positive 5 months or later after commencing treatment[Q] (Treatment failure) ▪ Patients who were smear negative at start of therapy and becomes smear positive after the 2nd month (treatment failure) ▪ Patient declared cured form any from of tuberculosis in the past after receiving on full course of chemotherapy and now has become sputum positive (Relapse) ▪ Patients who interrupt treatment for 2 months or more and returns sputum positive or clinically active tuberculosis (Defaulters)
Category III[Q]	▪ New cases of smear negative pulmonary tuberculosis with limited parenchymal involvement[Q] ▪ New cases of less severe forms of extrapulmonary tuberculosis like lymph node, unilateral pleural effusion, bone (excluding spine), peripheral joint or skin tuberculosis[Q].

Treatment regimens
- There are two treatment regimens sharing the common criteria classification which are:
  - WHO recommended regimes prescribed in 1997
  - Revised National Tuberculosis Control Program of the India recommended and followed in India.

WHO regimen [Treatment of tuberculosis: Guidelines, 4th Edition (2010) WHO Geneva]

Category	*Initial phase*	*Continuation phase*	*Duration*	*Comments*
I[Q]	2HRZE[Q]	4HR	6 months[Q]	Optimal
New	2HRZE	$4H_3R_3$	6 months	Acceptable if DOT ensured
Patient	$2H_3R_3Z_3E_3$	$4H_3R_3$	6 months	Acceptable if DOT ensure, and no HIV coinfection or its risk
II Previously treated patients pending	2HRZES + 1HRZE	5HRE	8 months	For patients with low/medium risk of MDR-TB
Drug sensitivity test result	Empirical (standardized) MDR regimen	Empirical (standardized) MDR regimen	18–24 or till DST result	For patient with high-risk of MDR-TB

RNTCP regimens

Category	*Initial phase*	*Continuation phase*	*Duration*
I	$2H_3R_3Z_3E_3$	$4H_3R_3$	6 months
II	$2H_3R_3Z_3E_3S_3 + 1H_3R_3Z_3E_3$	$5H_3R_3E_3$	8 months
III	$2H_3R_3Z_3$	$4H_3R_3$	6 months

(How to read the table:
- Each anti tubercular drug is given standard abbreviations.
  - Isoniazid (H): 600 mg
  - Rifampicin (R): 450 mg
  - Pyrizinamide (Z): 1500 mg
  - Ethambutol (E): 1200 mg
  - Streptomycin (S): 750 mg
- The number before a phase is the duration of that phase in months
- The number in the subscript is the number of doses per week. If there is no subscript number the drug is given daily)

b. Breaking the chain of transmission
- Done by concurrent disinfection of sputum collected in sputum cup half filled with 5% cresol or 8% bleaching powder or burning or disposing off paper towels used to receive sputum
- Belonging of the patient during the hospital stay are also disinfected
- Patient is advised to avoid indiscriminate spitting of sputum

c. Protection susceptible
  i. General measures
  - Health promotion
    - Improvement in general health of the individual to improve resisting power
    - Improvement in living conditions with good lightening and ventilation, personal hygiene, good food, adequate nutrition, exercise, etc.
  - Health education
    - Health education of community about the mode of transmission of the disease, its hazards and availability of drugs to cure it completely
    - Educate the mothers about importance of BCG vaccination
    - Motivate the tuberculosis patients and defaulters to take treatment regularly and continuously

  ii. Specific measures
  - Achieved by vaccination with BCG vaccine which is usually done at birth but up to 6 weeks
  - Chemoprophylaxis (children <6 years) who come in contact with sputum positive TB case

IF	AND	THEN	
Symptoms of TB	Clinician declare TB	Category I DOTS given	
No symptoms of TB	Tuberculin test not available	INH 5mg/kg for 6 months	
	Tuberculin test	INH 5 mg/kg for 3 months and then do the test	If induration <6 mm = stop INH, give BCG
			If induration >6 mm = continue INH for 3 more months

Significance

- Tuberculosis is not only a public health problem but also a social and an economic problem hence its prevention and control is of immense value
- WHO declared TB as Global Emergency in 1983[Q].

2. What are various methods of treatment and disposal technologies for health-care waste?

- Biomedical waste or health-care waste means any waste which generated during diagnosis, treatment or immunization of human beings or animals or in research activities pertaining thereto or in production or testing of biological and including categories as mentioned in schedule I. [Biomedical Waste (Management and Handling) Rules, 2015]

Composition of Hospital Waste[Q]

Paper[Q]	15%
Plastic[Q]	10%
Rags	15%
Metals (sharp[Q]), etc.	1%
Infectious waste	1.5%
Glass[Q]	4%
General waste[Q] (food waste, sweeping of premises)	53.5%

Categories of Biomedical Waste

Type of waste	*Component*	*Treatment and disposal*	*Container*
Yellow			
a. Human anatomical waste (1)	Human tissue, organs, body parts	Incineration/plasma pyrolysis/ deep burial	Yellow non-chlorinated plastic bags
b. Animal anatomical waste (2)	Animal tissues, organs, body parts, carcasses, bleeding parts, fluids, blood and experimental animals used in research, waste generated by veterinary hospitals, colleges, discharge from hospital, animal house	Incineration/plasma pyrolysis/ deep burial	Yellow non-chlorinated plastic bags
c. Soiled waste (6)	Items contaminated with blood and fluids including cotton, dressing, soiled plaster casts, linen, beddings, other material contaminated with blood	Incineration/plasma pyrolysis/ deep burial or Autoclaving/ microwaving/hydroclaving then Shredding/mutilation	
d. Discarded medicine and cytotoxic drugs (5)	Wastes comprising of outdated, contaminated and discarded medicines	Incineration/encapsulation/ plasma pyrolysis (>1200°C)	Yellow non-chlorinated plastic bags or Containers
e. Chemical waste (10)	Used in production of biologicals, for disinfections, etc.	Incineration/encapsulation/ plasma pyrolysis	Yellow non-chlorinated plastic bags or Containers
f. Chemical liquid waste (8)	Waste generated from laboratory and washing, cleaning, housekeeping and disinfecting activities	Disinfection by chemical treatment and discharge into drains	Separate collection system leading to effluent treatment system

Contd...

g. Beddings	Discarded linen, mattresses, beddings contaminated with blood or body fluids	Non-chlorinated chemical disinfection then Incineration/ plasma pyrolysis/ energy recovery or Shredding	Yellow non-chlorinated plastic bags or suitable packing material
h. Microbiology and biotechnology waste (3)	Waste from laboratory culture, stocks or specimens of microorganisms, live or attenuated vaccines, human and animal cell culture used in research and infectious agents from research and industrial laboratories, waste from production of biologicals, toxins, dishes and devices and for transfer of cultures	Pretreatment with non-chlorinated chemicals then Incineration	Disinfected plastic bag/conta ner
Red			
a. Contaminated recyclable waste (7)	Waste generated from disposable items other than waste sharps like tubing, catheters, IVs, etc.	Autoclaving/microwaving/ hydroclaving then Shredding/mutilation then Energy recovery/plastics to diesel or fuel oil/ road making	Red non-chlorinated plastic bags or containers
White (Translucent)			
a. Waste sharps^{Q} including metals (4)	Both used and unused needles, syringes, scalpels, blades, etc.	Autoclaving/dry heat Shredding/mutilation/ encapsulation then Iron foundries/sanitary landfills/ waste sharp pit	Puncture proof, leak proof, tamper proof containers
Blue			
a. Glassware (4) b. Metallic body implants		Sodium hypochlorite/ autoclaving/microwaving/ hydroclaving then Recycling	Cardboard box with blue colored marking

Treatment and Disposal Technologies for Health-care Waste

a. Incineration (mass burn technology)
   - Incineration is a high temperature dry oxidation processQ that reduces organic and combustible waste to inorganic matter thus converting waste into bottom ash and fly ash
   - Most widely used method
   - Significantly reduces waste volume and weight (by about 85–95%)
   - Offers direct disposal technology with zero occupational hazard
   - No chemical pretreatment is necessaryQ
   - Generation of smoke is biggest disadvantage.Q

Working of incinerator

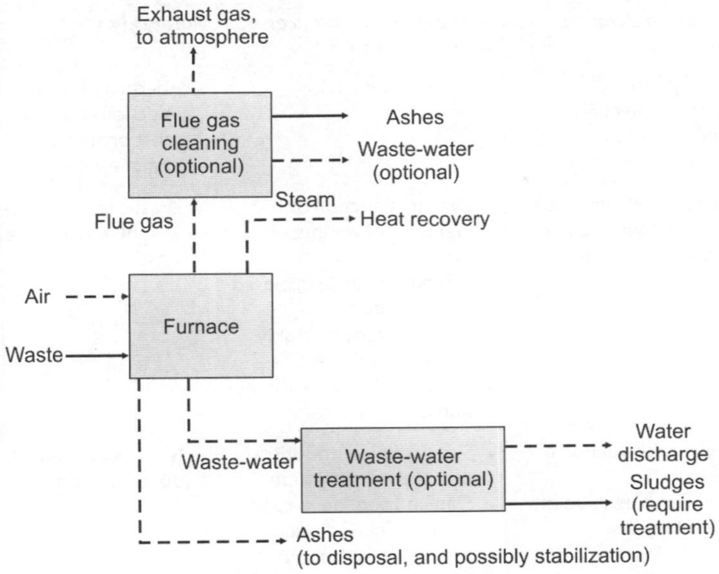

Fig. 1: Incinerator–working

Characteristic of ideal waste[Q]	*Application (used for)*	*Not suitable for*[Q]
▪ Low heating volume – >2000 Kcal/kg for single chamber incinerator – >3500 Kcal/kg for double chamber incinerator ▪ Combustible matter content >60% ▪ Noncombustible solid content <5% ▪ Noncombustible fines content <20% ▪ Moisture content <30%	▪ Waste that cannot be recycled, reused or disposed-off in a land fill	▪ Pressured gas containers ▪ Large amount of reactive chemical wastes ▪ Silver salts and photographic or radiographic wastes ▪ Haloganated plastics like PVC ▪ High mercury or cadmium containing wastes like broken thermometers, used batteries, lead lined wooden panels ▪ Sealed ampules or ampules containing heavy metals ▪ Sharps ▪ Cytotoxic drugs

Types

	Double chamber pyrolytic incinerator	*Single chamber furnaces with static grate*	*Rotary kilns*	*Drum or brick incinerator*
Features	▪ Especially designed to burn infectious health care waste ▪ Has pollution control device and also called controlled air incineration	▪ Preferred if double chambers are unaffordable ▪ Good to incinerate infectious waste including sharps, pathological waste and general health care waste	▪ Capable of causing decomposition of genotoxic substances and heat resistant chemicals at high temp ▪ Specifically used for chemical waste like infectious waste and pathological waste	
Temp range	800° ± 50°C in primary chamber[Q] & 1050° ± 50°C in secondary chamber[Q]	300–400°C	1200–1600°C	

	Double chamber pyrolytic incinerator	*Single chamber furnaces with static grate*	*Rotary kilns*	*Drum or brick incinerator*
Advantages	▪ Environment friendly ▪ Very high disinfection efficiency	▪ Good disinfection efficiency	▪ Adequate for all infectious waste and most pharmaceutical and chemical waste	
	▪ Adequate for all infectious waste, most chemical and pharmaceutical wastes	▪ Drastic reduction of weight and volume of weight ▪ Residues may be disposed off in landfills ▪ Does not require highly trained operatives' ▪ Relatively low investment and operative costs	▪ Drastic reduction of weight and volume of waste	▪ Very low investment and operative costs
Disadvantages	▪ Incomplete destruction of cytotoxics ▪ Relatively high investment and operating cost	▪ Significant contribution to atmospheric pollution ▪ Slag and soot need to be removed periodically ▪ Inefficient to destroy thermally resistant chemicals and drugs	▪ High investment and operative cost	▪ Only 99% microorganisms destroyed ▪ Inefficient destruction of many chemicals and pharmaceuticals ▪ Massive emission of smoke, ash, toxic gases and odors

b.. Chemical disinfection
- Consists of addition of chemicals to kill or inactivate pathogens
- Preferred method is treatment with 1% hypochlorite solution[Q]
- Commonly used chemicals include bleaching powder, glutaraldehyde, alcohols or quaternary ammonia compounds, etc.

Application (Used for)	*Advantages*	*Disadvantages*
▪ Treating liquid wastes like blood, urine, stools or hospital sewage ▪ Solid wastes like microbiological cultures, sharps, etc. (with certain limitations)	▪ Highly efficient under good operating conditions ▪ Requires highly trained technician	▪ Relatively inexpensive ▪ Requires comprehensive safety measures while using hazardous chemicals ▪ Inadequate for pharmaceutical, chemical and some type of infectious waste

c. Dry and wet thermal treatment (steam disinfection)
- Consists of non-burn, dry thermal disinfection by shredding of waste in heating it in rotating auger (screw feeding technology) which is followed exposure of shredded infectious waste to high pressure steam (15–51 psi) at high temperature (121–149°C[Q]) for considerable time (30–60 min) (autoclaving)

Application (Used for)	*Not suitable for*	*Advantages*	*Disadvantages*
▪ Infectious wastes and sharps	▪ Pathological, cytotoxic or radioactive wastes	▪ Environmentally sound ▪ Relatively low investment and operative cost	▪ Requires shredders which is subjected to frequent breakdown and poor functioning ▪ Requires qualified technician ▪ Inadequate for anatomical, pharmaceutical, chemical wastes and waste that is not readily steam permeable

d. Microwave irradiation
- Consists of heating water content of waste using microwaves of 12.24 nm at frequency of 2450 MHz[Q]

Advantages	Disadvantages
▪ Environment friendly ▪ Good disinfection efficiency under appropriate operating conditions ▪ Drastic reduction in waste volume (30–40%) ▪ Minimal occupational risk ▪ Cost effective ▪ Compact equipment ▪ Operation and maintenance problems ▪ Require routine efficiency checking through bacteriological and virological tests	▪ Relatively high investment and operative costs ▪ Operation and maintenance problems ▪ Require routine efficiency checking through bacteriological and virological tests ▪ Relatively high investment and operative costs

e. Land disposal (oldest method of waste disposal[Q])
   – Considered an acceptable disposal route if municipality or medical authority lacks means to treat waste before disposal.

   Types

Open dumps	Sanitary landfills
▪ Carries risk of people or animals coming in contact with infectious waste	▪ Geologically isolates wastes from environment ▪ Site is prepared with appropriate engineering to accept waste, i.e. has base is made impermeable using clay and pebbles with a grading to create leachate collection ▪ Operations are controlled by staff ▪ Deposition is organized and covered daily with earth and hay ▪ All bags completely pushed into landfill without getting opened up ▪ Area is sprayed with insecticides frequently

Advantages	Disadvantages
▪ Inexpensive ▪ Safe if access is restricted and natural infiltration is limited	▪ Potential risk of people or animals coming in contact with infectious waste

f. Inertization
   – Consists of mixing of cement and other substances with biomedical waste before disposal[Q] to minimize risk of migration of toxic substances in waste into surface or ground water.

Contents of mixture	Application (Used for)	Advantages	Disadvantages
▪ 65% pharmaceutical waste ▪ 15% lime[Q] ▪ 15% cement[Q] ▪ 5% water	▪ Pharmaceuticals and for incineration ashes with high metal content	▪ Inexpensive	▪ Not suitable for infectious waste

g. Hydroclave
   – Advanced autoclave method for treating infectious waste, using stream with much faster and more even heat penetration
   – Consists of steam sterilization under pressure at 121°C or 132°C causing fragmentation of waste[Q].

Application (Used for)	Not suitable for	Advantages
▪ Infectious waste, both liquid and solid	▪ Anatomical and cytotoxic waste	▪ Totally sterilizes waste ▪ Treats all infectious waste, including bulk liquid and pathological ▪ Volume reduction by 70% ▪ No harmful emissions ▪ Very low operating cost ▪ No loss steam (which returns back to boiler in form of clean, hot water to be reused)

Significance

- Biomedical waste is a unaccounted environmental pollutant which need to be controlled and disposed of safely considering potential harm to mankind

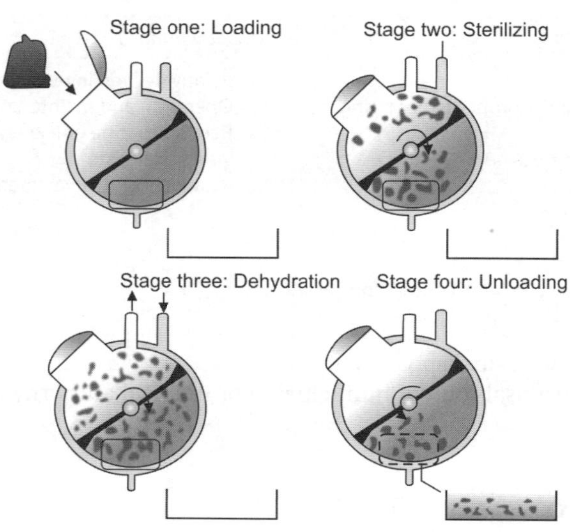

Fig. 2: Hydroclave (Treatment process)

- Biomedical waste management (Ministry of Health) provide regulatory framework for environmental management in health sector.

SHORT ESSAYS

3. Primary prevention of amoebiasis.

- Amoebiasis is condition of harboring protozoan parasite *Entamoeba histolytica* with or without clinical manifestations.

Primary Prevention

Objective

- Aimed at breaking chain of transmission by preventing contamination of water, food, vegetables and fruits with human feces.

Measures

a. Sanitation	▪ Proper sanitation measures like safe disposal of human excreta (sanitary barrier) ▪ Control of houseflies by keeping premises clean inside and around house ▪ Elementary sanitary practices likes washing hands after defecation and before eating, etc.
b. Water supply	▪ Preventing fecal contamination of water supplies (amoebic cysts survive for days and weeks in water) ▪ Filtration of drinking water using sand filters is effective method of removing amoebic cysts ▪ Regular chlorination does not kill amoebic cysts ▪ At domestic level, boiling of water should be carried out to prevent infection
c. Food hygiene	▪ Protection of food and drinks against fecal contamination ▪ Disinfection of uncooked vegetables and fruits with 5% acetic acid or full strength vinegar before consumption ▪ Periodic examination of food handlers and their treatment to prevent spread of infection
d. Health education	▪ Health education of community in regards to mode of spread of infection, preventive measures like boiling of water, sanitary practices, etc. go a long way in preventing amoebiasis ▪ Food handlers should be explained about their role in transmission of infection, early features of disease and sanitary practices to avoid spread of disease

Significance

- Amoebiasis is very common feco-oral disease with lots of public health importance considering its ability to cause extraintestinal infections but can be prevented by simple measures like healthy sanitary practices.

4. List out the indicators of MCH care.

- Various mortality and morbidity data is used as an indicator for quality of maternal and child health (MCH) care provided.

Indicator of MCH Care

Classification	*Magnitude of problem in India*
a. Maternal mortality i. Maternal mortality rate[Q]	212 per 100,000 live births[Q] (2012)
b. Mortality during infancy i. Perinatal mortality rate ii. Neonatal mortality rate iii. Postneonatal mortality rate iv. Infant mortality rate	 32 per 1,000 live births (2010) 29 per 1,000 live births (2012) 23 per 1,000 live births (2003) 42 per 1,000 live births[Q] (2013)
c. Mortality during childhood i. 1–4 years mortality rate ii. Under 5 mortality rate iii. Child survival rate	 5.1% of total deaths (2006) 59 per 1,000 live births (2012) 92.8% (2007)

a. Maternal mortality rate (MMR)
   - Maternal mortality or maternal death is defined as the death of a woman while pregnant or within 42 days of termination of pregnancy irrespective of the duration and site of pregnancy from any cause related to or aggravated by the pregnancy or its management but not from accidental or incidental causes.

$$\text{MMR} = \frac{\text{Total no. of female death due to complications of pregnancy childbirth or within 42 days of delivery from puerperal causes in an area during a given year}}{\text{Total no. of live births in the same area during the same year}^{Q}} \times 100{,}000$$

b. Perinatal mortality rate (PMR)
   - Number of deaths of newborn occurring during perinatal period, i.e. late fetal deaths (28 weeks of gestation) and early neonatal deaths (till 7 days after full-term)

$$\text{PMR} = \frac{\text{Late fetal deaths (28 weeks of gestation and more) + early neonatal deaths (first week) in one year}}{\text{Live births in the same year}} \times 1{,}000$$

   - Another formulae suggested by WHO expert committee for international comparison is

$$\text{PMR} = \frac{\text{Late fetal deaths (28 weeks of gestation and more) + early neonatal deaths (first week) weighing over 1,000 g at birth in one year}}{\text{Total live births weighing over 1,000 g in the same year}} \times 1{,}000$$

c. Neonatal mortality rate (NNMR)
   - Number of deaths of newborn occurring within 28 days after birth per 1,000 live births during a given year, in a given area[Q]

$$\text{NNMR} = \frac{\text{No. of deaths of newborn within first 28 days of birth in a year}^{Q}}{\text{Live births in the same year}} \times 1{,}000$$

d. Postneonatal mortality rate (PNNMR)
   - Number of deaths of infants from 28 day of life till the end of one year per 1,000 live births during a given year, in a given area

$$\text{PNNMR} = \frac{\text{No. of deaths of children between 28 days and one year of age in a year}}{\text{Live births in the same year}} \times 1{,}000$$

e. Infant mortality rate (IMR)
   - Rate of deaths of children under 1 year of age per 1,000 live births during a given year, in a given area

$$\text{IMR} = \frac{\text{No. of deaths of infants (children under 1 year of age) in a year}}{\text{Live births in the same year}} \times 1{,}000$$

f. 1–4 year mortality rate (Child death rate)
   – Number of deaths of children aged between 1–4 years per 1,000 children in the same age group in a given year, in a given area

$$\text{1–4 years mortality rate} = \frac{\text{No. of deaths of children between 1–4 years of age in a year}}{\text{Midyear population of children between 1–4 years of age}} \times 1{,}000$$

g. Under 5 mortality rate (Child mortality rate)
   – Number of deaths of children below age of 5 years per 1,000 live births in a year, in a given area

$$\text{CMR} = \frac{\text{No. of deaths of children under 5 years of age in a year}}{\text{Live births in the same year}} \times 1{,}000$$

h. Child survival index (Child survival rate)
   – Percentage of children surviving up to the age of 5 years

$$\text{CSR} = \frac{\text{1,000 – under 5 mortality rate}}{10}$$

Significance

- MCH indicator serve a good parameter to compare the health care delivery model of a country with another as well as they are considered the mirror the health status of the community.

5. What are the aims and objectives of under-fives' clinic?

Refer Question No. 2 December 2010 (RS2) Paper II.

6. Prevention and control of hepatitis-B.

Refer Question No. 1 December 2014 (RS2) Paper II.

7. Differential diagnosis of cholera and food poisoning.

- Food poisoning can be mistaken for cholera.

Differential Diagnosis of Cholera and Food Poisoning

Points of difference	*Cholera*	*Food poisoning*
a. Epidemiology		
– Occurrence	Occurs often in epidemic form associated with other cases in neighborhood	Often a single group of person who shared a common meal
– Secondary cases	Occurs	Does not occur
– Incubation	Few hours to 5 days	1–24 hours
b. Symptoms		
– Onset	With purging	With vomiting
– Nausea and retching	None	Present
– Vomiting	▪ Projectile, effortless and continuous ▪ Follows diarrhea	▪ Often single, violent and distressing ▪ Precedes diarrhea
– Vomitus	Watery	Mucus and blood streaked, never watery
– Stools	Copious rice watery, inoffensive	Frequent, may contain mucus and blood, offensive
– Tenesmus	None	Yes

Contd...

Contd...

Points of difference	*Cholera*	*Food poisoning*
– Muscular cramps	Constant and severe	Less constant
– Headache	None	Often
c. On examination		
– Abdominal tenderness	None	Yes
– Dehydration	Very marked	Distinct
– Surface temperature	Subnormal	Often upto 100–120°F
d. Laboratory investigations		
– Blood pH	Acidic	Alkaline
– Urine	Suppressed	Seldom suppressed
– Blood	Leukocytosis	Normal

Significance

- Since cholera is a notifiable disease, it is important to distinguish food poisoning from cholera.

8. What are major epidemiological types of malaria in India?

- Malaria is a communicable disease caused by plasmodium species of protozoa, transmitted from person-to-person by bite of infected female Anopheles mosquito.

Epidemiological Types of Malaria in India

Urban malaria	*Rural malaria*	*Project malaria (Industrial malaria)*	*Border malaria*	*Tribal malaria*
▪ Characterized by low endemicity, predominant *P. vivax* and focal transmission of *P. faciparum* and Anophelin culicifacies[Q] as main vector ▪ Account for 80% of cases reported under urban malaria scheme come from 15 cities including four metros	▪ Characterized by moderate to low endemicity, *P. vivax* in lean period and *P. falciparum* during periodic exacerbation and Anophelin culicfacies[Q] and Anophelin stephensi[Q] as main vectors ▪ Complicated by major irrigation projects	▪ Characterized by disproportionately high incidence of malaria compared to population size ▪ Results due to disturbed eco system because of temporary or seasonal migration of persons	▪ Characterized by existence of high endemic belts along international and state borders ▪ Difficult to control due to mixing of population and poor administrative control	▪ 50% of total falciparum cases come from tribal population which accounts only 5–6% of entire population ▪ Infants, young children and pregnant women constitute high risk groups followed by mobile tribal population engaged in forest related activities ▪ Morbidity and mortality is high due to poor health infrastructure, lack of drugs and malnutrition

9. Anthropometric measurements in children.

Refer Question No. 2 June 2010 (RS2) Paper I.

10. List out the sources of health information.

Refer Question No. 5 June 2013 (RS2) Paper I.

11. Stages of demographic cycle.

- Trends of population growth in a country undergo changes or variations in a stepwise manner and these variations are called the stages of demographic cycle or transition cycle.

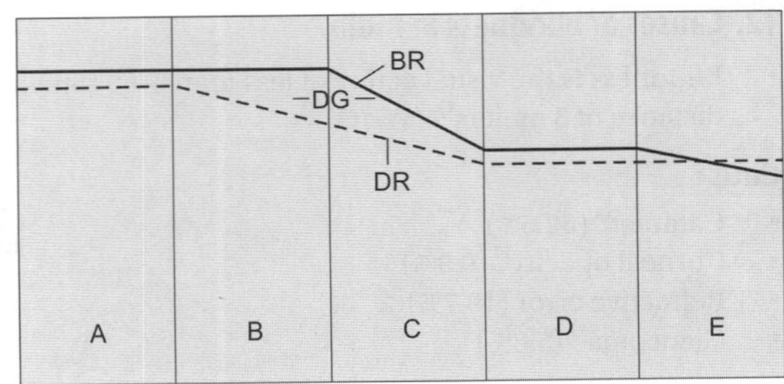

Fig. 3: Stages of demographic cycle

Stages

a. First stage (High stationary)
b. Second stage (Early expanding)

c. Third stage (Late expanding)
d. Forth stage (Low stationery)
e. Fifth stage (Stage of decline)

Stage	*Characteristics*	*Growth rate*	*Example*
a. First stage (High stationary)	▪ High birth rate and high death rate cancel each other ▪ Demographic gap is narrow ▪ Population remains stationary at high level ▪ Population composition is mostly young ▪ Age pyramid is pyramidal in shape	0.06%	India before 1920
b. Second stage (Early expanding)	▪ Death rate begins to decline and birth rate remains unchanged[Q] (high) ▪ Demographic gap starts increasing in early stage II and is maximum in late stage II[Q] ▪ Population grows slowly ▪ Population composition is mostly young ▪ Age pyramid is losing pyramidal shape	1.3%	India between 1921-30 Many countries in south Asia and Africa
c. Third stage[Q] (Late expanding[Q])	▪ Death rate decline further precipitously and birth rate starts declining[Q] ▪ Demographic gap starts declining in early stage III[Q] ▪ Population grows rapidly as birth rate exceeds death rate[Q] ▪ Population composition is mostly young ▪ Age pyramid is globular in shape	2%	India[Q], China, Singapore, Thailand, Korea, Philippines, Indonesia, Sri Lanka and some Latin American countries
d. Forth stage (Low stationery[Q])	▪ Birth rate falls rapidly and becomes equal to death rate ▪ Low birth rate and low death rate cancel each other ▪ Demographic gap is narrow ▪ Population remains stationary at low level ▪ Population composition is mixed ▪ Age pyramid is cylindrical in shape	0%	Australia, UK, Belgium, Denmark, Sweden in 1980s[Q]
e. Fifth stage (Stage of decline[Q])	▪ Death rate is higher than birth rate[Q] ▪ Demographic gap is in negative ▪ Population goes on declining[Q] ▪ Population composition is mostly aging ▪ Age pyramid is losing cylindrical shape	<0%	Germany and Hungary

Status of India

- India is late expanding stage of demographic cycle[Q]
- The crude death rate in India is declining rapidly from 16 (1970) to 8 (2007) where as crude birth rate has started slow decline from 38 (1970) to 23 (2007).

Significance

- Stages of demographic cycle occur sequentially and each stage lasts for several decades, thus it requires several centuries to undergo each cycle
- It is closely related to socioeconomic progress of a country.

12. Causes of blindness in India.

- Blindness is the visual acuity of less than 3/60 (Snellen)[Q] or its equivalent or inability to count fingers in daylight at distance of 3 meters[Q]. (WHO)

Causes

- Cataract[Q] (62.6%)
- Corneal opacity[Q] (0.9%)
- Refractive error (19.7%)
- Glaucoma[Q] (5.8%)

- Posterior segment pathology (4.7%)
- Others causes (6.2%)
  - – Retinopathy (diabetes, hypertension, prematurity)
  - – Retinal detachment
  - – Trachoma and associated infection
  - – Trauma
  - – Congenital disorders (rubella)
  - – Uveitis
  - – Tumors (retinoblastoma)
  - – Vitamin A deficiency.

Prevention and Control

a. Eye care
   i. Primary eye care
      - Targets the wide range of eye conditions like acute conjunctivitis, ophthalmia neonatarum trachoma superficial foreign bodies, xerophthalmia which can be treated or prevented at the grass root level
      - For this purpose local primary health workers are trained to identify these conditions and treat them. They are also trained to refer difficult cases such as corneal ulcers, penetrating foreign bodies painful eye conditions, etc. to the nearest PHC or district hospital
      - They are also supposed to promote personal hygiene, of the eye, good dietary habits rich in vitamin A and safety of eye
      - Besides training, they are provided essential drugs such as topical tetracyclines, vitamin A capsules, eye bandages shields, etc.
   ii. Secondary care
      - Comprises the definitive management of the common conditions like cataract, entropion, triachiasis, ocular trauma, glaucoma, etc. through PHCs and district hospitals
      - Besides PHCs and district hospitals, mobile eye clinics can also provide secondary care
      - PHC medical officer can also conduct eye camps in his area to provide specific protection and education making best use of local resources to provide inexpensive eye care to the population at the peripheral level
   iii. Tertiary care
      - Provides sophisticated eye care such as retinal detachment surgery, corneal grafting and other complex modes of management
      - These centers are located in the national or regional capitals and any case that cannot be handled by the PHC medical officer are transferred to these hospitals
b. Specific programs
   i. Trachoma control
      - Endemic trachoma and associated infections are a major cause of preventable blindness which can be cured by early diagnosis and treatment
      - Moreover, mass campaign with tropical tetracyclines and the improvement of socioeconomic conditions have reduced the severity of trachoma
   ii. School eye health services
      - School going children are screened and treated for refraction errors, squint ambylopia, trachoma, etc. as a part of school eye health services
      - They are also provided health education about good posture, proper lighting, avoidance of glare, proper distance and angle between the books and the eye and use of suitable type in textbook
   iii. Vitamin A prophylaxis
      - A child between age of 1– 6 years is administered 200,000 IV of vitamin A at ½ hourly interval to control xerophthalmia.
   iv. Occupational eye health services
      - Targets prevention or treatment of eye hazards in industries
      - Workers are educated about prevention of occupational eye hazards and use of protective devices
      - There should also be an attempt to improve the safety features of machines, proper illumination of the working area, pre-employment examination and encourage use of protective devices
c. Long-term measures
   - Aimed at improving the quality of life and modifying or attacking the factors responsibly for persistence of eye problems like poor sanitation lack of safe water supplies, diet poor in vitamin A, lack of personal hygiene
   - Health education is another measure to create community awareness, to motivate the community and to secure community participation
d. Rehabilitation
   - Provided to those who have become handicapped due to blindness in terms of physical, social, psychological and vocational
   - Comprises of providing specialized eye care (physical), removing social ostracism (social), psychological support (psychological) and training them for economically gainful employment (vocational)

Significance

- Early detection and prompt treatment of causes of preventable blindness can prevent loss of valuable vision in millions.

SHORT ANSWERS

13. Dynamics of typhoid fever transmission.

Refer Question No. 10 June 2010 (RS2) Paper II

14. What are the deformities occurring in the leprosy?

- Deformities are very common in leprosy and about 1/4th of patients who do not receive treatment at early stage develop deformities.

Pathogenesis

Due to disease process	*Resulting from paralysis of some muscles due to damage peripheral nerve trunk*	*Resulting from injuries and infections to hands and feet*
▪ Loss of eyebrows, other facial deformities	▪ Claw hand, foot drop, lagophthalmos	▪ Scar contracture of fingers, mutilation of hands and feet, corneal ulceration

Deformities

Face	*Nose*	*Ear*	*Eye*	*Hands*	*Feet*	*Others*
▪ Mask face ▪ Facies leonine ▪ Sagging face	▪ Perforated nose ▪ Depressed nose	▪ Deformities like nodules on ear ▪ Elongated lobule	▪ Lagophthalmos ▪ Loss of eye brow (superciliary madarosis) or eyelashes (ciliary madarosis) ▪ Corneal ulcers and opacities	▪ Claw hand ▪ Writ drop ▪ Ulcers ▪ Absorption of digits ▪ Thumb—web contracture ▪ Hallowing of interosseous spaces ▪ Swollen hand	▪ Plantar ulcers ▪ Foot drop ▪ Inversion of foot ▪ Clawing of toes ▪ Absorption of toes ▪ Collapsed foot ▪ Swollen foot ▪ Callosities	▪ Gynecomastia ▪ Perforation of palate

Classification

a. Hands and feet

Grade 0	No anesthesia and no visible deformity
Grade I	Anesthesia and but no visible deformity
Grade II	Visible deformity

b. Eyes

Grade 0	No eye problem, no evidence of loss of vision
Grade I	Eye problem due to leprosy but no loss of vision
Grade II	Severe visual impairment, lagophthalmos, iridocyclitis and corneal opacity

Significance

- Numerous deformities seen in a leprosy case is the main reason for the social ouster of a leprosy patient.

15. Disaster mitigation in health sector.

- Disaster mitigation involves measure designed either to prevent hazards or to lessen the likely effects of disaster.

Health Activities during Disaster Mitigation

i. Improving structural qualities of schools, houses and other building to minimize the number of medical casualty
ii. Ensuring safety of health facilities and public health services

iii. Improvement in water supply and sewage system
iv. Flood mitigation work
v. Appropriate land use planning
vi. Improved building codes
vii. Reduction or protection of population and structures
viii. Health education to disaster management teams and common man regarding first aid
ix. Vector control to prevent epidemics
x. Establishment of fully equipped health teams to handle casualties of disasters
xi. Linking of hospitals
xii. Provision of adequate supplies of essential drugs and other requirements.

16. Window period.

- Window period is the interval period between infection with HIV virus and appearance of antibodies in the serum
- This is the period where virus remains latent in the host cell for a short period of time during when no antibody can be detected in the blood.

Duration

- Usually 2–3 weeks but rarely longer than 6 months.

Significance

- The HIV infected person is most infectious in the window period when the diagnosis of HIV is not possible with standard antibody test thus he remains a potential source of infection to others and the transmission of infection cannot be controlled
- Though no antibodies can be detected in the blood, diagnosis of HIV infection in the window period can be done by detection of the virus in a small proportion of CD4 lymphocytes by DNA hybridization
- If report of a person highly suspected to have HIV comes negative for investigations, then the tests should be repeated after the 3 months.

17. Early neonatal care.

- Neonatal period is very crucial period in life of an newborn as newborn has to adapt itself rapidly and successfully to an alien external environment.

Early Neonatal Care

Objectives

- Provision of immediate and essential care of newborn
- Establishment and maintenance of cardiorespiratory functions
- Maintenance of body temperature
- Avoidance of infection
- Establishment of satisfactory feeding regimen
- Early detection and treatment of congenital and acquired disorders, especially infections.

Components

a. Clearing airway
   - Most important thing after birth of baby is establishment and maintenance of cardiorespiratory functions
   - To establish breathing, airways should be cleared of mucus and other secretions by positioning baby with his head low to help in drainage of secretions and application of gentle suction to remove mucus and amniotic fluid
   - If natural breathing fails, resuscitation measures like suction, application of oxygen masks, intubation and assisted respiration may be tried.

b. APGAR score
   - APGAR score is a scale designed to rate baby's survival chances based on important factors necessary for baby's survival

Sign	0	1	2
Heart rate	Absent	Below 100	Over 100
Respiratory effort	Absent	Slow, irregular	Good, crying
Muscle tone	Flaccid	Some flexion of extremities	Active movements
Reflex response	No response	Grimace	Cry
Color	Blue, pale	Body pink, extremities blue	Completely pink
Total score (10)	0–3 (severe depression)	4–7 (mild depression)	7–10 (no depression)

   - APGAR score is taken at 1 minutes and again at 5 minutes after birth
   - Score below 5 needs prompt action
   - Infants with APGAR score below 5 at 5 minutes after birth are at high-risk of complications and death during neonatal period.

c. Care of cord
   - Cord should be cut only after it has stopped pulsating thus permitting flow of about 10 mL of blood from mother to child
   - It should be cut with clean, sterile instrument to prevent neonatal tetanus
   - It should be tied with clean suture and antiseptic should be applied on cord stump and skin around base
   - It should be kept dry so that is shrivels up and separates by aseptic necrosis in 5–8 days.

d. Care of eyes
   - Lid margins of newborn should be cleaned with sterile wet swabs, one for each eye from medial to lateral side before opening eyes
   - Instill a drop of freshly prepared 1% silver nitrate solution or 1% tetracycline ointment to prevent gonococcal conjunctivitis
   - Any discharge from eye of infant is pathological and requires immediate treatment.

e. Care of nose and throat
   - Clear nose followed by throat using separate sterile gauze piece to establish airway.

f. Care of rectum
   - Ascertain patency of rectum to exclude imperforate anus
   - Expel meconium by inserting little finger with gloves into rectum for about 1/2 inch.

g. Care of skin
   - Newborn is bathed by nursing staff with soap and warm water within few hours to remove vernix, meconium and blood clots
   - Oil may be applied before bath if necessary

h. Maintenance of body temperature
   - Normal body temperature of a newborn is between 36.5–37.5°C
   - Newborns have little thermal control and can lose body heat quickly
   - Immediately after birth, most of heat is lost through evaporation of amniotic fluid from body of wet child therefore it is important to quickly dry newborn with clean cloth and wrap in warm cloth and given to mother for skin to skin contact and breastfeeding
   - Avoid putting newborn on cold surfaces such as metallic tray, rubber sheeting, etc. and placing them near cold walls, open windows.

i. Breastfeeding
   - Breastfeeding should be initiated within an hour of birth to establish feeding and bonding between mother child relationship
   - First milk called as colostrum is most suitable food for baby during this early period as it contains high concentration of proteins, other nutrients and rich anti-infective factors
   - Baby should be allowed to breast whenever it wants

Significance

- Importance of early neonatal care has been proved beyond doubt by fact that institutional deliveries where early neonatal care is imparted has shown very few neonatal deaths.

18. Voluntary health organizations.

Refer Question No. 10 December 2013 (RS2) Paper II.

19. Modes of transmission of rabies.

Refer Question No. 2 December 2008 (RS2) Paper II.

20. Life-expectancy.

- Life-expectancy or expectation of life is the average number of years a person is expected to live, according to the mortality patterns existing in that country
- Unless specified it always refers to life-expectancy at birth (LE_0)
- The life-expectancy at age 1 is the average number of years a 1 year old child is expected to live and it is higher than life-expectancy at birth as it excludes the risk of infant mortality
- It is a positive mortality indicator^Q.

Life-expectancy at Birth in India

	Male	*Female*
2015 (World Bank)	68.35 years	
2011	65 years	
2005^Q	62.3 years^Q	65.3 years^Q
At time of independence	32.45 years	31.66 years

Significance

- It is one of the best indicators of a country's level of development and of the overall health of its population
- It provides necessary information for the health policy makers to implement disease control measures in the country.

21. Spacing methods of contraception.

Refer Question No. 8 December 2010 (RS2) Paper II.

22. Growth chart.

- Growth chart or road to health chart or weight for age chart is a visible display of the child's physical growth and development
- Originally designed by David Morley^Q and later modified by WHO, and is recognized internationally
- It relies on the weight of the child to monitor the child's growth rather than height because
  - Weight is the most sensitive measure of growth and any deviation from normal can be detected by comparison with the normal reference curves
- Moreover, a child can lose weight but not height
- Growth chart is designed for longitudinal followup (growth monitoring) of a child
- It is generally plotted between weight and age^Q.

Design

- The chart is a graph showing horizontal X-axis and longitudinal Y-axis.
- The X-axis is divided into 5 main divisions, representing age from birth to 5 years, each division for one year. Further each division is divided into 12 subdivisions representing 12 months in a year. Thus in total there are 60 subdivisions on the X-axis.

- The Y-axis represents weight and has 22 solid lines indicating kilograms and interrupted lines in between for half kilograms
- The growth chart also exhibits reference curves
- These reference curves are provided for the purpose of comparison as these curves show the limits of normal growth
- These reference curves are based on extensive cross-sectional data of well-nourished healthy children and can be modified as per local needs and circumstance
- The WHO chart has 2 reference curves whereas the growth chart used in India have 4 reference curves
- WHO reference curves are based on NRHM standards[Q] (Best available standards[Q]) where as Indian reference curves are based on ICMR values
- Besides these details, there is also space provided for recording and presenting information about identification and registration, date of birth and birth weight, chronological age, history of sibling health, immunization procedures, introduction of supplementary foods, episodes of sickness, child spacing and reasons for special care.

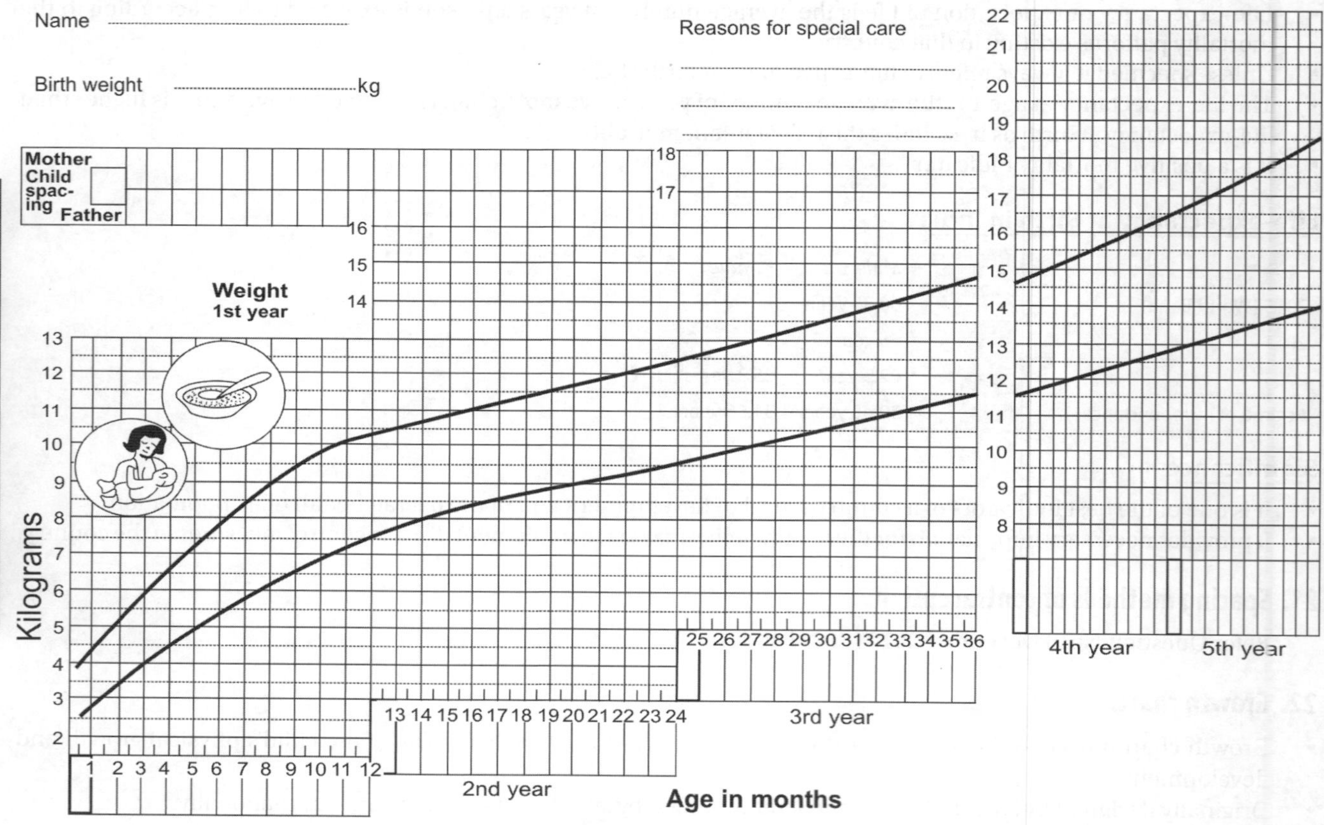

Fig. 4: WHO growth chart

Road to Health

- The space between the highest and next highest reference curve is called road to health[Q]
- This space indicates the weight of the 95% of the normal healthy children
- The weight of child if exceeds the highest reference curve, indicates obesity and similarly if it is less than the lowest reference curve then it is malnutrition
- The weight of the child is recorded monthly in infancy, once in two months during 2nd year and once in 3 months thereafter till 5 years and plotted on the growth chart and curve obtained by joining these dots constitutes growth curve of the child
- A normal growth is indicated by growth line which is below the highest reference curve and runs parallel to the reference curves.

- It is the direction of the growth curve that is important rather than position of the dots on the line, i.e. periodic weight record is more useful than single weight plot

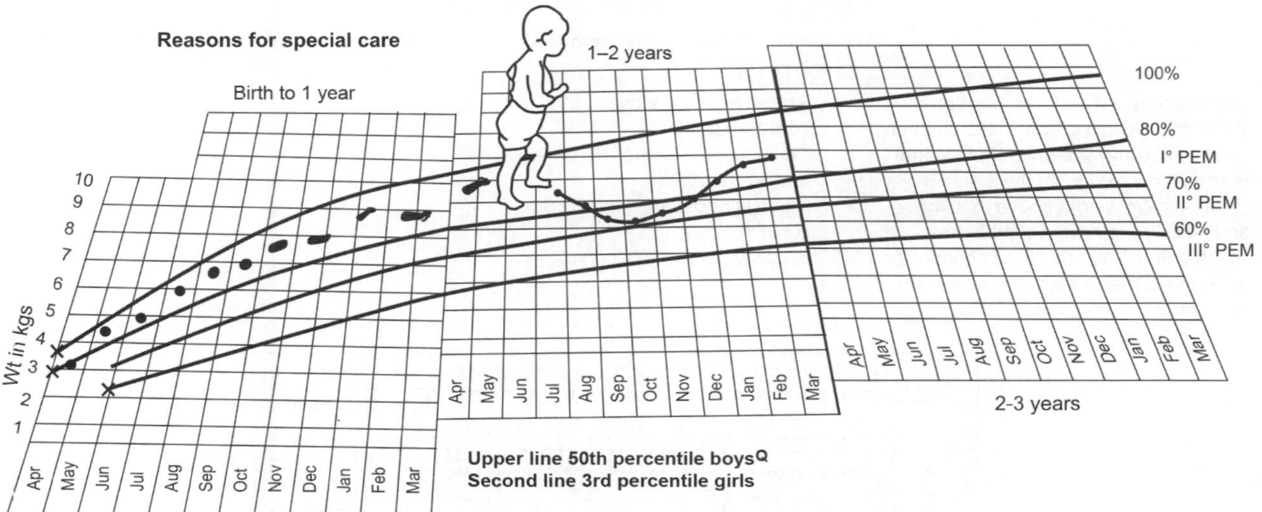

Fig. 5: Road to health

- Flattening of the curve indicates fall in child's weight and is the earliest sign of protein energy malnutrition^Q and precedes clinical signs by weeks or even months and such children need special care to keep their weight above the lowest reference curve
- If the growth curve falls in between the second and third reference curve, i.e. between the 80% and 70% of the 50th percentile then it is termed first degree malnutrition or mild malnutrition of Grade I and this can be managed by the mother at home
- If the growth curve falls in between the third and forth reference curve, i.e. between the 70% and 60% of the 50th percentile then it is termed second degree malnutrition or moderate malnutrition of Grade II and requires intervention by the medical professionals
- If the growth curve falls below the forth line, i.e. 60% of 50th percentile then it is termed third degree malnutrition or severe malnutrition of Grade III and requires hospitalization for investigation and treatment.

Various Health Charts

- There are numerous health charts used worldwide, and in India itself about 49 different growth charts are used.

WHO growth chart (Home-based charts)	*Growth chart used in India (Service charts) (49 types of growth charts used in India and they are separate for boys and girls)*	
	Government of India recommended growth chart	*ICDS growth chart (Based on WHO MGRS child growth standards 2006)*
▪ Has 2 reference curves^Q. ▪ Upper reference curve represents the median or 50th percentile for boys^Q starting at 3.5 kg at birth and ends at 18.5 kg at age 5 ▪ Lower reference curve represents the 3rd percentile for girls^Q beginning at 3.0 kg at birth and ends at 14.5 kg at age 5 ▪ Based on NCHS^Q (National Center for Health Statistics) USA, standards ▪ Used for both sexes	▪ Has 4 reference curves^Q. ▪ Topmost reference curve corresponds to the 80% of the 50th percentile of the WHO standard^Q ▪ Next lines in descending order represent 70%, 60% and 50% of the median, i.e. 50th percentile of WHO standard ▪ Also indicates 4 grades of malnutrition as recommended by the Indian Academy of Paediatrics^Q	▪ Has three reference curves^Q ▪ Topmost reference curve corresponds to the 50th percentile of the WHO standard considering it as 100% ▪ Next lines in descending order represent 2SD below of reference standards and 3SD below reference standard

Contd...

Contd...

WHO growth chart (Home-based charts)	*Growth chart used in India (Service charts) (49 types of growth charts used in India and they are separate for boys and girls)*	
	Government of India recommended growth chart	*ICDS growth chart (Based on WHO MGRS child growth standards 2006)*
▪ 50th percentile means the position of the 50th child in a group of 100 children of same age and sex when their weight is arranged in order, i.e. there are 50 children have weight above that line and 50 children have weight below the that line. Similarly only 3 children in 100 have their weight below the 3rd percentile	– Grade I or mild (Between 80% and 70% curves) – Grade II or moderate[Q] (Between 70% and 60% curves[Q]) – Grade III or severe[Q] (Below 60% curve[Q]) – Grade IV (Below 50% curve)	

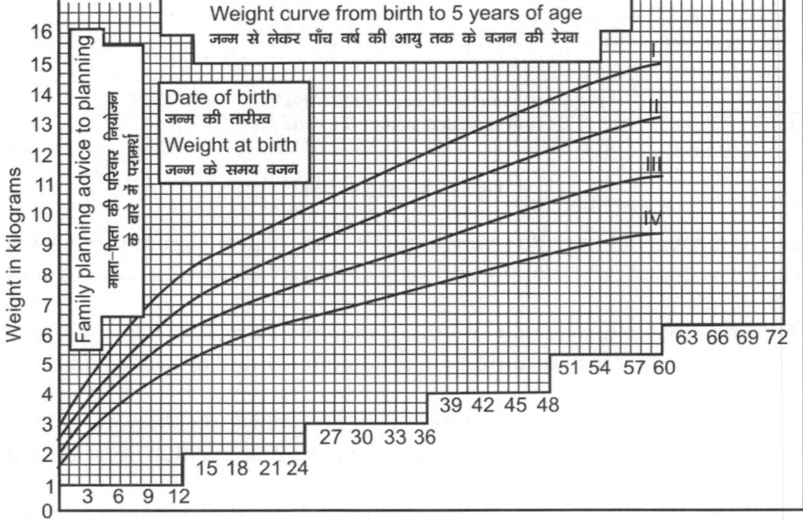

Fig. 6: Growth chart used in India

Growth Chart Used in India

Uses of growth charts

a. Growth monitoring tool	▪ Prime purpose of growth chart is monitoring the growth of child under age of 5 years which is very important for child health care
b. Diagnostic tool for identifying high-risk children	▪ Serves as a diagnostic tool for identifying high-risk children as it can detect malnutrition long before it becomes clinically evident
c. Planning and policy making	▪ By grading malnutrition, growth chart provides an objective basis for planning and policy making in relation to child health care at the local and central levels
d. Educational tool	▪ Because of visual nature of the growth chart, the mother can be educated to take care of her child and encourage her to participate more actively in growth monitoring
e. Tool for action	▪ Helps the health worker on the type of intervention needed thus helping the referrals easier
f. Evaluation of corrective measures and impact of program	▪ Provides a good method to evaluate the effectiveness of corrective measures and the impact of a program or of special intervention for improving child growth and development
g. Tool for teaching	▪ Can also be used for teaching important health tips like importance of adequate feeding, deleterious effect of diarrhea, etc.

Contd...

Contd...

h. Tool of information[Q]	▪ Growth chart contains numerous important information like i. Name of the child (identification and registration) ii. Birth date and birth weight iii. Chronological age iv. Weight for age v. Developmental milestones vi. Episodes of sickness vii. Immunization history viii. Introduction of supplementary foods ix. History of siblings health x. Child spacing (family planning method used by parents) xi. Reasons for special care

Merits	*Demerits*
▪ It can be easily understood by the mother as well as health care worker and thus provides them with a visual record of the health and nutritional status of the child	▪ It is meaningless under 6 months of age which is a more important period in terms of nutrition ▪ The presence of 3rd line which is very difficult for the auxiliary worker and its importance lies in undertaking a survey rather than measuring the progress of a child

Significance

- Growth chart is considered a Passport to child health care[Q].

MBBS PHASE III EXAMINATION

JUNE 2010

(Revised Scheme 2)

PAPER I

LONG ESSAYS

1. Write in detail about "Natural history of disease".

Refer Question No. 1 December 2007 (RS2) Paper I.

2. Describe various methods of nutritional assessment of a community with their merits and demerits.

- When the nutritional status of a group of persons or a community is undertaken, it is called nutrition survey.
- When the nutritional status of a group of people or community is assessed periodically, to monitor the success of a nutritional program, it is called nutritional surveillance.

Objectives	*Sample size*	*Methods*
To determine the extent of nutritional problems/diseases in a community and their contributing factors, so that nutrition programs can be implemented for the prevention and control of the nutritional diseases	Representative sample of 50–100 people	▪ Clinical examination ▪ Anthropometric examination ▪ Laboratory and biochemical examination ▪ Functional indicators ▪ Biophysical examination ▪ Vital statics ▪ Diet survey ▪ Assessment of ecological factors

Methods of Nutritional Assessment of a Community

A. Clinical examination
   - Consists of examination of an individual, clinically, from head to toe for the changes believed to be related to food consumption that can be seen or felt in the superficial tissues like hairs, eyes, skin, buccal mucosa, tongue, ears, nose, lips, teeth, gums, glands, nails, chest, abdomen and edema.
   - Conglomeration of signs helps in making the diagnosis of a specific disease and if the signs are absent, the subject is declared nutritionally healthy.
   - World Health Organization (WHO) expert committee classified signs used in nutritional surveys into three categories:
     - Not related to nutrition like alopecia, pyorrhea, pterygium
     - That need further investigations like malar pigmentation, corneal vascularization, geographic tongue
     - Known to be of value like angular stomatitis, Bitot's spots, calf tenderness, absence of knee or ankle jerks, enlargement of thyroid, etc.

Advantage	*Disadvantages*
Simplest, cheapest, very sound and most practical method of assessing the nutritional status	▪ Malnutrition cannot be quantified on the basis of clinical signs ▪ Many deficiencies are unaccompanied by physical signs ▪ Lack of specificity and subjective nature of most of the physical signs

B. Anthropometric examination
   - Consists of recording the body measurements, which are although genetically determined, they are profoundly influenced by the nutrition.

a. Weight[Q]
- Weight for age helps in assessing the nutritional status and also the growth, especially among children, when recorded periodically and plotted in "Road to Health" card
- It describes severity of malnutrition[Q]
  - Low weight for age is known as underweight[Q] (acute + chronic malnutrition[Q])
  - Low weight for height is known as nutritional wasting[Q] or emaciation[Q] (acute malnutrition[Q]).

Methods

i. In children
- Current weight (in kg) of the child is compared with the expected standard weight and the deficiency in percentage is expressed in terms of degrees of malnutrition
- Weight for age is also employed in Welcome's classification to assess Protein-energy malnutrition (PEM), as kwashiorkor, marasmus.
- Weight is measured using Salter's scale in field[Q]

ii. In adults (Body mass index)
- A composite index of the nutritional status of adults is called the body mass index (BMI)
- *Calculations*
- BMI is obtained by dividing the weight (in kg) of the individual by the height (in meters) squared

$$\text{BMI} = \frac{\text{Weight (in kg)}}{\text{Height}^2 \text{ (in meters)}}$$

- *Interpretation*

> 25	Obesity
18.5–25	Normal
<18.5	Chronic energy deficiency
18.5–17	First degree chronic energy deficiency
17–16	Second degree chronic energy deficiency
<16	Third degree chronic energy deficiency

- *Significance*
  - Weight reflect only present status
  - It is a single most reliable criterion of assessment of health and nutrition status[Q]
  - It is single most sensitive measure of growth[Q]
  - Along with rate of weight gain, it is single best parameter for assessment of physical growth[Q].

b. Height[Q]
- This is a linear dimension and is a measure of skeletal elongation
- Height for age gives an indication of duration of malnutrition and is best parameter of chronic malnutrition[Q]
- Low height for age is also known as nutritional stunting or dwarfing and it reflects past or chronic malnutrition[Q]
- It is an index of duration of malnutrition[Q]
- Height is a stable measurement of growth as opposed to weight
- It indicates events of past also.

c. Circumference of chest to head ratio
- Normally, at birth, the circumference of head is little more than that of the chest which become same by one year of age and crossing over takes after 1 year
- If the chest to head circumference ratio is less than 1 in preschool children, it is considered PEM.

d. Circumference of mid-arm[Q]
- This gives information about the muscle mass because muscle wasting is a cardinal feature of PEM especially during early childhood.

Mid-arm circumference	*Interpretation*
>13.5 cm	Well-nourished
12.5–13.5 cm	Mild to moderate malnourishment
<12.5 cm	Severe malnutrition

- For a quick nutrition survey, a bangle with an internal diameter of 4 cm can be used
- If it goes over the child's upper arm, it means the child is malnourished
- However, Shakir's tape is most commonly used[Q].

Disadvantages

- Child between 1 to 4 years of age will have almost the constant measurement

e. Skinfold thickness
- This gives information about the subcutaneous reserve of calories in the body
- Harpenden calipers are used for this and measurement of a thickness of a skin-fold is recorded over triceps of left arm or infrascapular region
- For a preschool child, 10 mm is taken as a cut-off point.

Advantages	*Disadvantages*
Anthropometric measurements can be recorded by non-medical personnel, given sufficient training	Anthropometric measurements by themselves are of little value unless they are analyzed with reference to age

C. Laboratory and biochemical examination

a. Laboratory test

i. Hemoglobin estimation and serum transferrin[Q]
- Most important laboratory test carried out in nutrition surveys
- Useful index of the overall nutrition

ii. Stools and urine
- Stool should be examined for intestinal parasites
- Urine is examined for albumin, sugar and urinary nitrogen[Q].

b. Biochemical tests
- Variations in the intake of nutrients in the diet are reflected by their concentration in the blood and urine thus, biochemical test helps to detect malnutrition much before the pathology has developed.

Nutrient	*Method*	*Normal value*
Vitamin A	Serum retinol	20 µg/dL
Thiamine	Thiamin pyrophosphate stimulation of RBC transketolase activity	1.00–1.23
Riboflavin	RBC glutathione reductase activity stimulated by flavine *adenine dinucleotide*	1.0–1.2
Niacin	Urine N-methyl nicotinamide	—
Folate	Serum folate	6.0 µg/mL
	Red cell folate	160 µg/mL
Vitamin B_{12}	Serum vitamin B_{12} concentration	160 mg/L
Vitamin C	Leukocyte ascorbic acid	15 µg/108 cells
Vitamin K	Prothrombin time	11–16 seconds
Protein	Serum albumin	35 g/L
	Transferin	20 g/L
	Thyroid binding pre-albumin	250 mg/L

D. Functional indicators

– Functional indices of nutritional status are emerging as important class of diagnostic tools

System	*Nutrient*
a. Structural integrity	
i. Erythrocyte fragility	Vitamin E, selenium
ii. Capillary fragility	Vitamin C
iii. Tensile strength	Copper
b. Host defense	
i. Leukocyte chemotaxis	P/E, zinc
ii. Leukocyte phagocytic capacity	P/E, iron
iii. Leukocyte bactericidal capacity	P/E, iron, selenium

iv. T cell blastogeneis	P/E, zinc
v. Delayed cutaneous hypersensitivity	P/E, zinc
c. Hemostasis	
i. Prothrombin time	Vitamin K
d. Reproduction	
i. Sperm count	Energy, zinc
e. Nerve function	
i. Nerve conduction	P/E, vitamin B_1 and B_{12}
ii. Dark adaptation	Vitamin A, zinc
iii. EEG	P/E
f. Work capacity	
i. Heart rate	P/E, iron
ii. Vasopressor response	Vitamin C

E. Biophysical examination
- Cytological examination of buccal mucosa is done to study the cornified cells
- Percentage of cornified cells increases with the degree of malnutrition
- In healthy children, the normal percentage of cornified cells is 30–40%.

F. Assessment of dietary intake (Diet survey)
- Diet survey or food consumption survey the study of the food consumption pattern in a group of individuals.
- Here the investigator makes home visits daily for 7 days, i.e. one dietary cycle[Q] and the data is recorded in a designed proforma and average for one day is calculated.

Methods

	Advantages	*Disadvantages*
Weighing raw food		
▪ Investigator visits the house hold and weighs all food which is going to be cooked and eaten as well as that which is wasted or discards ▪ Should be done for 1 to 21 days but usually is done for 7 days which makes one dietary cycle	▪ Practicable and hence most widely used ▪ Fairly accurate and reliable if carried out properly	▪ Weighs food that has to be discarded ▪ Long duration of survey ▪ Value obtained for whole family ▪ Deliberate addition of foods not meant for cooking
Weighing cooked food (recipe method)		
▪ Investigator visits the household and weighs all cooked food which is going to be consumed ▪ Left-over food is also weighed including platewaste	▪ Most accurate method ▪ Weighs food that is to be consumed	▪ Not easily accepted by the people ▪ Difficult and not practicable ▪ Give nutritive value of whole family
Questionnaire method		
▪ Study subject is asked about the food consumed in the previous 24–48 hours (recall method) or a literate person is asked to keep record of his diet for next 24–48 hours (record method) ▪ Quantity consumed is recorded in standard measures like cap and servings ▪ Quantity is converted to nutritive value of cooked food published in standard textbooks on nutrition	▪ Useful diet survey of large population ▪ Can be reliable (record method) ▪ Easy and consumes less time ▪ Can give seasonal variation in consumption pattern if repeated periodically ▪ Gives information about common food items and forms in which they are consumed ▪ Give nutritive information for each individual of family	▪ Less accurate especially recall method

Contd...

Contd...

	Advantages	*Disadvantages*
Food inventory or log book method		
▪ Quantity of food present in the house at the beginning of the survey is weighed and recorded ▪ An account of the food items purchased during one week of the study period should be kept by the head of the family and at the end of the week, the food items remaining unused is also weighed and recorded ▪ This gives information about the average food items consumed during one week and average for one day can be calculated	▪ Easy and simple ▪ Acceptable to families	▪ Cannot be employed in families with illiterate head of the family ▪ Requires cooperation from family ▪ Value obtained for whole family
Food list method		
▪ Investigator will have questionnaire containing a list of foods consumed by the family and the quantity of the food stated by the housewife are entered	▪ Easy and simple	▪ Have to rely on the housewife
Analysis of cooked food		
▪ Involves the actual analysis of the composite sample of each cooked food item for presence of various nutrients ▪ About 10% of by weight of the foods consumed by one individual is taken as sample and all the items are mixed and mashed in a fine paste and analyzed for nutrients present in the diet ▪ Analysis ▪ Data collected is converted into: – Mean intake in grams for each food, i.e. cereals, pulses, vegetables, fruit, eggs, etc. – Mean intake of nutrients per adult man, value or consumption unit	▪ Most accurate and reliable ▪ Provides value for individual ▪ Content of individual nutrient can be analyzed	▪ Time consuming ▪ Expensive ▪ Can be done in nutritional laboratories only

Significance

- Diet surveys provide information about dietary intake patterns, specific foods consumed, and estimated nutrient intake
- It indicates relative dietary deficiencies
- It provides information for planning health education activities
- Information obtained allows an assessment to be made of the extent and nature of the change needed in agriculture and food production industry.

G. Vital statistics

- Since malnutrition influences morbidity and mortality rates, three indicators of vital statistics are employed
  - i. Age specific death rate among 1 to 4 years (Infant mortality rate and mortality in the age group of 1 to 4 years).
  - ii. Cause specific death rate among under-fives (i.e. due to PEM)
  - iii. Proportional mortality rate among under-fives due to PEM.

H. Assessment of ecological factors

- Human malnutrition is an end result of multiple overlapping and inter-acting factors in the community's physical, biological and cultural environment
- Various influencing ecological factors are:

a. Conditioning infections and infestations	– Infections have deleterious effects on the nutritional status specially among children – There exists a vicious inter-relationship circle between infection and malnutrition. – Similarly associated infestation also affects the nutritional status

Contd...

Contd...

b. Cultural factors	– Different cultural factors which influence the nutritional status are food habits, customs, beliefs, traditions and attitudes – Family plays an important role and many times, the food habits pass from one generation to the other – Cultural factors make the individual to eat or not to eat a particular food item – These factors often affect the vulnerable groups – Religion has a powerful influence on the food habits of the people like Hindus do not eat beef and Muslims pork – Orthodox Hindus do not eat nonvegetarian food and all vegetarian items like onion and garlic – These are known as food taboos – Cooking practices like draining away the rice-water at the end of cooking, peeling of vegetables, etc. also affect the nutritional status – Child rearing practices such as premature weaning, bottle feeding, feeding artificial foods, etc. also affect – Habits like alcoholism have got a profound effect
c. Socioeconomic factors	– Important socioeconomic factors are income, education and the occupational status – These determine the quality-life, which in turn determines the nutritional status – Malnutrition is more among the poor
d. Food production	– Increased food production should lead to increased food consumption and better nutritional status
e. Food consumption	– It is obvious that the nutritional status of an individual is directly related to the quality and quantity of the food eaten – Under eating results in PEM and over eating results in obesity
f. Availability of health services	– Health services like nutritional services, immunization, family welfare services definitively improves nutritional status of a community

Significance

- Nutritional surveillance provides valuable input for program management and evaluation (to policy makers) and give timely warning and intervention (to prevent short-term food crisis) thus aid health development.

SHORT ESSAYS

3. Iceberg phenomenon of diseases meaning and application, with suitable examples.

- According to this concept disease in community can be compared with iceberg
- Also called as biological spectrum of disease
- In an iceberg very small portion of the iceberg is visible above the water surface and its large part is submerged below the water surface and hence is not visible
- The visible floating tip of iceberg represents what physician sees in the community, i.e. clinical cases and the vast submerged hidden portion represents the hidden mass of the disease, i.e. latent, inapperent, presymptomatic and undiagnosed cases and carriers in the community which are responsible for constant prevalence of disease in community and water surface is line of demarcation between apparent and inapparent infections and surrounding water is healthy population[Q]
- Epidemiologist is concerned with hidden portion of iceberg[Q] whereas clinician is concerned with the tip of iceberg[Q]
- Screening is done for the hidden portion of iceberg whereas diagnosis is done for the tip of the iceberg[Q]

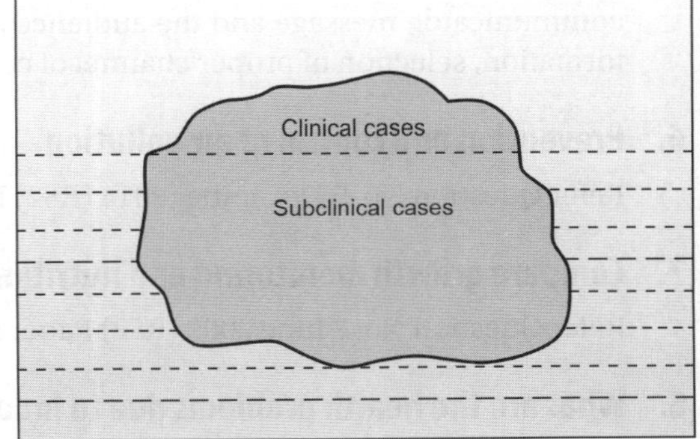

Fig. 1: Iceberg phenomenon

- This phenomenon is due to:
  - Mild cases taking treatment at home and cured
  - In some diseases very early stage cannot be diagnosed
  - In some instances persons harbor the organism but do not suffer from the disease (carriers).

Examples

- Communicable diseases: Gastroenteritis, cholera, hepatitis A[Q], polio[Q], diphtheria[Q], influenza[Q], AIDS[Q], etc.
- Noncommunicable diseases: Hypertension, diabetes, etc.
- Diseases not showing iceberg phenomenon: Rabies[Q], tetanus[Q], measles[Q], rubella[Q].

Significance

- The hidden part of the iceberg constitutes as important undiagnosed reservoir of infection or disease in the community and its detection and control is challenge[Q] to epidemiologist.

4. Classify occupational diseases with examples.

Refer Question No. 2 June 2016 (RS2) Paper I.

5. Barriers of communication in health education.

- They are four types of barriers of communication which are:

Barriers of Communication

Physiological	*Psychological*	*Environmental*	*Cultural*
▪ Mainly concerned with the person's ability to give good health education and to make the message palatable to the audience ▪ Examples: Difficulty in listening, visualization, speaking, expressing, habbits, stress and strain	▪ Main barrier between the health educator and his audience ▪ To become a good health educator, the psychological barriers must be broken between the audience and the communicator for which the audience should feel that the health educator is also one among them ▪ The emotional barrier between the communicator and the audience is eliminated ▪ Communicator should not feel nervous ▪ Examples: Mental tension, instability, lack of concentration, emotional disturbance, preoccupations	▪ Common barriers in giving health education to masses or groups ▪ Examples: Overcrowding, poor lightening, noise, thermal discomfort, bad odors, ill maintained channels of communication	▪ Common barriers the health educator feels difficult to remove therefore a health educator must understand the cultural background of the audience ▪ Health education should not hurt the sentiments of the people ▪ Examples: Poor knowledge of customs, practices, attitudes, habits, beliefs, language knowledge, confidence, level of understanding

Significance

- These barriers of communication can be identified before embarking on communication through the study of communicator, message and the audience and by importing training to communicator, finalizing a good message formation, selection of proper channel of communication, the audience can be effectively reached.

6. Prevention and control of air pollution.

Refer Question No. 5 December 2014 (RS2) Paper I.

7. Compare growth monitoring and nutritional surveillance.

Refer Question No. 7 June 2009 (RS2) Paper I.

8. What are the health problems due to industrialization?

Refer Question No. 1 December 2017 (RS2) Paper I.

9. Differentiate between case control study and cohort study.

- Case control and cohort studies are the two types of analytical epidemiological studies.

Difference between Case Control and Cohort Study

	Case control study	*Cohort study*
Direction	From effect to cause	From cause to effect
Starting point	Starts with the disease	Starts with people exposed to risk factors of suspected causes
Tests	Whether suspected case occurs more frequently in those with disease than among those without the disease	Whether disease occurs more frequently in those exposed than in those not similarly exposed
Application	▪ Usually first approach to testing of a hypothesis ▪ Useful for exploratory studies	Reserved for testing of precisely formulated hypothesis
No. of subjects	Fewer	Larger
Duration	Yields relatively quick results	Long follow-up period often needed, involving delayed results
Suitability	Suitable for the study of rare diseases	Inappropriate when the disease or exposure under investigation is rare
Yields	Only estimate of relative risk (odds ratio)	Incidence rates, relative risk as well as attributable risk
Diseases not involved in study	Cannot yield information about diseases other than that selected for study	Can yield information about more than one disease outcome
Cost	Relatively inexpensive	Expensive
Examples	Oral contraceptives and thromboembolic disease	Smoking and lung cancer, Framingham Heart study

10. Epidemic curve.

Refer Question No. 4 December 2016 (RS2) Paper I.

11. Integrated vector control measures.

- Integrated vector control is the utilization of all appropriate technological and management techniques to bring about an effective degree of vector suppression in a cost-effective manner
- It avoids the excessive use of any one method but tries to combine one or more methods whether they are directed towards only the larvae or adults or both, with a view to obtain maximum result with minimum inputs and also to prevent environmental pollution with toxic chemicals and development of resistance among vectors.

Components

a. Antilarval measures
   i. Environmental control
   ii. Chemical control
   iii. Biological control

b. Anti-adult measures
   i. Residual sprays
   ii. Space sprays
   iii. Genetic control

c. Protection against bites
   i. Mosquito nets
   ii. Screening
   iii. Repellants.

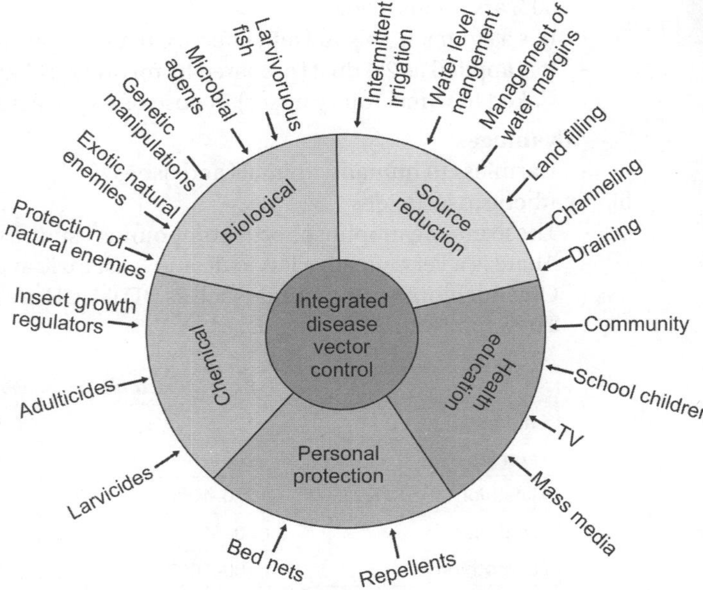

Fig. 2: Integrated management of vector—components

Integrated Vector Control Measures

A. Antilarval measures
   a. Environmental control
      - Also known as source reduction direction towards eliminating the mosquito breeding places
      - Source reduction methods generally permanent results.

      Components
      - Filling of low lying areas where water accumulation is possible (Anopheles)
      - Leveling or covering or drainage of cesspools ditches and sewers which are present near the houses (culex and anopheles)
      - Removal of water plants such as Pistia plants with herbicides (mansonia)
      - Clean-up the environment and get rid of water holding containers such as empty pots coconut shells discarded tins, broken bottles, etc. (Aedes)
      - Weekly emptying of household water collections intermittent irrigation, cultivation of banana plants where water accumulates near the house.

      Significance
      - Best approach to vector control[Q]
   b. Chemical control
      - Chemical control is the use of larvicides to kill the larvae
      - These larvicides may act as stomach poisons when it is ingested by larva while feeding or as contact poison which penetrate the body wall or respiratory tract
      - It is usually employed where source reduction is not feasible.
        i. Mineral oils[Q]
           - Diesel oil, fuel oil, kerosene when applied on water forms a thin film which cuts-off the air to the larvae and pupae[Q] and cause death within 1–2 hours of application
           - The oil is applied at rate of 40–90 L per heater simply by dipping from a bucket or pouring from a water can
           - However, mineral oil should be applied once in a week as the mosquito's life cycle is of 8 days.

           Disadvantages
           - Makes water unfit for human consumption and kills fishes.
        ii. Paris green[Q]
           - Paris green or copper acetoarsenite is an emerald green, micro crystalline powder containing more than 50% arsenious oxide
           - It is a stomach poison[Q] and effective mainly against Anopheles[Q] which are surface feeders
           - It is applied as 2% dust (prepared by mixing 2 kg Paris green in 98 kg diluents such as soapstone powder or slaked lime in a rotary mixer) in dose of 1 kg of actual Paris green per hectare of water surface.

           Advantages
           - Harmless to humans, animals and fishes.
        iii. Synthetic insecticides
           - These are organophosphorus compounds[Q] such as fenthion[Q], chlorpyrifos[Q], malathion, abate[Q], etc.
           - Abate is a very effective larvicide and least toxic at a concentration of 10 ppm
           - Organochlorine compounds such as DDT, HCH are not recommended because of their long residual effect.
           - They applied in following doses

	Dose (g/hectare)	*Duration of action*
Chlorpyriphos[Q]	10–20	3–17 weeks
Fenthion[Q]	20–110	2–12 weeks
Malathion[Q]	220–1000	1–2 weeks
Temephos	60–110	2–4 weeks
Fenitrothion	100–1000	2–11 weeks
Abate	60–100	2–4 weeks

Advantages
- Mosquitoes are destroyed before they disperse to human populations.
- Operations can be carried out in very short time.
- Widely available
- Can be applied by hand.

Disadvantages
- Temporary control and costly repetitions.
- Affection of other organisms
- Human toxicity.

c. Biological control
   i. Bacteria
   - Certain bacteria are useful to kill the larva of mosquitoes which are:
     o Bacillus sphaerizus 500–5,000 g/hr, acting for 1–2 weeks
     o Bacillus thiringiensis H14[Q]–100–6000 g/hr, acting for 2–8 weeks (Bt toxin)
   ii. Fishes
   - A wide range of small fish feed readily on mosquito larvae and best known among them are *Gambusia affinis*[Q], *Labister reticulatus* and *Poecilia*
   - These fishes can be used in burrow pits, sewage, oxidation ponds, cisterns and farm ponds.

B. Anti-adult measures
a. Residual sprays[Q]
- A long-acting insecticide is sprayed on walls[Q] and other surfaces where mosquitoes rest.
- Commonly used insecticides are:

	Dosage (g/m²)	*Duration of action*
Organochlorines		
DDT[Q]	1–2[Q]	More than 6 months
Lindane (BHC)	0.2–0.5	3 or more months
Organophosphrous		
Malathion[Q]	1–2	1–3 months[Q]
Fenitrothion	1–2	1–3 months
Methyl pirimphos	1–2	2–3 months
Carbamates		
Propoxus	1–2	2–3 months
Bendiocarb	0.2–0.4	2–3 months
Pyrethroids		
Permethrin	0.5	2–3 months
Cypermethrin	0.5	4 or more months
Deltamethrin	0.05	2–3 months

- Good residual insecticide should
  o Be toxic to target vector
  o Have long-lasting effect one a given surface
  o Be safe to human and domestic animals
  o Be acceptable to house owners
  o Be cost-effective
  o Be stable during storage and transport
  o Not be irritant or repellent to target insects to ensure that insects pick up a lethal dose
  o Mix well with water and be harmless to spraying instrument.

b. Space sprays
- Insecticidal formulations are sprayed into the atmosphere in the form of mist or fog to kill the insects which habitat outside the house

- Principle is to fill space with a mist of small droplets that are pick up by the insects when they fly
- Here a quick acting insecticide is usually used but residual insecticides such as malation[Q], fenitrothion are also used in form of ultra-low volume fogging[Q]
- Mist may contain either organophosphorus compounds like malation, fenitrothion, diazinon, cypermethrin, etc., and the fog contains *pyrethrum* extract from pyrethrum flower[Q] which contains pyrethrin as active principle a nerve poison. It is a surface acting insecticide which enters the mosquito through surface and used in dose of 10 z of spray solution per 1,000 cu feet
- Procedure carried out using a hand gun for domestic purpose or power sprayers or aerosol dispenser for large scale application.

Advantages	*Disadvantages*
▪ Has an immediate effect on adult population of insects and is therefore suitable for the control of disease outbreak ▪ Less laborious for a single application ▪ Large areas can be treated fairly quickly ▪ Uses less insecticide per application ▪ Kills mosquitoes that does not rest in house	▪ Temporary effect ▪ High recurrent cost therefore unsuitable for multiple application ▪ Costly equipment and costly maintenance ▪ Need for especially trained staff ▪ May cause contamination of non target areas and organisms and air pollution ▪ Non-acceptability due to pungent odor

c. Genetic control
- Genetic control comprises methods like sterile male technique, cytoplasmic incompatibility, chromosomal translocation, sex distortion and gene replacement.

Advantages
- Cheaper and more efficient
- No vector resistance

C. Protection against bite
a. Mosquito nets
- These offer protection against mosquito bites during sleep
- The mosquito nets should be white to allow easy detection of mosquitoes
- The size of the opening in the net should not exceed 0.0475 inch[Q] and number of holes per sq inch is usually 150[Q].

b. Screening
- Screening of building with copper or bronze gauze having 16 meshes to inch is recommended
- The diameter should not exceed 0.0475 inch
- It is a costly but effective method

c. Repellents[Q]
- Diethyltolumide (DEET) applied on skin[Q] remains active against culex mosquito for 18–20 hours
- Indalone, dimethyl phthalate, dimethyl carbate, etc. are also effective.

D. Health education
- An important component of integrated vector control
- People should be educated regarding the breeding places and life cycles of common insects and should be taught to take domestic measures such as source reduction, personal protection, etc.
- People should be informed to cooperate in regards to other measures of vector control such as space sprays, residual sprays, etc.

Significance

- Integrated vector control has successfully tackled the following problems
  - Technical problems like development of resistance to older insecticides
  - Financial problems like cost of newer insecticides
  - Environmental problems like environmental pollution by insecticides
  - Operational problems like lack of public cooperation for indoor spraying of insectides.

12. Describe briefly the methods of purification of water at household level.

Refer Question No. 2 December 2013 (RS2) Paper I.

SHORT ANSWERS

13. What is human development index?

Refer Question No. 3 December 2009 (RS2) Paper I.

14. Panel discussion.

Refer Question No. 2 June 2009 (RS2) Paper I.

15. Horrock's test.

Refer Question No. 6 June 2013 (RS2) Paper I.

16. What are the causes for occupational cancers?

Refer Question No. 8 December 2007 (RS2) Paper I.

17. Describe the reasons for the broken family.

- A broken family is one where the parents have separated/where death has occurred of one/both the parents or parent is absent because of imprisonment or enrollment in war
- Even if both parents are present, father or mother is considered as absent because of drunkenness, chronic disease, mental deficiency or drug addiction
- All the broken families are problem families.

Social Hazards of Broken Family

- Children who are victims of broken family early in their childhood have been found sometimes to display in later years psychopathic behavior, retardation of growth, speech and intellect
- They may also develop anti-social behavior, committing crimes
- They may drift away to prostitution, crime and vagrancy.

18. Census.

- Census is the total process of collecting, compiling and publishing demographic, economic and social data pertaining at a specified time or times to all persons in a country or delimited territory (United Nations).

Operation

- Census is massive undertaking to contact every member of the population in a given time and collect a variety of information
- It needs considerable organization a vast preparation and several years to analyze the results
- It is usually done under direct guidance and operation of Registrar General and Census commissioner of India[Q].
- The legal basis for census in India provided in Census Act of 1948[Q]
- It is usually held it the end of the first quarter of the first year in each decade, i.e., the last census was held in Feb – March 2011
- Conduced once every 10 years[Q]
- The first census in India was held in 1881[Q]
- It covers about 640 districts
- Nodal ministry overlooking census operation is Ministry of Home Affairs[Q].

Information obtained

Demographic	*Social and economic*
▪ Census is an important source of demographic information i.e. age/sex/religion/social classification, etc. at various levels.	▪ Census also provides information regarding religion, casts, housing, employment income, etc.

Types

De-facto (date system)	De-jure
In this system, a particular day is fixed and a person is counted at a place where he is found on that day	In this system, a person is counted at a place of his permanent residence irrespective of the place where he if found on the day of census
Practiced in India till 1931	Practiced in India till date since 1941
Tedious and unfeasible operation to be done in specified time	Easy compared to de-facto because the information can be obtained from any family member above age of 18
Conducted at night presuming that the person would beat place where belongs in nights	Conducted in daytime
Depends on the worker	Depends upon the information provided

Procedure

- Process is started as early as January and completed by February
- Population enumeration is done by 9th–28th February
- Houseless population enumeration is done on night of 28th February
- Census officially stops at 00.00 at 1st March[Q]
- Then form 1st March to 5th March Revision round is undertaken where the enumerator will go back to the respective houses and enquire about
  - Any births taken place since his/her last visit up to 1st March and if answer is positive then sex is noted down
  - Any deaths taken place since his/her last visit up to 1st March and if answer is positive then the name of the person is detected from the list
- Births and deaths occurring between 2nd to 5th March are ignored.

Problems of census operation	Disadvantages	Uses of census information
▪ Terms used in census proformas for collection of information may be misinterpreted ▪ Shortage of manpower can delay the collection and processing of information ▪ Data can be manipulated by dishonest or lazy workers ▪ False information by the general population ▪ Age is recorded in multiples of 5 thus correct age cannot be obtained. ▪ Infants are generally under-enumerated ▪ Many persons do not their exact age ▪ Old persons tend to add years to their actual age ▪ Information about handicapped person is incomplete ▪ Information about work status is distorted	▪ A costly affair requiring a huge manpower ▪ Depends totally on the information provided by the population ▪ Full results are not available quickly	▪ Provides demographic, social and economical date of the country ▪ Provides information on the composition (age and sex wise), size (total population) and distribution (density) of the population ▪ Helps to estimate the mid-year population which constitutes the important denominator to calculate morbidity, mortality and fertility rates ▪ Helps in calculation of growth rate ▪ Helps to access the trend of the population, through population projection, by comparing with that of previous decades ▪ Helps to formulate the population policies ▪ Helps to plan health and welfare measures ▪ Helps to compare with that of other countries ▪ Helps to formulate social security measures like Life Insurance, etc. ▪ Helps to access and evaluate population control programs ▪ Helps to know the quality of life of people

Significance

- Census is the backbone of demographic statistics considering all major health statistics are based on the midyear population
- It is also vital for planning any people directed services or programs.

19. Bar chart.

Refer Question No. 8 June 2017 (RS2) Paper I.

20. Attributable risk.

Refer Question No. 1 December 2016 (RS2) Paper I.

21. Food adulterants.

- Adulteration is practice of mixing, substituting, removal, concealing the quality, selling of decomposed products, misbranding addition of toxicants done by traders for greed for money.

Examples (Food Adulterants)

Food stuff	*Common adulterant*
Cereals	Stone, sand, grit
Dals	Kesari dal
Milk	Water, starch
Ghee	Vanaspati
Butter	Starch, animal fat
Turmeric powder	Lead chromate powder
Black pepper	Dried seeds of papaya
Chilli powder	Brick powder
Tea leaves	Husk of blackgram, resuse of tree leaves
Coffee seeds	Tamarind seeds
Baking powder	Citric acid
Honey	Sugar, jaggery
Sugar	Chalk
Mustard seed	Seeds of *Argemone*
Edible oil	Mineral oil
Ice cream	Starch, cellulose, washing powder
Sweets	Non-permitted colors
Hing	Resins, gums

Disadvantages for Consumers

- He is paying more money for a food stuff of lower quality
- He is at risk of ill health like epidemic dropsy, paralysis, allergy, gastritis and sometime even death.

Significance

- Adulteration is a social evil and punishable offence under Prevention of Food Adulteration Act, 1954.

22. Migration studies.

- Migration studies are study aimed to find out changes in disease frequency among migrants.

Methods

Comparison with original population	*Comparison with local population*
▪ Comparison of disease and death rate for migrants with those of their kin who have stayed at original location ▪ This permits study of genetically similar groups but living under different environmental conditions or exposure	▪ Comparison of disease and death rate for migrates with people local to geographic region ▪ This provides information on genetically different groups living in similar environment

Applications	*Limitations*
▪ To study varying pattern of disease in geographic locations ▪ To indicate duration of residence necessary to acquire susceptibility to diseases in question ▪ To find out specific environmental factors or life style change needed for disease to occur	▪ Lack of random assignment under observation ▪ Migration bias ▪ Action of specific environmental factors at certain critical point or certain specific age

Significance

- Migration studies have yielded a mine of information about role of possible genetic and environmental factors in regards to geographical variation of diseases.

MBBS PHASE III EXAMINATION

JUNE 2010

(Revised Scheme 2)

PAPER II

LONG ESSAYS

1. Discuss multicausation in diabetes. How do you control diabetes in district?

- Diabetes is a heterogeneous group of diseases, characterized by a state of chronic hyperglycemia resulting from diversity of etiologies, environmental and genetic acting together.

Clinical Classification

<table>
<tr><th colspan="9">A. Clinical cases</th><th colspan="2" rowspan="2">B. Statistical risk classes (Subjects with normal glucose tolerance but substantially increased risk of developing diabetes)</th></tr>
<tr><th colspan="5">I. Diabetes mellitus</th><th colspan="3">II. Impaired glucose tolerance (IGT) and impaire fasting glucose (IFG)</th><th rowspan="3">III. Gestational diabetes mellitus (GDM)</th></tr>
<tr><td rowspan="2">Insulin dependant diabetes mellitus (IDM. Type-1)</td><td colspan="2">Non-insulin dependant diabetes mellitus (NIDDM. Type-2)</td><td rowspan="2">Malnutrition related diabetes (MRD)</td><td rowspan="2">Other types of diabetes (associated with certain diseases as pancreatic disease, hormonal), drug induced, etc.</td><td rowspan="2">Non-obese</td><td rowspan="2">Obese</td><td rowspan="2">Associated with certain diseases</td><td rowspan="2">Previous abnormality of glucose tolerance</td><td rowspan="2">Potential abnormality of glucose tolerance</td></tr>
<tr><td>Non-obese</td><td>Obese</td></tr>
</table>

Epidemiology (Multicausation)—Epidemiological Determinants

Agent factors	
a. Insulin deficiency, either absolute (IDDM) and partial (NIDDM) due to	Pancreatic disorders ▪ Congenital, inflammatory, neoplastic, traumatic, surgical Defects in formation of insulin ▪ Synthesis of abnormal, biologically less active insulin Destruction of beta cells ▪ Viral infections, chemical agents Decreased insulin sensitivity ▪ Due to decreased numbers of adipocyte and monocyte insulin receptors Genetic defects ▪ Mutation of insulin gene Auto immunity

Contd...

Contd...

Host factors (Risk factors)	
a. Age	▪ Diabetes occurs at any age but prevalence rises steeply with age ▪ Type 1 diabetes is common among younger age group below 30 years whereas type 2 is among middle aged and elderly ▪ Younger the age at diagnosis, worse the prognosis
b. Sex	▪ Type 1 diabetes is common among men whereas type 2 among women
c. Genetic factors	▪ NIDDM is entirely genetic in origin (90%) but IDDM is not totally genetic in origin (50%) ▪ Susceptibility to diabetes is function of a defective gene, inherited as recessive Mendelian pattern
d. Genetic markers	▪ IDDM is associated with HLA-B8 and B15 and more powerfully with HLA-DR3 and DR4 ▪ NIDDM is not HLA associated
e. Immune mechanism	▪ Certain individuals exhibit both cell-mediated and humoral immunity against islet cells of pancreas
f. Obesity	▪ Obesity, particularly central obesity is a major risk factor for NIDDM and is related to both degree and duration of obesity however it has no role in IDDM pathogenesis ▪ Obesity increases insulin resistance and/or reduces number of insulin receptors on target cells
g. Maternal diabetes	▪ Children born to mothers with gestational diabetes are at higher risk of developing type 2 diabetes at early age ▪ Children of diabetic mothers are at 3times more risk of developing diabetes
Environmental factors	
a. Sedentary lifestyle[Q]	▪ An important risk factor for NIDDM by altering interaction between insulin and its receptors
b. Diet	▪ Intake of high saturated fat is associated with higher risk of impaired glucose tolerance, higher fasting glucose and insulin levels ▪ Diet rich in unsaturated fatty acids reduces risk of type 2 diabetes by lowering fasting and 2 hour glucose levels
c. Dietary fiber	▪ High intake of dietary fibers (through non-starch polysaccharides) reduces blood glucose and insulin levels in people with type 2 diabetes
d. Malnutrition[Q]	▪ Malnutrition in early infancy and childhood may result in partial failure of beta cells functions
e. Alcohol[Q]	▪ Excess alcohol intake increases risk of diabetes by damaging pancreas and liver and promoting obesity
f. Viral infections	▪ Viral infections like rubella, mumps, human coxsackie virus may trigger immunogenic reaction in susceptible individuals resulting in beta cells destruction
g. Chemical agents	▪ Chemical agents like alloxan, streptozotacin, etc. are toxic to beta cells
h. Stress and strain	▪ Stress situations like surgery, trauma, etc. may predispose to diabetes
i. Other factors	▪ Diabetes is also linked to other factors like occupation, marital status, religion, economic status, education, urbanization and changes in lifestyle

Screening Tests

- Commonly employed screening test for diabetes mellitus are urine and blood examination for presence of sugar in target population or high-risk groups.

Target Population

High-risk	*Routine*
▪ Age over 40 years ▪ Obesity ▪ Family history of diabetes ▪ Sedentary workers with lack of exercise	▪ Weight gain of more than 3 kg body weight in any one month of pregnancy ▪ Premature atherosclerosis ▪ Complaints of polyuria, polyphagia, polydypsia, sudden loss of weight, repeated infections, non-healing ulcer ▪ Expectant mothers at antenatal check-up ▪ Patients undergoing surgery ▪ Industrial recruits ▪ History of babies weighing more than 4.5 kg

Methods of Screening

a. Urine examination
   - Testing urine for glucose 2 hours after a meal using Benedict's test is commonly used screening test for diabetes and all the cases with glycosuria are considered diabetic unless otherwise proved by a standard oral glucose tolerance test
   - This method detects more of the milder cases of diabetes than a fasting urine specimen
   - Sensitivity of this test varies between 10–15% and specificity of the test is over 90%
   - Therefore, this test is not considered an appropriate tool for case finding or epidemiological surveys of the population.

Advantages	*Disadvantages*
Simple, easy and economical	Yields false positive and false negative depending upon the renal threshold

b. Blood sugar testing
   - Estimation of blood sugar level 2 hour after administration of 75 g glucose orally (postprandial) alone or with fasting value is used for epidemiological purposes
   - This test is also known as GTT.

Glucose tolerance test
- Glucose tolerance test or GTT is the gold standard test in diabetes screening (Confirmatory test)

Procedure
- Prior to the test patient is on a carbohydrate rich diet for 3 days
- For the test the patient is starved overnight
- A sample of blood and urine (fasting) are taken in morning
- A solution of glucose 75 g (1–1.5 g/kg body wt) in 250 mL of water is given to drink slowly to avoid vomiting
- Blood and urine samples are collected at ½ hour intervals for 2 ½ hours
- Glucose content of blood is determined by O-toluidine method and urine is checked for presence of glucose by Benedict's reagent.

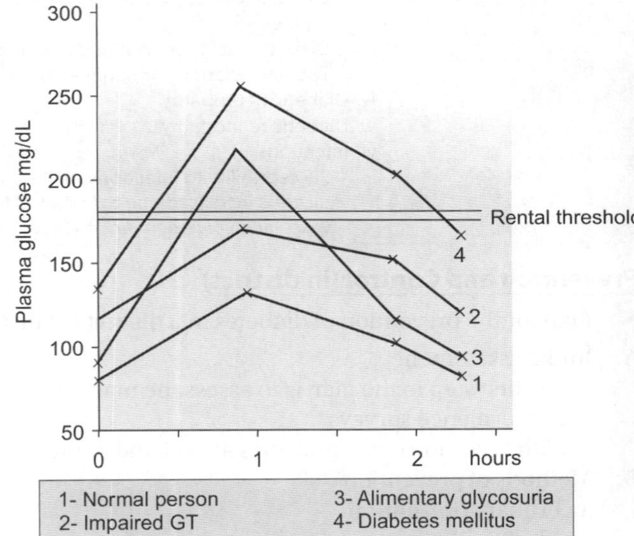

Fig. 1: Glucose tolerance test

Interpretation
- Criteria for diagnosis is prescribed by World Health Organization (WHO) is

	Glucose level (in mg/dl)			
	Whole blood		*Plasma*	
	Venous	*Capillary*	*Venous*	*Capillary*
Diabetes mellitus				
Fasting value[Q]	≥120Q	≥120Q	≥140	≥140
2 hours after glucose load	≥180	≥200	≥200	≥200
Impaired glucose tolerance				
Fasting value	<120	<120	<140	<140
2 hours after glucose load	120–180	140–200	140–200	160–220
Impaired fasting glucose				
Fasting value	≥100 but <110		≥110 but <126	

- Testing of blood for sugar level has become the cornerstone of diagnosis of diabetes.

Significance

- Early detection of diabetes through prompt screening can help control it and can prevent the complications (disability) arising due it.

Complications

- Complications of diabetes are seen in almost every tissue and organ of the body due to biochemical and structural alterations as a result of hyperglycemia.

Classification

Acute metabolic complications	*Late systemic complications (Seen in either type, after 15–20 years and responsible for morbidity and mortality)*
i. Diabetic ketoacidosis ii. Hyperosmolar nonketotic coma iii. Hypoglycemia	i. Atherosclerosis ii. Diabetic microangiopathy iii. Diabetic nephropathy – Diabetic glomerulosclerosis which are diffuse and nodular lesions of glomerulosclerosis – Vascular lesions such as hyaline arteriosclerosis of afferent and efferent arterioles and atheromas of renal arteries – Diabetic pyelonephritis and necrotizing renal papillitis – Tubular lesions or Armanni—Ebstein lesion iv. Diabetic neuropathy v. Diabetic retinopathy vi. Infections – Susceptibility to infections such as tuberculosis, pneumonias, pyelonephritis, otitis, carbuncles and diabetic ulcers is increased due to impaired leukocyte function, reduced cellular immunity, poor blood supply due to vascular involvement and hyperglycemia per se

Prevention and Control (in district)

- Plan for the prevention of diabetes in a district (or PHC) is formulated and executed as follows.

A. Initial assessment
  - The first step in the plan is to assess the magnitude, geographical distribution and causes of diabetes in the region by prevalence surveys
  - With this knowledge priorities are set and appropriate intervention program is developed

B. Methods of prevention
  a. Primary prevention
    i. Population strategy
      - In this strategy, the efforts are directed towards the children and adults from harmful lifestyles, so that there will be elimination or modification of risk factors
      - This done through mass education on following issues
        - Improvements in the nutritional habits like avoiding sweets, fatty foods, alcohol, and regular intake of proteins, dietary fiber rich foods
        - Maintenance of body weight by doing moderate exercise.
    ii. High-risk strategy
      - People at high-risk should be screened for diabetes by urine and blood examination

High-risk people	*Preventive care*
▪ Age over 40 years ▪ Obesity ▪ Family history of diabetes ▪ Sedentary workers with lack of exercise ▪ Weight gain of more than 3 kg body weight in any one month of pregnancy ▪ Complaints of polyuria, polyphagia, polydypsia, sudden loss of weight, repeated infections, non-healing ulcer ▪ Expectant mothers at antenatal check up ▪ History of babies weighing more than 4.5 kg	▪ Correction in obesity ▪ Avoiding over nutrition and alcohol ▪ Changing lifestyle ▪ Regular exercise ▪ Maintenance of normal body weight ▪ Avoidance of oral contraceptives and steroids ▪ Reduction of factor promoting atherosclerosis like hypertension, smoking, cholesterol level, etc.

b. Secondary prevention
   i. Early diagnosis and treatment
      - High risk screening in people at risk for early diagnosis
      - Treatment of diagnosed cases.

      Objectives
      - To maintain blood glucose levels as close within the normal limits as is practicable
      - To maintain ideal body weight.

      Treatment regimens
      - Diet alone: Small balance meals with plenty of raw vegetables and less cereals more frequently and no fast and no feast
      - Diet and antidiabetogenic drugs: Restriction of diet along with antidiabetic drugs for type II DM
      - Diet and insulin: Restriction of diet along with insulin for type I DM and uncontrolled type II DM and in emergency situations.
   ii. Self-care
      - Self-care in diabetes mellitus means that the diabetic should take a major responsibility for his own care with medical guidance.

      Components of self-care

a. Personal hygiene	▪ Maintain a high standard of personal hygiene from head to toe. ▪ Take protective care of the feet as follows: – For changes in color, temperature, swelling, cracks and wounds – To always use diabetic footwear while walking – To keep the feet clean, dry and warm – To file the nails and not to cut them – To change the socks daily – To ensure that there are no stone/nails inside the footwear
b. Habits	▪ Avoid smoking (predisposes to coronary artery disease), alcohol (predisposes to obesity and damages liver and pancreas) and steroids (lowers immunity)
c. Exercise	▪ Do moderate exercise regularly
d. Diet	▪ Strict prohibition of sweets, bakery products, fatty foods and junk foods ▪ Unrestricted intake of leafy vegetables and dietary fibers ▪ Restricted intake of beet root, potato, sweet potato and refined cereal products like maida, noodles, etc. ▪ Adequate intake of proteins ▪ Avoidance of egg yolk ▪ Small but frequent balanced meals ▪ No fast and no feast
e. Treatment	▪ Should take the treatment daily and regularly ▪ Should administer insulin by self
f. Self-examination	▪ Of urine for sugar and protein ▪ Of blood sugar

      Significance
      - Self-care is a crucial element in secondary prevention of diabetes mellitus and has yielded rewarding results.

c. Tertiary prevention
   i. Disability limitation
      - Consists of giving an intensive treatment in diabetic clinics in diabetic person who comes late with complications
   ii. Rehabilitation
      - Directed towards disabled and handicapped due to complications resulting in blindness, amputation of leg, etc.
      - They are rehabilitated physically, mentally, socially, psychologically and vocationally.

C. Long-term measures
   – These measures are aimed at improving the quality of life and modifying or attacking the factors responsibly for persistence of diabetes like sedentary lifestyle, obesity, etc.
   – Health education is another measure to create community awareness, to motivate the community and to secure community participation.

D. Evaluation
 - Evaluation should be done to measure the extent to which diabetes has been controlled, asses the manner and degree of activities carried out determine the nature of other changes produced.

Significance

- Diabetes is an "iceberg" disease
- There is increase in both the prevalence and incidence of type 2 diabetes, which could be attributed to the increased susceptibility of Indians to diabetes mellitus.

2. Discuss briefly the functions and organizational aspects of ICDS scheme.

- Integrated Child Development Services (ICDS) scheme was initiated by the Government of India in Ministry of Social and Women's welfare in 1975[Q]
- However, nodal ministry for ICDS scheme is Ministry of Human Resource Development[Q]
- It is a centrally sponsored program[Q].

Objectives

- To improve the nutritional and health status of children in age group of 0–6 years and mothers[Q]
- To lay foundations for proper psychological physical and social development of the child
- To reduce incidence of mortality, morbidity, malnutrition in children and mothers and reduce school dropout rate
- To reduce the incidence of low birth weight babies
- To provide non-formal preschool education to children in age group of 3–6 years
- To achieve effective coordination of policy and implementation amongst the various departments to promote child development
- To enhance capability of mothers to look after the normal health and nutritional needs of the child through education regarding health and nutritional needs of children.

Strategy

- Simultaneous delivery of primary health care services in an integrated package consisting of:
  - Supplementary nutrition[Q]
  - Immunization[Q]
  - Health check-ups[Q]
  - Medical referral services
  - Nutrition and health education for women
  - Non-formal education[Q] of children up to age of 6 years and pregnant and nursing mothers in rural, urban and tribal areas.

Organization Structure

(*See* Fig. 2)

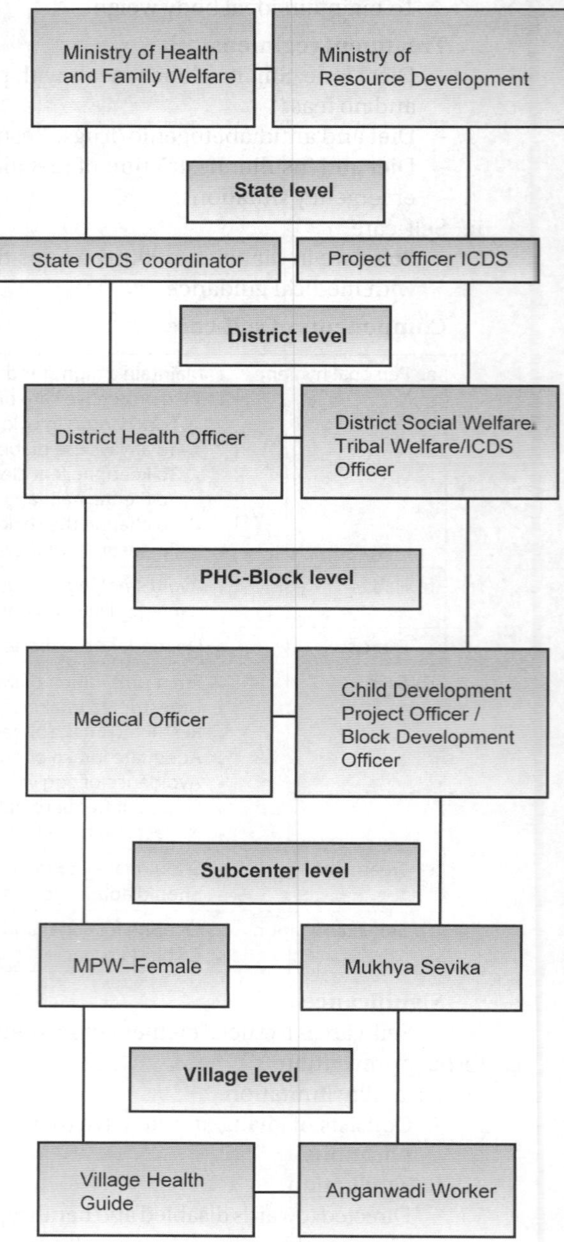

Fig. 2: Organization structure of ICDS

Abbreviations: ICDS, Integrated Child Development Service; MPW, Multipurpose worker

Revised Scheme 2

ICDS Program – Organization Structure

Level	*Personnel*	*Functions*
National	Secretary to Department of Social Welfare	▪ National coordinator
State	Director of health services	▪ State coordinator
District	District health officer	▪ Chief Program officer (District coordinator)
Block (Community development block per 100000 population[Q] covering about 100 villages or tribal development block per 35000 population[Q] covering about 50 villages. It is administrative unit of ICDS program in rural area[Q])	Child development project officer ▪ Qualified medical graduate, trained for 2 months at National Institute for Public Cooperation and Child Development at Delhi in child development, accounting, finance management, survey techniques and community organization ▪ As per Govternment of India proposal, this post should be held by a woman	▪ Chief administrative officer incharge of 100 Anganwadi centers ▪ In-charge of 4 Mukhya sevika ▪ He guides, supervises, directs and monitors the program ▪ He submits the report periodically to the District coordinator
Sector	Mukhya sevika (Lady health assistant) ▪ Graduate lady with training in Department of Social Welfare for 3 months	▪ Supervisor of 20–25 anganwadi centers ▪ Acts as mentor to anganwadi workers ▪ Assists in record-keeping, visits of health personnel and organizing community visits ▪ Provides on the job training to anganwadi workers
Village (Anganwadi is the nucleus or heart[Q] of the ICDS program, located in the rural, tribal and urban slums at the rate of one Anganwadi for every 400–800 rural and urban slum population[Q] and 300–800 tribal population[Q]. It is managed by one anganwadi worker and one helper. One mini anganwadi center covers population of 150–500 (rural and urban) or 150–300 (tribal)	Anganwadi Worker (focal of ICDS service delivery) ▪ A multipurpose agent selected from the local community, usually studied up to atleast 10th std ▪ She is trained for 4 months in PHC in various aspects of health, nutrition, immunization, family planning, child development, record-keeping, community work and survey techniques ▪ She is a part-time worker[Q] and is paid an honorarium of ₹ 1500/- per month as stipend ▪ She is provided with a helper. ▪ She caters to about 170 children in 0–6 years age group and 30 expecting and 15 lactating mothers	▪ Anganwadi worker is in-charge of the anganwadi and provides the services under ICDS scheme to the population covered by the anganwadi ▪ She prepares the food daily and distributes among beneficiaries ▪ Records the weight of children once a month and thus monitor growth of children ▪ Plots the road to health card thus detects malnutrition[Q] early and manages 1st degree malnutrition by educating mother and refers 2nd, 3rd and 4th degree malnutrition to PHCs ▪ Gives health education and nutrition education to mothers and non-formal education to children ▪ Provides immunization to children and pregnant women ▪ She provides vitamin A syrup and iron and folic acid tablets ▪ Assists her supervisor and health worker female in carrying out their work ▪ Maintains the record of all her activities ▪ Attends monthly meetings and submits the report to Child Development Project Officer (DPO) ▪ Thus, she works at the grass root level constituting the link between the community and the health system

Beneficiaries (Irrespective of income of family[Q])

Beneficiaries	*Services*
i. Pregnant women	▪ Health check-up ▪ Immunization against tetanus[Q] ▪ Supplementary nutrition ▪ Nutrition and Health Education
ii. Nursing mothers	▪ Health check-up ▪ Supplementary nutrition ▪ Nutrition and Health Education
iii. Other women of 15-45 years	▪ Nutrition and Health Education
iv. Children below 3 years of age	▪ Supplementary nutrition ▪ Immunization ▪ Health check-up ▪ Medical referral services

Contd...

Contd...

Beneficiaries	*Services*
v. Children in age group of 3–6 years	▪ Supplementary nutrition ▪ Immunization ▪ Health check-up ▪ Medical referral services ▪ Non-formal education
vi. Adolescent girls in age group of 11–18 years	▪ Supplementary nutrition ▪ Nutrition and health education

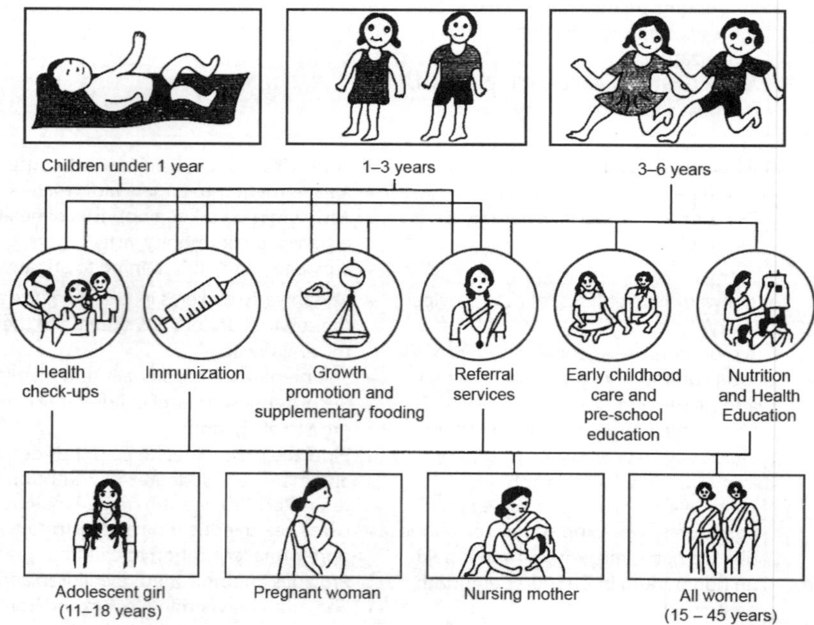

Fig. 3: ICDS program—beneficiaries and services

Services Provided (Activities of Anganwadi Center)

a. Supplementary nutrition[Q]
   - Supplementary nutrition is provided to children below 6 years and nursing and expectant mothers from low income group
   - Type of food depends upon the local availability, type of beneficiary, location, etc.
   - Supplementary nutrition is provided 300 days in a year[Q] and 65 days are vacation days.

Calorie and protein provision

Beneficiary	*Calories*	*Proteins*
Child 0–1 years	500 cal[Q]	12–15 g[Q]
Child 1–6 years	500 cal[Q]	12–15 g[Q]
Adolescent girls	500 cal	20–25 g
Pregnant and nursing mother	600 cal[Q]	18–20 g[Q]
Malnourished child	800 cal	20–25 g

   - For children with 1st degree malnourishment, their mothers are provided nutrition education and health education
   - Children with 2nd and 3rd degree malnourishment are provided therapeutic food
   - Children with 4th degree malnourishment are referred for hospitalization.

b. Nutrition and Health Education[q]
   – Education on nutrition and health care is given to all the women in age group of 15–45 years with priority to nursing and expectant mothers through specially organized courses in village during home visits by anganwadi workers.
c. Immunization[Q]
   – Children below age of 6 years are immunized for vaccine preventable diseases as per National Immunization Program and the expectant mothers are immunized against tetanus.
d. Health check-up
   i. Antenatal care of expectant mothers
      - Tetanus toxoid immunization
      - Iron and folic acid tablets
      - Protein supplementation
      - Referral of high-risk mothers to higher centers for special care
   ii. Postnatal care of nursing and care of newborn
   iii. Health care of children under 6 years
      - Record weight and height of children at periodical intervals
      - Watch over developmental mile stones
      - Immunization
      - General check-up every 3–6 months to detect diseases, malnutrition, etc.
      - Treatment of diseases like diarrhea, dysentery, respiratory tract infections, etc.
      - Deworming
      - Prophylaxis against vitamin A deficiency and anemia
      - Referral of serious cases to hospital.
e. Non-formal preschool education[Q]
   – Children between age group of 3–6 years are provided non-formal preschool education in each village with about 1,000 population
   – It is provided 3 hours per day in the form of play, toys, games, songs, pictures, etc.
   – There is no rigid curriculum of learning.

   Objectives
   – To provide opportunities to develop desirable attitudes, values and behavior pattern among children
   – To prepare the child for future school
   – To prevent future school dropouts
f. Kishori Shakti Yojana
   – It is renamed version of adolescent girl scheme of ICDS

Objectives	*Beneficiary*	*Strategy*	*Services*
▪ To improve the nutritional and health status of adolescent girls ▪ To promote self-development, health awareness, hygiene, nutrition and family life and child care	▪ Adolescent girls aged 11–18 years	i. Adolescent girls scheme I – For girls aged 11–15 years – Girls to girl approach is used ii. Adolescent girls scheme II – For girls aged 11–18 years – Balika mandals provide services	▪ Supplementary nutrition ▪ Health education of preventive health, hygiene and nutrition ▪ Family life education ▪ Participation in creative activities, working of anganwadi ▪ Skill development or vocational training ▪ Learn about significance of education and life skills, personal hygiene, environmental sanitation, nutrition, home nursing, first aid, communicable diseases, VPDs, family life, child care and development, constitutional rights and their impact on quality of life

   Significance
   – Kishori Shakti Yojana covers about 2000 ICDS projects
g. Supportive services
   – Other supportive services like family planning, safe drinking water supply, sanitation, functional literacy for adult women, etc. are encouraged.

Achievement

- Establishment of 5,78,457 anganwadi centers
- About 403 lakhs of children under 6 yeas of age provided supplementary nutrition
- About 24 lakhs adolescent girls covered under Kishori Shakti Yojna
- About 81.05 lakhs of pregnant and nursing mothers covered.

Significance

- ICDS program is a unique, single, largest, multisectorial, outreach National Program in the world for welfare of the mother and children of our country with an in build monitoring system
- Currently, it is most important scheme in field of child welfare making both a preventive and a developmental effort
- It is one of the world's largest program for early childhood development[Q].

SHORT ESSAYS

3. Describe the IPPI (Intensified Pulse Polio Immunization) program.

Refer Question No. 1 June 2014 (RS2) Paper II.

4. Assessment of obesity.

- Obesity is defined as an excess of adipose tissue that imparts health risk, a body of 20% excess over ideal weight for age, sex and height is considered health risk[Q1]
- It is commonly defined as a body mass index of 30 kg/m^2 or higher.

Assessment of Obesity

- Although obesity can be easily identified on vision but a precise assessment requires measurements and reference standards.

a. Body weight
   - Body weight though not an accurate measure of excess fat, but is the most widely used index
   - + 2 standard deviations from the median weight is considered cut-off point for obesity in epidemiological studies.

b. Ponderal index[Q]

$$\text{Ponderal index}^{Q} = \frac{\text{Height (cm)}^2}{\text{Cube root of body weight (kg)}^2}$$

c. Corpulence index[Q]

$$\text{Corpulence index} = \frac{\text{Actual body weight of the individual}}{\text{Expected body weight}}$$

   - Corpulence index of 1.2 or more is considered as obesity[Q]
   - It height independent criterion for obesity[Q]
   - The expected body weight for an individual is calculated by two methods.
     i. Broca's method
        - Expected weight (kg) = Height (cm) – 100
     ii. Lorentz's methods

$$\text{Expected weight (kg) in males} = \text{Height (cm)} - 100 - \frac{\text{Height (cm)} - 150}{4}$$

$$\text{Expected weight (kg) in females} = \text{Height (cm)} - 100 - \frac{\text{Height (cm)} - 150}{2}$$

d. Body mass index[Q]
   - Body mass index (BMI) is widely used and internationally most accepted indicator of obesity
   - It is also called Quetelet's index[Q], named after a Belgium scientist Lambert Adolph Jacques Quetelet.

Calculations[Q]

- BMI is based on the weight and height of the individual.

$$\text{Body mass index} = \frac{\text{Weight (kg)}}{\text{Height}^2\ \text{(m)}}$$

- BMI above 25 is considered obese and higher the BMI, higher the risk of morbidity[Q].

Interpretation

- Body mass index is used for classification of obesity as follows:

BMI (kg/m²)	*Classification*
<16.0	Grade III underweight
16.0–16.99	Grade II underweight
17.0–18.49	Grade I underweight
<18.5[Q]	Underweight[Q]
18.5–24.9[Q]	Normal range[Q]
>25[Q]	Over weight[Q]
25–29.9[Q]	Pre-obese[Q]
30–34.9[Q]	Obese class I[Q]
35–39.9[Q]	Obese class II[Q]
>40[Q]	Obese class III[Q]

Merits

- Universally accepted and most widely used indicator of obesity[Q]
- Independent of age
- Same for both sexes.

Demerits

- Does not distinguish between the weight associated with muscle and weight associated with muscle and weight associated with fat. As a result the relationship between BMI and body fat content may vary according to body build and proportion. Therefore, a given BMI may not correspond to the same degree of fatness across the populations
- Percentage of body fat mass increases with age group up to 60–65 years in both sexes and is higher in women than men of equivalent BMI.

Significance

- BMI helps in comparison of weight status within and between populations, helps in identification of at risk groups, for implementation of intervention programs and also for evaluation of program.

e. Skinfold thickness[Q]

- Based on the principle that a large proportion of body fat is located just under the skin and since it is most accessible, this method is most used method[Q].

Calculations

- Several varieties of calipers are available for measuring the skinfold thickness
- Herpenden skin calipers are good for estimation of skin fold thickness[Q]
- The measurements are taken at four sites namely, mid-triceps[Q], biceps[Q], subscapular[Q] and suprailiac regions
- Single best site is mid triceps[Q].

Interpretation

- The sum of the four measurements should not exceed 40 mm in boys and 50 mm in girls
- Skinfold thickness >18 mm in boys and >12 mm in girls at mid triceps indicate obesity

Merits

- Rapid and noninvasive method
- Easy and most accessible site of measurements.

Demerits

- Standards for comparison does not exist

- Poor repeatability
- Difficult to measure in extreme obesity.

f. Waist circumference
- Helps to measure abdominal fat
- Is an approximate index of intra-abdominal adipose tissue and total body fat.

Calculations
- Measured at the midpoint between the lower border of the rib cage and the iliac crest.

Interpretation
- In India, cut-off for waist circumference is 90 cm in males and 80 cm in females[Q].

Merits
- Convenient and simple measurement
- Not related to height and closely corresponds to BMI and waist-hip ratio
- Changes in waist circumference reflect changes in risk factors for cardiovascular diseases and other forms of chronic disorders like diabetes mellitus.

g. Waist-hip ratio
- Measures abdominal fat accumulation.

Interpretation
- Waist hip ratio of >1.0 in men and >0.85 in women indicates obesity[Q].

h. Waist height ratio
- WHO has declared waist height ratio as best indicator of cardiovascular risk.

Interpretation
- Cut-off is 0.5.

Merits
- Age and sex independent.

i. Others
- Measurement of total body water, of total body potassium and of body density are three other well-established and more accurate measurements used for estimation of body fat but are not used for routine purpose because of their complex nature.

Ref:
1. World Health Organization (2000); Technical report series 894: "Obesity: preventing and managing the global epidemic." (PDF), Geneva: World Health Organization. *ISBN 92-4-120894-5* dated 28th Aug. 2008.

5. Describe the natural family planning methods.

- Natural family planning methods are contraceptive measures without using any barriers or chemicals
- With this knowledge, a couple can avoid pregnancy, by abstaining from sex or by using a barrier method during the fertile time.

Failure rate	*Merits*	*Demerits*
▪ 5–20 per 100 WYE	▪ Simple, safe, effective, economical and immediately reversible	▪ Requires a long time of about 6 months to know the shortest and longest cycle ▪ Requires continuous cooperation and commitment of both the partners ▪ Hard to use if the woman has fever, vaginal infection or after child birth during breastfeeding ▪ Not effective in irregular cycles ▪ Does not protect against STDs including HIV/AIDS

Natural Family Planning Methods

a. Abstinence
- Only method of birth control which is completely effective[Q]
- Complete abstinence is easy to say but difficult to practice
- It amounts to repression of a natural biological necessity which may result in temperamental changes and even nervous breakdown.

b. Coitus interruptus (withdrawal method)
- Oldest method of voluntary fertility control[Q]
- In this method, during the act of intercourse, the male partner withdraws his organ at the time of climax, so that deposition of semen into the vagina is prevented.

Failure rate	*Merits*	*Demerits*
▪ 25 per 100 WYE	▪ Better than not using any method at all	▪ Difficult to practice ▪ Precoital secretion may contain sperms and result in pregnancy ▪ Delay in withdrawal results in pregnancy ▪ High failure rate

c. Rhythm method (calendar method, safe period method)
- Was described by Ogino[Q]
- In this method, the couple should avoid sex during the fertile period
- Before relying on this method, the woman records the number of days in each menstrual cycle for at least 6 months[Q].

Calculations
- First day of bleeding is counted as day 1
- Thus she should record the period of shortest and longest cycle
- Ovulation occurs from 12 to 16 days before the onset of menstruation with an average of 14 days
- Suppose, intercourse takes place on 10th day, and ovulation takes place on 12th day, fertilization can occur, because sperms live for 2 days
- Similarly if ovulation occurs on 16th day, even if sexual intercourse is performed on 17th day, fertilization can take place, because ovum lives for 1 day
- Thus period form 10th to 17th day is fertile period, provided her cycle is of 28 days regularly
- In case of variations in the cycle, to know the fertile period, subtract 18 from the length of the shortest cycle to get the estimated first day of the fertile period
- Then subtract 11 days from the length of the longest cycle[Q] to get the last day of the fertile period
- Couple should avoid sex or use condom during the fertile period.

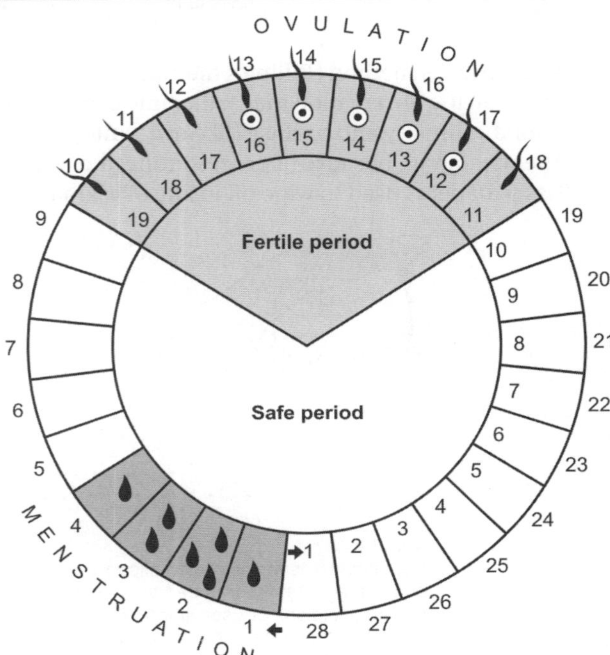

Fig. 4: Rhythm method

Failure rate	*Merits*	*Demerits*
▪ 21 per 100 WYE	▪ Simple ▪ Safe ▪ Effective ▪ Economical ▪ Immediately reversible	▪ Requires a long time of about 6 months to know the shortest and longest cycle ▪ Requires continuous cooperation and commitment of both the partners ▪ If the cycles are irregular (as in most of the women) it is difficult to predict fertile period and safe period ▪ If the couples are illiterate, it is difficult to practice ▪ Compulsory abstinence during the fertile period or condom to be used ▪ Not applicable during postnatal period ▪ High failure rate ▪ Not effective in irregular cycles ▪ Does not protect against STDs including HIV/AIDS ▪ Medical complications like ectopic pregnancies and embryonic abnormalities

d. Basal body temperature
- Depends upon an event that basal body temperature rises by about 0.3–0.5°C on the day of ovulation[Q], because of an increase in the progesterone level[Q]
- Woman should record her temperature daily in the morning, at the same time, before she gets out of the bed

- Method is reliable if the couple avoid sex or use condom from the first day of the cycle till the day the woman's temperature is raised and also if the couple restrict the intercourse to the post-ovulatory safe period, commencing 3 days after the rise of basal body temperature.

Failure rate	Merits	Demerits
▪ 20 per 100 WYE	▪ Simple ▪ Safe ▪ Effective ▪ Economical ▪ Immediately reversible	▪ Difficult to practice, if couples are illiterate ▪ Practically difficult to record the temperature daily and adopt ▪ Compulsory abstinence during the entire preovulatory period or condom to be used ▪ Hard to use if the woman has fever, vaginal infection ▪ High failure rate ▪ Does not protect against STDs including HIV/AIDS

e. Cervical mucus method (Billing's method[Q]/ovulation method[Q])
   - Based on the observation that at the time of ovulation, the cervical mucus becomes watery, can be stretched, clear, smooth, slippery and profuse (like egg white)
   - After ovulation, because of progesterone, the mucus thickens and lessens in quantity
   - Tissue paper is used to wipe off inside of vagina and mucus is analyzed.

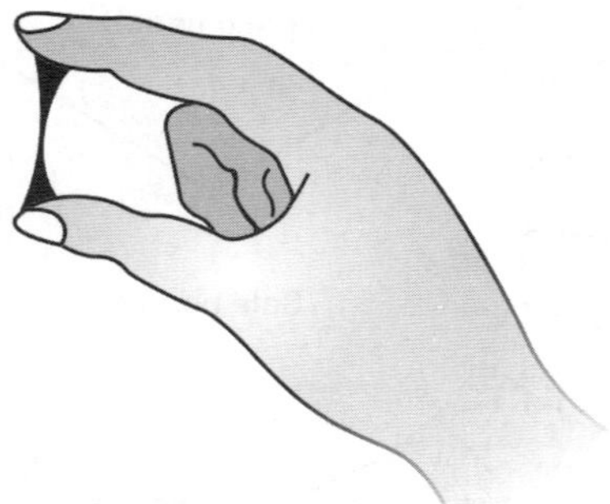

Avoid sex
Secretions – especially when slippery, wet, and can be stretched – mean the couple should avoid sex or use withdrawal or a barrier method until the 4th day after the peak day.

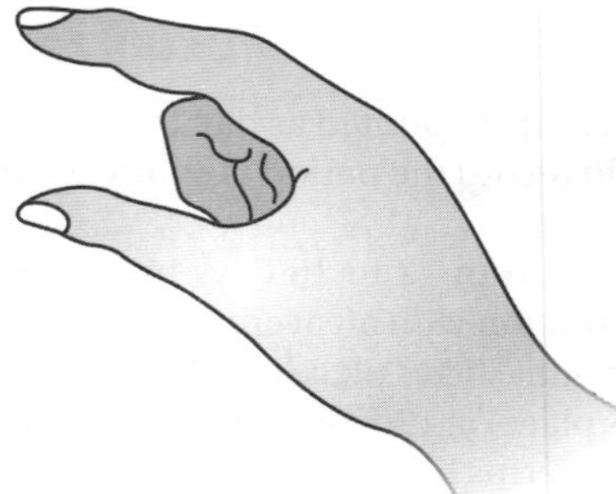

Can have sex
No secretions – mean the women probably cannot become pregnant. She can have unprotected vaginal sex

Fig. 5: Cervical mucus method

Merits	Demerits
▪ Simple ▪ Safe ▪ Effective ▪ Economical ▪ Immediately reversible	▪ Requires a high degree of motivation to the women ▪ Difficult to practice, if couples are illiterate ▪ High failure rate ▪ Does not protect against STDs including HIV/AIDS

f. Feel of the cervix
   - As the fertile time begins, the cervix opens slightly and cervix is felt soft and moist
   - During the remaining period the cervix is firm and closed.

g. Symptothermal method (Multiple indicator method)
   - This method consists of a combination of basal body temperature and Billing's method[Q] and also rhythm method and feel of the cervix
   - More effective than Billing's method.

h. Lactational amenorrhea method
   - This method is based upon the beneficial effect of exclusive breastfeeding in a lactating mother, because exclusive breastfeeding is associated with increased prolactin level, which prevents ovulation, thus protecting the mother from pregnancy, in a natural way

– Thus this method is effective when:
  - Mother practices exclusive breastfeeding
  - Her menstrual periods have not returned
  - Her child is less than six months of age
– When weaning is started, protection from pregnancy decreases because of decrease in prolactin level thus this method is very effective up to first six months
– However, if she keeps breastfeeding more frequently, protection from pregnancy may last even longer.

Failure rate	*Merits*	*Demerits*
▪ 0.5–2 pregnancies per 100 WYE	▪ Simple, safe and effective, especially during the first six months after child birth ▪ Encourages scientific practice of breastfeeding ▪ No direct cost for family planning ▪ No hormonal side effects ▪ Child gets all the benefits of exclusive breastfeeding ▪ Encourages the mother to start a follow on method after 6 months	▪ Effectiveness after 6 months is not certain ▪ Frequent feeding is difficult for working mothers ▪ Does not protect against STDs including HIV ▪ If the mother is HIV positive, there is a risk of transmission to the baby

6. Describe the purpose and recommendations of Shrivastav Committee.

- Shrivastav Committee or "Group on Medical Education and Support Manpower[Q]" was appointed by the Government of India in 1974 under the chairmanship of Dr JB Srivastav; Director General of Health Services; Government of India
- The committee submitted its report in April 1975.

Objectives

- To study the medical education and health care delivery system in India
- To devise a suitable curriculum for training a cadre of health assistants so that they can serve as a link between the qualified medical practitioners and the multipurpose workers thus forming an effective team to deliver health care, family welfare and nutritional services to the people
- To suggest steps for improving the existing medical education processes as to provide due emphasis on the problems particularly relevant to national requirements
- To make any other suggestions to realize above objectives and matters incidental thereto.

Recommendations

- **Creation of band of paraprofessional and semiprofessional health workers from within the community[Q]** itself like teachers, postmasters, gram sevaks, etc. to provide simple preventive, promotive and curative services to the community
- Establishment of 2 cadres, namely multipurpose health workers[Q] and health assistants[Q] between community health workers and medical officers at Primary Health Centers
- Development of a referral services complex[Q] by establishing proper linkage between the primary health center and higher referral and service centers
- Establishment of Medical and Health Education Commission[Q] for planning and implementing reforms needed in health and medical education on lines of University Grants Commission
- Reorientation of Medical Education (ROME) to medical students and health workers[Q]
- Introduction of village health guide (community health worker) scheme[Q]
- Establishment of 3 tier rural health infrastructure[Q] (Panchayat - Panchayat Samiti - Zila Parishad).

Significance

- The current three tier health care delivery system in rural area is based on recommendation of Shrivastav Committee[Q].

7. Write short notes on National Health Policy.

- National Health Policy was formulated by the Ministry of Health and Family Welfare in 1982[Q] and was approved by the India parliament in 1983[Q]

- The goal of this policy was to achieve health for all by 2000 AD
- In the year 2002, this policy was revised to new National Health Policy 2002
- The revised goals of this policy were to achieve a level of health that will enable every individual a protective life (Primary Health Care[q]).

Salient points	*Objectives which received more attention were*
▪ Implementation of the program was given more importance under 5 year plans and 20 points program	▪ Training and support to voluntary health guides ▪ One Anganwadi worker and one trained dai per every 1,000 population ▪ Establishment of one subcenter per every 3,000 population in tribal areas and one per every 5,000 in plain areas ▪ Establishment of 1 PHC per every 30,000 population in plain area and 1 PHC per every 20,000 population in tribal areas ▪ Establishment of 1 community health center per every 100,000 120,000 population to provide specialist care

Goals

For 2005	▪ Eradication of polio and yaws by 2005[Q] ▪ Elimination of leprosy by 2005[Q] ▪ Establish integrated system of surveillance, health statistics and health accounting by 2005 ▪ Increase health sector spending from 5.5% to 7% of budget
For 2007	▪ Achieving zero level growth of HIV infection by 2007[Q]
For 2010	▪ Elimination of Kala azar by 2010[Q] ▪ Reduce prevalence of blindness to 0.5% by 2010[Q] ▪ Reduce mortality by 50% on account of tuberculosis, malaria, and other water-borne and vector-borne disease by 2010[Q] ▪ Reduction of IMR <30/1000 and MMR to 100/lakh by 2010[Q] ▪ Control of communicable diseases[Q] ▪ Increased utilization of health care facilities by the people from present 20% to >75% by 2010 ▪ Increased health expenditure of present 0.9% in GDP to 2% by 2010 ▪ Increase share of central grants to constitute >25% of total health spending ▪ Further increase state sector health spending to 8% of budget
For 2015	▪ Elimination of lymphatic filariasis by 2015[Q]

8. Briefly discuss the services of UNICEF.

- UNICEF (United Nations International Children's Emergency Fund) is one of the specialized agencies of the United Nations established in 1946[Q].

Aim

- Development of the child as a whole.

Offices

Headquarters	New York[Q]
Regional offices	
▪ Europe	Geneva
▪ Eastern and Sothern Africa	Nairobi
▪ West and Central Africa	Abidjan
▪ America and Caribbean	Bogota
▪ East Asia and the Pacific	Bangkok
▪ Middle East and North Africa	Amman
▪ South Asia	Kathmandu
▪ Japan	Tokyo
Central and Eastern Europe, Commonwealth of Independent states and Baltic states	Geneva

- It was renamed United Nations Children Fund in 1953 but still retaining the same abbreviation
- The Chief executive officer of UNICEF is the Executive director who is appointed by the Secretary General of United Nations
- UNICEF works in Close association with other UN agencies like WHO, UNDP, FAO and UNESCO.

Activities of UNICEF in India

a. Child health[Q] and Immunization[Q]
   - UNICEF has provided substantial support for the production of the vaccines and sera
   - It has supported India's BCG vaccination program[Q]
   - It has assisted creation of a penicillin plant near Pune, donated a DDT plant, and two plants for manufacturing of DPT and iodized salt
   - It has also assisted environmental sanitation program emphasizing safe and sufficient drinking water for drinking and household use in rural India
   - It is focused on providing primary health care to mother and child through emphasis on immunizations, safe water and adequate sanitation
   - These services are delivered economically at the village level through resident volunteers or part time primary health workers
   - The purpose is to reduce child illness and death but more importantly to improve the quality of life in villages.

b. Child nutrition[Q]
   - UNICEF gives high priority to improving child nutrition
   - It developed a low cost protein rich mixture for supplementing child feeding
   - In collaboration with FAO, it aids "applied nutrition" program through community development, agricultural extension, schools and health services to help the rural population to grow and eat the foods required for better child nutrition
   - UNICEF has supplied equipments for modern dairy plants in various parts of India
   - It also provided specific aid for intervention against nutritional deficiency disorders inform of large doses of vitamin A, iodine enrichment of salt and provision of iron and folate supplements
   - In 1991, UNICEF promoted the baby friendly hospital initiative to create awareness and promotion of breastfeeding practices and for this in collaboration with WHO it has formulated ten steps to successful breastfeeding
   - It association with FAO and WHO, it is encouraging development of national food and nutrition policies to make provision for child nutrition.

c. Family and child welfare
   - Care of the children is improved both within and outside their homes by means of parent education day—case centers, child welfare and youth agencies and women's clubs
   - These services are carried as part of health, nutrition and education[Q] or home economics extension programs
   - In September 1990, it organized Rights of the Child convention to spell out civil, political, economic and cultural rights of the child
   - Some of these rights are right to life, right to survival, right to development, right to highest standard of attainable health and right to constitute into an association or union.

d. Formal and nonformal education
   - UNICEF, in association with UNESCO is assisting Indian in the expansion and improvement of teaching science.
   - Science laboratories equipment, workshop tools library books, audio-visual aids are provided to educational institutions
   - Emphasis is on the kind of schooling relevant to the environment and future life of the children.

e. GOBI-FFF[Q]
   - GOBI is the new campaign of the UNICEF promoted to encourage 4 strategies for a child health revolution.

     G: Growth charts to better monitor child development
     O: Oral rehydration to treat all mild and moderate dehydration[Q]

B: Breastfeeding
I : Immunization against measles, diphtheria, polio, pertussis, tetanus and tuberculosis.

– Of late 3F's have been added to this campaign.
F: Family welfare (Fertility regulation)
F: Female literacy
F: Food supplementation

f. Urban basic services
- Since 1979, UNICEF is participating in urban basic services to upgrade basic services like health, nutrition, water supply, sanitation and education especially of children and women
- Overall objective is to improve the degree and quality of survival and development of the children of urban low – income families.

Significance

- UNICEF provides greater attention to the concept of Whole Child, i.e. long-term personal development of the child and to the development of the country in which they live
- This approach is known as Country Health Programming.

9. Describe the strategies adopted by the National AIDS Control Program.

Refer Question No. 2 June 2015 (RS2) Paper II.

10. Write about the epidemiological features of typhoid fever.

- Typhoid fever is acute infectious disease of small intestine, caused by *Salmonella typhi*, transmitted through fecal contaminated water, food and vegetables.

Epidemiological Features

Agent factors	
i. Agent	▪ Typhoid fever is caused *Salmonella typhi*, a Gram-negative, capsulated, flagellated, actively motile bacilli ▪ Salmonella paratyphi A and Salmonella paratyphi B are relatively infrequent causes ▪ Salmonella typhi possess 3 types of antigens – Group specific somatic or O antigen – Type specific flagellar or H antigen – Capsular or Vi antigen related to virulence ▪ Organism is sensitive to heat and chemicals ▪ Readily killed by heat at 60°C for 15 minutes and also by routine disinfectants like chlorine, bleaching powder, $KMnO_4$, cresol and formalin ▪ Commensal of human intestine but can also survive in environment like food, water, sewage, ice cream, soil, etc.
ii. Reservoir of infection	▪ Only known reservoir of infection are humans, either case or carrier ▪ A case may be an active clinical case or sublinical case ▪ Carriers may be classified into incubatory, convalescent (excrete bacilli for 6-8 weeks) or chronic (excrete bacilli for >1 year after clinical attack) carriers and into temporary or chronic and into intestinal, urinary or biliary carriers ▪ Carriers may shed organisms continuously or intermittently ▪ These carriers constitute submerged portion of ice in iceberg phenomenon
iii. Source of infection	▪ Main source of infection is feces of infected person and to some extent urine also ▪ Secondary sources are fecal contaminated water, food and fruits and vegetables, finger and flies
iv. Infective material	▪ Feces of cases and feces and/or urine of carriers
v. Incubation period	▪ 10–14 days[Q]
vi. Period of communicability	▪ Varies from several days to months or even years

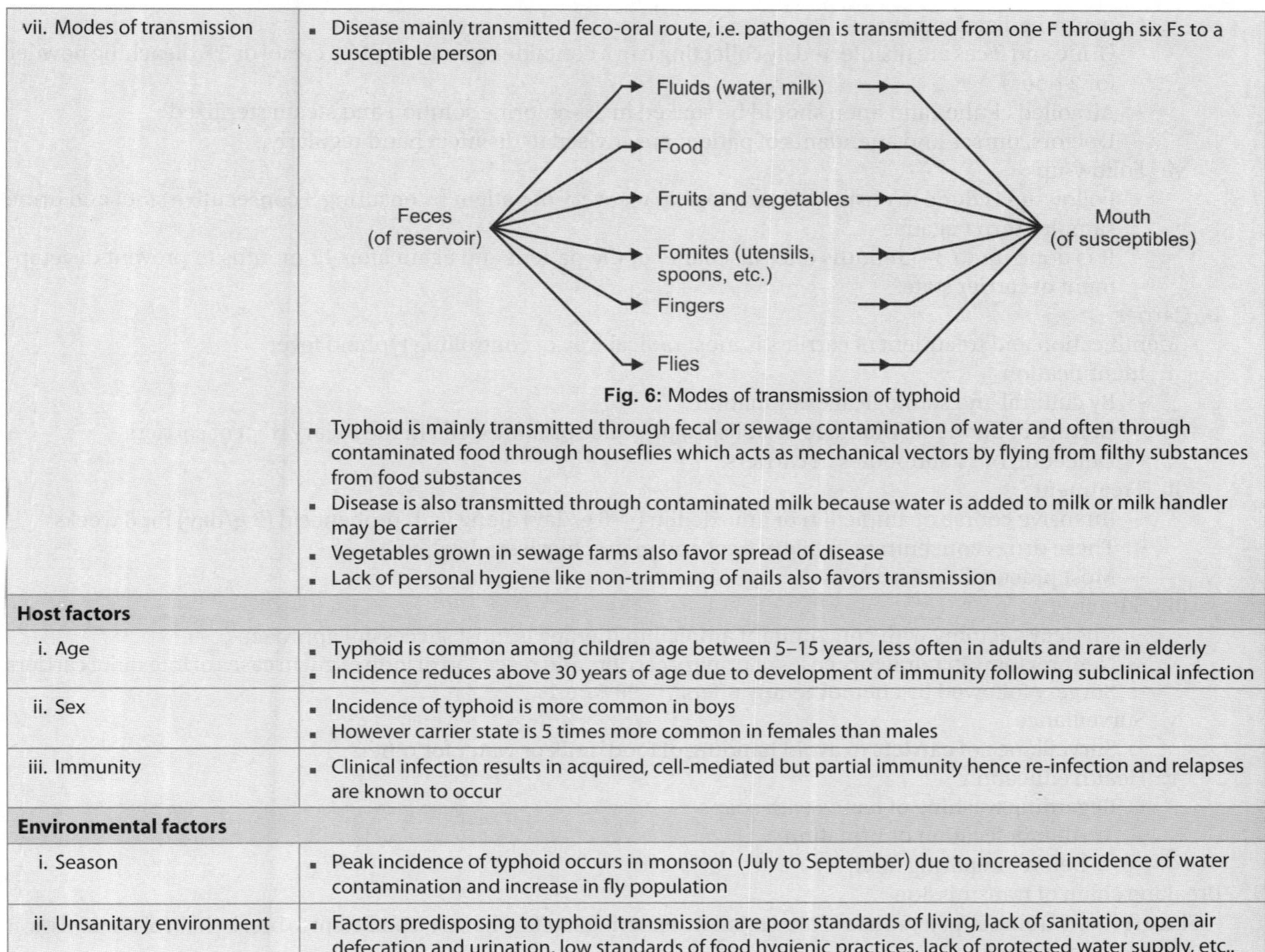

vii. Modes of transmission	▪ Disease mainly transmitted feco-oral route, i.e. pathogen is transmitted from one F through six Fs to a susceptible person **Fig. 6:** Modes of transmission of typhoid ▪ Typhoid is mainly transmitted through fecal or sewage contamination of water and often through contaminated food through houseflies which acts as mechanical vectors by flying from filthy substances from food substances ▪ Disease is also transmitted through contaminated milk because water is added to milk or milk handler may be carrier ▪ Vegetables grown in sewage farms also favor spread of disease ▪ Lack of personal hygiene like non-trimming of nails also favors transmission
Host factors	
i. Age	▪ Typhoid is common among children age between 5–15 years, less often in adults and rare in elderly ▪ Incidence reduces above 30 years of age due to development of immunity following subclinical infection
ii. Sex	▪ Incidence of typhoid is more common in boys ▪ However carrier state is 5 times more common in females than males
iii. Immunity	▪ Clinical infection results in acquired, cell-mediated but partial immunity hence re-infection and relapses are known to occur
Environmental factors	
i. Season	▪ Peak incidence of typhoid occurs in monsoon (July to September) due to increased incidence of water contamination and increase in fly population
ii. Unsanitary environment	▪ Factors predisposing to typhoid transmission are poor standards of living, lack of sanitation, open air defecation and urination, low standards of food hygienic practices, lack of protected water supply, etc..

Prevention and Control of Typhoid Fever

A. Elimination of reservoir
- Cases and carriers are major reservoir of typhoid bacilli.

a. Cases

i. Early diagnosis
- Early diagnosis of cases of utmost importance as early symptoms are non-specific
- Blood and stool cultures are vital investigations to diagnose cases.

ii. Notification
- Notification of outbreak should be done wherever it is mandatory.

iii. Isolation
- Since, typhoid is very infectious and has prolonged courses, it is always ideal to isolate cases
- Cases are isolated by hospitalization for about 2 weeks, i.e. till 2–3 consequent stool and urine cultures become negative.

iv. Chemotherapy
- Chemotherapy reduces duration of illness from 3–4 weeks to 3–4 days
- Cefotaxime (drug of choice) 200 mg BD for adults and 100 mg BD for children for about 10 days
- Severely ill patients can also receive hydrocortisone 100 mg IM daily for 3–4 days
- Symptomatic treatment.

v. Concurrent disinfection
- Urine and feces are disinfected by collecting it in a container containing 10% cresol or 8% bleaching powder for 2 hours
- All soiled clothes and linen should be soaked in 2% chlorine solution and steam sterilized
- Doctors, nurses and attendants of patient are advised to disinfect hand regularly.

vi. Follow-up
- Follow-up is done to ensure bacteriological recovery of patient by ensuring 3 consecutive stool and urine samples turn negative
- It is done up to 3–4 months after discharge of the patient and again after 12 months to prevent development of carrier state.

b. Carrier
- Identification and treatment of carriers is most radical way of controlling typhoid fever

i. Identification
- By cultural and serological examination
- Culture of duodenal drainage establishes presence of salmonella in the biliary tract of carriers
- Detection of Vi antibodies in carriers.

ii. Treatment[Q]
- Intensive course of ampicillin or amoxicillin (4–6 g/day) along with probenecid (2 g/day) for 6 weeks[Q]
- These drugs concentrate in bilary tract and may achieve eradication
- Most practical method[Q].

iii. Surgery
- Cholecystectomy with concomitant ampicillin therapy is most successful approach[Q]
- Nephrectomy in refractory cases of urinary carriers and resection of loop of gut in cases of intestinal carriers
- Surgery followed by chemotherapy offers 70–90% cure.

iv. Surveillance
- Surveillance of carriers to avoid handing of food, milk or water for others.

v. Health education
- Regarding washing of hands with soaps
  - o After defecation or urination
  - o Before preparing food.

B. Breaking chain of transmission
– Since feco-oral route is major mode of transmission, ensuring sanitary barrier is sufficient to break chain of transmission

a. Control of sanitation
- Construction and utilization of sanitary latrines prevents access of pathogen from feces to 6F's

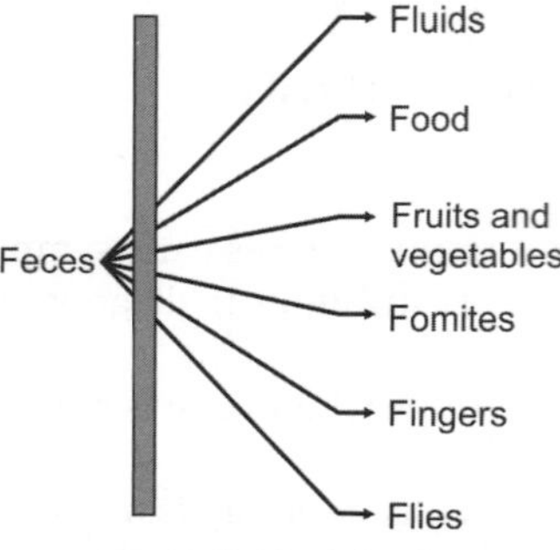

Fig. 7: Sanitary barrier

b. Other measures
- Chlorination of water for drinking purpose
- Pasteurization of milk
- Adoption of food hygienic measures
- Disinfection of fruits and vegetables with potassium permanganate
- Disinfection of fomites like utensils, and plates

- Adopting high standard of personal hygiene measures like trimming of nails, hand washing with soap after defection and before eating
- Control of houseflies by maintaining clean environment.

C. Protection of susceptible
  a. Health promotion
    - Provision of safe and chlorinated water
    - Sanitary disposal of sewage
    - Health education regarding
      - Use of sanitary latrines
      - Mode of spread of disease
      - Washing of hands after defection to act as sanitary barrier
      - Improvement in living conditions
      - Sanitation in and around the house
      - To maintain personal hygiene
      - To use protected water for drinking and cooking purpose
      - Disinfection of water on short scale, i.e. use of boiled and cooled water.
  b. Specific protection
    - Immunization is only specific protection against typhoid and is used as a complementary approach for prevention of typhoid.

Anti-typhoid vaccines

- Anti-typhoid vaccines offer active immunity against the typhoid fever.

Indications	*Efficacy*	*Types*
• General population in endemic areas • Household contacts • High-risk groups like school children, hospital staff • Travelers to endemic areas • Attendees of yatras and melas	85%[Q]	a. Killed (not longer used) i. Monovalent anti-typhoid vaccine ii. Bivalent anti-typhoid vaccine iii. TAB vaccine b. Live i. Ty21a vaccine c. Subunit i. Vi polysaccharide vaccine

Killed vaccines	*Live vaccines*	*Subunit vaccine*
	Ty21a vaccine[Q] (marketed as Typhoral[Q])	Typhim Vi polysaccharide vaccine
Contents		
a. Monovalent anti-typhoid vaccine – Contains only *S. typhi* (major cause of typhoid fever in India) – It is an agar grown, heat killed and phenol preserved vaccine containing 1,000 millions of *S. typhi* per mL – Known as AKD (acetone killed and dried) vaccine if it is prepared by inactivation of the organism with acetone b. Bivalent anti-typhoid vaccine – Contains S. typhi and S. paratyphi AQ – Killed vaccine containing 1,000 million and 500 million organism of S. typhi and *S. paratyphi* A respectively per mL which are killed by heating at 54°C for one hour and preserved by addition of 0.5% phenol – Can also be prepared by inactivation of organism with acetone in dried form c. TAB vaccine – Trivalent organism containing 1,000 million organisms of *S. typhi*, 500–750 million organisms of *S. paratyphi* A and 500–750 million organisms of *S. paratyphi* B per mL – However, they are been recommended by WHO for discontinuation due to their doubtful effectiveness and enhanced reactions due to paratyphoid A and B proteins	• It is an enteric coated capsule of lyophilized vaccine containing $>10^9$ viable organisms of the attenuated *S. typhi* strain of Ty21aQ • This registered strain is completely devoid of pathogenicity due to an irreversible change in cell wall biosynthesis	• Purified Vi capsular polysaccharide from Ty2 *S. typhi* strain • Each mL contains 50 µg of antigen

Contd...

Contd...

Killed vaccines	*Live vaccines*	*Subunit vaccine*
Storage (in refrigerator)		
• 2°–4°C but should not be frozen	• 2°–8°C	• 2–8°C
Shelf life (stability)		
• 18 months	• 14 days at 25°C	• 6 months at 37°C and 2 years at 22°C
Formulations		
–	• Capsules (for individuals ≥ 5 years) • Liquid (for young children >2 years)	• Liquid
Route of administration		
• Subcutaneously at outer aspect of upper arm, behind the posterior border of the deltoid muscle	• Oral	• Subcutaneously or intramuscularly
Dosage and Schedule		
i. Primary immunization – 2 doses, each of 0.5 mL for adults and 0.25 mL for children between 1 to10 years given at an interval of 4–6 weeks – Immunity develops in 10–21 days and offers protection for atleast 3 years[Q] ii. Booster doses – Recommended every 3 years – If booster is lapsed for more than 3 years then repeat the full primary course	i. Primary immunization – One capsule administered on days 1, 3 and 5[Q] irrespective of age for adults and children above 6 years of age one hour before a meal with cold or lukewarm milk or water – Protection commences 2 weeks after taking the last capsule and offers immunity for 3 years[Q] ii. Booster dose – Recommended every 3 years	i. Primary immunization – Single dose of 0.5 mL (25 µg of antigen) – Protection starts within 7days and lasts up to 3 years ii. Booster doses – Recommended every 3 years
Reactions		
• Local reactions—usual – Pain, swelling and tenderness • Constitutional symptoms—very frequent – Malaise, headache and pyrexia but usually subsides in 36 hours • To avoid reactions, it is advised to take late in afternoon or evening	• Nil	• Rare and include local pain, tenderness, swelling and pain
Contraindication[Q]		
• Late pregnancy[Q]	• Congenital or acquired immunodeficiency including treatment with immuno-suppressants and antimitotic drugs • Acute febrile illness and acute intestinal infection *Caution* • Do not administer oral antibiotics during the course as they may destroy the live vaccine strain	• Children below 2 years (does not illicit adequate immune response) • Acute febrile illness • Hypersensitivity reaction to vaccine components
Remarks		
• Discontinued since strong side effects	*Advantages* • Can be given simultaneously with other vaccines including live vaccines • Can be administered in HIV positive, asymptomatic individual with CD4 count >200/mm^3	*Advantages* • Can be coadministered with other vaccines recommended for international travel and routine childhood immunization • Safe for HIV infected individuals *Immune response* • T cell independent IgG response that is not boosted by additional doses • Does not illicit adequate immune response in children aged less than 2 years

Significance

- Typhoid is a very common communicable disease present in almost all over India in small endemic foci with regular epidemic outbreaks
- Tendency to turn chronic or carrier state are major reasons, that efforts should be directed to control and prevent spread of typhoid.

11. Discuss briefly about various levels of health care services.

- Health care services are delivered at three different levels involving varying degrees of complexity.

Level of Health Care Services

Primary care level	*Secondary care level*	*Tertiary care level*
▪ First level of contact[Q] of individuals, family and community where primary health care is provided *Infrastructure and manpower* ▪ Primary health centers and their subcentres[Q] along with their multipurpose health workers, village health guides, anganwadi workers and trained dais *Advantages* ▪ Close to people, where most of their health problems can be dealt with and resolved ▪ Bridges cultural and communication gap between rural population and organized health sector *Significance* ▪ Primary care level provides most effective health care in context of area's need and limitations ▪ To achieve Health for All by 2000, primary health care system has been reorganized and strengthened to make it more effective	▪ Intermediate level of health care dealing with more complexes problems ▪ Essentially curative services are provided ▪ Is first referral level of health care in India[Q] *Infrastructure* ▪ Taluka hospitals and community health centers	▪ Highest level of health care providing specialized care through specific facilities and highly qualified health workers ▪ Is second referral level of health care in India[Q] *Infrastructure* ▪ District hospitals and regional or central level institutions like Medical College Hospitals, All India Institutes, etc.

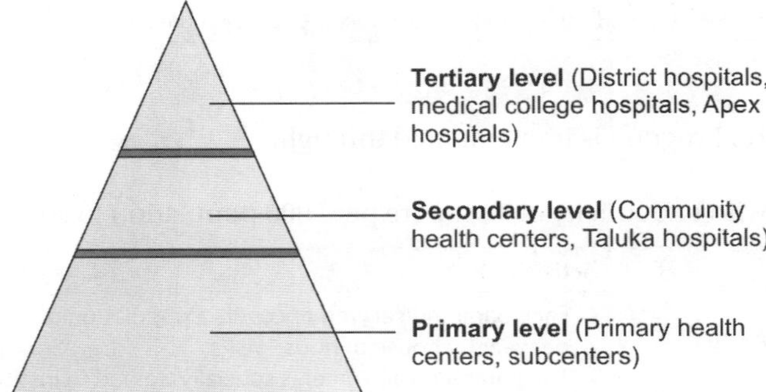

Fig. 8: Levels of health care

Significance

- Sound referral system through various levels of health delivery system is fundamental and necessary function of health care system
- This ensures continuity of care and inspire confidence of patient into health care services.

12. Describe the National Leprosy Control Program.

- National Leprosy Eradication Program, started by Government of India in 1983[Q] is a continuation of National Leprosy Control Program to eradicate leprosy from India by 2000AD by introducing multidrug therapy.

Components	Goals	Targets (by March 2017)	
▪ Dencentralized integrated leprosy services through general health care system ▪ Capacity building of all general health services functionaries ▪ Intensified information, education and communication ▪ Prevention of disability and medical rehabilitation ▪ Intensified monitoring and supervision	▪ Elimination of leprosy, i.e. prevalence of <1 case per 10,000 population[Q] in all districts ▪ Strengthen disability prevention and medical rehabilitation of leprosy affected person ▪ Reduction in level of stigma associated with leprosy	Prevalence rate (<1/10,000)	642 districts (100%)
		Annual new case detection rate (<10/100,000)	642 districts (100%)
		Cure rate of MBL	>95%
		Cure rate of PBL	>97%
		Grade II disability rate in new cases	1.98%
		Stigma reduction	50% over NSS report

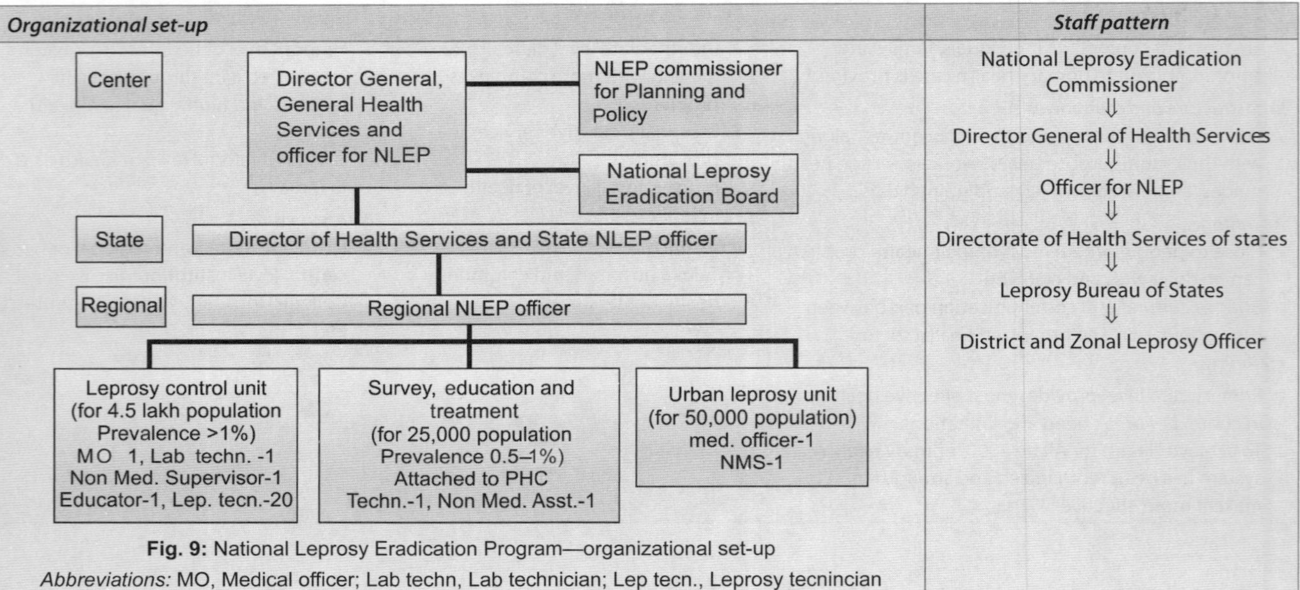

Fig. 9: National Leprosy Eradication Program—organizational set-up

Abbreviations: MO, Medical officer; Lab techn, Lab technician; Lep tecn., Leprosy tecnincian

Health Infrastructure

- National Leprosy Eradication Program is implemented through.

a. Leprosy control unit
   - It is established in areas with endemicity of 5 or more per 1000 population to cover population of 4.5 lakh[Q]

Organization pattern	Activities
▪ 20 paramedical workers ▪ 2 non-medical supervisors ▪ 1 medical officer	▪ Each paramedical worker covers a population of 20,000 and should visit 8000 persons per year by house to house visits ▪ The paramedical worker is specially trained to institute domiciliary treatment

b. SET (Survey, Education, Training) centers
   - There is one SET center for a population of 20,000–25,000[Q] in the endemic areas with prevalence rate less than 5 per 1,000 population[Q].
   - They are attached to the primary health center

Organization pattern	Activities
▪ One paramedical worker for each SET center ▪ One nonmedical supervisor for every 4–5 paramedical worker	i. Survey – Paramedical worker surveys the whole population to detect cases of leprosy including the school children – He looks for hypopigmented patches for loss of sensation over the body, in good day light with minimum clothes and palpates nerves for thickening

Contd...

Contd...

Organization pattern	Activities
▪ Medical officer of the PHC is the administrative and controlling head	– Such cases are referred to medical officer for confirmation ii. Education – Paramedical worker gives health education to the patient that leprosy is curable and he should take treatment correctly and completely – He educates the family that not all cases are infectious, it is caused by bacteria, there is treatment and that the patient should be shown sympathy and should not be thrown out of the family iii. Treatment – He provides the multidrug therapy for all paucibacillary cases with a combination of dapsone and rifampicin and all multibaciilary cases with dapsone, rifampicin and clofazinine iv. Contact tracing and their chemoprophylaxis

Significance

– SET centers are component of horizontal approach of National Leprosy Eradication Program in low endemic areas.

c. Urban leprosy unit (Under Urban Leprosy Control Program)
   – It is established in urban areas to cover population of 100,000[Q]

   Organization pattern
   – One nonmedical supervisor who functions under the supervision of the medical officer.

d. Mobile leprosy treatment units
   – It provides services to leprosy patients in nonendemic areas.

   Organization pattern
   – One medical officer
   – One nonmedical officer
   – One nonmedical supervisor
   – Two paramedical workers
   – One driver.

Strategies

Integrated leprosy services

a. Intensification of early case detection by
   – Population surveys (done if prevalence is 10/1000[Q])
   – School surveys
   – Contact information
   – Voluntary referral
b. Regular treatment with Shrut Course Chemotherapy with multidrug therapy

Type of leprosy	Drug	Adult dose	10–14 year child dose	Frequency of administration	Duration	Follow-up
Multibacillary (6 or more skin lesions and/or >1 nerve involvement)	Rifampicin[Q]	600 mg	450 mg	Monthly under supervision	12 months[Q]	Once a year for 5 years[Q]
	Dapsone[Q]	100 mg[Q]	50 mg	Daily self-administered[Q]		
	Clofazimine[Q]	300 mg	150 mg	Once monthly supervised		
		50 mg	50 mg*	Daily self-administered		
Paucibacillary[Q] (1–5 or more skin lesions and/or 1 nerve involvement)	Rifampicin[Q]	600 mg	450 mg	Monthly under supervision[Q]	6 months[Q]	Once a year for 2 years[Q]
	Dapsone[Q]	100 mg	50 mg	Daily self-administered[Q]		
Single skin lesion	Rifampicin	600 mg	450 mg	Single dose	Single dose treatment of ROM	
	Ofloxacin	400 mg	200 mg	Single dose		
	Minocycline	100 mg	50 mg	Single dose		

* Alternate days

Note: ROM therapy is discontinued and single skin lesion patients are treated at par with paucibacillary leprosy

June 2010 (Paper I)

d. Accompanied MDT
   - If patient is unable to come to collect his/her MDT from clinic, any responsible person from family or village can collect it[Q].

   Significance
   - Designed to help patients who have to interrupt their treatment due to any unavoidable reason
   - Especially useful for irregular patients
   - Gives patients a choice.

e. Health education of the patients, their families and the community about leprosy and its curability
f. Rehabilitation of cured patients
g. Prevention of deformities.

Newer Initiatives Under NELP

Focused leprosy elimination plan (2005)	*SAPEL and LEC[Q]*	*Accompanied MDT[Q]*
▪ Priority areas – Prevalence >3 per 10,000 ▪ Increased efforts on IEC, training and integrated service delivery ▪ Week long block leprosy awareness campaign	▪ Special action project for elimination of leprosy (SAPEL) in rural areas and leprosy elimination campaigns (LEC) in urban areas to cover population residing in difficult/inaccessible areas, which are not generally covered by regular program activities	

Achievements

- Cured cases (2011) — 90% (MBC)–95% (PBL)
- Indicators
  - Annual case load (2004) — 2.2 lakh
  - Prevalence rate of leprosy (2011) — 0.68 per 10,000 population
- Infrastructure (1995)
  - Number of leprosy control units — 781
  - Number urban leprosy units — 906
  - Number SET centers — 5,739
  - Number of mobile leprosy treatment units — 347

Significance

- With commitment by the Government for eradication of this crippling social disease, National Leprosy Eradiat on Program achieved the Leprosy Elimination Targets by December 2005[Q] in 15 states.

SHORT ANSWERS

13. Management of dengue hemorrhagic fever.

Refer Question No. 12 June 2012 (RS2) Paper II.

14. Secondary prevention of hypertension.

Refer Question No. 10 December 2012 (RS2) Paper II.

15. Prevention of measles.

Refer Question No. 1 December 2010 (RS2) Paper II.

16. Write briefly on cancer registries.

Refer Question No. 9 June 2012 (RS2) Paper II.

17. Enumerate the objectives of school health services.

Refer Question No. 4 December 2013 (RS2) Paper II.

18. What is network analysis?

Refer Question No. 6 December 2011 (RS2) Paper II.

19. How training of local dais is given?

- Traditional birth or local dais are the women which conduct the deliveries in rural India.
- They are called untrained dais until they are when they are as trained birth.
- They cater to a population of 1,000 people[Q].

Selection

- Should be female
- Should be the permanent resident of the area
- Should be acceptable to all sectors of the community.

Training

- Dais are trained in PHC or subcenters or MCH centers by the lady medical officer
- She is receives training for 30 working days and receives and 300 rupees during this training period
- Per week she spend 2 days at training center studying anatomy of the reproductive system, physiology of pregnancy and labour, observation for danger signals warranting referral, proper and aseptic precautions while conducting delivery and understanding when not to interference or understanding of their own limitations
- Main emphasis is on asepsis by following 5 cleans, i.e. clean hands, clean surface, clean blade, clean thread and clean stump
- For the rest of 4 days of week, they will accompany health assistant female to the villages, preferably the dais own village to gain on field experience, assist and conduct deliveries
- During the training period, the dai is required to conduct at least 2 deliveries under the guidance and supervision of the health worker female, ANM or health assistant female
- After completion of training, she receives a certificate and delivery kit containing sterile gauze, sterilized cotton thread, new razor blade, soap, polythene sheet and iodine.

Duties Assigned

- Conduct safe, aseptic deliveries[Q] in her village, for which receives ₹ 10/- for every registration[Q] in subcenter or PHC and she also receives ₹ 3/- for every newborn registered to her, however she is free to charge her fees for conducting delivery
- Promote family planning methods[Q]
- Refer complicated cases to PHCs or other higher centers.

Importance of Training Dais

- Age old practice of conducting delivery by dais is still prevalent
- Their skills are accepted by the people
- Not only rural people but also some of the urban areas take their help
- Female health worker may not be available all the time to conduct deliveries in her area
- About 90% of all deliveries are normal and do not require the services of the specialists
- Dais can be trained locally in PHCs
- Their training would improve the quality of MCH services
- This helps in community participation.

Significance

- Traditional birth attendants have reduced significant case of maternal morbidity and mortality and it is proposed to have all the deliveries conducted in village to be conducted by them.

20. How will you prevent juvenile delinquency?

Refer Question No. 10 December 2012 (RS2) Paper I.

21. Influenza vaccine.

- Influenza is an acute, febrile, highly infectious, respiratory viral disease characterized by sudden onset of fever, non-specific respiratory symptoms, malaise, headache and myalgia.

Influenza vaccine

- There are three types of influences vaccines available.

a. Killed vaccine (inactivated influenza vaccine)

Types	*Saline vaccine*	*Oil adjuvant vaccine*
	▪ Most commonly used	▪ Better than saline vaccine but less preferred
▪ Contents	▪ 15 µm of H antigen per dose in aqueous solution	▪ 15µm of H antigen per dose in oil emulsified preparation
▪ Dose	▪ 0.5 mL for adults and children above 3 years ▪ 0.2 mL for children above 6 months up to 3 years	▪ 0.2 mL
▪ Schedule	▪ 2 doses of 4 weeks apart ▪ Revaccination is recommended every year	▪ 2 doses of 4 weeks apart ▪ Revaccination is recommended every year
▪ Route of administration	▪ Subcutaneously or intramuscularly	▪ Subcutaneously
▪ Immunity	▪ 6 months	▪ 1 year
▪ Efficacy	▪ 70–90%	–
▪ Complications	▪ Fever, local inflammation at site of injection ▪ Hypersensitivity ▪ Guillain-Barre syndrome[Q]—very rare	▪ Sterile abscess and painful nodules

b. Live attenuated vaccine
   – Based on temperature sensitive (ts) mutant.

Route of administration	*Advantages*	*Disadvantages*
▪ Intranasally as nasal drops[Q]	▪ Induces both local and systemic immunity[Q]	▪ Difficult to produce effective new vaccine for every new antigenic mutation

c. Newer vaccines

Split virus vaccines[Q]	*Surface antigen vaccine*	*Neuraminidase specific vaccine*	*Recombinant vaccine[Q]*
▪ Highly purified subunit vaccine ▪ Also known as subvirion vaccine ▪ Recommended for children Advantages ▪ Fewer complications Disadvantages ▪ Require several injections because lesser antigenic	▪ Subunit vaccine containing only surface antigens H and N	▪ Subunit vaccine containing N antigen Advantages ▪ Reduces virus replication in respiratory tract and ability of virus to transmit ▪ Significantly reduces clinical symptoms ▪ Provides lasting immunity by permitting subclinical infection Disadvantage ▪ Induces antibody formation only to neuraminidase	▪ Vaccine containing desirable antigenic properties of virulent strain (artificial hybrid virus) prepared by recombinant technique

Significance

- Influenza vaccine at present offers best prospect of controlling of influenza however considering changing antigenic characteristic of virus, there is always a need for newer vaccine
- These newer vaccine to be effective should contain both H and N component of prevalent strains to keep it up-to-date.

22. Enumerate the health problems of the aged.

Refer Question No. 2 June 2009 (RS2) Paper II.

MBBS PHASE III EXAMINATION

DECEMBER 2010

(Revised Scheme 2)

PAPER I

LONG ESSAYS

1. Define screening. List and briefly describe the criteria for a good screening test. List and briefly describe the features of a disease which make it suitable for screening.

- Screening for disease is defined as the search for unrecognized disease[Q] or defect by means of rapidly applied tests, examinations or other procedures in apparently healthy individuals[Q].

Aims	*Objectives*
To sort out those having the disease and those not having the disease from a group of apparently healthy individuals	To provide treatment to those detected person, so that the disease is controlled in the community

Flowchart 1: Screening—procedure

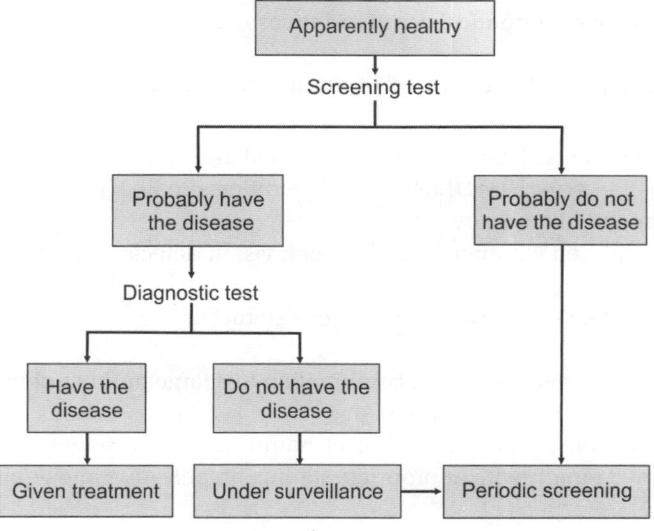

Methods

	Descriptive screening	*Prospective screening*
▪ Definition	▪ People screened for own benefit	▪ People screened for other's benefit
▪ Purpose	▪ Case detection	▪ Disease control
▪ Request	▪ No specific request	▪ Request from authority
▪ Examples	▪ Neonatal screening ▪ PAP smear ▪ Urine for diabetes mellitus	▪ Screening of immigrants ▪ Screening of HIV in sex workers

Types

a. Mass screening
   - Screening of a whole population or a subgroup
   - Offered to all irrespective of the particular risk individual carries of contracting the disease is question
   - Indiscriminate mass screening is not a useful preventive measure
   - Should be backed up by suitable treatment that will reduce the duration of illness or alter its final outcomes.

b. High-risk or selective screening
   - Screening if applied to selectively high-risk groups is most productive[Q]
   - For example, screening of lower socioeconomic group population for Ca. Cervix will yield more number of newer cases as it is more common in them
   - More recently instead of population, risk factors or the factors which apparently antedata the development of actual disease are screened
   - For example, people with elevated serum cholesterol have high risk of developing coronary artery disease
   - Advantage of screening for risk factors especially those of pathophysiological nature such as serum cholesterol and blood pressure is that these risk factors are amenable to effective intervention and this way preventive measure can be applied before the disease occurs
   - Other advantages are effective economical use of resources.

c. Multipurpose screening
   - Screening of a group of population by application of two or more tests, at one time to detect more number of diseases.

   Example
   - Screening of pregnant mothers with blood for Hb%, venereal disease research laboratory (VDRL), enzyme-linked immunosorbant assay (ELISA) for HIV, HBSAg, blood grouping and Rh typing
   - Urine for albumin, sugar and microscopy
   - Screening of all school children with height and weight, vision defects, hearing impairments, dental problems, congenital anomalies
   - Screening of elderly for diabetes, hypertension, cancer, cataract, etc.

d. Multiphase screening
   - Application of two or more screening tests in combination to a large number of people at one time than to carry out separate screening fests for single disease
   - Procedure may include a health questionnaire, clinical examination and a range of measurements and investigations
   - All these can be performed rapidly with appropriate staffing organization and equipment.

e. Opportunistic screening
   - Also called case finding screening where the screening is done for a patient who consults the doctor for some other purpose.

Flowchart 2: Multiphase screening

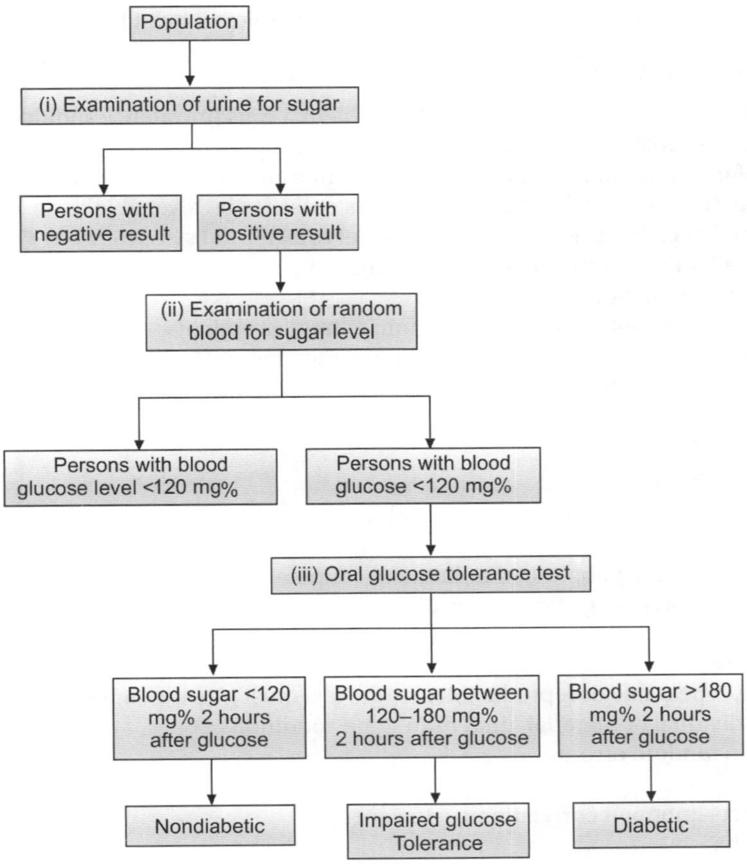

Population

(i) Examination of urine for sugar

Persons with negative result

Persons with positive result

(ii) Examination of random blood for sugar level

Persons with blood glucose level <120 mg%

Persons with blood glucose <120 mg%

(iii) Oral glucose tolerance test

Blood sugar <120 mg% 2 hours after glucose

Blood sugar between 120–180 mg% 2 hours after glucose

Blood sugar >180 mg% 2 hours after glucose

Nondiabetic

Impaired glucose Tolerance

Diabetic

Application

For case detection	*For control of disease*	*For research purpose*	*For educational purpose*
▪ People are screened for their own benefit ▪ Done so that disease can be detected early and treated early so that complications are prevented ▪ Such type of screening is also called prescriptive screening ▪ For example, screening of the newborn, of the pregnant mother for bacteriuria, detection of cancer cervix, diabetes, hypertension, etc.	▪ People are screened for the benefit of others, i.e. by early diagnosis and early treatment, further spread in the community can be prevented ▪ Such type of screening is called prospective screening ▪ For example, screening of the immigrants for HIV or pulmonary tuberculosis and syphilis ▪ It thus helps in reducing morbidity and mortality	▪ Screening helps to know more about the natural history of the disease ▪ For example, initial screening helps to know about the prevalence of disease and subsequent screening, the incidence ▪ Also gives information about risk factors and risk groups	▪ Screening procedure creates awareness among the people about the disease, thus educating the public

Significance

- Screening is an important component of primary level of intervention for early diagnosis of the diseases.

Criteria for Screening (Principles of Screening—WHO)

- Before initiating a disease screening program, the ethical, scientific and economical factors should be looked into for which the disease to be screened and the screening test to be employed must fulfill certain criteria.

Criteria for Diseases to be Screened

a. The condition sought should be an important health problem, i.e. its prevalence should be high[Q].
b. There should be a recognizable latent or early asymptomatic phase.
c. The natural history of the condition, including development from latent to declared disease should be adequately understood so that we can know at what stage the process ceases to be reversible.
d. There is a test that can detect the disease prior to the onset of signs and symptoms.
e. Facilities should be available for confirmation of the diagnosis.
f. There is an effective treatment for the condition.
g. There should be an agreed on policy concerning whom to treat as patients.
h. There is good evidence that early detection and treatment reduces morbidity and mortality.
i. The expected benefits of early detection exceed the risks and costs.

Criteria for Screening Test

a. Simplicity and applicability
   - It should be simple, safe, cheap and rapidly applicable.
b. Acceptability
   - It should be acceptable by the people so that they can cooperate
   - If the test is painful, embarrassing and causing discomfort like injection, per-rectal or per-vaginum examination, people will not cooperate.
c. Repeatability/Reliability
   - It should be reliable, repeatable or reproducible, i.e. the test must give the same results even after doing it repeatedly on the same individual or material, under the same conditions
   - Is inversely related to random errors
   - Measured by
     i. Pearson product—moment correlation coefficient
     ii. Cronbach's alpha
        - Depends upon

i. Observer variations	• Intraobserver or within observer variations – Variation observed in the test result, when the same observer applies the test on one individual at different times under identical situations – Can be overcome by taking average of several readings – Example: Recoding of blood pressure. • Interobserver or between observer variations – Variation observed in the test result when two or more observer apply the same test on one individual under identical conditions – Can be minimized by standardization of the procedures, intensive training of the observers and using of two or more observers for independent assessments; however, it is difficult to eliminate it completely – Example: Differential leukocyte count
ii. Biological variations (Subject variation)	• Variation observed in the test result in the same individual, when applied under identical conditions • May be due to changes in the parameters observed, variations in the way patients perceive their symptoms and answer and regression to the mean • Can be overcome by repeat measurements over time • Example: Variations in pulse rate.

Contd...

Contd...

iii. Mechanical variations	• Variation observed in the test result due to defect in the machine or procedure • Large number of such errors may limit the repeatability and single test results may be unreliable • Can be overcome by checking the machine or the procedure • For example: Defective instrument, erroneous calibrations, faulty reagents, etc.

d. Validity (accuracy)
   - Ability of a test to correctly identify those with disease form those without the disease among the apparently healthy population
   - Refers to what extent the test actually measures which it is supposed to measure[Q].

   Components
   - Sensitivity[Q]
   - Specificity[Q].

   Sensitivity and Specificity
   - Sensitivity and specificity are the measures used to evaluate a screening test
   - Sensitivity is inversely proportional to specificity.

Sensitivity	*Specificity*
Definition	
▪ Ability of a test to identify correctly and those who have the disease, that is true positive[Q] ▪ In other word sensitivity is the ability of the test to detect disease in those who actually have it, i.e. it gives usefulness of a screening test ▪ It is a statistical index of diagnostic accuracy ▪ Expressed in percentage ▪ A 90% sensitivity means that 90% of the patients screened people would give true positive result and remaining 10% a false negative result $\text{Sensitivity} = \frac{\text{Persons with disease detected by the screening test}}{\text{All persons with disease detected by diagnostic test}}$	▪ Ability of a test to identify correctly those who do not have the disease, that is true negative[Q] ▪ In other words specificity is the ability of the test to detect absence of disease in those who actually do not have it ▪ Expressed in percentage ▪ A 90% specificity means that 90% of non-diseased persons will give true negative results, 10% of non-diseased people screened will be wrongly classified as diseased when they are not $\text{Specificity} = \frac{\text{Persons without disease detected by the screening test}}{\text{All persons without disease detected by diagnostic test}}$

Calculations

Screening test results	Diagnosis: Diseased	Diagnosis: Not diseased	Total
Positive	a (true +ve)	b (false +ve)	a + b
Negative	c (false -ve)	d (true -ve)	c + d
Total	a + c	b + d	a + b + c + d

Hence
- Sensitivity = a/a + c x 100[Q]
- Specificity = d/b + d x 100[Q]

Relationship between sensitivity and specificity
- Sensitivity and specificity are inversely related, i.e. sensitivity may be increased only at the cost of specificity and vice versa

Significance

- An ideal screening test should be 100% sensitive and 100% specific which seldom occurs.

2. Discuss in detail about the various agents used for disinfection.

- Disinfection is process of destruction or removal of pathogenic organisms outside body by direct exposure to chemical or physical agents

Points of difference	Disinfection	Sterilization
▪ Definition	Disinfection is the process of destruction or removal of pathogenic organism outside the body, usually inanimate objects, and not necessarily the spores and not necessarily all the microbes but reduction of their numbers to such a low level that is not harmful to health	Sterilization is the process of destruction only the vegetative forms of the bacteria but also their spores, fungal spores and viruses
▪ Target	All pathogenic organism	Vegetative forms and spores
▪ Outcome	Reduction in the number to nonharmful level	Complete destruction of pathogenic organisms
▪ Methods used	Chemicals like phenol, cresol, bleaching powder	Various methods like heating, autoclaving, drying, filtration, etc.

- Total number of microorganism contained within or upon surface of item prior to its being disinfected or sterilized is called as bioload or bioburden.[Q]

Types of Disinfection

Prophylactic disinfection[Q] (Pre-current disinfection[Q])	*Concurrent disinfection (Concomitant disinfection)*	*Terminal disinfection*
Objective ▪ As a preventive measure, to prevent the onset of the disease *Example* ▪ Chlorination of water[Q], pasteurization of milk[Q], sterilization of the vaccines, scrubbing and washing the hands before surgery and after examining the patient, sterilization of the instruments before using for surgery	▪ Consists of immediate destruction of the pathogens, as soon as they come out of the infected person's body, through the body fluids *Objective* ▪ To prevent further spread of the disease and is carried out throughout the period of illness, i.e. as long as the patient is in the hospital ▪ Procedure ▪ Undertaken to disinfect the infectious material of the patients and articles used by them like – Infectious material like saliva, sputum, urine, vomitus, feces and other body discharges – Linen, clothes, towels, dressings, utensils and bedding used by them – Instruments, gloves, aprons, bowls and such others used during interaction with these patients	▪ Carried out after the death or discharge of the infectious patients ▪ Complementary to the process of concurrent disinfection ▪ Consists of disinfection of not only all the articles left behind in the ward by the patient, but also includes disinfection floor, walls, furniture, curtains, etc. of the ward

Disinfection Agents

- Disinfectants are substances used for disinfection, i.e. kill bacteria[Q].

Classification

A. Natural agents	
a. Sunlight	▪ Direct and continuous exposure to ultraviolet rays of sunlight is lethal to bacteria and some viruses ▪ Acts by coagulation of protoplasm of bacteria *Used for* ▪ Linen, bedding and furniture
b. Air	▪ Open air acts by drying or evaporation of moisture is lethal to most bacteria
B. Physical agents	
a. Dry heat	▪ No power of penetration ▪ Destroys spores alos
i. Burning (incineration)	▪ An excellent method of disinfection ▪ Should not be done in open air, best done in incinerator *Used for* ▪ Inexpensive items like contaminated dressings, rags and swabs and also for feces ▪ Health care waste (in incinerators)

Contd…

Contd…

ii. Hot air	▪ Done in hot air oven at 160–180°C for atleast 1 hour *Used for* ▪ Glasswares, syringes, swabs, dressings, french chalk, oils, vaseline and sharp instruments *Disadvantage* ▪ Unsuitable for plastics, rubber, other delicate substance (as they are destroyed at high temperature) and bulky articles like mattresses (due no penetrating power of hot air)
iii. Flaming	▪ Done by holding article over flame *Used for* ▪ Wire loops, needles
b. Moist heat	
i. Boiling below 100°C	▪ Water is boiled below boiling point *Used for* ▪ Pasteurization of milk ▪ Sterilization of vaccine
ii. Boiling at 100°C	▪ Provides an effective method of disinfection by providing atmosphere of boiling and steam ▪ Boiling for 5–10 minutes kills bacteria but not viruses and spores ▪ Effectiveness can be enhanced by 1% soap and 0.3% washing soda *Used for* ▪ Small instruments and tools, utensils, bedpans, rubber goods, etc. ▪ Linen stained with feces, pus or blood (after washing in cold water and treated with 2.5% cresol) *Disadvantage* ▪ Slow process, unsuitable for thick bedding and woolens
iii. Autoclaving	▪ Most widely used sterilization method in hospitals and laboratory ▪ Destroys all forms of life including spores using saturated steam under pressure ▪ Has greater power of penetration and gives off latent heat *Types* ▪ Single chamber ▪ Double chamber *Used for* ▪ Linen, dressings, gloves, syringes, certain instruments and culture media *Disadvantage* ▪ Not suitable for plastics and sharp instruments
c. Radiation	▪ Most effective, viable, safe and economic method ▪ Uses gamma radiation from Cobalt-60 which has great penetration power ▪ Items need to placed in plastic bag before sterilization *Used for* ▪ Bandages, dressings, condoms, catgut and surgical instruments *Disadvantages* ▪ Expensive
d. Filtration	▪ Liquids are passed through filters to remove pathogens ▪ Most of them retain bacterial but viruses pass through *Types of filters* ▪ Earthenware ▪ Asbestos ▪ Sintered glass ▪ Membrane of cellulose and other polymers *Used for* ▪ Water at domestic level ▪ Heat labile liquids
C. Chemical agents	▪ Preferred for articles not suitable for physical sterilization ▪ Commonly used for disinfection of feces, urine and other contaminated materials *Ideal chemical disinfectant* ▪ Should be safe, cheap and effective ▪ Should kill all pathogens but not harmful to man ▪ Should be readily soluble, highly penetrable, consistently reliable, low in toxicity and rapid in action

Contd…

Contd...

	▪ Should neither corrode metals nor bleach or stain articles ▪ Should be stable and not have unpleasant smell ▪ Should act in both acidic and alkaline medium ▪ Should not be influenced by organic matter
a. Phenol and related compounds	
i. Phenol (carbolic acid)	▪ Not an effective disinfect ▪ Acts by protoplasmic poisonous activity ▪ Only used as a standard to compare germicidal activity of other disinfectant[Q] ▪ Rideal Walker Coefficient of Phenol is 1 *Disadvantage* ▪ Produce skin burns
ii. Crude phenol	▪ Mixture of phenol and cresol ▪ Effective against Gram-positive and gram-negative bacteria and certain viruses ▪ Not readily inactivated by organic matter but efficacy weakened by dilution *Used for* ▪ Disinfection of feces (>10%) ▪ Mopping floor and cleaning drains (5%) ▪ As bacteriostatic (0.2–1%) *Disadvantages* ▪ Only slowly effective against spores and acid fast bacilli
iii. Cresol	▪ All purpose general disinfectant ▪ 3–10 times more powerful than phenol ▪ No significant activity against bacterial spores[Q] *Used for* ▪ Feces and urine (5–10%)
iv. Cresol emulsions	▪ Contains cresol emulsified with soap (saponified cresol) *Examples* ▪ Lysol (5–10 times more powerful than phenol) ▪ Izal (8 times more powerful than phenol) ▪ Cyllin (17 times more powerful than phenol) ▪ Powerful disinfectants *Used for* ▪ Feces and urine (2% lysol) ▪ Hands and clothes ▪ Drains and latrine
v. Chlorhexidine (hibitane)	▪ Most useful skin antiseptic ▪ Highly active against vegetative Gram-positive organism and moderately active against Gram-negative microbes *Used for* ▪ Hand lotions (0.5% aqueous or alcoholic solution) ▪ Burns and hand disinfection (1% creams or lotions) ▪ Mouth wash, neonatal bath *Disadvantages* ▪ Inactivated by soaps and detergents
vi. Hexachlorophene	▪ Highly active against Gram-positive organisms but less active against Gram-negative organisms *Used for* ▪ Soap preparations (for its cumulative action on skin) ▪ Deodorizer *Disadvantages* ▪ Slow in action
vii. Dettol (chloroxylenol)	▪ Active against streptococci but worthless against some Gram-negative bacteria ▪ 70 times powerful than phenol *Used for* ▪ Instruments and plastic equipments (5% dettol for 15 minutes) *Disadvantages* ▪ Easily inactivated by organic matter

Contd...

Contd…

b. Quaternary ammonia compounds	
i. Cetrimide (cetavlon)	▪ Active against vegetative gram positive organisms but less active against gram negative organism *Used for* ▪ Disinfection of injuries (1–2%) ▪ Surgical instruments, gloves ▪ Utensils
ii. Savlon	▪ Combination of 3% cetavlon and 0.3% hibitane[Q] *Used for* ▪ Plastic appliances (20 min contact) ▪ Thermometers (1 in 6 spirit for 3 min)
iii. Zephiran	▪ All purpose disinfectant and antiseptic ▪ Active against Gram-positive cocci and less active against Gram-negative bacteria *Used for* ▪ Preoperative skin disinfectant ▪ Douche for irrigating mucous cavities ▪ Surgical instruments
c. Halogens and their compounds	
i. Bleaching powder (chlorinated lime)	▪ Most widely used disinfectant in public health practice ▪ Cheapest disinfectant ▪ Kills most of organisms ▪ Rapid action but brief ▪ Contains 33% available chlorine *Used for* ▪ Water (2.5 g for 1000 L) ▪ Feces and urine (5% solution for 1 hour) ▪ Deodorant in bathrooms and latrines *Disadvantages* ▪ Unstable content and loses its chlorine content ▪ Efficacy reduced by organic content
ii. Sodium hypochlorite (liquid bleach)	▪ Provides 80,000–80,000 ppm of chlorine *Used for* ▪ Infant's feeding bottle *Disadvantages* ▪ Corrodes metals
iii. Halazone tablets	▪ Chlorine tablets containing 25% chlorine *Used for* ▪ Water (1 tablet containing 4 mg halazone for 1 liter of water for 30–60 minutes)
iv. Iodine	▪ Most effective skin antiseptic ▪ Cheap, readily available and quick in action *Used for* ▪ Plastic appliance (1/2500 aqueous solution) ▪ Water (1 drop in emergency) *Disadvantages* ▪ Stains skin ▪ Produce sensitivity in some people
v. Iodophors	▪ Complexes of iodine and solubilizers which release iodine ▪ Nonirritant and do not stain skin ▪ Acts by oxidizing microbial protoplasm and precipitating proteins ▪ Possess sporocidal action *Used for* ▪ Antiseptic *Disadvantages* ▪ Rapidly inactivated by organic matter

Contd…

Contd...

d. Alcohols	▪ Widely used antiseptics and disinfectants ▪ Commonly used are ethyl alcohol and isopropyl alcohol ▪ Active in range of 50–70% strength ▪ Lethal to nonsporing bacteria and inactivates viruses *Used for* ▪ Skin disinfection ▪ Hand washing *Disadvantages* ▪ Expensive ▪ Inflammability
e. Formaldehyde	▪ Active against vegetative bacteria, fungi and many viruses ▪ Slowly effective against bacterial spore and acid fast bacilli ▪ Acts by precipitation and destruction of proteins ▪ Does not bleach textiles or damage metals *Used for* ▪ Rooms, walls and furniture (by spraying 2–3% solution or gaseous fumigation) ▪ Blankets, beds, books and other valuable articles (gaseous fumigation) *Disadvantages* ▪ Highly inflammable, irritating and toxic gas ▪ Potentially carcinogen
f. Hydrogen peroxide	▪ Oxidizing liquid ▪ Acts by releasing nascent oxygen which removes pus, slough and loosens dead necrotic matter *Used for* ▪ Cleansing suppurative wounds and ulcers ▪ Mouth gargles
g. Miscellaneous	
i. Lime	▪ Cheapest ▪ Used in form of fresh quick lime (dry) or milk of lime (10–20% aqueous suspension) *Used for* ▪ Feces and urine (2:1 ratio and 2 hours contact) ▪ Treating walls as lime wash ▪ Deodorant in cattle sheds, stables, urinals and latrines
ii. Potassium permanganate	▪ Good oxidizing agent but weak disinfectant *Used for* ▪ Fruits and vegetables ▪ Water (rarely) *Disadvantage* ▪ Causes reddish discoloration of water and metallic taste
iii. Ethylene oxide	▪ Effective against bacteria, spores and viruses ▪ Used in mixture with 12% CO_2 and water vapors *Used for* ▪ Heat sensitive articles ▪ Fabrics, plastic equipment, cardiac catheters, books, etc *Disadvantages* ▪ Explosive ▪ Difficult to control process

Disinfection Procedures

a. For feces and urine	▪ Excreta should be collected in impervious vessels and broken with sticks to allow proper disinfection ▪ Then equal quantity of disinfectants is added and allowed to stand for 1–2 hours – 8% bleaching power solution – 10% crude phenol – 5% cresol[Q] (ideal for chloric stool[Q]) – 10% formalin – Equal amount of milk of lime ▪ After disinfection, the excreta is emptied into a water closet or buried in the ground

Contd...

Contd...

	▪ Bed pans and urine cans should ideally be steam disinfected or disinfected with 2.5% cresol for an hour after cleaning with boiling water ▪ If none is available, they can as well be washed with soap and water ▪ Burning a cotton ball soaked in spirit inside a bed pan is useful in a field/emergency situation
b. For sputum	▪ This is received in the gauze or paper handkerchiefs and destroyed by burning[Q], autoclaving[Q] or it is buried[Q] in the earth far from human habitation ▪ Alternatively, sputum may be received in a cup half filled with 5% cresol and when full it is allowed to stand for one hour and the contents are emptied and disposed off
c. For room (operation theater/isolation ward)	▪ The isolation ward needs to be disinfected after discharge or death of the patient ▪ The doors and windows are kept open for several hours for good aeriation ▪ Then the room is disinfected usually by all the three methods—mopping, spraying and fumigation ▪ Floors and hard surfaces may be mopped with formalin solution (10%) or cresol (2.5%) or phenol (5%) and washed after a contact period of 4 hours ▪ Furniture items may also be mopped with 5% formalin solution ▪ Blood spills disinfected with sodium hypochloride[Q] ▪ The room as a whole may be disinfected by fumigation with formaldehyde gas, when the room is kept closed for preferably 24 hours as a contact period ▪ Alternatively, the room may be disinfected by spraying it with formalin solution ▪ Care must be taken to spray the walls from below upwards to prevent running down of the liquid disinfectant along the walls of the rooms
d. Articles used by patients	▪ Articles such as linen, clothes, etc. soiled with blood or dejecta, are disinfected by soaking them in a solution of formalin (10.0%) or cresol (2.5%) or 5% phenol and then after the contact period, washed with soap and water followed by sun drying and ironing ▪ Alternatively such linen and clothes are disinfected by boiling for half an hour or by steaming ▪ Damageable goods of fur and leather and also woolen and silk fabrics may be disinfected by exposure to formaldehyde gas ▪ Paper, books and woolen materials can be disinfected with hot air ▪ Utensils and crockery items can be disinfected by boiling for 5–10 minutes ▪ Cutlery items especially knives, which may get blunt on boiling may be disinfected by immersion in 10% formalin or 2% lysol for 10 minutes before being washed and cleaned
e. Clinical instruments used	▪ Clinical thermometer is disinfected either by keeping it in surgical spirit or dettol or savlon solution ▪ Disposable items like tissue paper, gauze pieces[Q], cotton swabs[Q] and rags may be directly disposed of by burning or incineration[Q] ▪ Do not detach the needles from the syringes after use; aspirate disinfectant fluid into the syringe; Immerse the syringe with attached needles in the disinfectant fluid horizontally in flat metal or glass tray or puncture proof plastic container and keep them immersed in the disinfectant fluid for at least 30 minutes; The needles and syringes are then removed from the tray and destroyed mechanically before disposal ▪ Alternatively, all the disposable material[Q] can be put in the hot air oven at a temperature of 160°C for 30–60 minutes[Q] to ensure that there will not be any possibility of its reuse ▪ If incineration is not available, the only next best alternative is deep burial in controlled landfill sites ▪ Sharp instruments disinfected using hot air oven[Q]

Significance

- Proper sterilization and disinfection is essential for reducing morbidity and mortality from iatrogenic and nosocomial infections and right of every patient.

SHORT ESSAYS

3. Measures of central tendency.

- Central tendency is the tendency of the values of observation in a continuous series to aggregate in the center of the distribution series
- This central value is called statistical average
- It lies somewhere in the middle of values of data and majority of values tend to cluster around it
- It represents the majority of the values in the data.

Measures of Central Tendency

	Mean[Q]	*Median*[Q]	*Mode*[Q]
	▪ Sum of scores divided by the number of cases[Q] ▪ Arithmetic mean unless otherwise specified ▪ Like center of gravity of a series of data	▪ Middle most point in a distribution with an equal number of cases on the either side of it[Q]	▪ Most frequently occurring observation in a series[Q] ▪ In a frequency polygon, the mode can be calculated from the point, where the curve takes a turn from increase to decrease ▪ It corresponds to mean and median in a normal frequency distribution
Calculation	$\text{Meam} = \frac{\text{Sum of all observations}}{\text{Number of observations made}}$ ▪ Represented symbolically $\bar{x} = \frac{\sum x1}{n}$ Where $\chi 1$ = value of each observation in the data $\bar{x}$ = mean Σ = Sum of n = number of observations in the data	▪ Individual measures are arranged in ascending or descending order[Q] ▪ In a distribution with odd number, the middle value is taken as median ▪ In a distribution with even number, the average of two central values is taken as median	▪ Mode can also be calculated from the relationship i.e. Mode = Mean – 3(Mean – Median) ▪ There can be more than one mode for a series of data e.g. Bimodal distribution has two modes ▪ In bimodal series – Mode = 3 median – 2 means
Examples	The systolic blood pressure in mm of Hg of ten individuals are as follows: 116, 118, 122, 120, 120, 124, 122, 116, 118, 124 $\text{Mean } \bar{x} = \frac{1200}{10} = 120 \text{ mm of Hg}$	▪ Calculate the median of number of days of stays of patient in a hospital ward 13, 42, 8, 9, 7, 3, 5, 6, 52, 8, 2, 11, 11, 10, 9 ▪ Arrange these values in ascending order 2, 3, 5, 6, 7, 8, 8, 9, 9, 10, 11, 11, 13, 42, 52 ▪ The total number of observations is 15 then the median is value at 8th position ▪ Median = 9 days	▪ Calculate the mode of the following ages of 10 students 18, 18, 19, 19, 20, 20, 20, 21, 22, 23 ▪ Mode = 20 years
Advantages	▪ Easy to calculate and understand ▪ Most commonly used in statistics	▪ Easy to calculate and understand ▪ Easily detected ▪ Not influenced by extreme values	▪ Easy to calculate and understand ▪ Least influenced by extreme of values
Disadvantages	▪ May be unduly influenced by an abnormal value in the distribution, i.e. extreme value	▪ Not suitable for mathematical treatment	▪ Often not clearly defined ▪ May not exist in a small group of values ▪ Cannot be subjected to mathematical treatment

Significance

a. Central tendency in various distribution

Distribution	*Central tendency*
▪ Normal (Gaussian) distribution	Mean = Median = Mode
▪ Right (positive) skew distribution	Mean > Median > Mode
▪ Left (negative) skew distribution	Mean < Median < Mode

b. In distribution with extreme values (Outliers)
- Most affected measure of central tendency—Mean
- Least affected measure of central tendency—Mode
- Most preferable measure of central tendency—Median

4. Pneumoconiosis.

Refer Question No. 2 June 2012 (RS2) Paper I.

5. Pasteurization of milk.

Refer Question No. 6 December 2009 (RS2) Paper I.

6. Explain the various methods of mosquito control.

Refer Question No. 11 June 2010 (RS2) Paper I.

7. Describe the various occupational cancers.

Refer Question No. 8 December 2007 (RS2) Paper I.

8. Radiation hazards.

- Workers employed in industries using radium and other radioactive substances are exposed to hazards of radiation
- These industries are:
  - Mining of radioactive ores, monozite sand workers and handling these products.
  - Use of X–rays[Q]
  - UV rays in arc and other electric welding processes.
  - Infrared rays in welding, glass blowing, foundry work, etc.
- Maximal permissible exposure to radiation is 5 rem/year[Q] for workers and 0.5 rem/year for general public.

Hazards of Radiation

- Pregnant women and children are more prone to radiation hazards
- Extent of damage depends upon.

Tissue involved	*Types of radiation*	*Area of the body exposed*
▪ Lymphocytes, bone marrow cells and gonadal cells are highly sensitive to radiation.	▪ Both α and β rays are harmful if injected or inhaled. ▪ β particles can affect skin also ▪ X–rays have high penetrating power and affect skin as well as internal organs ▪ γ–rays cause even more damage	▪ Irradiation of large area of the body may lead to death in days to weeks because of bone marrow depression

Hazards

a. Acute exposure	▪ Massive doses of penetrating radiation such as X–rays and γ–rays may cause death in a few hours or days ▪ In less severe cases, loss of appetite, nausea and vomiting occur within one hour or two ▪ Symptoms may subside after a day or two weeks but reappear after a latent period in form of diarrhea, fever, bleeding and ulceration of mucus membranes, fall in blood pressure, increased susceptibility to infections, epilations, amenorrhea, increased capillary fragility and marked decrease in blood cells especially lymphocytes and polymorphs
b. Chronic exposure	
i. Malignancy	▪ Various types of cancer may be induced, particularly of lung, blood and skin ▪ Leukemia is a frequent result of repeated exposure, a significantly higher rate being noted among radiologists
ii. Genetic effects	▪ X–rays are known to induce genetic mutations ▪ Radiation mutations beings recessive, the chance of its manifestations in future generations is small ▪ In 95% cases, the offspring dies during gestation or soon after. In remaining, the mutations are mainly in chromosomes other than sex chromosomes
iii. Shortening of life span	

Contd...

Contd...

iv. Skin lesions	▪ β particles and low energy X – rays are responsible for most of the damage to skin because they are absorbed at the surface ▪ High energy X–rays and γ–rays penetrate readily, hence the skin is usually spared ▪ The skin reactions appear after a latent period of a week or two as erythema, edema, pruritus, blisters, sloughing of epidermis and ulcerations ▪ Healing is slow ▪ Delayed effects include hyperkeratosis, atrophy of sweat and sabaceous glands and eventually epidermoid carcinoma
v. Cataract	▪ This is common with particulate type of radiations especially neutrons

9. Nutritional surveillance.

Refer Question No. 2 June 2010 (RS2) Paper I.

10. What are the medical benefits under ESI Act?

Refer Question No. 4 December 2012 (RS2) Paper I.

11. Differentiate between health education and health propaganda.

- Health education is not health propaganda but more than it
- To educate means to cause or facilitate learning whereas propaganda means to spread particular systemized doctrine.

Difference between Health Education and Health Propaganda

Health education	*Health propaganda or publicity*
▪ Knowledge and skill actively acquired	▪ Knowledge is passively acquired, i.e. it is instilled in the minds of people
▪ It makes people think for themselves before acting	▪ It prevents or discourages thinking because of readymade slogans or information
▪ It disciplines primitive desires	▪ It arouses and stimulates primitive desires
▪ It develops reflective behavior and trains people to used judgment before acting	▪ It develops reflexive behavior and aims at impulsive actions
▪ It appeals to reason	▪ It appeals to emotions
▪ It develops individuality, personality and self-expression	▪ It develops a standard pattern of attitudes and behaviors according to the mould used
▪ Knowledge is acquired through self-reliant activity	▪ Knowledge is spoon fed and passively received
▪ The process is behavior centered	▪ The process is information centered
▪ It aims at developing favorable attitudes, habits and skills	▪ It does not aim for change in attitude or behavior
▪ It aims at improvement of health	▪ It aims to derive profit
▪ It is mainly concerned with betterment of life	▪ It is mainly concerned with the sale of the product
▪ It has long-lasting effect	▪ It has temporary effect
▪ It is costly but cheap in long run	▪ It is cheap but not cost effective

12. Role of culture in health with suitable examples.

- All people, whether rural or urban, have their own beliefs and practices concerning health and disease.

Sociocultural Factors in Health

A. Concept of etiology and cure
   - Majority of rural people considered a disease is caused by supernatural powers or physical factors

a. Supernatural causes
   i. Wrath of Gods and Goddesses
      - There are good many people (even among the educated) who believe that certain diseases are due to the wrath of some God or Goddess
      - Smallpox and chickenpox are outstanding examples and are respectively known as Bari Mata (Sitla Devi) and Chhoti Mata
      - Where the disease is considered to be due to the wrath of Gods and Goddesses, administration of drugs is considered harmful
      - Cases are not notified and pujas are made to appease the gods.
   ii. Breach of taboo
      - Breach of taboos is believed by some people to be responsible for certain diseases
      - Venereal diseases are believed by some to be due to illicit sexual intercourse with a woman of low caste, or a woman during menstruation.
   iii. Past sins
      - Diseases such as leprosy and tuberculosis are believed by some to be due to their past sins.
   iv. Evil eye
      - A widely held belief throughout the country is the effect of evil eyes
      - Children are considered to be most susceptible to the effect of evil eyes
      - In order to ward off the effects of the evil eye, charms and amulets are prescribed and incantations recited by the exorcist.
   v. Spirit or ghost intrusion
      - Some diseases such as hysteria and epilepsy are regarded as due to a spirit or ghost intrusion into the body. The services of an exorcist are sought to drive away the evil spirit or ghost.

b. Physical causes
   i. Weather
      - Exposure to heat during summer is responsible for an attack of 100 (heatstroke)
      - The folk remedies consist of application of oil and ghee on the soles of feet and administration of mangophool (prepared by keeping unripe mangoes under hot ashes for a few minutes, and extracting the pulp in cold water) with a pinch of salt.
   ii. Water
      - Impure water is associated with disease.
   iii. Impure blood
      - Skin diseases, viz. boils and scabies are considered to be due to impure blood
      - Eating neem leaves and flowers is considered to purify blood.

B. Environmental sanitation

a. Disposal of human excreta
   - Majority of the people in rural areas use open fields for defecation
   - They are ignorant that feces is infectious and pollutes water and soil and promotes fly breeding

b. Disposal of wastes
   - The average villager is not aware that mosquitoes breed in collections of waste water and it is permitted to flow into the streets
   - The solid waste (refuse) is invariably thrown in front of the houses where it is permitted to accumulate and decompose
   - Periodically, it is removed to the fields and used as manure
   - The animal dung (cow dung) is allowed to accumulate and is used sometimes as manure and often times pressed into cakes, sun-dried and used as fuel.

c. Water supply
   - Well occupies a pivotal place in the cultural environment of villages
   - It a common meeting place of men and women of the village, a place where people bathe and wash their clothes, a place where animals are washed and given a drink
   - These cultural practices lead to the pollution of well water
   - Tanks and ponds are used for washing, bathing, ablution and sometimes even as a source of drinking water
   - Some rivers are considered holy and people go on pilgrimage to these rivers to have a dip and also drink the raw water which they consider sacred
   - Epidemics of cholera and gastroenteritis have been due to these cultural practices.

d. Housing
- Rural houses are usually kutcha and damp, ill-lighted and ill-ventilated with no windows
- Absence of a separate kitchen, latrine, bathroom and drainage are characteristic features of an average rural house
- Infrequently, human beings and animals live under one roof
- Houses are generally kept clean inside, regularly white-washed or plastered with mud and cowdung.

C. Food habits
- Food habits have deep psychological roots and are associated with love, affection, warmth, self-image and social prestige
- Vegetarianism is given a place of honor in Hindu society and even among vegetarians, the pattern of eating is not the same; some do not take onions and garlic on religious grounds
- Muslims abhor pork, and Hindus beef—these food habits have a religious sanction from early days
- The concept of hot and cold food is widely prevalent in the country
- Foods such as meat, fish, eggs, and jaggery are considered to generate heat in the body; foods such as curd, milk, vegetables and lemon are considered to cool the body
- Adulteration of milk is a common practice because of a deep-rooted belief that if pure milk is boiled the milk secretion of the donor animal may dry up
- Muslims observe fasts during Ramzan and Hindus on several occasions as important adjuncts to religion. Drinks and drugs are among the food habits of the people
- Alcoholic drinks are tabooed by Muslims and high caste Hindus
- Ganja, bhang and charas are frequently consumed by sadhus
- Eating and drinking from common utensils is considered as a sign of brotherhood among Muslims
- Hindu women often take food left over by their husband
- In some societies, men eat first and women last and poorly
- Some people do not eat unless they have taken a bath
- Thus, food is a subject of widespread customs, habits and beliefs, which vary from country-to-country, and from one region to another.

D. Mother and child health
- Mother and child health is surrounded by a wide range of customs and beliefs all over the world
- Marriage is universal in Indian society, and family is incomplete without the birth of a male child
- Various customs in field of maternal and child health (MCH) have been classified as good, bad, unimportant and uncertain.

a. Good
- Prolonged breastfeeding, oil bath, massage and exposure to sun are good customs.

b. Bad
- Some foods (e.g. eggs, meat, fish, milk, leafy vegetables) are forbidden during pregnancy, deliveries conducted by the traditional untrained dai or birth attendant whose methods of conducting delivery are far from safe, the child is not put to the breast during the first 3 days of birth because of the belief that colostrum might be harmful; instead the child is put on water, and sugar solution, branding of the skin, administration of opium and drastic purgatives.

c. Unimportant
- Punching the ear and nose, application of oil or a paste of turmeric on the anterior fontanelle.

d. Uncertain
- Practice of applying kajal or black soot mixed with oil to the eyelids partly for beautification and partly for warding off the effects of evil eye.

E. Personal hygiene
- Indians have an immense sense of personal cleanliness, much of which is closely interwoven with ideas of ritual purification.

a. Oral hygiene
- Many people in the countryside use twigs of neem tree as a tooth brush; some use ashes; and some charcoal
- The educated and those who have come in contact with urban life use tooth brushes
- Eating pan leaves smeared with lime with/without tobacco is a common social custom.

b. Bathing
- Bathing naked is a taboo
- Apart from regular baths of which Indians are very fond, there are baths fixed on special occasions

- The women after menstruation must have a purifying bath; after childbirth, there may be two or three ceremonial baths, the time for which is fixed upon the advice of the priest
- The practice of an oil bath is a good Indian custom
- Womenfolk in the countryside use a paste consisting of gram, mustard oil and turmeric powder and rub it on the body before a bath.

c. Shaving
- In country side, this is done by the traditional barber who does not sterilize the instruments used, as he does not have any idea of microorganisms.

d. Smoking
- Smoking hukka is a social custom in some parts of the country. It can spread tuberculosis
- Smoking with the burning end of the cigar in the mouth, which is a common custom among some villagers in Andhra Pradesh, is associated with oral cancer.

e. Purdah
- Muslims and some high caste Hindu women observe purdah
- The incidence of tuberculosis is reported to be high amongst those who observe purdah, which also deprives them of the beneficial effect of the sunrays.

f. Sleep
- Many people in the villages sleep on the ground for reasons of poverty, and they are exposed to insect bites.

g. Wearing footwear
- The transmission of hookworm disease is associated with bare feet.

h. Circumcision
- This is a prevalent custom among Muslims and Jews which has a religious sanction.

F. Sex and marriage
- Sexual customs vary among different social, religious and ethnic groups
- For certain religious groups menstruation is a time of uncleanness when women are forbidden to pray or have intercourse
- Orthodox Jews are forbidden to have intercourse for seven days after the menstruation ceases
- These customs have an important bearing in family planning
- It is the usual social custom in India to perform marriages early, at about the age of puberty because it is considered a sound and desirable practice because late marriages may create problems in adjustments especially in joint family systems
- Because of the universality of marriage in India, there are no problems such as unmarried mothers and of illegitimate births
- Monogamy is the most universal form of marriage however polygamy or polyandry is found in certain communities
- The high rate of venereal diseases in Himachal Pradesh is attributed to the local marriage customs.

Significance

- Cultural factors are deeply involved in all the affairs of man, including health and sickness and not all customs and beliefs are bad
- Some are based on centuries of trial and error and have positive values, while others may be useless or positively harmful
- Some of these cultural factors, hallowed by centuries of practice, have stood in the way of implementing health programs.

SHORT ANSWERS

13. What is sentinel surveillance?

Refer Question No. 5 June 2012 (RS2) Paper I.

14. What are the indices of air pollution?

Refer Question No. 5 December 2014 (RS2) Paper I.

15. Differentiate between the term endemic and epidemic.

	Epidemic	*Endemic*	*Sporadic*	*Pandemic*
Definition	Unusual occurrence in a community or region of disease, specific health related behavior or other health-related events clearly in excess of expected occurrences	Constant presence of a disease or infections agent within a geographical area or population group without importation from outside[Q]	Irregular haphazard occurrence of cases from time to time and generally infrequently	Epidemic affecting a large proportion of population in a wide geographic area (section of a nation entire nation, a continent or the world)
Examples	Polio outbreaks	Malaria, leprosy	Chickenpox	AIDS
Relation with other cases	Yes, exhibit common source of infection	May exhibit common source of infection	Show little or no connection with each other nor a recognizable common source of infection (because cases are few and separated widely in space and time)	May exhibit common source of infection
Epidemicity	Yes	May be the starting point of an epidemic under favorable conditions	May be the starting point of an epidemic under favorable conditions	Yes
Geographical location	Large	Small	Small	Very large
Temporal clustering	Yes	No	No	Yes
Spatial clustering	Yes	Yes	No	No

16. Write short notes on aflatoxins.

- Aflatoxins are a group of mycotoxins produced by fungi, *Aspergillus flavus* and *Aspergillus parasiticus* which infest foodgrains like ground nut, maize, parboiled rice, sorghum, wheat, rice, cotton seed, etc. when stored under improper conditions, i.e. moisture level above 16% and temperature ranging from 11°–37°C
- They are brightly fluorescing furanocoumarin compounds
- Of the various toxins produced, B_1 and G_1 are most potent hepatotoxins[Q] and are carcinogenic
- Infestation by aflatoxin is called aflatoxicosis
- It is characterized by hepatitis (jaundice), ascitis, portal hypertension, liver cirrhosis and hepatocellular carcinoma.

Prevention and Control

- Drying and proper storage to keep the moisture level below 10%
- Detoxification of affected food by ammonia process (but fit only for animal consumption)
- Contaminated food should not be consumed
- Health education of the population is also essential.

Significance

- Aflatoxin exposure and HBV infection are the main risk factors accounting for high incidence of hepatocellular carcinoma.

17. What are the methods of sewage disposal?

- Sewage is a mixture of human excreta, urine, wash water, liquid waste coming from bathrooms and kitchen, surface water and industrial waste water
- It is liquid waste containing excreta[Q]
- It consists of 99.9% water and 0.1% solids[Q] (organic and inorganic).

Methods of Sewage Disposal

Sewage treatment	*Sewage dilution*	*Sewage lagoon (oxidation pond^Q or ditches)*	*Sewage farming (land treatment^Q)*
Stage wise handing of sewage, i.e. anaerobic digestion followed by aerobic oxidation	Discharging sewage directly into a large body of water like river (river outfall^Q) or sea (sea outfall)	Subjecting sewage to biological oxidation in oxidation pond involving algae, aerobic bacteria, oxygen and sunlight	Disposal of sewage in porous land through broad irrigation

Significance

- Sewage is dirty water with unpleasant sight and smell, which if not disposed off, can contaminate source of drinking water and food resulting in diseases.

18. List the warning sign of poor mental health.

Refer Question No. 6 June 2009 (RS2) Paper I.

19. Write briefly on case fatality rate.

Refer Question No. 4 December 2007 (RS2) Paper I.

20. Enumerate the various community nutrition programs.

- The Government of India has initiated several large scale supplementary feeding progams and programs aimed at overcoming specific deficiency diseases through various Ministries to combat malnutrition.

Community Nutrition Programs

		Ministry
a. Programs to improve overall nutritional status		
i.	Special Nutrition Program	Ministry of Social Welfare
ii.	Balwadi Nutrition Program	Ministry of Social Welfare
iii.	Integrated Child Development Services (ICDS) Program^Q	Ministry of Social Welfare^Q
iv.	Mid-day Meal Program	Ministry of Education
b. Programs to combat specific deficiencies		
i.	Vitamin A prophylaxis program	Ministry of Health and Family Welfare
ii.	Prophylaxis against Nutritional anemia	Ministry of Health and Family Welfare
iii.	Iodine deficiency disorders control program	Ministry of Health and Family Welfare

21. What is the contribution to medical sciences by. (a) Robert Koch, (b) John Snow, (c) James Lind

a. Robert Koch
   - Robert Koch (1843–1910) was is a German practitioner
   - He is known as Father of Medical Microbiology.

Contributions

- He introduced staining techniques for bacteria
- He introduced methods of obtaining bacteria in pure culture using solid media (agar)
- He isolated first bacteria (anthrax bacilli) in pure culture
- He discovered the bacillus of tuberculosis and the cholera vibrio
- He perfected idea of steam sterilization along with his assistant
- He produced new tuberculin
- He demonstrated Koch phenomenon which is a hypersensitivity reaction seen in a guinea pig already infected with the tuberculous bacilli when the tubercle bacillus or its protein is injected into it.

- He proposed the Koch's postulates which are the criterion or conditions laid down by Koch to accept a microorganism as the causative agent of an infectious agent. They are:
  - The bacterium should be constantly associated with the lesions of the disease
  - It should be possible to isolate the bacterium in pure culture from the lesions
  - Inoculation of such pure culture into suitable laboratory animals should reproduce the lesions of the disease
  - It should be possible to reisolate the bacterium in pure cultures from the lesions produced in the experimental animals.
- He introduced Atoxyl for treatment of sleeping sickness
- We won Nobel Prize for medicine in 1905 for investigation and discoveries in relation to tuberculosis.

John Snow

- John snow was a British doctor practicing in London
- He is often called Father of Epidemiology/Modern Epidemiology for his study of cholera
- He is also known as Greatest Doctor.

Contributions

- He studied epidemiology of cholera in London (1848–1854)
- He established causative role of polluted water in spread of cholera
- He devised system of methodological observations of natural events or experiments
- He studied and calculated dosage for use of ether and chloroform as surgical anesthesia.

James Lind

James Lind (1716–1794) was a Scottish naval surgeon who by his work influenced practices of preventive medicine and good nutrition among British soldiers.

Contribution to Community Medicine

a. Contribution to epidemiology
   - James Lind was the first ever to conduct a clinical trial for his study to find treatment of scurvy.

b. Treatment of scurvy[Q]
   - James Lind performed a human experiment in which he added different substances to diet of 12 soldiers who were suffering from scurvy
   - He divided his patients into 6 pairs and supplemented the diets of each pair with cider, elixir, vitriol, vinegar, sea water; a mixture of nutmeg, garlic, mustard and tamarind in barley water; and two oranges and one lemon daily
   - All the subjects were studied for 6 days and it was the observed that the limeys recovered from scurvy
   - Thus, he advocated the intake of fresh fruit and vegetables for prevention of scurvy.

c. Naval hygiene
   - He advocated practice of naval hygiene like
     - Drying of ships by using better ventilation
     - Improvement in clothing and cleanliness of sailors
     - Fumigation of ships with sulfur and arsenic.

22. Write briefly on epidemiological triad.

- Epidemiological triad is a model developed to explain the disease causation which was insufficiently explained by the germ theory
- According to this model, a state of equilibrium exists between the agent[Q], host[Q] and environment[Q]
- When an agent reaches a susceptible host in favorable environment it results in disease state
- When an agent reaches a semi-resistant host and when the agent is not much virulent, then it results in carrier state
- In this concept, the agent can be a microorganism, a chemical or physical agent and environment includes external and internal environment.

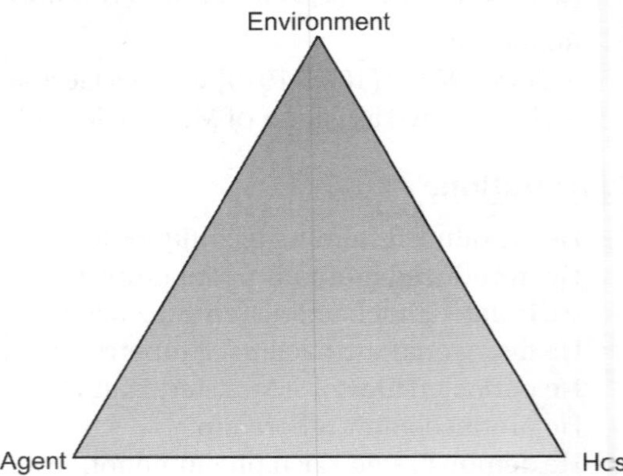

Fig. 3: Epidemiological triad

Epidemiological Triad

a. Agent factors – Disease agent is a substance, living or non–living or a force, tangible or intangible the excessive presence or relative lack of which may initiate or perpetuate a disease process – A disease may be caused by a single agent, a number of alternative agents or a complex of two or more factors.	
i. Biological agents	▪ Living agents, i.e. bacteria, viruses, parasites, fungi, etc. which exhibit certain host-related biological properties like – Infectivity: Ability of an infection agent to invade and multiply in host – Pathogenicity: Ability to induce clinically apparent illness – Virulence: Ability to produce severe clinical manifestations
ii. Nutrient agents	▪ Any excess or deficiency of proteins, fat, carbohydrates, vitamins, minerals and water
iii. Physical agents	▪ Heat cold, humidity, pressure, radiation, electricity sound, etc.
iv. Chemical agents	▪ Endogenous: Urea, serum bilirubin, ketone bodies, uric acid, etc. ▪ Exogenous: Allergens, metal fumes, dust gases, etc.
v. Mechanical agents	▪ Friction, pressure impact, etc.
vi. Physiological agents	▪ Hormones, enzymes, nutrients, absence of organ or part of it, chromosomal abnormality, immunological abnormality
vii. Social agents	▪ Poverty, smoking, drug abuse, alcoholism, unhealthy lifestyles, social isolation, parental deprivation
b. Host factors	
i. Demographic characteristics	▪ Age, sex, ethnicity
ii. Biological characteristics	▪ Genetic factors, blood levels of important substances, blood groups, enzymes, cellular components of blood, immunological factors, physiological functions of organs
iii. Social and economic characteristics	▪ Socio-economic status, education, occupation, stress, marital status, housing, etc.
iv. Lifestyle factors	▪ Personality traits, habits, nutrition, physical exercise, alcohol, tobacco and drug use behavioral pattern
c. Environment factors	
i. Physical environment (All nonliving things)	▪ Air, water, soil, housing, climate, geography, heat, light, noise, radiation, etc.
ii. Biological environment (All living things)	▪ Microorganisms, insects, rodents, plants animals ▪ May act as disease producing agents, reservoirs of infection, intermediate hosts and vectors of disease
iii. Psychosocial environment	▪ Cultural values, customs, habits beliefs, attitudes, morals, religion, education, lifestyles, community life, health services, social and political organization

Significance

- Epidemiological triad considered the role of host as well his immediate surrounding besides the causative agent in disease causation.

MBBS PHASE III EXAMINATION

DECEMBER 2010

(Revised Scheme 2)

PAPER II

LONG ESSAYS

1. Describe epidemiology, prevention and control of measles.

- Measles is an acute highly infectious disease of childhood caused by a specific virus of myxovirus^{Q} group and is clinically characterized by fever and catarrhal symptoms of upper respiratory tract followed by a typical rash
- Also called Rubeola.

Epidemiological Factors

a. Agent factors	
i. Agent	▪ Measles is caused by a single stranded RNA virus belonging to paramgyxovirus group^{Q} ▪ There is only one serotype^{Q} ▪ Virus cannot survive outside the human body for any length of time^{Q} ▪ But it can retain infectivity when stored at sub–zero temperature
ii. Reservoir of infection	▪ Measles is disease of human beings only and only a case of measles the reservoir of infection^{Q} ▪ Carrier states are not known to occur^{Q} and is not important in transmission of disease^{Q}
iii. Infective material	▪ Secretions of the nose, throat and respiratory tract during the prodromal period and the early stage of the rash
iv. Incubation period	▪ 10–14 days^{Q}
v. Period of communicability	▪ Measles is highly infections during the prodromal period^{Q} and at the time of eruption ▪ Communicability declines rapidly after the rash appears^{Q} on the 4th day^{Q} ▪ Period communicability is approximately 4 days before and 5 days after the appearance of rash^{Q}
vi. Secondary attack rate	▪ Over 80%^{Q} among susceptible household contacts. (high secondary rate^{Q})
vii. Mode of transmission	▪ Is by droplet infection and droplet nuclei
b. Host factors	
i. Age	▪ Affects everyone in infancy or childhood between 6 months and 3 yrs in developing countries and over 5 years in developed countries
ii. Sex	▪ Equal in both sexes
iii. Immunity	▪ No age is immune if there is no previous immunity ▪ One attack confers lifelong immunity^{Q} and second attacks are rare ▪ Maternal antibodies protect the infant for 6 months after birth^{Q} ▪ Immunity after vaccination is also long lasting^{Q}
iv. Nutrition	▪ Malnourished child presents with very severe form of disease carrying 400 times higher risk of mortality^{Q}. ▪ It is related to the poor cell mediated immunity response ▪ Malnourished children tend to excrete the virus for longer period ▪ Measles may also precipitate malnutrition in a healthy well nourished child
c. Environmental factors	▪ Measles is a winter disease in temperate climates ▪ Epidemics are common in winter and early spring ▪ Epidemicity is not affected by population density and movement ▪ Low socioeconomic condition also favour the disease ▪ Measles show cyclic trends, increasing every 2–3 years

Clinical Features

- Disease progresses through three stages

Prodromal stage	*Eruptive phase*	*Post measles stage*
▪ Also called pre-eruptive stage or catarrhal stage ▪ Begins 10 days after infection and lasts until 14th day ▪ Characterized by fever, coryza with sneezing and nasal discharge, cough, red eyes, lacrimation and photophobia giving child the appealing woebegone expression on face, characteristic of measles ▪ Koplik spots[Q] pathognomonic of measles appear on buccal mucosa opposite 1st and 2nd lower molars around the orifice of Stenson's duct ▪ They innumerable, small, bluish white spots on a red base, smaller than head of a pin appearing like table salt crystals against red background	▪ Also called exanthematous stage ▪ Characterized by typical, dusky red, velvety, macular or maculopapular rash ▪ It begins on 4th day of fever, behind ears and spreads rapidly in a few hours over face and neck, extending down body till lower legs within 2–3 days ▪ Rash often becomes confluent and blotchy though may remain discrete ▪ At this stage, temperature is very high but reduces after onset of rash[Q] ▪ Lesions and fever disappear in another 3–4 days signaling end of disease ▪ Rash fades in same order of appearance leaving a brownish discoloration which may persists for 2 months or more	▪ Child loses weight and remains weak for number of days ▪ There may be failure to recover and gradual deterioration into chronic illness ▪ Complications include growth retardation, diarrhea, cancrum oris, pyogenic infection, candidiasis, reactivation of pulmonary tuberculosis, etc.

Complications of Measles

a. Respiratory	
i. Croup	▪ Metallic cough is metallic along with laryngeal stridor and respiratory distress
ii. Pneumonia	▪ Post measles bronchopneumonia is caused by bacteria (medical emergency)
iii. Tuberculosis	▪ If there is latent infection of primary complex, it often flares up to into active tuberculosis
iv. Otitis media[Q]	▪ Occurs due to secondary infection – MC complication in young children[Q]
b. Gastrointestinal	▪ Acute gastroenteritis (most common and dreadful) associated with severe dehydration and malnutrition— MC cause of post measles death[Q]
c. Neurological	
i. Febrile convulsions	▪ Occurs when the temperature is very high
ii. Encephalitis	▪ 1 in 1000 with 40% mortality rate
iii. Subacute Sclerosing Pan Encephalitis (SSEP)[Q]	▪ Also know as Dawson's disease or Dawson's encephalitis ▪ A rare complication[Q] seen 7 in millions[Q] cases and develops many (7–10 years) years after the initial measles infection ▪ The virus trapped in brain exists as latent infection, activating after years resulting in progressive mental deterioration leading to paralysis, blindness, decerebrate rigidity and death
iv. Other rare complications	▪ Multiple sclerosis, retrobulbar neuritis, toxic encephalopathy, etc.
d. Ophthalmic	
i. Conjunctivitis	▪ Common in all cases and becomes more severe due to secondary bacterial infection
ii. Corneal ulceration	▪ Seen in malnourished children

Preventive and Control Measures

WHO measles elimination strategy	*Accelerated measles mortality reduction strategy (WHO-UNICEF)*
Components a. Catch up vaccination[Q] – One time, nationwide vaccination campaign targeting usually all children aged 9 months to 14 years regardless of history of measles disease or vaccination status b. Keep up vaccination[Q] – Routine services aimed at vaccinating more than 95% of each successive birth cohorts[Q] c. Follow-up vaccination[Q] – Subsequent nationwide vaccination campaign conducted every 2–4 years targeting usually all children born after catch up campaign	▪ 2 doses of measles containing vaccine to all children through routine and supplementary immunization activities

Preventive Measures

a. Active immunization
   - Active immunization is done with the measles vaccine.

Measles Vaccine

Nature	▪ Live virus vaccine of single antigen and is freeze dried[Q]
Composition	▪ Each dose of 0.5 mL contains not less than 1000 TCID 50 live attenuated, Edmonston Zagreb (EZ) strain[Q] of measles virus propagated on human diploid cells ▪ Reconstituted vaccine should be used within 1 hour[Q]
Storage	▪ 2–8°C[Q] ▪ Vaccine remains potent for 2 years if cold chain is maintained ▪ It is both thermolabile and thermostable[Q]
Efficacy[Q]	▪ 85%[Q]
Dose	▪ 0.5 mL
Route of administration	▪ Subcutaneously[Q] in the upper arm or anterolateral surface of the thigh
Schedule	▪ One dose during 9th month of infancy ▪ Because given before 9 months, it will be rendered ineffective by the maternal antibodies and given after 9th month, the child runs risk of contracting measles ▪ However in case of epidemics, the vaccine can be given as early as 6th month, and such children are reimmunized during 15–18 weeks[Q]
Immunity	▪ Develops 10–12 days after vaccination[Q] and lasts life long
Reaction	▪ After 5–10 days of immunization, the virus multiplies in the body inducing mild measles illness manifesting as fever and rash lasting for 1–3 days
Indications	▪ For active immunization of infants against measles ▪ For contact of measles case (provides protective effect within 7 days[Q])
Contraindications	▪ Acute febrile illness ▪ Diseases of central nervous system, convulsions[Q] ▪ Immunosuppressive therapy
Adverse effects	▪ Mild measles illness in 15–20% vaccines ▪ Encephalitis 1 in 1 million vaccines ▪ Anaphylactic shock is very rare ▪ Toxic shock syndrome is most dreadful adverse effect produced due to contamination of vaccine by Staphylococci[Q]
Uses	▪ Measles vaccine is used for active immunization against measles in a dose of 0.5mL administered subcutaneously at 9 months ▪ However, it can be administered above 6 months of age also if there is measles outbreak in the community and such infants should receive booster dose at age of 9 months provided there is a 4 weeks gap between the two doses[Q] ▪ At least 80% of population should be vaccinated to eradicate measles[Q]

b. Passive immunization
   - Passive immunization is done by human normal immunoglobulin
   - It is not specific immunoglobulin.

Indications	▪ Recommended in people where vaccine is contraindicated in case of outbreak
Dose	▪ 0.25 mL/kg body weight intramuscularly[Q] (WHO)
Schedule	▪ Within 3–4 days of exposure
Immunity	▪ Immunity last 3 weeks ▪ Person passively immunized should be vaccinated 8–12 weeks later

Control Measures

- Isolation of the patient for 7 days after onset of rash
- Immunization of contacts within 2 days of exposure or immunoglobulin within 3–4 days of exposure
- Prompt at the beginning of an epidemic is essential to limit the spread.

Significance

- Measles is on WHO list of diseases for elimination
- However, major challenges for measles elimination include:
  - Weak immunization system
  - Highly infectious nature
  - Inaccessible population
  - Refusal to immunization
  - Changing epidemiology (increased transmission among adolescent and adults)
  - Need to provide catch up immunization to >130 million children in India
  - Gaps in human and financial resources at country/regional/global level.

2. Define infant mortality rate. Describe role of under fives clinics to reduce infant mortality.

Infant Mortality Rate

- Infant mortality rate (IMR) is the rate of deaths of children under 1 year of age per 1000 live births during a given year, in a given area

$$\text{IMR} = \frac{\text{No. of deaths of infants (children under 1 year of age) in a year}}{\text{Live births in the same year}} \times 1000$$

Under Five Clinics

- Under five clinics is a new concept which combines prevention, treatment, health supervision, nutritional surveillance and education into a system of comprehensive health care within the resources available in the country making use of non-professional auxiliaries, thus making the service not only economical but also available to a larger proportional of children in the community
- It is conducted one afternoon every week at subcenter or primary healthcare center (PHC) whereas the pediatric OPD at a hospital functions as under five clinic every day.

Aim	*Objectives*
▪ To provide comprehensive health care to under five through non-medical person, in an economical manner ▪ Most effective worker in under five clinic is mother of the child	▪ Maintenance of the positive health of the child by regular health check-up ▪ Growth monitoring ▪ To detect childhood disorders like infections, nutritional deficiencies ▪ To provide preventive, promotive and curative services to maximum number of children ▪ To cover all the children with timely immunization ▪ Promotion of physical, mental and social well-being of the children

Components

- The five components of under five clinic[Q] can be explained on the basis of the symbol for under five clinic
- It is a triangle subdivided into four equilateral triangles.

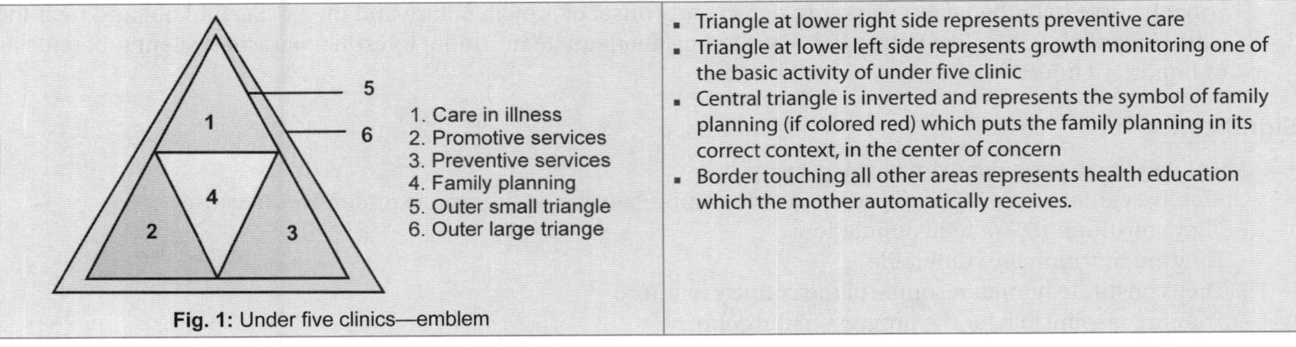

Fig. 1: Under five clinics—emblem

- Triangle at lower right side represents preventive care
- Triangle at lower left side represents growth monitoring one of the basic activity of under five clinic
- Central triangle is inverted and represents the symbol of family planning (if colored red) which puts the family planning in its correct context, in the center of concern
- Border touching all other areas represents health education which the mother automatically receives.

Activities of Under five Clinics

a. Care in illness
  i. Diagnosis and treatment
    - Acute illness
    - Chronic illness including physical, mental, congenital and acquired abnormalities
    - Disorders of growth and development.
  ii. X-ray and laboratory service.
  iii. Referral services.
  iv. Training of nurses and auxiliary health worker to a handle care responsibly.

b. Preventive care
  i. Immunization
    - Immunization of child against big six infections diseases of childhood, namely diphtheria, whooping cough, tetanus, measles, polio and tuberculosis as per the universal immunization program.
  ii. Nutritional surveillance
    - Its purpose is to identify subclinical nutrition because under five age group is at more risk of all major nutritional disorders like PEM, anemia, rickets, nutritional blindness
    - Food supplements or on site feeding its important components
    - Vitamin A prophylaxis is done through 5 mega doses of vitamin A syrup
    - Nutritional anemia is prevented by distribution of iron and folic acid tablets containing 20 mg of iron and 0.1 mg of folic acid.
  iii. Health check-ups
    - A child is provided physical examination and appropriate laboratory test every 3–6 months
    - A special card called as child health card is provided to children with particulars of their regular check ups
    - Its purpose is to identity at risk children and bring them under special care.
  iv. Oral rehydration
    - Its purpose is to reduce child deaths and malnutrition by home use of ORT
    - In a poor community a child on an average suffers an attack of diarrheal infection between 2–6 times per year
    - Each episode lowers the child's nutritional level and caries risk of death due to dehydration.
  v. Family planning
    - The mother is given counseling with regard to family planning because family planning is in center of concern for the health and well being of the child.
  vi. Health education
    - A mother is educated how to keep the child clean, how and what to feed and when she should bring the child for immunization which will be of great help to her in rearing the children.

c. Growth monitoring
  – One of the basic activities of under five clinic growth monitoring with help of a growth curve
  – A child is weighed periodically at monthly intervals during 1st year every months during 2nd year and every 3 months thereafter up to age of 5 years
  – Weight is then plotted against the age of the child on a growth chart to obtain a growth curve
  – Growth curve help the health worker to detect early onset of growth failure and the he has find out and treat the cause of growth failure like failure in breastfeeding, inadequate nutrition, intestinal parasites, silent tuberculosis or important infections.

Significance

- Absolute growth is seen maximally in 1–4 years[Q]
- Under five clinics are very important to provide comprehensive health care to under fives because
  – They constitute 15% of total population
  – They are nutritionally vulnerable
  – They constitute human resource of the country in future
  – They are responsible for the progress of the country.

SHORT ESSAYS

3. Write a note on planning cycle.

Refer Question No. 8 June 2008 (RS2) Paper II.

4. Enumerate national demographic goals to be achieved by 2010.

Refer Question No. 7 December 2007 (RS2) Paper II.

5. Enumerate the soil-transmitted helminthes and diseases caused by them.

- Soil-transmitted helminths are commonly known as intestinal worms
- Infections caused by them are called soil-transmitted helminthiasis.

Examples

Helminth	*Diseases*	*Route of transmission*
a. *Ascaris lumbricoides*	Ascariasis	Ingestion of eggs from contaminated soil
b. *Ancylostoma duodenale* and *Necator americanus* (Hookworms)	Ancylostomiasis (Hookworm infection)	Active penetration of skin by larvae in soil
c. *Trichuris trichura*	Trichuriasis (Whipworm infection)	Ingestion of eggs from contaminated soil

- Soil-transmitted helminths produce a wide range of symptoms including intestinal manifestations (diarrhea, abdominal pain), general malaise and weakness, that may affect working and learning capacities and impair physical growth
- Hookworms cause chronic intestinal blood loss that results in anemia.

Significance

- Infections by soil-transmitted helminths are most common infections worldwide affecting most deprived communities hence preventive measures against them are very important.

6. Explain rule of halves in hypertension.

Refer Question No. 12 December 2008 (RS2) Paper II.

7. List warning signals of cancer, with examples.

Refer Question No. 12 December 2007 (RS2) Paper II.

8. Write a note on benefits of barrier contraceptives, with examples.

- A contraceptive method is a one which helps the woman to avoid unwanted pregnancy resulting from coitus.

Barrier Methods (Conventional Contraceptive)

- These are the methods, which act as barrier between the sperms and the ovum
- It is a temporary method of contraception (non-terminal or spacing method)
- They are also called contraceptive method, i.e. methods that requires action at the time of sexual intercourse[Q], e.g. condoms, spermicides, diaphragm, etc.

Types

A. Physical methods
B. Chemical methods
C. Combined methods (Physical + Chemical)

Physical Methods (Barrier Method)

- The devices employed for physical barrier methods are condom, diaphragm, cervical cap, vault cap and vimule cap.

a. Condom
  - 2 types, male condom and female condom.
    i. Male condom
      - It is a sheath made up of latex, a kind of plastic
      - It is cylindrical shaped measuring 15–20 cm length, 3 cm diameter, and 0.003 cm thick
      - It is closed at one end with a teat-end and open at the other end, with an integral rim
      - It is electronically pre-tested and pre-sterilized by gamma-radiation and made available in packs
      - Storage over three years can weaken latex and increase chances of breakage.

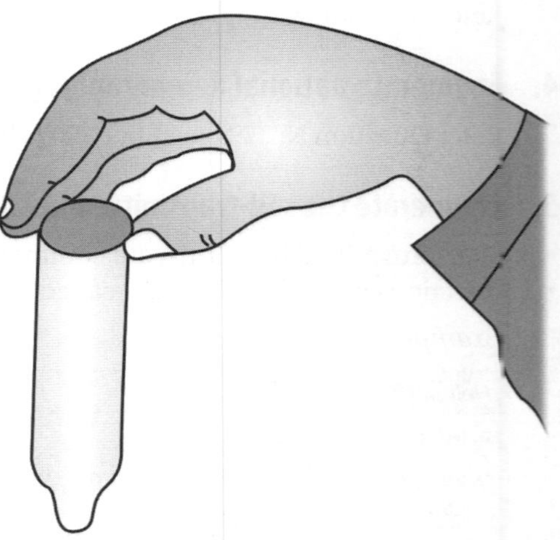

Fig. 2: Condom

Method to use
- It is used by the male partner to cover erect penis during coitus
- Before wearing, the air from the teat-end is expelled to make room for the collection of semen, by pressing it and if air from the teat-end is not removed, it may tear due to force of ejaculation
- Keeping the teat-end pressed, it is rolled over the erect penis up to the base
- After climax and before losing his erection, the person should hold the rim of the condom against penis and he should withdraw, so that the condom does not slip and the semen is not spilled
- Promoting proper use of condom is an important measure of prevention of STDs/ AIDS
- After use, it should be wrapped in a piece of paper and thrown in dustbin and not commode of the latrine
- A new condom must be used for each sexual act
- About 72 condoms are required for protection for 1 year[Q].

Varieties

Dry types (nonlubricated)	*Deluxe types (lubricated)*	*Super deluxe types*
▪ Nirodh, Durapac, Kohinoor ▪ Lubricants can be applied over this, such as glyceline, spermicide and even water ▪ Oil based lubricants should never be applied such as cooking oil, coconut oil, mineral oil, petroleum jelly, Vaseline, cream, lotion, butter, etc. because they weaken the latex rubber very quickly	▪ Adams, Fiesta, Kamasutra, Durex, Kohinoor-pink, etc.	▪ Share, Rakshak, etc. ▪ They are colored, thinner varieties lubricated with spermicides

Failure rate	*Merits*	*Demerits*
▪ 15–20 per 100 women years of exposure (WYE)[Q] ▪ This can be decreased by using it in conjunction with a spermicidal jelly, inserted into the vagina before intercourse	▪ Simple ▪ Safe ▪ Effective ▪ Cheap ▪ Easily available ▪ Without side effects and contraindications ▪ Protects against not only pregnancy, but also against STDs including AIDS[Q] (biggest advantage) ▪ Easy to use ▪ Does not require medical supervision ▪ Light, disposable, available without prescription and harmless ▪ Often prevents premature ejaculation and help the man last longer during sex play	▪ If not properly used, it may slip off or tear during sex play ▪ Interferes with sex sensation but many get used to it ▪ Rarely allergic reaction can occur to latex ▪ Becomes weak when stored for long time ▪ Cannot be used more than once ▪ Causes little embarrassment to buy, to put on, to take off and throwaway ▪ Contraindications ▪ Allergy to condom

Non-contraceptive benefits
- Prevention of HIV and STI transmission.[Q]

ii. Female condom
- It is also a sheath made up of thin, transparent, soft plastic, closed at smaller end and opened at the wider end
- Invented by Danish MD Lasse Hessel[Q]
- There are stiff and flexible rings at both the ends
- It is available in India now but is costly.

Method of use
- Before sex the woman places the closed end of the sheath high up in vagina and larger open end stays outside the vulva
- During sex, the man's penis goes inside the female condom
- Effectiveness is similar to male condoms
- It is meant for one time use only.

Types	*Failure rate*	*Merits*	*Demerits*
▪ FC–made of polyurethane ▪ FC2–made of nitrile polymer ▪ Latex	▪ 5–21 per 100 woman years of exposure	▪ Controlled by woman ▪ Prevents both pregnancy and STDs, including AIDS[Q] ▪ No apparent side effects ▪ No allergy ▪ No contraindications	▪ Expensive ▪ Not impressive ▪ Woman must touch her genitals

Significance
- Only tool for HIV prevention that woman can initiate and control[Q].

b. Diaphragm (Vaginal Diaphragm, Dutch Diaphragm)
- It is also known as Dutch cap
- It is a shallow, soft rubber cup, with a stiff but flexible rim, made up of coiled spring, which helps in retention
- Size varies from 5–10 cm in diameter and the required size for a woman can be determined by inserting two fingers in the posterior fornix and noting how far on the finger the symphisis pubis comes and this distance indicates the approximate diameter of the diaphragm, required for that woman.

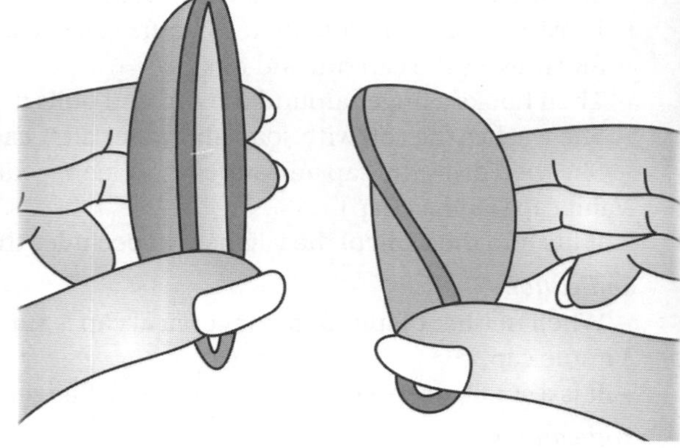
Fig. 3: Diaphragm

Method of insertion
- She holds the diaphragm with the dome down, like a cup, with a tablespoonful of spermicide jelly into the cup
- She then presses the opposite sides of the rim together and pushes the diaphragm into the vagina as far as it goes and makes sure that is covers the cervix with her fingers
- When it is inserted, it lies snugly between the sacrum and the pubic symphisis
- It is held in position partly by the tension of the spring and partly by the tone of the vaginal muscles
- It is to be inserted just before the intercourse
- It must remain there at least for 6 hours after the act[Q]
- For each additional act of intercourse during these 6 hours, she must use spermicide to be more effective
- It should not be retained for more than 24 hours
- She should not douche for at least 6 hours after sex.

Method of removal
- She should hook the rim from behind the pubic symphisis and pull out carefully
- After removal, it should be washed with soap and water
- Meanwhile she checks for holes either by filling it with water or by holding against light
- After drying, it should be stored in a cool, dark and clear place.

Contraindications	Failure rate	Merits	Demerits
▪ Prolapse of uterus ▪ Cystocoele ▪ Too long or too short cervix	▪ 10–20 per 100 women years of exposure ▪ Can be reduced to 2 per HWYE by using alongwith the spermicidal jelly	▪ Simple ▪ Safe ▪ Effective ▪ Easy to use ▪ Protection against pelvic inflammatory disease and human papilloma virus[Q]	▪ Requires services of a medical or paramedical person for the demonstration of using it ▪ May tear while removing, if not careful ▪ May rarely result in toxic shock syndrome if left in the vagina for a long time (if left in situ >24 hours[Q]) ▪ Increased risk of UTI, yeast infection and bacterial vaginosis

c. Cervical cap
   - It is thimble shaped
   - It is like diaphragm but smaller
   - It covers the vaginal portion of the cervix, thus acting as a barrier
   - The woman inserts the cervical cap with spermicide, in the proper position in the vagina before having sexual intercourse
   - She fills the dome of the cap 1/3 full with spermicidal jelly or cream

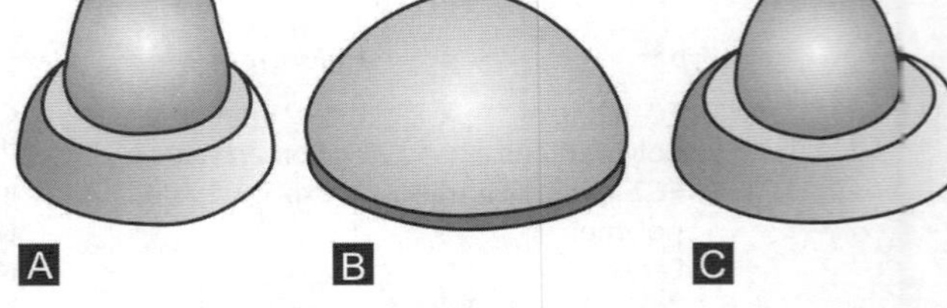

Figs 4A to C: Cervical cap

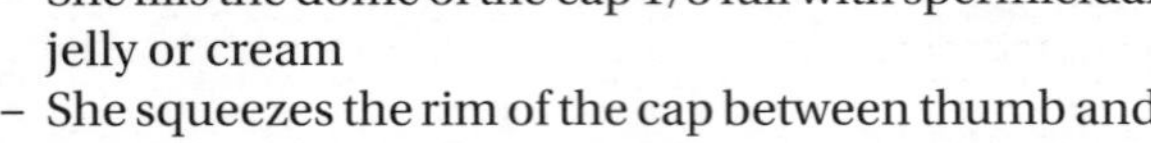

   - She squeezes the rim of the cap between thumb and index finger and with the dome side towards the palm of the hand, slides the cap into the vagina and presses the rim around the cervix
   - She leaves the cap for at least 6 hours after the act
   - She should not douche for at least 6 hours after the sex
   - Leaving in situ for more than 48 hours can cause bad odour and may increase the risk of toxic shock syndrome
   - She presses the cap rim and tilts
   - Then hooks a finger around the rim and pulls it
   - She washes the cap with soap and water after each use, then, checks for holes as in diaphragm
   - She then dries the cap and stores in a clean, cool and dark place.

d. Vault cap (Dumas Cap)
   - It fits into the vault of the vagina and occludes the cervix.

   Indications
   - When neither diaphragm nor cervical cap is suited to the woman.

e. Vimule cap
   - It is a small, deep, cup-like device with a flanged base, because of which it fits firmly on the cervix.

   Indications
   - Woman, with lax vaginal walls and cannot use diaphragm.

Chemical Methods

- These are the contraceptives that a woman places in her vagina shortly before sex
- These are all spermicides.

Classification

- Foams
- Creams, jellies, pastes
- Suppositories
- Soluble films.

a. Foams/sponge
   - The foam tablets contain the spermicide Chloramin T or Phenyl mercuric acetate
   - A few drops of water are poured on it and then introduced high up in the vagina
   - Foam is produced and spreads to all parts of vagina

– Foam aerosols are better than foam tablets because dissolve better than tablets
– The commercial name is Today[Q] which contains 1000 mg of Nonoxynol-9 spermicide[Q], which paralyses the sperm[Q]
– The effect lasts for about 1 hour
– It is inserted vaginally prior to intercourse and must be placed over the cervix to be effective[Q]
– It must be left in place for 6hrs after intercourse[Q]
– All sponges must be removed within time specified by the manufacture (For Today, it is 24 hours)

Failure rate	*Demerits*
▪ Parous woman—20–40 per 100 WYE[Q] ▪ Nulliparous woman—9–20 per 100 WYE[Q]	▪ No protection from STDs ▪ Can lead to toxic shock syndrome[Q] ▪ Increased risk of *Candida* + urinary tract infection

b. Creams, pastes and jellies
– Creams and pastes have soap base where as jelly has an aqueous base
– They are supplied along with the applicator, which is like a syringe with screw
– They also contain Chloramine T or Phenyl mercuric acetate.

Example	*Failure rate*	*Merits*	*Demerits*
▪ Delfen cream, volper cream, orthogynol jelly, perception jelly, etc.	▪ 25 pregnancy per 100 WYE ▪ Can be reduced by using it in conjunction with physical barriers	▪ Simple, safe and easy to use ▪ Offer contraception just when needed ▪ Do not require medical assistance ▪ Free from systemic toxicity	▪ Burning or irritation and messiness ▪ Local allergic reaction and urinary tract infection ▪ Have to be used at each act of sex

Significance

- Barrier method is most commonly used method of contraception due to its ease of use
- However, most important advantage it offers over all others methods of contraception is protection against STDs and HIV.

9. Mention the objectives of antenatal care.

- Antenatal care is the care of the woman during pregnancy
- Ideally, it should start soon after conception and continue till onset of labor.

Aim	*Objectives*
▪ To achieve healthy mother and a healthy baby at the end of the pregnancy	▪ To promote, protect and maintain the health of the mother during pregnancy[Q] ▪ To preserve the physiological aspects of pregnancy ▪ To detect high-risk cases and given them special attention ▪ To foresee complications and prevent them ▪ To remove anxiety and dread associated with delivery and prepare her physically and mentally ▪ To reduce maternal and infant mortality and morbidity ▪ To teach the mother elements of child care, nutrition, personal hygiene and environmental sanitation[Q] ▪ To prepare her for breastfeeding ▪ To sensitize the mother to the need for family planning, including advice to cases seeking medical termination of pregnancy ▪ To attend to the under fives accompanying the mother

Components

a. Antenatal registration and maintenance of antenatal card
– The mother's name is registered in antenatal register after confirmation of pregnancy clinically in the hospital and after 12 weeks of amenorrhoea in rural areas
– An antenatal card is prepared by writing the registration number, identifying data and details of previous and present health history including present complaints if any
– Preparation of the card not only helps in enumeration of mothers to the calculate IMR and MMR, it also helps in evaluation of other mother and child health and family planning services.

b. Antenatal history

Obstetric history	*Gynecological history*
▪ Age at marriage ▪ Duration of married life ▪ Age at first pregnancy ▪ Details of previous pregnancies and deliveries including gravid status ▪ Number of viable deliveries ▪ Abortions, still birth if any ▪ Number of living children and dead children	▪ Age at menarche ▪ History of menstrual cycles ▪ Date of last menstrual period to calculate duration amenorrhoea and to calculate the expected date of delivery (Expected date of delivery = Last menstrual period + 7days – 3 months)

c. Antenatal examination

i. Physical examination	▪ To look for built, nourishment, anemia, BP, height and weight and position of the nipple
ii. Systemic examination	▪ Consists of examination of various systems like central nervous system (CNS), cardiovascular system (CVS), respiratory system (RS), alimentary and genitourinary system to find out any systemic disease if any
iii. Abdominal examination	▪ To monitor the progress of pregnancy, fetal growth, fetal lie, position, presentation and fetal heart sounds
iv. Pelvic examination	▪ Done in the last check-up to exclude cephalopelvic disproportion

d. Antenatal investigations

i. Urine examination	▪ Albumin to exclude toxemia and urinary infections ▪ Sugar to exclude diabetes ▪ Microscopy to exclude urinary infections
ii. Blood examination	▪ Hb% to know the severity of anemia ▪ Venereal disease research laboratory (VDRL) to exclude syphilis ▪ Blood grouping to arrange for blood if necessary and prevent erythroblastosis fetalis ▪ Tridot to exclude HIV infection ▪ Hepatits B surface antigen to exclude HBSAg carrier state
iii. Stool examination	▪ For ova and cyst
iv. Other investigations	▪ USG scanning, ECG, etc.
v. Prenatal diagnosis of congenital anomalies	▪ Alfa fetoprotein estimation in maternal blood to detect neural tube defects ▪ Ultrasound examination to visualize the fetus and its congenital anomalies ▪ Amniocentesis in second trimester to detect Down's syndrome, neural tube defects, Rh status of the fetus ▪ Chorionic villi biopsy during 10th week of pregnancy to detect the chromosome status

e. Antenatal advice
- During pregnancy, mother is very receptive and constitutes a captive audience, thus health education becomes effective
- She is advised on.

i. Nutrition	▪ No restrictions in the diet ▪ Balanced diet providing 2200 Kcal/day[Q] ▪ No food or fruit is abortifacient ▪ Should consume more green leafy vegetables ▪ Should avoid spicy foods because of physiological acidity during pregnancy ▪ Should gain weight at the rate of 1.5 kg per month[Q] as to get 3.0 kg newborn baby
ii. Personal hygiene	▪ Daily bath, not to be very particular about nipples ▪ Oral hygiene to be maintained ▪ Should wear clean, light and loose clothes
iii. Rest and sleep	▪ 2 hours after lunch and 8 hours during night
iv. Exercise	▪ Light household work can be done ▪ Walking in the morning and evening is preferred ▪ Excessive physical labor to be avoided

Contd...

Contd...

v. Drugs and Radiations	▪ She should not take any drugs without consulting the doctor, i.e. should avoid self medication ▪ Doctors should not prescribe tetracycline, steroids, lysergic acid diethylamide (LSD), streptomycin, thalidomide, gastric irritants like nonsteroid anti-inflammatory drugs (NSAIDs) because they affect fetal growth and development ▪ X-rays should be avoided because of radiation hazards
vi. Habits	▪ Alcohol and smoking are strictly prohibited because alcohol affects fetal growth and development and smoking results in low birth weight
vii. Sexual relation	▪ Restricted during third trimester ▪ Prohibited if there is history of miscarriage or premature delivery ▪ Can be indulged if position is comfortable and pressure free
viii.Warning signs	▪ Mother should be advised to report any of the following signs and symptoms in her ▪ Bleeding per vagina ▪ Blurring of vision ▪ Convulsions ▪ Loss of fetal movements ▪ Severe headache or giddiness ▪ Any other unusual symptoms

f. Antenatal services (Specific protection)

i. Nutritional services	▪ Under Integrated Child Development Services Scheme, all rural expectant malnourished mothers are given a supplementary food daily providing 500 Kcals of energy including 25 g of proteins for 300 days in a year to prevent malnutrition among mothers
ii. Immunization services	▪ Against tetanus – To prevent neonatal tetanus, first dose of TT should be given to the mother in the first antenatal visit and second dose after one month – If she has conceived within 5 years of previous complete immunization, only one booster dose is given – If the mother comes late in pregnancy atleast one dose should be given ▪ Against erythroblastosis fetalis – If the mother is Rh negative and the fetus is Rh positive, mother is given Rh anti-D immunoglobulin during 28th week and 34th week to prevent erythroblastosis fetalis – If the newborn is Rh positive then mother is given another dose after delivery ▪ Against rubella – Single dose of rubella vaccine has to be given to all potential mothers but not to pregnant mothers ▪ Against Hepatitis B – If the pregnant mother is HBsAg negative, she should be Hepatitis B vaccine course
iii. Medicinal services	▪ Under National Anemia Control Program, the expectant mothers are provided a pack of 100 iron and folic acid tablets during the last trimester, each tablet containing 100 mg of elemental iron and 0.5 mg of folic acid with instruction to take one tablet per day after food ▪ If the mother is anemic, then she is advised to take 2 tablets per day to control anemia ▪ Antihelmithic drugs should be given once during the second trimester to deworm her ▪ Benzathine Penicillin 24–48 lakh units is given to mother to prevent congenital syphilis if she is suffering from primary or secondary syphilis
iv. Family welfare services	▪ If the mother is primgravid, she is sensitized about different contraceptive methods and if she wants to have a second child, she is motivated for spacing with an intrauterine contraceptive device after delivery ▪ If she is second gravid, she is motivated for sterilization
v. Educational services	▪ Mothers are educated to seek medical care in case of any health problem ▪ She is taught the art of mother craft, i.e. art of child care ▪ She is provided health education regarding physiology of pregnancy and child birth, breastfeeding, different family welfare methods ▪ Mothers are allowed to talk freely and frankly, so that all her doubts are cleared, thereby the fear-borne out of ignorance is removed and the anxiety and tension associated with delivery are also relieved i.e. she is prepared mentally for pregnancy and delivery ▪ She is educated about breastfeeding practices such as initiation of breastfeeding within ½ hour of birth, feeding colostrums, avoiding prelacteal feeds, exclusive breastfeeding up to 6 months and strict prohibition of bottle feeding

g. Pediatric component
   - A pediatrician should be in attendance at all antenatal clinics to attend the health care needs of the under fives accompanying their mothers.

   Strategy
   - Antenatal care is provided through antenatal visits by female health worker[Q].

Timing	*Services offered*		
	First visit (at 20 weeks)	*Second visit (at 32 weeks)*	*Third visit (at 36 weeks)*
▪ Antenatal visits should be done regularly and periodically as follows ▪ Once a month, till 28 weeks of pregnancy ▪ Then twice a month till 32 weeks of pregnancy ▪ Then once a week, till delivery ▪ If these visits are not possible, then atleast 3 visits are recommended[Q] respectively at 20 weeks, 32 weeks and 36 weeks	▪ Confirmation of pregnancy ▪ Registration of mother ▪ Detection of high risk pregnancy ▪ Immunization with first dose of TT ▪ Providing antenatal advice	▪ Deworming the mother ▪ Immunization with second dose of TT detecting position and presentation of the fetus ▪ Providing antenatal advice ▪ Deciding place of delivery ▪ Education regarding warning signals	▪ Exclusion of cephalopelvic disproportion ▪ Providing antenatal advice ▪ Distributing disposable delivery kit to the mother in the rural areas

Significance

Antenatal care is an important tool of Maternal and Child Health (MCH) strategy as it has impact on both maternal and infant mortality and morbidity.

10. List the functions of anganwadi worker.

Refer Question No. 2 June 2010 (RS2) Paper II.

11. Briefly describe the role of NGOs in health care (Nongovernmental organization).

- Nongovernmental organization are nonprofit organization working for betterment of society through voluntary work and donations.

Role of NGOs in Health Care

a. Innovation and initiation	▪ Official channels of health care delivery have limited scope for innovation and initiation due to rigid framework of their working atmosphere ▪ However, NGOs work in rather flexible manner thus permitting them innovate and initiate new scheme Example: ▪ Village health guide scheme , training of dais, conducting peripheral eye camps in peripheral areas were first initiated by NGOs which were later adopted by government health agencies
b. Supplementation	▪ It is impossible for healthcare delivery system to reach everybody in everywhere at all times ▪ This vacuum of health care delivery is filled in effectively by NGOs Example: ▪ Central Social Welfare Board, plays a leading role in coordinating NGOs in field of social welfare and informal education of under fives ▪ Tuberculosis association of India has undertaken task of training doctors and paramedics in antituberulosis activities ▪ Indian Red Cross Society has established chain of blood banks
c. Health education	▪ Health education in their respective field is one of main objective of all NGOs ▪ Health education imparted by NGOs provide a wider base and bring element of variety ▪ They also bring closeness amongst formal healthcare system and beneficiaries by acting as a link between them
d. Evaluation	▪ One of prime function of NGOs is acting as watch dog on performance of governmental health agencies ▪ They have proved to be very valuable in bringing out some useful changes in National Health Programs
e. Working as pressure group	▪ NGOs often have worked as pressure groups for drafting various policy decisions Example: ▪ Various legislations like MTP Act, Organ Transplantation Act, prenatal sex determination, etc. were due to pressure from NGOs

Significance

- NGOs are very crucial element of healthcare delivery system in India, which besides supplementing government efforts, provide innovative modalities of for government agencies to work eventually resulting in better health care of community.

12. Write advantages of program evaluation review technique.

Refer Question No. 6 December 2011 (RS2) Paper II.

SHORT ANSWERS

13. Enumerate functions of UNICEF.

Refer Question No. 8 June 2010 (RS2) Paper II.

14. Enumerate health problems of old age.

Refer Question No. 2 June 2009 (RS2) Paper II.

15. Enumerate indicators of child health care.

Refer Question No. 4 December 2009 (RS2) Paper II.

16. What is total fertility rate?

Refer Question No. 10 December 2008 (RS2) Paper II.

17. Enumerate the important zoonatic diseases.

- Zoonotic diseases are infections or infectious diseases transmitted from vertebrates to man.

Examples

	Diseases in man	*Animal principally involved*
Bacterial	i. Anthrax[Q]	Herbivores, pigs
	ii. Brucellosis[Q]	Cattle—sheep, goats, camels, pigs, dogs, horses, and buffaloes
	iii. Ornithosis	Wild and domestic birds
	iv. Q fever	Cattle—sheep, goats and wild animals
	v. Tuberculosis[Q]	Cattle—sheep, goats, pigs, cats and dogs
	vi. Plague[Q]	Rodents
	vii. Leptospirosis[Q]	Rodents
	viii. Tulareia[Q]	Rodents
Viral	i. Cowpox	Cattle
	ii. Monkeypox	Monkeys and rodents
	iii. Eastern equine encephalitis	Horses, rodents
	iv. Ross river fever	Cattle— horses, goats, sheep, dogs, rats, bats and pigs
	v. Yellow fever	Monkeys
	vi. Japanese encephalitis[Q]	Wild birds
	vii. Lassa fever	Mulitmammate rat
	viii. Rabies[Q]	Dog, fox, shunk, mongoose, bat and jackal

Contd...

Contd...

	Diseases in man	*Animal principally involved*
Protozoan	i. Leishmaniasis	Dogs, cats and swine
	ii. Toxoplasmosis	Cats, mammals and birds
	iii. Trypanosomiasis	Game animals and cattle
	iv. Babesiosis	Cattle
Helminthic	i. Clonorchiasis	Dogs, cats, swine, wild mammals and fish
	ii. Fasciolopsis	Swine and dogs
	iii. Schistosomiasis	Rodents
	iv. Teniasis	Cattle
	v. Trichinellosis	Swine, rodents, wild carnivores and marine mammals

18. Define new case, relapse, failure with reference to tuberculosis.

Definitions according to Revised National Tuberculosis Control Program (RNTCP)

New case[Q]	*Relapse*	*Failure*[Q]
New case is a patient with patient with sputum positive pulmonary tuberculosis[Q] who has never had treatment for tuberculosis or has taken antituberculosis drugs for less than 4 weeks	Relapse is a patient who returns smear positive having previously been treated for tuberculosis and declared cured after completion of his treatment	Failure is a patient who was initially smear positive, who began treatment and who remained or became smear positive again at five months or later during course of treatment[Q]

19. What is a population pyramid?

Refer Question No. 18 December 2008 (RS2) Paper II.

20. Write in brief principles of School Meal Program.

- Mid-day School Meal Program was started in 1962 on recommendations of School Health Committee[q]
- Also called school lunch program.

Objectives	*Principles*	*Model menu*
▪ Attract more children to school ▪ Prevent dropouts ▪ Combat malnutrition and improve health of school going children ▪ Incorporating nutrition education into the curriculum ▪ Improving school attendance as well as educational performance of the pupils	▪ An ideal mid day meal should supply at least 1/3 of calorie requirement and ½ of the protein requirement of the child[Q] ▪ It should be a supplement not a substitute to home diet i.e., it should be provided at "no profit no loss" basis in school canteen to those cannot afford to bring their tiffin from home ▪ Menu should be such that it can be easily prepared in school without any complicated cooking process ▪ Use of locally available food should be encouraged ▪ Menu should be changed frequently to avoid monotony ▪ A child should receive 250 feeds per year	▪ Cereals and millets—75 g ▪ Pulses—30 g ▪ Oils/fats— 8 g ▪ Leafy Vegetables—30 g ▪ Non leafy Vegetables—30 g

Significance

- Mid-day meal should not be limited only to school feeding, but should also try to reorient the eating habits of the children and encourage use of local commodities.

21. Enumerate functions of a manager.

- A manager in healthcare services is the one, who manages the activities of an organization efficiently in various capacities, as a captain and achieves the objectives.

Functions

a. Planner	▪ Planning the healthcare project work in such a way as to achieve the objective
b. Promoter	▪ Promoting the concerned persons of health team in carrying out their activities efficiently
c. Organizer	▪ Organizing the work with good resources such as manpower, money and materials like equipment, transport supplies, etc.
d. Director	▪ Directing the entire team members properly by describing their nature of work and placing the right person for the right job to work efficiently
e. Coordinator	▪ Coordinating all members as to carryout activities smoothly without any hurdles
f. Controller	▪ Controlling entire health team through proper direction
g. Monitor	▪ Preparing the budget, monitoring the activities and investment and assessing financial performances
h. Evaluator	▪ Evaluation of activities periodically by going through the records and reports
i. Innovator	▪ Coming out with new ideas for efficient functioning of the organization

Significance

- Manager is the heart of any organization and efficient manager equals efficient organization
- Medical officer of Primary Health Center is a good example of manager.

22. Enumerate human factors in accidents.

Refer Question No. 2 June 2016 (RS2) Paper II.

MBBS PHASE III EXAMINATION

JUNE 2011

(Revised Scheme 2)

PAPER I

LONG ESSAYS

1. What are the modes of intervention? Discuss briefly about them by giving suitable examples.

Refer Question No. 1 December 2007 (RS2) Paper I.

2. What are the host defense mechanisms? Describe briefly about the various components of the host defense mechanisms.

- Host defense mechanism is specific set of reaction stimulated in host when exposed to any infectious agent by virtue of which host is able to recognize, destroy and eliminate antigenic material forting to his own.

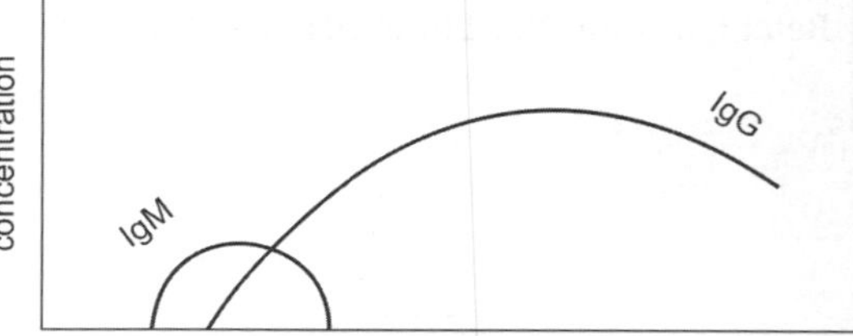

Fig. 1: Primary response

Classification

- Local and systemic
- Specific and nonspecific
- Humoral and cellular.

Components

Primary response	*Secondary response or booster response*
▪ Primary response is first immune response when body is exposed to infectious agent for first time *Stimulus* ▪ Exposure to an antigen for first time *Mechanism* ▪ After exposure to antigen, there is latent period of induction of 3–10 days before appearance of antibody i. IgM type of response – First antibody to appear is IgM which rises steadily during next 2–3 days or more and reaches peak level to decline almost as fast as it developed ii. IgG type of response – If antigen stimulation is strong, then IgM type of response is followed by appearance of IgG in few days which reaches peak in 7–10 days and then gradually falls over a period of weeks or months *Outcome* ▪ Education of reticuloendothelial cells ▪ Production of memory cells or primed cells by B and T lymphocytes which are responsible for immunological memory	▪ Secondary response is a subsequent immune response when body is exposed to known antigen *Stimulus* ▪ Exposure to an antigen subsequently after primary response *Mechanism* ▪ B and T cell collaborate to initiate secondary response ▪ Involves production of IgM and IgG antibodies ▪ IgM production is brief but IgG production is much larger and more prolonged *Features* ▪ Shorter latent period ▪ Rapid production of antibodies ▪ Abundant antibodies ▪ Antibody response maintained at higher levels for a longer period of time ▪ Antibody elicited tends to have a greater avidity or capacity to bind to antigen

Contd...

Contd...

Primary response	*Secondary response or booster response*
Factors determining primary response i. Dose of antigen – Small dose of antigen only induces IgM type of response – Antigenic dose for production of IgG type of response is 50 times that of IgM type of response ii. Route of administration iii. Adjuvants iv. Nutritional status *Significance* ▪ Immunization produces a classical primary response	*Significance* ▪ Immunological memory developed during primary response is responsible for secondary response

SHORT ESSAYS

3. What is the difference between generation time and incubation period?

Point of comparison	*Generation time*	*Incubation period*
Definition	Time taken for a person from receipt of infection to develop maximum infectivity[Q]	Time interval between invasion by an infectious agent and appearance of first sign or symptom of disease in question
Remarks	Roughly equal to incubation period of disease[Q] but may be shorter (mumps) or longer (measles)	Median incubation period is time required for 50% of cases to occur following exposure
Applicability	Transmission of infections whether clinical or subclinical	Infections that result in manifest disease

4. What are the benefits to the employees under the ESI Scheme?

Refer Question No. 4 December 2012 (RS2) Paper I.

5. What is residual chlorine? Is it necessary to have residual chlorine?

- Free or residual chlorine is the chlorine which appear in the water after the chlorine demand of water is met, i.e. any chlorine added beyond the break point appear as hypochlorons acid (HOCI) and OCl (free chlorine).

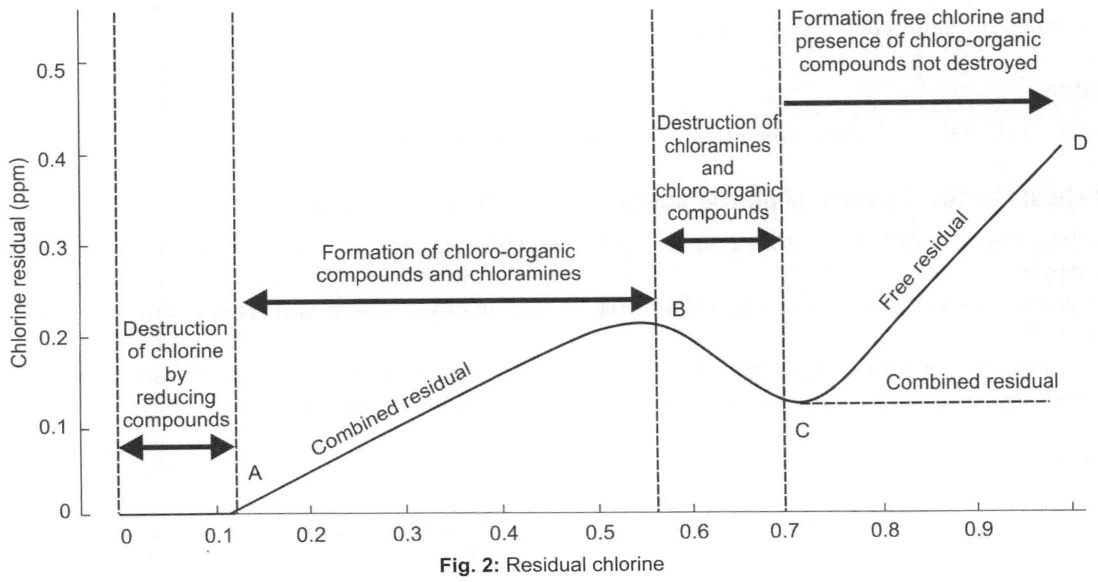

Fig. 2: Residual chlorine

Role of Free Residual Chlorine

- Chlorine is only agent which possess residual germicidal effect when used for disinfection of water[Q]
- Free residual chlorine remaining in water acts as a powerful germicide, killing pathogenic bacteria, but has no effect on spores cysts, ova and viruses of polio and viral hepatitis
- However for this action takes place there should be atleast 0.5 mg of free residual chlorine per liter for 1 hour of contact period[Q]
- Therefore for chlorination, total chlorine dose is calculated by chlorine demand of water +0.5 mg/L of chlorine
- The minimum concentration of free residual chlorine for drinking purpose should be 0.5 mg per liter, i.e. 0.5 ppm for 1 hour[Q] but postdisaster this should be 0.7 ppm for 1 hour
- The level of free residual level in water can be obtained by orthotoluidine test[Q] where the reading is taken 10 seconds after adding 0.1mL of tolidine dissolved in 10% HCl to 1 mL of water[Q] which turns yellow.

Significance

- Free residual chlorine is the insurance providing a margin of safety against further contamination of water which is likely to occur during storage and distribution.

Testing (by Orthotoluidine test)

- Orthotoluidine test is a test done to measure free and combined chlorine in water[Q].

Principle

- Orthotoluidine is converted into yellow compound by chlorine present in water.

Requirements	Procedure	Observation	Inference
• Chloroscope[Q] (chlorotex apparatus) containing – Reagent—orthotoluidine dissolved in 10% HCl – 2 graduated measuring cylinders – Pipette – Stirring rod – Reference chart showing range of color for concentration of free chlorine	• Take 1 mL of reagent using pipette in a graduated cylinder • In another graduated cylinder, take 10 mL of water to be tested • Slowly pour water from 2nd cylinder into 1st cylinder containing reagent while mixing slowly with stirring rod • Allow mixture to stand for 1 minute exactly	• Yellow color is produced which is compared with reference chart • Also note time for development of yellow color	• Intensity of yellow color developed corresponds to concentration of free chlorine • Time taken for yellow color to develop varies with presence of free chlorine and residual chlorine • If color appears immediately within 10–15 seconds, indicates presence of free chlorine • If color appears slowly after 15–20 minutes, indicates presence of both free and combined chlorine

Fallacies

- Development of yellow color if water contains iron, manganese and nitrites.

Significance

- Orthotoluidine test is a simple, rapid and accurate tool to measure free chlorine in water.

6. What should be the thickness of plastic bags should they be permitted? Why?

- Plastic bags has become indispensible item for any household for matter of economy and convenience to both retailer and shopper
- Its increasing use has created a very heavy adverse impact on environment and also directly on health of humans and animals
- Thus to control this ever growing menace, Ministry of Environment and Forest has passed Plastic Waste (Management and Handling) Rules of 2011 which has laid down rules in regards to use of plastic.

Minimum thickness	Reason
▪ Not less than 40 microns[1]	▪ Plastic bags less than 40 microns can not be recycled therefore they are banned ▪ Plastic bags having less than 40 micron will not degrade naturally if it is buried in the ground ▪ Moreover, as a general tendency people reuse thicker plastic bags whereas thinner bags are disposed off

Significance

- As doctors, its our duty to educate general population in regards to adverse impact of plastic on our health and we ourselves should start using jute or cloth bags whenever we go shopping.

Ref:

1. Plastic Waste (Management and Handling) Rules of 2011.

7. What is spurious association? How do you prevent it during research studies?

Refer Question No. 12 December 2017 (RS2) Paper I.

8. What are secular trends? How are they useful to the doctors?

Refer Question No. 1 June 2015 (RS2) Paper I.

9. What are illusions, delusions and hallucinations?

- Illusions, delusions and hallucinations are errors in perception of stimuli.

Illusion	*Delusion*	*Hallucinations*
▪ Illusion is a false interpretation by senses of an external object or stimulus which has a real existence ▪ *Example:* A person imagines a rope to be a snake	▪ Delusion is a false belief in something which is not a fact and which persists even after its falsity has been clearly demonstrated ▪ *Example:* Delusion of persecution (Person imagines that attempts are being made to poison him or kill him by his nearest relatives like wife, son or parents)	▪ Hallucinations are a false sense perception, without any external object or stimulus to produce it. They are purely imaginary and may affect any or all the special senses. ▪ *Example:* Auditory hallucinations (patient hears voice or sound without any source or any such thing)

Significance

- Even a sane person can have these errors of perception but is capable of correcting it by his reasoning power by his past experience and by being convinced by others but an insane continues to believe in illusion even though the real facts are clearly pointed out
- These errors of perception are symptoms of a brain disease.

10. What are alcoholic beverages? Can they give 'empty calories'? Why?

- Alcoholic beverages are drinks containing ethyl alcohol varying from 5–45%
- Example: Beer, whisky, rum, gin, etc.

Empty Calories

- Empty calories describes foods high in calories but low in nutritional values
- Alcoholic beverages provide about 7 kcal/g^{Q} which mostly comes from glucose
- However, these calories are low on nutrition, i.e. they do not contain any macronutrients
- Most alcoholic drinks contain traces of vitamins and minerals, but not usually in amounts that make any significant contribution to our diet
- In addition, alcohol interferes with fat metabolism, i.e. liver breaks down alcohol for energy first, causing a build-up of fatty acids
- Moreover, calories from alcohol tend to be stored as fat in abdomen.

Significance

- Alcohol is known to be addictive but this aspect of empty calories is not well-known fact and should be informed to every individual.

11. What are the different sources of health information? What are the disadvantages of hospital records?

For Different sources of Health Information

Refer Question No. 5 June 2013 (RS2) Paper I.

Hospital Records

- Hospital records are the records maintained by a hospital of the patients treated by it.

Advantages (Uses)	*Disadvantages*
▪ Provide information about healthcare activities and utilization ▪ Contains useful information on diagnosis, therapeutic and diagnostic procedures, complications, length of stay, laboratory parameter, etc. ▪ Furnishes information in regards to – Geographic sources of patients – Age and sex distribution of different disease and duration of stay in hospital – Distribution of diagnosis – Association between different diseases – The period between different diseases – The period between disease and hospital admission – The distribution of patients according to different social and biological characters – The cost of hospital care ▪ Helps to derive indices such bed occupancy rates, duration of stay, cost effectiveness of treatment of treatment which useful in monitoring the use of hospital facilities ▪ Provides valuable information for planning healthcare services	▪ Constitute only tip of the iceberg, i.e. they provide information on only those who seek medical care but not on a representative sample of the population[Q] ▪ Admission policy may vary[Q] from hospital to hospital, thus the statistics tend to differ ▪ Population served by hospital (population at risk) cannot be defined[Q] because there no precise boundaries to the catchment area of a hospital

Significance

- Hospital records should be considered as an integral and basic part of National Statistical Program (WHO)
- In developoing countries where other sources of health information are defective or unreliable, hospital records constitute a basic and primary source of information about disease prevalence.

12. Why human fecal matter needs to be treated before disposal?

- Human fecal matter is source of infections like enteric fever, dysnteries, diarrheas, cholera, hookworm disease, ascariasis, viral hepatitis and similar other intestinal infections and parasitic infestations
- It is an important source of environment pollution in form of soil pollution and water pollution
- It propagates flies which then act as vectors of disease transmission
- These diseases not only add burden of sickness to community but also cause mortality and a low expectation of life
- Moreover, it is a basic deterrent to social and economic progress
- Therefore, proper disposal of human excreta is a fundamental environmental health service for improvement in state of community health.

SHORT ANSWERS

13. Sporadic diseases.

- Sporadic diseases are diseases which occur irregularly, haphazardly, from time to time and generally infrequently in a community in singles
- Sporadic = scattered about

Features	*Examples*
▪ Cases are very few and separated widely in space and time ▪ Cases do not exhibit any connection with each other nor a recognizable common source of infection	▪ Chickenpox, polio, tetanus, herpes zoster

Significance

- Sporadic disease though occur in singles, but under favorable conditions, may become starting point of an epidemic

14. Attrition.

- Attrition is a major disadvantage of cohort study
- It means reduction in numbers of individuals

- It may be seen in study subjects due to migration, dropout or death and also in investigators due to loss of interest or poor pay.

Significance

- If attrition in a cohort study is >10–15% then study is considered invalid.

15. Methylene blue test.

Refer Question No. 6 December 2009 (RS2) Paper I.

16. Institute.

- An institute is a permanent organization body created for a certain purpose
- Often it is a research organization created to do research on specific topics
- An institute can also be a professional body
- Word comes from latin word institutum meaning facility or habit; from instituere meaning build, create, raise or educate.

17. Cancer in dye industries.

- Occupational cancer is serious occupational hazards.

Common cancers seen in dye industries	*Prevention*
▪ Skin cancers ▪ Bladder cancer	▪ Personal cleanliness ▪ Substitution of process ▪ Periodic medical examination ▪ Health education

18. Mention tick-borne diseases.

- Ticks are ectoparasites of vertebrate animals.

Tick-borne Diseases

Hard tick transmits	*Soft tick transmits*
▪ Tick typhus ▪ Viral encephalitis ▪ Viral fevers (Colorado tick fever) ▪ Viral hemorrhagic fevers (Kyasanur forest disease[Q]) ▪ Tularaemia ▪ Tick paralysis ▪ Human babesiosis	▪ Q fever[Q] ▪ Relapsing fever[Q] ▪ Kyasanur forest disease[Q]

19. Difference between epidemic and outbreak.

Points of comparison	*Epidemic*	*Outbreak*
▪ Definition	▪ Unusual occurrence of a disease in a community or region clearly in excess of expected occurrence	▪ Occurrence of more cases of disease than normally expected within a specific place or group of people over a given period of time
▪ Number of cases	▪ Very large	▪ Small
▪ Geographical location	▪ Large	▪ Limited
▪ Death rate	▪ Above average	▪ Below average
▪ Loss	▪ Human, animal and economic	▪ Human
▪ Reporting	▪ Mandatory	▪ Optional

20. Mode of action of hand-wash gels.

- Hand-wash gels are latest innovations in disinfectives.

Components	*Mode of action*	*Method of use*
▪ Antimicrobial agents ▪ Surfactants ▪ Alcohol	▪ Components of hand wash gels effectively denature microbial proteins and denature enzymes of metabolic pathways ▪ Moreover, alcohol is a very effective antimicrobial agent when compared to soaps or other disinfects	▪ Apply product to the palm of one hand ▪ Rub hands together ▪ Rub the product over all surfaces of hands and fingers until hands are dry

Significance

- With introduction of hand wash gels, it has become very easy to maintain personal hygiene, thus can reduce chances of infections.

21. Write the formula for the calculation of relative risk.

Refer Question No. 1 December 2016 (RS2) Paper I.

22. Physical quality of life index (PQLI).

Refer Question No. 16 December 2007 (RS2) Paper I.

MBBS PHASE III EXAMINATION

JUNE 2011

(Revised Scheme 2)

PAPER II

LONG ESSAYS

1. Define population explosion. What are the demographic trends in India? What measures do you suggest for the control of population explosion?

- Population explosion or population bomb is the rapid the growth of the population to an extent that the natural resources of the country are unable to support and provide the basic needs
- This phenomenon is seen when the growth rate exceeds 2%[Q].

Demographic Trends in India

- Population of India according to last census (2011) is 1,210 million growing at annual growth rate of 1.64%
- India, is currently 2nd most populous country in world, next to China
- In India, 16.87% of world population inhabits on only 2.4% of land area of world
- Since 1921, population of India has steadily increased
- At time of Independence (1947), population of India was 34 crores which become 68 crores by 1981 (in just 34 years) adding a Second India
- In another decade, it rose to 91 crores and since then 2 crores people are added to population every year
- India crossed 1 billion mark (100 crores) by 2001
- At this rate, we would soon overtake China to become world number 1 in population.

Factors Responsible for Population Explosion in India

High birth rate (causes)	*Low death rate (causes)*
▪ Early onset of puberty (between 11–13 years among girls) ▪ Universality of marriage (everyone must and should get many and prove their fertility) ▪ Early age at marriage (60% of girls in India get marry before 19 years of age and early marriage results in too early pregnancy, too many pregnancies and too frequent pregnancies) ▪ High proportion of young adults (potential parents) ▪ Social and cultural factors, such as poverty, illiteracy, ignorance, poor standard of living, lack of knowledge about family planning, religious fetters against birth control (children are God's gift), and belief to have a son	▪ Decreased frequency of natural calamities like earthquakes, floods, famines, epidemics and pandemics[Q] ▪ Advancement in the medical science ▪ Development of health consciousness among people[Q] (extensive use of chemotherapeutic antibiotics and insecticides) ▪ Availability of better healthcare facilities through Primary Healthcare Centers (PHCs) ▪ Launching of various National Health Programs ▪ International Aid, etc.

Hazards of Population Explosion

Physical	*Psychological*	*Social*	*Miscellaneous*
▪ Housing (Eruption of slums with poor living conditions)	▪ Behavioral disorders ▪ Mental illness (neuroses and Psychoses)	▪ Alcoholism ▪ Broken homes ▪ Corruption	▪ Malnutrition ▪ Infections ▪ STDs including AIDS

Contd...

Contd...

Physical	*Psychological*	*Social*	*Miscellaneous*
▪ Environmental pollution (air, soil, water, etc.) ▪ Vector problems	▪ Anxiety (due to stress and strain) ▪ Tension, worries	▪ Divorces ▪ Drug abuse ▪ Gambling, unemployment problems ▪ Anti-social activities ▪ Theft, murder, robbery ▪ Sex-crimes (rape, prostitution), child abuse, juvenile delinquency	▪ Accidents ▪ Epidemics ▪ Hypertension due to stress and strain, etc.

Population Stabilization

- Population stabilization means measures to control population explosion which could be achieved by either reducing birth rate or increasing death rate
- Since, death rate cannot be increased, only method of stabilizing population is to reduce birth rate to a level lower than death rate such that birth rate will negate death rate thus stabilizing population.

Reduction of Birth Rate

a. Birth control measures	▪ Includes family planning methods like promoting use of contraceptives, sterilization, etc.
b. Nonbirth control measures	▪ Includes social welfare methods as follows
i. Raising age at marriage	▪ Raising age at marriage stabilizes population by lengthening generation gap and increasing doubling time ▪ For example, if girl marries at 15 years of age, population doubles every 16 years but if she get married at 25 years, doubling occurs after 26 years
ii. Raising literacy level	▪ Fertility rates and family size is lower in literate women in comparison to illiterate women, hence efforts should be directed to raise literacy level in females through – Establishment of Anganwadi centers – Enrolment of all children, esp female children for primary education – Retention of enrolled children, i.e. reducing drop out rate – Providing free education to female children – Establishment of primary schools at rate of 1 per 200 children – Encouraging adult literacy
iii. Improvement in economic status	▪ By sanctioning loans (for education, agriculture, home industries) ▪ By encouraging self-employment programs ▪ By encouraging job oriented training courses (Jawahar Rozgar Yojana) ▪ By providing guaranteed income (Rajiv Gandhi Gramin Rozgar Yojana)
iv. Raising housing standards	▪ By allotment of free sites to poor ▪ By sanctioning house loans
v. Improving status of women	▪ By giving equal job opportunities and pay ▪ By legislation ▪ By information, education and communication
Vi. Adopting one child norm	▪ By massive educational campaign
Vii. Improving quality of health services	▪ Especially maternal and child health services

Significance

- Population explosion is not only a health problem, but also a social problem, economic problem and demographic problem
- Hence, population stabilization should be national priority.

2. How many infants are dying in India? Why? How do you prevent these deaths?

- Infant mortality is the death of a child within 1 year since its birth.

Infant Mortality Rate

- Infant mortality rate (IMR) is the ratio of deaths of children under 1 year of age per 1000 live births during a given year, in a given area

$$\text{IMR} = \frac{\text{No. of deaths of Infants (children under 1 year of age}^{Q}\text{) in a year}}{\text{Live births in the same year}} \times 1000$$

- It is expressed as rate per 1,000 live births.[Q]

Current Rate

- Current IMR in India is 34 per 1000 live births[Q] (SRS September 2017).

Causes (2 components)

Neonatal mortality causes (0–28 days)—70%	*Post neonatal mortality causes (1–12 months)*
▪ Low birth weight and prematurity[Q] (MC- 57%) ▪ Birth injury and difficult labor ▪ Congenital anomalies ▪ Hemolytic disease of newborn ▪ Conditions of placenta and cord ▪ Diarrheal diseases ▪ Acute respiratory infections ▪ Tetanus ▪ Sepsis	▪ Diarrheal diseases ▪ Acute respiratory infections ▪ Other communicable diseases ▪ Malnutrition ▪ Congenital anomalies ▪ Accidents
Current rate (SRS 2015) ▪ Early neonatal mortality rate—19 ▪ Late neonatal mortality rate—6	Current rate (SRS 2015) ▪ Post neonatal mortality rate—12

Factors Affecting IMR

a. Biological factors	
i. Birth weight	IMR greater in birth weight <2.5 kg and >4.0 kg
ii. Age of mother	IMR is greater in age <19 years and >35 years
iii. Birth order	IMR greatest for birth order 1 and least for 2 It increases from birth order 3 onwards[Q]
iv. Birth spacing	IMR reduces with wider birth spacing
v. Multiple births	IMR increases in multiple births
vi. Family size	IMR increases as family size increases
vii. High fertility	IMR increases with high fertility
b. Economic factors	
i. Socioeconomic status	IMR is higher in lower socioeconomic status
ii. Cultural and social factors	Few social and cultural factors increase IMR
iii. Breastfeeding	IMR is higher in early weaning and bottle fed infants living in poor hygienic conditions
iv. Religion and caste	IMR is affected by patterns, habits, customs, child care, etc
v. Early marriages	IMR is higher in teenage pregnancy
c. Other factors	
i. Sex of the child	IMR in girls > IMR in boys[Q]
ii. Quality of mothering	IMR is low in good quality mothering
iii. Quality of health care	IMR is high in improper obstetric and pediatric care

Contd...

Contd...

iv. Maternal education	IMR is low in mother with high literacy rate
v. Broken family	IMR is higher
vi. Illegitimacy	IMR is higher
vii. Brutal habits and customs (not feeding colostrums, applying cow dung to umbilical stump, faulty feeding techniques)	IMR is high
viii. Untrained dai	IMR is high
ix. Bad environmental sanitation	IMR is high

Preventive Measures

a. Prenatal feeding	▪ Improvement in state of maternal nutrition even in a small amount goes a long way in improving the birth weight of babies ▪ It is also an important component of ICDS
b. Prevention of infection	▪ Infection diseases like tetanus, measles are major causes of death in neonatal age group which can be prevented by immunization ▪ Therefore, universal immunization program aims to protect child from 6 vaccine preventable diseases and ensure greater child survival
c. Breastfeeding	▪ Safeguard against gastro intestinal and respiratory infections and PEM
d. Growth monitoring	▪ All infants should be weighed periodically at least once a month and their growth. Charts maintained ▪ hese health charts help to identify children at risk of malnutrition early ▪ Special health care is given to babies who do not thrive or show growth failure to pull them on the road to heath
e. Family planning	▪ Family limitation and spacing of births contribute of reduce infant mortality
f. Sanitation	▪ Exposure to infections through contaminated food and polluted water lack of elementary hygiene, flies and poor housing and other environmental factors could be prevented by proper sanitation
g. Provisions of primary health care	▪ All health workers involved in maternity care should collaborate and work together as a team ▪ Prenatal care must be improved to defect mothers with high risk factors and those with prenatal conditions associated with high risk and such mothers should be hospitalized and treated ▪ Special care body units for babies weighing less than 2000 g ▪ Proper referral services
h. Socioeconomic development	▪ Spread of nutritional standards ▪ Provision of safe water and basic sanitation ▪ Improvement of housing conditions ▪ Growth of agriculture and industry ▪ Availability of commerce and communication ▪ All round health and social development of the community
i. Education	▪ Educated mothers generally do not have early pregnancies are able to space their pregnancies, have better access to information related to personal hygiene and care of their children and make better use of health care services

Significance

- Infant mortality rate is a rate
- Infant death account for 18.7% of total death of country[Q]
- Infant mortality rate reflects socioeconomic progress of a country[Q] (2nd best indicator)
- It is a sensitivity parameter of combined pediatric and obstetric care in a country[Q]
- It is more universally accepted indicator of health status of whole population and their socioeconomic condition[Q]
- It is a sensitive indicator of availability, utilization and effectiveness of health care particularly perinatal care
- It is amongst best predicator of state failure[Q]
- IMR is the most important indicator of health status of community, level of living and effectiveness of MCH services in general.

Revised Scheme 2

SHORT ESSAYS

3. What is congenital rubella syndrome? How do you assess the probability of its occurrence? Is it possible to prevent it by immunization? How?

- congenital rubella syndrome refers to infants born with defects secondary to intrauterine infection or who manifest signs and symptoms of intrauterine infection sometime after birth
- Classical triad consists of deafness, cardiac malformations (most common—PDA[Q]) and cataract
- If associated with glaucoma, retinopathy, microcephalus, cerebral palsy, intrauterine growth retardation, hepatosplenomegaly, mental and motor retardation, it is termed expanded rubella syndrome
- Congenital rubella syndrome is said to have occurred if:
  - Infant has IgM rubella antibodies shortly after birth
  - IgG antibodies persist for more than 6 months.

Etiopathogenesis

- Congenital rubella syndrome occurs due to maternal infection with rubella in first trimester pregnancy[Q] (most disastrous time)
- Rubella virus inhibits cell division resulting in multiple structural defects
- Once infected, fetus remains infected through period of gestation and for many months or years after birth.

Probability of Occurrence

- Probability of occurrence is dependent upon gestational age at which maternal infection occurs which is also a major determinant of extent of fetal damage
- In other words, infection early in pregnancy result in extensive damage to fetus.

Stage of gestation	*Probability of occurrence*	*Manifestations*
▪ 4–8 weeks[Q]	80%	Abortion, still births, skin lesions (blueberry muffin lesions[Q])
▪ 8–12 weeks[Q]	25%	Classical triad
▪ 12–16 weeks	10%	Deafness (only)
▪ >17 weeks	00%	No major abnormalities

Prevention

- It is possible to prevent congenital rubella by preventing maternal infection by active and passive immunization.

a. Active immunization

i. Monovalent rubella vaccine

Type	▪ Live attenuated, freeze dried vaccines, supplied with diluents
Examples	▪ Wistar RA 27/3 vaccine[Q] (virus propagated on human diploid fibroblasts) ▪ Cendehil vaccine (virus propagated on rabbit kidney cells) ▪ HPV-77, DE-5 vaccine (virus propagated on duck embryo cells) ▪ Japanese to 336 vaccine ▪ Leningrad 8/23 vaccine
Efficacy	▪ 95%
Immunity	▪ 15 years
Dose	▪ 0.5 mL
Route of administration	▪ Subcutaneously at left upper arm
Indications	▪ 15–18 months of age ▪ Women aged 15–49 years[Q] (1st priority)
Adverse effects	▪ Malaise, fever, mild rash and transient arthralgia
Contraindications	▪ Pregnancy ▪ Infants
Remarks	▪ If female vaccinated for rubella, advice against pregnancy for next 3 months[Q]

ii. Combined vaccine

Type	▪ Live attenuated, freeze dried vaccines, supplied with diluents
Example	▪ Measles mumps and rubella (MMR)
Indication	▪ 15–18 months of age

b. Passive immunization
   – Done using human normal immunoglobulins.

Indications	▪ Infected mothers ▪ At risk individuals, i.e. close contacts
Timing	▪ Within 2–3 days of exposure
Dose	▪ 20 mL
Route of administration	▪ Intramuscularly

Significance

- Best way to prevent congenital rubella is immunization of girls of marriageable age which is substantiated by saying that "Best gift to a girl at engagement is a shot of rubella vaccine".

4. What is blood safety? How do you ensure blood safety? What is the current policy regarding blood donation?

- Blood safely program is component of National AIDS Prevention and Control Policy.

Objectives	*Components*	*Strategy (Current policy)*
▪ To ensure safe collection, processing, storage and distribution of blood and blood products	▪ Setting of blood transfusion councils at national and state levels ▪ Establishment of zonal blood testing centers top provide linkage with blood banks affiliated to public, private and voluntary sectors which test blood samples from attached blood banks and report HIV test results ▪ Strengthening the existing blood transfusion services ▪ Developing facilities for component separation in medical colleges ▪ Strengthening quality control of blood and blood products through regular monitoring of Government and Private Blood Banks	▪ Professional blood donation is prohibited since 1st April 1998 ▪ Encouragement of voluntary blood donation ▪ Licensing of blood banks and permitting only licensed blood banks to operate ▪ Mandatory testing of donated blood for HIV, HBV, HBC, malaria and syphilis

5. Write the formula for the calculation of maternal mortality rate. What are the problems that kill mothers in India?

Refer Question No. 2 June 2012 (RS2) Paper II.

6. How many millennium development goals are related to the health of the community? What are they? Write about any one of them.

Refer Question No. 2 December 2013 (RS2) Paper II.

7. Write the names of five bacterial agents that can cause acute respiratory infections among children. What is the dose schedule of cotrimoxazole for the treatment of pneumonia among children below 5 years of age, as per the ARI control program?

- Acute respiratory infections (ARI) is a complex and heterogenous group of disease, caused by number of etiological agents.

Etiological Agents

Bacteria	*Virus*	*Other agents*
▪ *Bordetella pertussis* ▪ *Corynebacterium diphtheriae* ▪ *Haemophilus influenzae* ▪ *Klebseilla pneumoniae* ▪ Legionenella pneumophila ▪ *Staphylococcus pyogenes* ▪ *Streptococcus pneumoniae* ▪ *Streptococcus pyogenes*	▪ Adenovirus ▪ Enterovirus ▪ Corona virus ▪ Measles ▪ Rhino virus ▪ Influenza virus ▪ Respiratory synctial virus	▪ *Chlamydia* type B ▪ *Coxiella burntii* ▪ *Mycoplasma pneumoniae*

ARI Control Program

- Under ARI control program, each health worker is trained to diagnose and assess severity of pneumonia and are provided with cotrimoxazole tablet to be administered to moderate cases of pneumonia
- It is preferred to other drugs because it can be safely used by health workers in field and by mothers at home.

Composition of Cotrimoxazole

Drug	*Tablet*	*Syrup/5 mL or tablespoon*
▪ Sulfamethoxazole	▪ 100 mg	▪ 200 mg
▪ Trimethoprim	▪ 20 mg	▪ 40 mg

Dose Schedule

Age	*Tablet*	*Syrup*	*Duration*
▪ <2 months (Weight 3–5 kg)	▪ 1 tablet BD	▪ ½ tablespoon BD	▪ 5 days
▪ 2–12 months (Weight 6–9 kg)	▪ 2 tablets BD	▪ 1 tablespoon BD	▪ 5 days
▪ 1–5 years (Weight 10–19 kg)	▪ 3 tablets BD	▪ 1½ tablespoon BD	▪ 5 days

Precautions

- In children below months, cotrimoxazole is not routinely used but should be initiated before referral
- Cotrimoxazole should not be given to premature babies and cases of neonatal jaundice.

Significance

- Cotrimoxazole is a drug of choice for acute respiratory infection because it is effective with high cure rate, few side effects and less expensive.

8. How do you manage a case of dengue hemorrhagic fever in a primary health center?

Refer Question No. 12 June 2012 (RS2) Paper II.

9. Is it necessary to universally breastfeed the babies? Why?

- It is necessary to universally breastfeed babies as breast milk is ideal food for infant under any circumstances
- Infant does not need additional feed besides breast milk till 6 months of age
- Besides nutrition, breast milk offers numerous benefits to infant and mother in particular and family and community in general
- WHO recommends breastfeeding for minimum 24 months[Q].

Benefits of Breastfeeding

a. Benefits to baby
   - Mother's milk is most complete food available in nature
   - Provides all essential nutrients in desired quantities

- Nutrients are present in easily digestible and assimilable form for both normal and premature babies
- Besides nutrients, also contains hormones, enzymes, protective antibodies
- Also contain other protective substances
  - Leukocytes which fight infection
  - Lactoferrin which binds iron and prevents growth of pathogen requiring iron
  - Antistreptococal factors protects against necrotising enterocolitis
  - Lysozymes which destroy pathogens
  - Bifidus factor which helps *Lactobacillus bifidus* to grow in intestine, which in turn prevents growth of pathogen causing diarrhea
- Bacteriologically clean and pure, hygienic
- Cost effective, easily obtainable, 24 × 7 and at suitable temperature
- Improves intelligent quotient and visual acuity of child due to presence of special fatty acids
- Prevents childhood obesity
- Prevents or postpones onset of diseases like diabetes, cancer and hypertension
- Protects against respiratory, alimentary diseases and also allergies, eczema and asthma due to presence of anti-infective factors
- Exercise while sucking help in development of jaws and teeth and also gives child chubby cheek appearance
- Prevents malnutrition and reduces infant mortality
- Provides several biochemical advantages like prevention of neonatal hypocalcemia and hypomagnesemia
- Thus, it promotes overall growth and development of child, i.e. physical, psychological, social, motor and mental development.

b. Benefits to mother
   - Exclusive breastfeeding is a natural contraceptive method thus allowing spacing between children
   - Prevents breast cancer, ovarian cancer and osteoporosis
   - Boosts mother's immune system
   - Acts as antidiabetogenic factor, by reducing requirement of insulin in diabetic mothers
   - Adds beauty and complexion to mother
   - Helps in restoration of original physique
   - Helps in quick and early involution of uterus and reduces postpartum bleeding and anemia.

c. Benefits to both baby and mother
   - Breastfeeding helps in establishment of bonding between infant and mother which is permanent and psychologically beneficial to both.

d. Benefits to family and nation
   - Saves money, time, conserves energy
   - Reduces infant morbidity and mortality.

Significance

- Universally accepted facts about breastfeeding are:
  - It is best start to life
  - It is unique
  - It provides umpteen number of benefits to both mother and baby
  - It is gold standard of infant feeding
  - It is safe, sound and sustainable
  - It is foundation for fulfilling rights of child
  - It is specific species and eco-friendly.

10. How do you calculate annual parasite incidence? What is the current API in India?

- API or annual parasite incidence is a parameter used for measurement of malaria in the eradication era
- It is calculated as follows:

$$\text{API} = \frac{\text{Confirmed cases of malaria during one year}}{\text{Population under serveillance}} \times 1000$$

- It based on intensive active and passive surveillance and cases are confirmed by blood examination
- It is parasitological in nature.

Current API in India

- Current API in India is 0.89.[1]

Significance (Role of API in Malaria Control)

- API is the most important malaria indices used as criteria to classify area to direct the preventive measures.

Categories	*API*	*Strategy phase*
Category 0	Zero indigenous cases of malaria	Prevention of re-establishment phase
Category 1	API <1 per 1000 population at risk in all districts	Elimination phase
Category 2	API <1 per 1000 population at risk but few districts reporting API >1 per 1000 population	Pre-elimination phase
Category 3	API >1 per 1000 population	Intensified control phase

Control Strategies

<table>
<tr><th>Control strategy in areas with API <1</th><th>Control strategy in areas with API >1</th></tr>
<tr><td>
i. Spraying
– These areas will not be under regular insecticidal spraying, however focal spraying with DDT or malathion is to be taken up only around the P. falciparum cases detected during surveillance[Q]
ii. Surveillance
– Active and passive surveillance is to be carried out vigorously every fortnight[Q]
iii. Treatment
– All detected cases should receive radical treatment as prescribed
iv. Follow-up[Q]
– Follow up blood smear are to be collected from all positive cases on completion of radical treatment and thereafter monthly for a year[Q]
v. Epidemiological investigation
– All malaria positive cases are to be investigated including mass surveys
</td><td>
i. Spraying
– All these areas are brought under regular insecticidal spray at 6 week interval[Q] in following insecticides in order of priority depending upon the resistant of vector
<table>
<tr><th>Insecticide</th><th>No. of round</th><th>Dosage (g/m² surface)</th></tr>
<tr><td>DDT</td><td>2</td><td>1.0</td></tr>
<tr><td>Malathion (Resistant to DDT)</td><td>3</td><td>2.0</td></tr>
<tr><td>Pyrethrin (Resistant to DDT and malathion)</td><td>2 (6 weeks apart)</td><td>0.25</td></tr>
</table>
ii. Entomological assessment
– Entomological teams carry out susceptibility tests periodically and suggest appropriate insecticides to be used in particular area
iii. Surveillance
– Active and passive surveillance is carried out fortnightly.
v. Treatment of cases
– Great emphasis is laid on presumptive and radical treatment of cases
</td></tr>
</table>

Ref:

1. Govt of India, National framework for malaria elimination in India (2016–2030); p. 36.

11. Why do we take night blood smears? What is the rationale in mass drug administration?

Night Blood Smears

- Night blood examination is a component of filarial survey
- Here the examination of the population for filariasis is done at night.

Principle	*Protocol*
▪ Based on the fact that microfilaria of *W. bancrofti* and *B. malayi* occurring in India display nocturnal periodicity, i.e. they appear in large number at night and retreat from the blood stream during the day	▪ Timing ▪ Between 8.30 pm—12.00 midnight ▪ Procedure

Contd...

Contd...

Principle	Protocol
▪ Maximum density is reported between 10 pm–2 am ▪ This is a biological adaptation to the nocturnal biting habits of vector mosquitoes	▪ 20 cc of blood is collected by a deep finger prick under aseptic conditions and a thick smear is prepared with it on a glass slide ▪ Age, sex and other factors are recorded on the survey card or register along with slide number ▪ Next day the blood films are dehemoglobinized, dried, fixed with methyl alcohol, stained with Giemsa stain and examined microscopically for microfilaria

Significance

- Night blood examination offers definitive diagnosis of lymphatic filariasis by demonstration of living parasites in the human body.

Mass Drug Administration

- Mass therapy is one of approach of filarial control where DEC is given to almost everyone in community irrespective of whether they have microfilaremia, disease manifestation or no signs of infection
- This approach is indicated in highly endemic areas but is abandoned in India.

Objective	Indications	Rational (advantages)	Disadvantages
▪ To reduce morbidity by treating cases ▪ To reduce transmission by treating carriers of microfilariae ▪ To interrupt transmission by elimination of parasite from human population	▪ Indicated in high and hyperendemic areas ▪ Almost everyone in the community, irrespective of their symptoms except children below 2 years, pregnant women and very sick patients	▪ As effective as 12 days therapy for public health measure ▪ Cost effective ▪ Avoids cost of blood examination ▪ Improves patient—drug compliance ▪ Has eliminated lymphatic filariasis in other countries ▪ Can be integrated into primary health care system	▪ Requires intensive efforts of educating the people for their cooperation

Significance

- Filariasis is a major public health problem which besides efforts of health workers, require compliance of general population to offer night blood samples and taken drugs irrespective of infective status.

12. Define tuberculosis control in the community. Name at least two countries that have controlled TB. How could they do it?

- Tuberculosis control is defined as when prevalence of natural infection in age group of 0–14 years is of order of 1%[Q]
- It means reduction in prevalence and incidence of disease in community.

Countries that have controlled TB	Reason
▪ United States of America ▪ United Kingdom ▪ Canada ▪ Switzerland ▪ Australia ▪ New Zealand	▪ These countries have contained tuberculosis long before advent of BCG or chemotherapy by: – Changing nonspecific determinants of disease such as improvements in standards of living and quality of life of people – Application of available technical knowledge and health resources

SHORT ANSWERS

13. Mantoux test.

Refer Question No. 1 December 2009 (RS2) Paper II.

14. Mention three gametocidal drugs in malaria control.

- Antimalarials drugs which kill gametocytes of malarial parasite in blood are called gametocidal.

Revised Scheme 2

Gametocidals

Drugs	P. falciparum	P. vivax
▪ Chloroquine	–	+
▪ Quinine	–	+
▪ Primaquine	+	+
▪ Artemisinin	+	+

Significance

- Gametocidal drugs do not offer any benefit to patient being treated but used to reduce transmission to mosquito.

15. What is the dose of vitamin A solution for a 9-month-old child? Why?

- According to National Vitamin A Prophylaxis Program.

Dose at 9 months	Reason
▪ 100,000 IU (55 mg) orally of retinol palmitate	▪ Dose at 9 months is given along with measles vaccine so that parents need not come separately for vitamin administration

16. What are the common side effects of DPT immunization?

- DPT is combination of diphtheria toxoid, whole cell killed pertussis vaccine and tetanus toxoid
- It is popularly known as triple antigen.

Efficacy
- Two toxoids are highly immunogenic and antibodies to them are almost completely protective
- Pertussis vaccine, given in 3 doses, has a protective efficacy of about 70–80% only
- Pertussis component enhances potency of diphtheria toxoid[Q]

Nature
- Killed, bacterial liquid vaccine

Types
- Plain
- Absorbed (on a mineral carrier like aluminum phosphate/hydroxide) WHO recommended
  - Aluminum salts have adjuvant effect[Q]

Composition (per 0.5 mL)

Components	Glaxo	Kasauli
• Diphtheria toxoid (Ramon and Glenny, 1923)	25 Lf[Q]	30 Lf
• Tetanus toxoid (Ramon and Zoeller, 1927)	5 Lf	10 Lf
• Killed *Bordetella pertussis* (Madsen, 1923)	20,000 million	30,000 million
• Toxoids adjuvanted (Aluminum hydroxide/phosphate)	2.5 mg	3.0 mg
• Preservative (Thiomersal)	0.01%	0.01%

Storage
- 4–8°C[Q]
- DPT vaccine supplied as liquid, store refrigerated
- Aluminum adjuvanted vaccines should not be frozen
- Vaccine remains potent if cold chain is maintained

Dose
- 0.5 mL

Route of administration
- Deep intramuscularly, preferably anterolateral aspect of thigh

Contd...

Contd...

Schedule

• Primary course (along with OPV)	DPT_1— 6th week DPT_2—10th week DPT_3—14th week
• 1st booster	10th month
• 2nd booster (DT only)	5th year

Indications

- For active immunization of infants against diphtheria, pertussis and tetanus simultaneously.

Contraindications

Absolute	*Relative*
• Severe hypersensitivity reaction to previous dose (collapse or shock like state, persistent screaming, fever >40°C, convulsions, neurological symptoms and anaphylactic shock) • Progressive neurological disease (Example, Active epilepsy) (However, DPT can be given in epilepsy controlled on antiepileptics and cerebral palsy)	• Acute febrile illness • History of convulsions

Adverse Effects (Reactions)

- Pain, fever and mild local reaction on next day (due to toxoid component)—2–6%
- Swelling and induration or pain for more than 48 hours—5–10%
- Anaphylactic shock
- Encephalitis, prolonged convulsions, infantile spasms, Reye's syndrome (due to pertussis component)—rarely
- Convulsions (rare and earliest signs of incipient neurological disease in infant)
- Provocative reaction—very rarely.

Precautions

- Shake the vial before use and discard if turbidity or floccules seen (Shake test)
- Use before date of expiry
- Avoid exposure to direct sunlight when in use[Q]
- Half used vials should not be put back into the cold chain after session[Q]

Uses

- DPT vaccine is used for simultaneous active immunization against diphtheria, pertussis and tetanus in 3 doses of 0.5 mL each administered deep intramuscularly at 4 weekly interval starting 6th week
- If an unimmunized child aged more than 2 years reports, he is immunized with two primary doses of DT at 4 week interval, followed by booster dose with DT at 5th year.

17. Fernandez reaction.

- Fernandez reaction is first positive response of lepromin test
- Also called as early response of lepromin test
- It is a delayed type of hypersensitivity response[Q] induced by soluble component of leprosy bacilli (Lepromin).

Observation	*Interpretation*			*Merits*
▪ Erythema and induration at the site of inoculation developing in 24–48 hours and usually remaining for 3–5 days ▪ Read at 48 hours[Q] ▪ Redness >10 mm indicates positive test	*Diameter of redness*	*Inference*	*Type of leprosy*	▪ Superior to late response (Indicates whether or not a person has been previously sensitized by exposure to and infection by the leprosy bacilli)
	<10 mm	Negative (–)	Lepromatous leprosy	
	10–15 mm	Mild/weak positive (+)	Borderline leprosy	
	15–20 mm	Moderate positive (++)	Indeterminate leprosy	
	>20 mm	Strongly positive (+++)	Tuberculoid leprosy	

Significance

- Lepromin test is used for detection of cell-mediated immunity against lepra bacilli
- It is analogous to the tuberculin reaction[Q], is poorly defined and carries little significance.

18. Which vitamin deficiency can cause psychosis? Why?

- Deficiency of thiamine (vitamin B_1) can cause Korsakoff's psychosis.

Reason

- Active form of thiamine is thiamine diphosphate which plays a major role as cofactor or coenzyme for enzymes associated with CAC cycle, and catalyze oxidation of pyruvate, alphaketoglutarate and branched chain amino acids
- This leads to accumulation of pyruvic acid and lactic acid in parts of brain leading to atrophy of specific regions of the brain, especially mamillary bodies, anterior region of thalamus, medial dorsal thalamus, basal forebrain and median and dorsal raphe nuclei.

19. How do you manage postpartum hemorrhage in a community health care?

- Postpartum hemorrhage is bleeding more than 500 mL after birth of child.

Types

	Primary PPH	*Secondary PPH*
Definition	▪ Bleeding within 6 hours of delivery	▪ Bleeding between 5th to 10th day
Cause	▪ Atonia of uterus ▪ Retained placenta ▪ Laceration of cervix or vagina	▪ Retention of bits of placenta
Treatment	▪ Injection ergometrine, bimanual compression of uterus and blood transfusion (uterine atonia) ▪ Stitching laceration followed by vaginal pack and blood transfusion (lacerations)	▪ Exploration and evacuation of uterus under general anesthesia

Significance

- Community health center have obstetricians hence cases of postpartum hemorrhage can be well-managed and do not require referral to higher centers.

20. Write the formulae for calculation of sensitivity and specificity.

Refer Question No. 1 December 2010 (RS2) Paper I.

21. What is the duration of training of a local dai? What does she learn during her training?

Refer Question No. 19 June 2010 (RS2) Paper II.

22. Write six uses of cancer registry.

Refer Question No. 16 June 2010 (RS2) Paper II.

MBBS PHASE III EXAMINATION

DECEMBER 2011

(Revised Scheme 2)

PAPER I

LONG ESSAYS

1. What are the laws meant for the protection of industrial workers? Write in detail about Factories act 1948.

Legislative Measures

- The important legislative measures available for to safeguard the health, safety and welfare of the industrial workers and prevention of occupational disease in India are:
  i. The Factories Act, 1948
  ii. Employees State Insurance Act, 1948
  iii. Workmen's Compensative Act, 1923
  iv. Mines Act
  v. Tea Plantation Act
  vi. Atomic Energy Act
  vii. Minimum Wages Act, 1948
  viii. Maternity Benefit Act
  ix. Dock Laborer's Act
  x. Industrial Dispute Act
  xi. Employees Provident Fund Act, 1952
  xii. Family Pension and Deposit Linked Insurance Fund Act.

Significance

- The standards laid down by these acts if complied by the employer will go a long way in prevention of occupational diseases and promote the health, safety and welfare of the employees.

Indian Factories Act

- The first Indian Factories Act was passed in 1st July 1881 and since then revised and amended 7 times, latest in 1987.
- The act has 9 chapters.

Chapter I: Preliminary—Scope and definitions

a. Section 1: Scope—The act extends to the whole of India except the state of Jammu and Kashmir
b. Section 2: Definitions
  - Child—an individual who has not completed 15 years of age
  - Adolescent—an individual who has completed 15 years of age but not 18 years of age
  - Young person—an individual who is either child or adolescent
  - Adult—an individual who has completed 18 years of age
  - Factory—an establishment employing 10 or more workers where power is used and 20 or more persons where power is not used[Q]
  - Worker—a person employed, whether for wages or not, in any manufacturing process
  - Power—an energy transmitted mechanically and is not generated by human agency.

Chapter II: The inspecting staff

a. Section 8: Inspectors
   - The State Government may appoint Chief Inspectors and Additional Inspectors of factories
   - Every District Magistrate shall be an Inspector for his district.
b. Section 9: Powers
   - An inspector can enter any factory, within his local limits and make an examination of premises, machineries or records which he may consider necessary.
c. Section 10: Certifying Surgeons
   - The State Government may appoint a qualified medical practitioner to be the certifying surgeon.

Chapter III: Health

- This chapter makes provisions for the sanitary environment for the protection and promotion of health of the workers.
  a. Section 11: Cleanliness
  b. Section 12: Disposal of refuse
  c. Section 13: Ventilation and temperature
  d. Section 14: Dust and fumes
  e. Section 15: Artificial humidification
  f. Section 16: Over crowding
  g. Section 17: Lighting
  h. Section 18: Drinking water
  i. Section 19: Latrines and urinals
  j. Section 20: Spittoons.

Chapter IV: Safety

- This chapter prescribes the precautions to be taken for safety of the workers against accidents and injuries
- These safety precautions include casing of machinery, devices for cutting off the power, hoist and lifts, cranes and other lifting devices, protection for eyes and precautions against dangerous fumes, explosives and inflammable materials
- It states provision of a minimum 500 cubic feet of air space per worker[Q]
- The act also advices appointment of a "Safety officer" for a factory involving 1000 or more workers.

Chapter V: Welfare measures

- Facilities for washing, drying and storing clothes
- Facilities for rest and recreation
- Canteen if there is more than 250 workers
- Crèches, for the children of women workers, if there are more than 30 women workers
- First aid appliances, at the rate of 1 box for every 150 workers
- A Welfare Officer, if there are more than 500 workers.

Chapter VI: Working hours[Q]

- Weekly hours: Not more than 48 hours in a week[Q] and not more than 60 hours including overtime
- Weekly holiday: One day in a week, preferably on Sunday
- Daily hours: Not more than 9 hours, with half an hour rest after 5 hours of continuous work
- Women: No women shall be allowed to work between 7 PM and 6 AM
- Adolescents: Adolescents shall work only between 6 AM to 7 PM and for 4½ hours per day.

Chapter VII: Employment of young persons

- No child who has not completed 14 years of age shall be allowed to work in any factory[Q]
- 15–18 years adolescents should be duly certified by the certifying surgeon regarding their physical fitness for work and the certificate has to be renewed every year.

Chapter VIII: Annual leave with wages

- Besides weekly holidays and general holidays, every worker is entitled to leave with wages after 12 months of continuous service at the rate of 1 day for every 20 days of work and the leave can be accumulated up to 30 days.

Chapter IX: Special provisions

a. Section 88
   - Certain accidents, including death or serious injuries should be notified by the manager to District Magistrate and Police Enquiry should be conducted in every fatal accident.

b. Section 89
   - It gives a schedule of Notifiable diseases and occurrence of such a disease should be notified by the manager to the chief factory inspector and certifying surgeon
   - About 29 diseases are notifiable under Factories Act[Q].

Significance

- Legislation to protect workers have been formulated and implemented since industrial revolution because happy labor force means more productivity and more productivity means increased income which indirectly translates into better health care.

2. Define health education. Explain the principles of health education giving examples.

- Health education is a process aimed at encouraging people to want to be healthy, to know how to stay healthy, to do what they can individually and collectively to maintain health and to seek help when needed. (Declaration of Alma Ata)
- Health education is the process by which individuals and groups of people learn to behave in a manner conducive to the promotion, maintenance or restoration of health (John M Last).

Aims and objectives	*Goal*
▪ To encourage people to adopt and sustain health promoting lifestyle and practices ▪ To promote the proper use of health services available to them ▪ To arouse interest, provide new knowledge, improve skills and change attitudes in making rational decisions to solve their problems ▪ To stimulate individual and community self-reliance and participation to achieve health development through individual and community involvement at every step from identifying problems to solving them	▪ To make realistic improvement in the basic quality of life

Strandfeild's principles of health education (Seven Is)
▪ Identification ▪ Involvement ▪ Indigenization ▪ Indoctrination ▪ Integration ▪ Influencers ▪ Innovation

Principles[Q]

a. Credibility	▪ Degree to which the message to be communicated is perceived as trustworthy by the audience ▪ Unless the people have trust and confidence in the communicator, no desired action will ensue after receiving the message
b. Interest	▪ Psychological principle that people are unlikely to listen to those things which are not to their interest ▪ Salutary to remind ourselves that health teaching should relate to the interests of the people ▪ Health educators must find out the real health needs (felt needs) of the people[Q] and people will happily participate If a health program is based on these "felt needs" and only then it will be a people's program ▪ If the felt needs are not known due to some reasons like illiteracy then the health educator has to bring about recognition of the needs before he proceeds to tackle them
c. Participation[Q]	▪ Based on the psychological principle of active learning ▪ Health education should aim at encouraging people to work actively with health workers and others in identifying their own health problems and also in developing solutions and plans to work them out ▪ A high degree of participation tends to create a sense of involvement, personal acceptance and decision—making and provides maximum feedback ▪ Participation of community is important for a health program to succeed
d. Motivation[Q]	▪ Process of awakening the fundamental desire to learn in a person *Types* i. Primary motives (e.g. sex, hunger, survival) are driving forces initiating people into action; these motives are inborn desires ii. Secondary motives are based on desires created by outside forces or incentives like praise, love, rivalry, rewards and punishment, and recognition ▪ In health education, motivation is an important factor; and is used to change behavior ▪ Motivation is contagious, i.e. one motivated person may spread motivation throughout a group

Contd...

Revised Scheme 2

Contd...

e. Comprehension	▪ Involves knowing the level of understanding, education and literacy of people to whom the teaching is directed because one of the barrier to communication is using words which cannot be understood ▪ Therefore in health education, always communicate in the language people understand, and never use words which are strange and new to the people and limit the teaching within the mental capacity of the audience[Q]
f. Reinforcement[Q]	▪ Repetition of health education at intervals because if there is no reinforcement, there is every possibility of the individual going back to the pre-awareness stage ▪ If the message is repeated in different ways, people are more likely to remember it
g. Learning by doing	▪ Learning is an action process; not a "memorizing" one in the narrow sense ▪ The Chinese proverb "If I hear, I forget; if I see, I remember; if I do, I know" illustrates the importance of learning by doing
h. Known to unknown	▪ In health education the rules of teaching are to proceed "from the concrete to the abstract"; "from the particular to the general"; "from the simple to the more complicated;" "from the easy to more difficult"; and "from the known to the unknown" i.e. start where the people are and with what they understand and then proceed to new knowledge
i. Setting an example	▪ Health educator should set a good example in the things he is teaching ▪ For example if he is explaining the hazards of smoking, he will not be very successful if he himself smokes
j. Good human relations	▪ A good relation makes sharing of information, ideas and feelings very easy
k. Feedback	▪ One of the key concepts of the systems approach and it is of paramount importance for effective communication ▪ In light of feedback, the educator can modify the elements of the system
l. Leaders	▪ Learning is best when the instructor is someone whom we respect and regard ▪ Leader are agents of change and they be made use of in health education program[Q] ▪ If the leaders are convinced first then the rest of the task of program implementation becomes easy ▪ A good leader understands the needs and demands of the community, provides proper guidance, takes the initiative, is receptive to views and suggestions of the people, identifies himself with the community, selfless, honest, impartial, considerate and sincere, easily accessible to the people, able to control and compromise various fractions in the community, possesses the requisite skill and knowledge of eliciting cooperation and achieving coordination of various organizations

Approaches to health education[Q]

Regulatory approach (managed prevention)	*Coercive or Legislative approach*	*Service approach*	*Health education approach*	*Primary health care approach*
• Defined as any governmental intervention	• Useful in times of emergency	• Providing health services at people's door steps • Not based on felt needs	• Slow but enduring results	• Radically new approach[Q] • Community involvement and intersectoral coordination • Helps individuals become self-reliant in health

Contents

- The scope of health education extends beyond the conventional health sector and should cover every aspect of family and community health
- Thus the content of health education can be as follows:

a. Human biology
   - It involves study of structure and functions of the body; how to keep physically fit—the need for exercise, rest and sleep; the effects of alcohol, smoking and drugs on the body; cultivation of healthy lifestyles, etc.
   - Understanding of the human biology is important if one wants to learn about health
   - UNICEF's has drawn up a basic list of health information comprising about child spacing, breastfeeding, safe motherhood, immunization, weaning and child growth, diarrheal disease, respiratory infections, house hygiene which it believes, every family has a right to know and would enable them to bring about significant improvements in their own and their children's health
   - The best place to teach human biology is the school as only the school, through its sequential health curriculum, which can provide continuous in-depth learning experiences for millions of students and provision of information and advice on human biology and hygiene is vital for each new generation

b. Nutrition
   - The aim of nutrition education is to guide people to choose optimum and balanced diets, remove prejudices and promote good dietary habits
   - Nutritional education can best solve the nutritional problems such as ignorance about the value of breastfeeding beyond the first year of life, misconceptions about proper weaning, ignorance of the appropriateness of certain diets for infants and pregnant women, traditional food allocation pattern within the families, etc.
   - Nutrition education is a major intervention for the prevention of malnutrition, promotion of health and improving the quality of life

Contd...

Contd...

c. Hygiene

Personal hygiene	*Environmental hygiene*
• Aim of personal hygiene is to promote standards of personal cleanliness within the setting of the condition where people live and it includes bathing, clothing, washing hands and toilet; care of nails, feet and teeth; spitting, coughing, sneezing, personal appearance and inculcation of clean habits in the young • Training in personal hygiene should begin at a very early age and must be carried through school age	• Domestic hygiene • Comprises that of the home, use of soap, need for fresh air, light and ventilation; hygienic storage of foods; hygienic disposal of wastes, need to avoid pests, rats, mice and insects • Community hygiene – Comprises of improvement of basic sanitary services consisting of water supply, disposal of human excreta, other solid and liquid wastes, vector control, food sanitation and housing which are fundamental to health

e. Family health
   - Family is the first defence, and health largely depends on the family's social and physical environment and its lifestyle and behavior
   - Role of the family in health promotion and in prevention of disease, early diagnosis and care of the sick is of crucial importance
   - Health education should target to promote the family's self-reliance, especially regarding the family's responsibilities in child-bearing, child rearing, self-care and in influencing their children adopt a healthy lifestyle
f. Disease prevention and control
   - Without health education, a person may fall sick again and again from the same disease because drugs alone will not solve all health problems
   - Education of the people about the prevention and control of locally endemic diseases is the first of eight essential activities in primary health care
g. Mental health
   - Aim of education in mental health is to help people to keep mentally healthy and to prevent a mental breakdown
   - It has become very important as there is a tendency to an increase in the prevalence of mental diseases when there is a change in the society from an agricultural to an industrial economy, and when people move from the warm intimacy of a village community to the isolation found in big cities
   - People should enjoy their relationships with others and learn to live and work without mental breakdown
   - There are certain critical periods of life when external pressure tends to breakdown mental health for example mother after child birth; child at entry into school for the first time, school child entering the secondary school, decision about a future career, starting a new family and at the time of widowhood
   - Health workers should help people achieve mental health by showing sympathy, understanding and by social contact
h. Prevention of accidents
   - Accidents are a feature of the complexity of modern life
   - In the developed countries, they are taking an increasing toll of life and limb
   - Accidents occur in three main areas: the home, road and the place of work and safety education should be directed to these areas
   - The predominant factor accidents is carelessness and the problem can be tackled through health education
i. Use of health services
   - Many people particularly in rural areas do not know, what health services are available in their community, and many more do not know what signs to look for that indicate a visit to the doctor is necessary
   - One of the declared aims of health education is to inform the people about the health services that are available in the community and how they can utilize them (e.g., screening programs, immunization, family planning services etc.) and use the health care resources

Planning a Health Educational Session or Campaign

A. Research and planning
   a. Situational analysis
      i. National policy and organizational structure
         - Study of existing policies at that time about the health of the study group
         - Need for advocacy to change policies should also be assessed
         - Study the organizational structure existing at that time and how best to utilise this organizational structure for the improvement of IEC activities
      ii. Philosophy
         - By understanding the philosophy the approach to the target groups could be decided
         - This will entail a decision on concerned education
         - Here, too, it is necessary to not disturb the delicate balance between promotion of traditional values and practical progamme to meet the needs of people
      iii. Examining the existing data
         - By analyzing the existing data target group could be understood, key influencers of the target group can be known
         - These reports may indicate the habit preferences of target groups and the effectiveness of different media on target groups
         - This date can be used to
            o Stratify the target groups
            o Develop the suitable messages
            o Ensure participation and involvement of youth in the design of message and developing of communication tools
            o Identify and use peer groups as communicators
            o Identify suitable media (to reach target groups)
            o Develop appropriate school curriculum
            o Develop cocurricular activities

Contd...

Contd...

b. Identification of target groups
- If AIDS is taken as an example the identified target group will be youth (both males and females)
- This group can be further segmented into:
  - Youth in schools (urban and rural)
  - Youth out of school (urban and rural)
  - Street children
  - University students
  - Here, each group has different levels of literacy, and knowledge behavior, so, different approaches are needed for different groups
  - It is also important to include parents and teachers

c. Establishment of objectives, goals and targets (indicators)
- Here goal is defined as the ultimate desired state towards which objectives and resources are directed
- In the example under study, the desired behavior goals may be stated as follows:
  - Delay sexual initiation
  - Reduce number of sexual partners
  - Increase use of condoms
  - Discuss sexual matters openly
  - Actively seek information on sexual matters and sexual counseling
  - Seek STD services (when needed, without fear)
  - Promote healthy lifestyles
- Objectives should be precise and to achieve the goal some objectives are formulated but whether objectives are achieved or not, final aim is to achieve the goals
- Target often refers to a discrete activity and is measurable, such as number of condoms dispersed, number of people attending STD clinic, taking sexual counseling, number of disposable syringes, etc.
- So as far as possible, the goals and objectives should be quantified (or expressed in measurable terms) and then specific indicators should be developed, which are useful in collecting appropriate information

B. Preparatory activities and material development

a. Linkages with existing organizational structure and other organizations
- Close and active collaboration with other agencies is vital for the success of any IEC activity
- Here collaboration should be established with educational authorities and educational institutions (e.g. ministries of education, youth, women and child welfare, tourism, information and broadcasting, transportation, etc.)
- Linkages should also be sought with youth clubs and sports organisations
- NGOs and voluntary organisations could play an important role because of the commitment and dedication and their better rapport with young people, their ability to reach out to school youth and street children
- Linkage with entertainment industry is also beneficial for many IEC activities
- Linkage with the existing organizational structure such as STD and Family Planning Services is very much useful

b. Arrange support services
- The supporting services for this target group includes:
  - Counseling (which is of special relevance for this age group)
  - Condom distribution
  - STD/health services
  - Information services
  - Advocacy

c. Conduct training
- Effective implementation of IEC activities needs effective training of manpower to improve their knowledge and skills
- Development of appropriate training material should be part of total program
- The training measures should be:
  - Long-term measures: Such as incorporation of IEC components into the curriculum of basic training programs for health and health related workers, teacher's training, etc.
  - Short-term measures: Such as in-service training to special groups (e.g. health and health related workers, teachers, NGO workers, volunteers, leaders, peer groups from high risk population and vulnerable groups)
  - Material development

d. Conduct targeted research
- Rapid research among specific target groups is needed to know the needs of target groups, their attitudes, knowledge, behavior, practice of a particular problem, where and how to intervene by giving health education
- By this effective IEC material can be formulated and IEC activities can be done effectively

e. Design and pretest the targeted message
- Now the message for the targeted group is designed for mass health education (such as posters, matter for TV, radio, etc.), for health education at personal level, family level and for groups and message for communication (two-way process) and interactive sessions
- In many cases, folk media such as puppetry, drama and story-telling can be used quite effectively and it is highly cost-effective medium also
- Targeted message should be pretested first on a small number of targeted group and if it is not found sufficient it may be revised and pretested again to produce it

Contd...

Contd...

f. Choose appropriate media and channels of communication
   - Next step is choosing the appropriate media for IEC activities, which should be cost effective
   - Resources are always scarce, so the affordabi1ity and cost-benefit analysis is a must
   - Traditional media (including puppetry, songs and traditional theatre) and interpersonal communication tools (such as flip-charts and flash cards) are often neglected, though they are generally cost effective. So, special efforts should be made to use traditional media whenever they are more suitable

g. Develop IEC material
   - After taking decisions about message, media and channels of communication (to be used for delivery to each target group), IEC material should be prepared
   - Material may consist of radio or TV spots, booklets, posters, hand-outs, hoardings, etc.
   - IEC material also contains tools for use in interpersonal communication (it must be kept in mind that IEC materials are only tools to support the activities)
   - Pretesting of the material is one of the most important steps
   - It prevents the wastage of resources by ensuring that materials are effective
   - Once materials are developed, they are carefully reviewed with small groups selected from target groups
   - IEC material for non-literate audience must be prepared carefully and separately

C. Dissemination and utilization of material
   - Planning effective ways to make sure that materials reach their target audience
   - It is often the case that costly and good quality materials never reach those who need them

D. Monitoring
   - Monitoring can be defined as the on-going process of collecting and analysing information about implementation of the program and it involves regular checking to see programmed activities are being carried out correctly or not
   - It allows managers to follow the progress, to identify problems, to get feedback and solve the problems

E. Evaluation
   - Evaluation is the process of collecting and analysing information at regular intervals about the effectiveness and impact of the program
   - At a given point of time, evaluation can answer the following questions (IEC program on AIDS)
     - Availability and utilization of condoms
     - What proportion of health workers are providing health education?
     - What proportion of prostitutes report the correct and consistent use of condoms?
     - What proportion of general population can answer at least two acceptable ways to protect themselves from HIV infection?
     - What proportion of women have been advised on risks of HIV infection?
     - What proportion of general population who are sexually active can report that they are practicing safer sex?
   - Evaluation should include not only the impact on the target audience, but must also cover an evaluation of other activities, such as training, utilization of services, etc..

Factors Influencing the Success of IEC Campaign (6 Cs)

1. Communicator	• Should be trustworthy and should speak the dialect and style the audience understands
2. Context	• Should be relevant to the audience
3. Clarity	• Message to be given should be in simple terms
4. Consistency	• Message must be consistent to penetrate into the minds of the audience
5. Channels	• Existing channels of communications should be used
6. Capability of audience	• Audience must be capable of understanding what is told

Significance

- Health education is still art rather than a science and each community and country should develop tailored techniques to meet their own needs.

SHORT ESSAYS

3. Explain iceberg phenomenon in diseases giving example.

Refer Question No. 3 June 2010 (RS2) Paper I.

4. Bias in case control study.

Refer Question No. 6 June 2014 (RS2) Paper I.

5. Role of family in health and disease.

- Family is defined as a group of biologically-related individuals living together and eating from a common kitchen.

Role of Family in Health and Disease

- Family performs numerous functions but there are certain functions which are relevant to health and health behavior.

a. Health perception	▪ A traditional, rural, Indian family perceives health as a token of divine benevolence and disease as a curse or punishment from almighty ▪ Illness among the children is considered a result of a spell cast by an evil eye ▪ These beliefs and taboos are deep rooted amongst rural and tribal families who seek appeasement of gods by performing poojas and homas by giving prey ▪ Such irrational misbeliefs cause stigmatization of diseases like leprosy and interfere with control measures
b. Child rearing	▪ Physical care of the dependent young in order that they may survive to adulthood and perpetuate the family is an important function of family ▪ The child rearing practices have profound influence on the health of growing children like breastfeeding practices, eating habits, feeding habits, sleeping habits, etc. ▪ The child care is determined by tradition and varies from society-to-society and from time-to-time depending upon the factors such as capital resources, level of knowledge, state of technology and system of values ▪ The patterns of child care are passed on from one generation to another
c. Socialization	▪ Socializing means teaching the young the values of society and transmitting information, culture, beliefs, general codes of conduct, by example and precept, in order to make them fit for membership in the wider society of which the family is a part ▪ The young are persuaded, given punishments, rewards for good behavior—all these vary from time-to-time. In some societies, the young are given freedom to develop into individuals who are freely able to take initiatives
d. Personality formation	▪ The capacity of an individual to withstand stress and strain and the way in which he interacts with other people is to a large extent determined by his early experience in the family, mainly with the father, mother and siblings who provide the earliest and most immediate component of the child's external environment ▪ The family acts as a "placenta" excluding various influences, modifying others that pass through it and contributes some of its own in laying the foundation of physical, mental and social health of the child
e. Care of the dependents	
i. Care of the sick and injured	▪ In all forms of society, adults may become dependent either through injury, illness or because of basic biological limitation for performing functions normally expected by adults ▪ The family is charged with the responsibility of care of such individuals ▪ The family is expected to provide the front-line care, particularly the mother ▪ Much depends upon her understanding of illness and the extent she believes herself capable of providing nursing care ▪ Usually family does more nursing than the hospital
ii. Care of women during pregnancy and child birth	▪ Pregnancy and childbirth is an important function of the family ▪ The attitude of society to pregnancy and child-bearing may have an important bearing on the infant deaths, maternal morbidity and mortality, premature and stillbirths ▪ In many societies today, women are given financial help, maternity leave facilities, diet and nutritional supplements and decreased responsibilities during pregnancy and puerperium
iii. Care of the aged and handicapped	▪ The increased number of aged and infirm people has created new problems in terms of long-term care and specialist facilities ▪ Without the support of the family, no amount of medical care can succeed. In India, the joint family provides for such support
f. Stabilization of adult personality	▪ In situations of stress and strain like injury, illness, births, deaths, tension, emotional upsets, worry, anxiety, economic insecurity, etc. the family provides an opportunity, both for adults and children, for release of tension so that the individual can attain mental equilibrium and strive to maintain a stable relationship with other people ▪ Thus, the family has an important function in the stabilization of the personality of both adults and children and in meeting their emotional needs
g. Familial susceptibility to diseases	▪ The members of a family share a pool of genes and common environment and together, these decide the susceptibility to disease ▪ Certain diseases such hemophilia, color blindness, diabetes and mental illness are known to run through families ▪ Schizophrenia, psychoneurosis and some forms of mental deficiency are also known to have familial incidence ▪ The family is often the playground also for such communicable diseases as tuberculosis, common cold, scabies, diphtheria, measles, mumps, rubella, chickenpox, dysentery, diarrhea, and enteric fever ▪ These diseases are known to spread rapidly in families because of the common environment which the family members share ▪ It is generally agreed that the incidence of congenital malformation is higher among offsprings of consanguineous as compared with nonconsanguineous marriages

Contd...

Contd...

h. Housing condition	▪ A poor housing condition with ill ventilation and ill lighted rooms, often associated with overcrowding and with livestock, with lack of drainage facilities, lack of sanitary latrine, lack of clean water supply, kitchen without smoke vent, infested with cockroaches, rodents and flies, etc. predispose to air-bone and vehicle-borne infections
i. Personal hygiene	▪ Certain traditional practices like oil bath, women massaging with turmeric powder is a healthy practice ▪ Brushing teeth with neem twig is believed to promote oral hygiene ▪ Nevertheless, certain practices like chewing pan, tobacco, smoking, alcohol consumption have serious effects ▪ Certain religious practices like circumcision and belief that coitus during menses is sinful are justified with regards to hygiene
j. Lifestyle	▪ Certain unhealthy, traditional practices are responsible for prevalence of disease in community – Walking barefoot and indiscriminate defecation for ankylostomiasis – Defecation on the banks of river, lakes, ponds, etc. for lack of unprotected water supply contributing to water-borne diseases – Poor housing with dampness of floor and walls, burning of fuels for cooking increases prevalence of respiratory infections – Smoking, alcoholism and chewing pan increases predisposition to certain cancers
k. Dietary practices	▪ Dietary practices are responsible for prevalence of malnutrition in India amongst the high-risk groups, i.e. mother and children ▪ Strict vegetarian diet deprives the individual from first class proteins ▪ Mild adulteration decreases its nutritious value ▪ Food faddism like consuming meat, egg during pregnancy increases heat during pregnancy deprives expectant mother from proteins ▪ Poverty, illiteracy and ignorance about food taboos also predispose to malnutrition ▪ Higher position of earning member of family makes him rightful of eating first, resulting in women and children getting leftovers ▪ Practice fasting also affects the nutritional status
l. Disposal practices	▪ Habit of accumulating solid waste near dwelling, promotes breeding of flies and attracts roaches and rodents ▪ It promotes insanitation ▪ Habit of open air defecation promotes soil pollution, water pollution and fly breeding ▪ Bathing in pond, lakes, rivers causes water pollution
m. Reproductive behavior	▪ Early marriage for girls predisposes to higher fertility and consequence of teenage pregnancy ▪ Polygamy and polyandry increases the risk of sexually transmitted diseases in the society ▪ Gender preference exposes the women to repeated pregnancies
n. Broken families	▪ A broken family is one where the parents have separate or where death has occurred of one or both the parents ▪ Separation of the child from its father (paternal separation) and separation of the child from both of its parents (dual-parental separation) are important factors in child development ▪ Children who are victims broken families early in their childhood have been found sometimes to display in later years psychopathic behavior, immature personality and even retardation of growth, speed and intellect. Children from these families may drift away to prostitution, crime and vagrancy
o. Problem families	▪ Problem families are those which lag behind the rest of the community ▪ In these families, the standards of life are generally far below the accepted minimum and parents are unable to meet the physical and emotional needs of the children ▪ The home life is utterly unsatisfactory ▪ The underlying factors in most problem families are usually those of personality and of relationship, backwardness, poverty, illness, mental and emotional instability, character defects and marital disharmony. These families are recognized as problems in social pathology ▪ Children who are reared in such an environment are victims of prostitution, crime and vagrancy ▪ Problem families may be found in all social classes but are more common in the lower social classes ▪ The health visitor, the health inspector, the midwife, the social worker, the medical officer of health, all can render useful service in rehabilitating such families in a community

Significance

- The family is the fulcrum of health service and plays an important part both in health and disease—in the prevention and treatment of individual illness, in the care of children and dependent adults, and in the stabilization of the personality of both adults and children.

6. Tests of significance.

Refer Question No. 4 June 2008 (RS2) Paper I.

7. Carriers of disease.

Refer Question No. 1 June 2009 (RS2) Paper I.

8. Write in brief about types of screening giving examples.

Refer Question No. 1 December 2010 (RS2) Paper I.

9. Causes and prevention of lead poisoning.

- Chronic lead poisoning is also called as plumbism, Saturnism or Painter's colic[Q]
- Lead poisoning is the most common toxic metal poisoning[Q] occurring during the course of occupation because of the wide application of lead in various industries.

Sources of Lead

Occupational source	*Non-occupational sources*
▪ Mines of lead ores ▪ Industries of glass, paint and storage batteries ▪ Printing and potteries ▪ Plumbing works (pipe fitting)	▪ Exhaust from automobiles using leaded petrol[Q] (greatest source of lead poisoning) ▪ Drinking water conveyed through lead pipes or drinking wine contaminated with lead because the lid made up of lead ▪ Eating fruits sprayed with insecticides containing lead ▪ Chewing lead-paint by nibbling of toys coating with lead paint, chewing on window sills, keeping lead-pencils in the mouth, etc. (in children) ▪ Contaminated hands

Absorption, Storage and Elimination

- Poisoning occurs mainly by inhalation[Q] and often by ingestion
- Can also occur by absorption through the skin[Q] of only organic compounds such as alkyl lead
- Normal average lead ingestion is about 0.2–0.3 mg/day largely from food and beverages of which 90% is excreted in the feces and only 10% is absorbed
- But regular intake can increase the amount of lead in the body
- Lead is mainly stored in the bones and to some extent in the liver and kidneys. It is a cumulative poison.

Mechanism of Action

- Lead exerts its toxic action by combining with "SH" group of certain enzymes involved in porphyrin synthesis in RBCs and suppresses it and it also suppresses carbohydrate metabolism.

Clinical Features

Inorganic lead poisoning	*Organic lead poisoning (involvement of central nervous system[Q])*
▪ Anemia (microcytic hypochromic[Q]), anorexia, arthralgia, amenorrhea ▪ Blue (or black) line on the gums (Burton's or Burtonian line[Q]) – Lead sulfide line on upper jaw ▪ Colicy abdomen (cramps) ▪ Diarrhea ▪ Encephalopathy ▪ Fatigue ▪ Giddiness, growth failure among children ▪ Headache ▪ Insomnia, irritability ▪ Joint pains ▪ Kidney damage (Chronic nephritis) ▪ Lassitude	▪ Insomnia ▪ Headache ▪ Mental confusion ▪ Irritability ▪ Nervousness ▪ Anxiety ▪ Convulsions ▪ Delirium ▪ Coma ▪ Death

Contd...

Contd...

Inorganic lead poisoning	*Organic lead poisoning (involvement of central nervous system[Q])*
▪ Myalgia, mental retardation ▪ Nausea, nervousness ▪ Oliguria ▪ Paralysis (Lead palsy: wrist drop[Q] due to paralysis of extensor muscles of hand) ▪ Pallor, pica (Facial pallor is earliest and most consistent sign[Q]) ▪ Seizures, sterility ▪ Tremors ▪ Vertigo, vomiting ▪ Weakness	

Other Epidemiological Features

- Occupational inorganic lead poisoning is common among adults and non-occupational organic lead poisoning is common among young children
- Children suffering from pica, are at a risk of plumbism
- Chronic respiratory and intestinal infections predispose to plumbism
- Pregnancy increases susceptibility to plumbism
- Not only the pregnant mother but also the fetus is at risk of intrauterine growth retardation and mental retardation
- Predisposing personal factors are alcoholism, lack of personal hygiene, nail baiting and wearing work uniform outside the factory
- Children with plumbism will develop growth failure, progressive mental retardation, low I-Q, aggressive behavior, lack of concentration, etc.

Diagnosis

- History of occupational exposure to lead
- Clinical symptomatology
- Laboratory investigations
  - Hemoglobin percentage—to know the severity of anemia
  - Peripheral blood smear—shows microcytic hypochromic picture and basophilic stippling of RBCs
  - RBC count—decreased
  - Reticulocyte count—increased
  - Blood level of lead and urinary level of lead, coproporphyrin and aminolevulinic acid
  - Coproporphyrin level in urine is a useful screening test for lead poisoning[Q].

Parameters for Lead Poisoning[Q]

Parameters	*Normal value*	*Dangerous value*
Blood lead[Q]	25–40 µg/dL	>70 µg/dL[Q]
Urinary lead	0.2–0.8 mg/L	>0.8 mg/L
Urinary ALA	5 mg/L	60 mg/L
Urinary coproporphyrin	<150 µg/L	>250 µg/L

Management

- Prevention of further exposure to lead absorption by change of job
- Saline purge helps in the removal of unabsorbed lead from gut
- Promotion of lead excretion in the urine from the soft tissues by giving chelating agents such as Ca-EDTA and d-penicillamine.

Prevention and Control

a. Health promotion	▪ Preplacement examination to rule out the presence of contraindications if any such as pallor, blue line of gums, etc. ▪ Improvement in the sanitation by mandatory good house-keeping (i.e. wet mopping of floors), ventilation and cleanliness ▪ Control of dust ▪ Use of unleaded petrol for automobiles ▪ Health education of all employees about maintenance of personal hygiene for plumbers and for those working with paints, to change the work-uniform after leaving the factory ▪ Substitution of lead compounds by less toxic materials wherever possible
b. Specific protection	▪ Use of gloves among painters ▪ Use of respirators and masks for those exposed to dust and fumes
c. Early diagnosis and treatment	▪ Periodical examination of at-risk population for early detection and treatment with chelating agents like Ca-EDTA and d-penicillamine
d. Disability limitation	▪ Development of further disability in a case presenting late, by aggressive treatment followed by change of the job
e. Rehabilitation	▪ For those with wrist drop (lead palsy) or neurological deficits following lead encephalopathy

Significance

- Plumbism is a notifiable disease[Q] under Indian Factories Act 1948 and a compensatable disease under Workmen's Compensation Act 1959.

10. Oxidation pond.

- Oxidation pond or waste stabilization pond or redox pond or sewage lagoon is a cheap and old method of purifying sewage[Q].

Principle

- Working principle of oxidation pond is the purification of sewage by forces of nature which are:

Bacteria feeding on organic matter	*Algae*	*Sunlight*
▪ Bacteria are aerobic and degrade (oxidize) the organic matter to carbon dioxide ammonia and water ▪ However, there is also a bottom layer of anaerobic bacteria which work even in absence of sunlight	▪ Algae utilize the carbon dioxide, water and inorganic matter for their growth by means of photosynthesis and produce oxygen ▪ This oxygen is utilized by the bacteria for aerobic oxidation. Thus, there exists a symbiotic relation between the bacteria and algae ▪ However some amount of oxygen is also derived from environment	▪ Another important factor for proper functioning of oxidation pond which aids photosynthesis of algae

Structure

- Oxidation pond is an open, shallow pool of depth of 1–1.5 m with an inlet for waste (sewage and industrial effluents) and an outlet for effluent
- The length and breadth of pond depends on the size of the community to serve
- The pond surrounding should be free from vegetation and weeds to avoid mosquito menace.

Parts

- An oxidation pond ideally consists of 3 sequential ponds for differentiate treatment of waste.

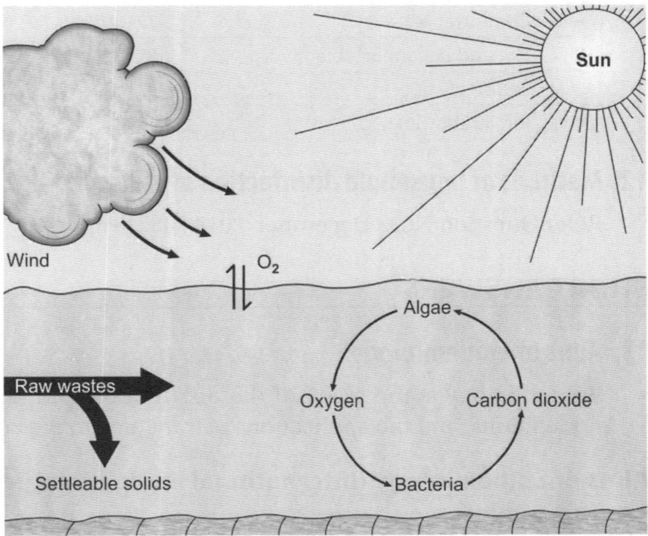

Fig. 1: Oxidatin pond

Anaerobic pond	*Facultative pond*	*Maturation pond*
▪ It is 2–5 m deep which receives strong raw waste ▪ If functions are an open septic tank carrying out anaerobic digestion	▪ It is 1–2 m deep and receives waste from anaerobic pond ▪ In upper layer of pond aerobic digestion takes place whereas in deeper layer the digestion takes place anaerobically	▪ It is 1–2 m deep and receives effluent from facultative pond ▪ Its main function is aerobic reduction of excreted pathogens and nutrients ▪ Overall retention time for effluent in oxidation pond is at least 20 days ▪ Effluent obtained from the oxidation pond can be used for irrigation or may be discharged into river or sea after appropriate treatment

Advantages

- It is a cheap and efficient method of sewage treatment especially for small communities[Q]
- The effluent from oxidation pond can be used for irrigation
- It may also be used for fish farming
- There is no odor associated with properly maintained pond
- Water hyacinth, a plant used in oxidation pond can also be used for production of manure rich in nitrogen, phosphorus and potassium.

11. Thermal comfort zone.

- Comfort zone is the range of effective temperature over which the majority of adults feel comfortable
- Comfort zone is expressed in range because comfort is complex subjective experience depending upon the physical physiological and psychological factors
- So, comfortable thermal conditions are those under which a person can maintain normal balance between production and loss of heat at normal body temperature and without sweating.

Ranges of Corrective Effective Temperature

- Corrective effective temperature is an arbitatory index combining the effects of air temperature, velocity humidity and mean radiant heat into single value obtained using a globe thermometer
- Corrective effective temperature is an index of comfort zone
- Comfort zones are expressed in corrected effective temperature

Comfort zones	*Ranges of corrected effective temperature*
i. Pleasant and cool	69°F
ii. Comfortable and cool[Q]	69–76°F[Q]
iii. Comfortable[Q]	77–80°F[Q]
iv. Hot and uncomfortable	81–82°F
v. Extremely hot	83+°F
vi. Intolerably hot	86+°F

12. Methods of household disinfection of water.

Refer Question No. 2 December 2013 (RS2) Paper I.

SHORT ANSWERS

13. Aims of epidemiology.

- Epidemiology is the study of the distribution and determinants of health-related states or events in specified populations, and the applications of this study to the control of health problems.

Aims of Epidemiology (International Epidemiological Association)

a. To describe the distribution and magnitude of health and disease problems in human populations
b. To identify etiological factors or risk factors in the pathogenesis of disease

c. To provide the data essential to the planning implementation and evaluation of services for prevention, control and treatment of disease and to the setting up of priorities among the services
d. To lead to effective action
   - To eliminate or reduce the health problem or its consequences
   - To promote the health and well-being of society as a whole.

14. Quarantine.

Refer Question No. 5 December 2016 (RS2) Paper I.

15. Record linkage.

Refer Question No. 12 June 2014 (RS2) Paper I.

16. Audio-visual aids used in health education.

- Audio-visual aids are the aids used in health education for making it more effective and impressive by:
  - Simplifying unfamiliar concepts
  - Bringing about understanding where word fail
  - Reinforcing learning by appealing to more than one sense
  - Providing dynamic way of avoiding monotony.

Classification

Auditory aids	*Visual aids*		*Combined audio-visual aids*[Q]
	Not requiring projection	*Requiring projection*	
▪ Radio ▪ Tape recorder ▪ Microphones ▪ Earphones ▪ Amplifier	▪ Black board and chalk ▪ Leaflets ▪ Posters ▪ Charts ▪ Models ▪ Exhibits ▪ Specimens ▪ Health museum, etc.	▪ Slides ▪ Film strips ▪ LCD ▪ Transpierces (OHP sheets)	▪ Television ▪ Sound films ▪ Slide tape combination

Advantages	*Disadvantage*
▪ Since they are close to being natural, they create interest among the people ▪ They make learning easy and permanent ▪ The pictures are impressed in the mind of the people and stimulate thinking ▪ People are able to see the things which they are unable to see otherwise	▪ A knowledge of the advantages, disadvantages and limitations of each audio-visual aid besides their operating mechanism is necessary in order to make proper use of them

Significance

- Audio-visual aids occupy the central role in health education practice.

17. Stabilized bleach.

- Stabilized bleach is a stable preparation of bleaching powder
- Freshly prepared bleaching powder is an unstable compound which rapidly loses its chlorine content (33%) on exposure to air, light and moisture making it storage difficult
- Stabilized bleach retains strength of available chlorine.

Preparation

- It is prepared by mixing it with excess of lime in ratio of 4:1
- Stabilized bleach is available in market as pittchlor, penchlor, etc.

Advantages

- Stabilized bleach can be stored for longer period of about an year without losing its strength.

18. Relative risk.

Refer Question No. 1 December 2016 (RS2) Paper I.

19. Occupational risk to farmers.

Refer Question No. 5 June 2009 (RS2) Paper I.

20. Population genetics.

- Population genetics is the study of distribution and determinants of gene frequencies in the population and it deals with the etiology distribution and control of genetic disorders in the population
- In short, it is the application of the principles of epidemiology to genetics
- Hardy and Weinberg in 1908 proposed a law for distribution of genotypes which is known as "Hardy–Weinberg law[Q]" according to which if the mating is random, the genotypes are distributed in the proportion of gene frequencies in the population and remain constant from generation to generation.

Factors Affecting Gene Frequencies

- Hardy–Weinberg law assumes that human population is static but in reality human population and consequently human gene pool is never static
- There are various factors which influence the human gene pool.

a. Mutation	▪ Mutation is the emergence of the new gene ▪ Though in strict sense, any change in the genetic material is mutation but in practice a genetic change which is not due to chromosomal re-arrangement is called mutation ▪ Most mutations are lethal and less likely to be carried to the next generation
b. Natural selection	▪ Natural selection is the process of elimination of harmful genes from gene pool and preservation of favorable genes and passing on to the off-springs ▪ This theory proposed by Darwin is best till date to explain the process of evolution
c. Population movements	▪ With advancement of technology there has started a new trend of migration, migration from rural parts to urban areas migration from one country to another for search of better living ▪ This resulted in changes in the distribution of genes, affecting both the areas of immigration and emigration ▪ The intermixing of people makes new genetic combinations possible ▪ A chance fluctuation in the gene frequency in a small group is called genetic drift ▪ Introduction of new genes in an ethnic group by another group is called gene flow
d. Mating systems	▪ Hardy–Weinberg law has a pre-requisite of random mating ▪ A random mating means that a genotype has a purely random probability of combining with any other genotype at that locus. ▪ However, individuals in any ethnic group mostly follow in group marriages than marrying out of the group and such mating are non–random and are called assortive mating
e. Public health measures	▪ Advance in medicine has increased the life span of an individual thus giving a chance for those genes to transmit to next generation which could not be transmitted earlier

21. Warning signals of poor mental health.

Refer Question No. 6 June 2009 (RS2) Paper I.

22. Sullivan's index.

- Sullivan's index or indicator describes expectation of life free of disability[Q]
- Also know as disability free life expectancy[Q] (DFLE).

Calculations

- It is calculated by subtracting the probable duration of disability, i.e. bed ridden and inability to perform major activities from the life expectancy according to the cross-sectional data from the population surveys

Sullivan's index = Life expectancy – Probable disability duration (bed disability and inability to perform major activities)

Significance

- It is one of the most advanced indicator currently available and a commonly used indicator.

Revised Scheme 2

MBBS PHASE III EXAMINATION

DECEMBER 2011

(Revised Scheme 2)

PAPER II

LONG ESSAYS

1. Write about risk factors and complications of diabetes mellitus. Add a note on prevention of diabetes mellitus.

Refer Question No. 1 June 2010 (RS2) Paper II.

2. Define perinatal mortality. What are the factors responsible for high perinatal mortality rate in developing countries and how can these factors be controlled?

- Perinatal mortality includes later fetal deaths (still births) and early neonatal deaths, i.e. deaths occurring during 28th week of gestation to 7th day after birth
- But according to WHO, perinatal period is from 22 completed weeks gestation to 7th completed day of life.

Criteria

- Babies included in perinatal mortality statistics should
  - Be above a minimum birth weight of 1000 g at birth[Q] (normal weight at 28 weeks of gestation[Q])
  - Should have completed at least 28 weeks of gestation
  - Should have at least 35 cm of body length.

Perinatal Mortality Rate (PMR)

- Perinatal mortality is the number of deaths of newborn occurring during perinatal period, i.e. late fetal deaths (28 weeks of gestation) and early neonatal deaths (till 7 days after full term)

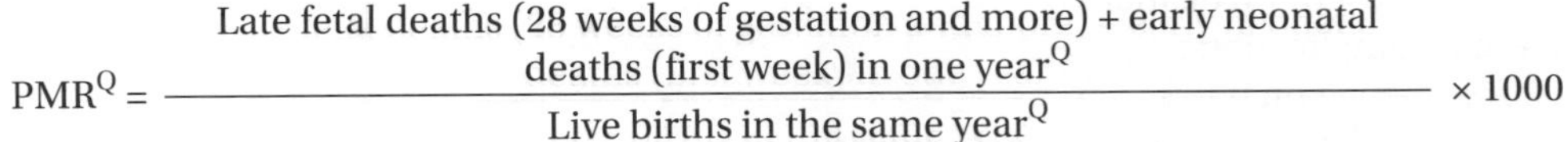

$$\text{PMR}^{Q} = \frac{\text{Late fetal deaths (28 weeks of gestation and more) + early neonatal deaths (first week) in one year}^{Q}}{\text{Live births in the same year}^{Q}} \times 1000$$

- Another formula suggested by WHO expert committee for international comparison is:

$$\text{PMR} = \frac{\text{Late fetal deaths (28 weeks of gestation and more) + early neonatal deaths (first week) weighing over 1000 g at birth in one year}}{\text{Total live births weighing over 1000 g in the same year}} \times 1000$$

Magnitude

- Maximum number of death in children occur in first 7 days[Q]
- PMR in India currently 23 per 1000 live births (SRS 2015)
- It is usually reported on an annual basis.

Causes

a. Medical causes		
Antenatal causes	*Intranatal causes*	*Postnatal causes*
– Maternal diseases—hypertension, cardiovascular disease, diabetes, tuberculosis anemia – Pelvic diseases—uterine myomas, endometriosis, ovarian tumours – Anatomical defects—uterine anomalies, incompetent cervix – Endocrine imbalance and inadequate uterine preparation – Blood incompatibilities – Malnutrition – Toxemia of pregnancy – Antepartum hemorrhages – Congenital defects – Advanced maternal age	▪ Birth injuries (cranial fractures, visceral rupture, massive subdural hematoma) ▪ Birth asphyxia[Q] (most common cause) ▪ Obstructed labor ▪ Prolonged labor ▪ Birth infections ▪ Obstetric complications	▪ Prematurity and/or low birth weight ▪ Acute respiratory distress syndrome ▪ Respiratory infections ▪ Alimentary infections ▪ Congenital anomalies ▪ Neonatal tetanus
b. Miscellaneous causes		
Placental causes	*Fetal causes*	
– Placenta previa – Placental insufficiency syndrome – Placental anomalies – Aburptio placenta	▪ Fetal malformations ▪ Multiple pregnancies ▪ Hydramnios	
c. Socioeconomic causes (predisposing factors)—factors responsible for high perinatal mortality rate in developing countries		
– Low socioeconomic status. – High maternal age (Age >35 years) – Low maternal age (Age <16 years) – High parity (5th and subsequent pregnancies) – Heavy smoking (10 or more cigarettes daily) – Maternal height (short statue) – Short interval between pregnancies (less than 24 months) – Poor past obstetric history (one or more previous still births and neonatal deaths, one or more premature live birth – Malnutrition and severe anemia – Multiple pregnancy		

Interventions of Reducing Perinatal Mortality

i. Advice of avoid pregnancy in women with medical problems till health improves.
ii. Birth spacing[Q].
iii. TT immunization in antenatal period[Q].
iv. Iron and folic acid tables for prevention of anemia[Q].
v. Early treatment of maternal complications.
vi. Institutional delivery for women at high risk.
vii. Immediate referral and appropriate case of emergency obstetric complications.
viii. Safe and clean delivery practices.
ix. Essential newborn care
x. Resuscitation of newborn without spontaneous cry at birth.

Preventive Measures

a. Prenatal feeding	▪ Improvement in the state of maternal nutrition even in a small amount goes a long way in improving the birth weight of babies ▪ It is also an important component of Integrated Child Development Services (ICDS)
b. Prevention of infection	▪ Infection diseases like tetanus, measles are major causes of death in neonatal age group which can be prevented by immunization ▪ Therefore universal immunization program aims to protect child from 6 vaccine preventable diseases and ensure greater child survival

Revised Scheme 2

c. Breastfeeding	▪ Breastfeeding is a safeguard against gastrointestinal and respiratory infections and PEM
d. Family planning	▪ Family limitation and spacing of births contribute of reduce infant mortality
e. Sanitation	▪ Exposure to infections through contaminated food and polluted water lack of elementary hygiene, flies and poor housing and other environmental factors could be prevented by proper sanitation
f. Provisions of primary healthcare	▪ All health workers involved in maternity care should collaborate and work together as a team ▪ Prenatal care must be improved to defect mothers with high-risk factors and those with prenatal conditions associated with high-risk and such mothers should be hospitalized and treated ▪ Special care body units for babies weighing less than 2000 g ▪ Proper referral services
g. Socioeconomic development	▪ Spread of nutritional standards ▪ Provision of safe water and basic sanitation ▪ Improvement of housing conditions ▪ Growth of agriculture and industry ▪ Availability of commerce and communication ▪ All round health and social development of the community
h. Education	▪ Educated mothers generally do not have early pregnancies are able to space their pregnancies, have better access to information related to personal hygiene and care of their children and make better use of healthcare services

Significance

- Perinatal mortality rate is a very sensitive indicator of obstetric and neonatal care, i.e. the quality of healthcare available to the mother and the newborn
- Since decrease in infant mortality rate in developed countries, perinatal mortality rate has assumed a greater importance as yardstick of obstetric and neonatal care
- It is a major marker to assess the quality of healthcare delivery[Q]
- Inclusion of still birth and early neonatal are included under one term as perinatal rate because the factors responsible for these two types deaths is often similar.

SHORT ESSAYS

3. Integrated vector control.

Refer Question No. 11 June 2010 (RS2) Paper I.

4. Functions of Voluntary Health Agencies.

Refer Question No. 10 December 2013 (RS2) Paper II.

5. Measles vaccine.

Refer Question No. 1 December 2010 (RS2) Paper II.

6. Management techniques based on behavioral sciences.

- Management is defined as purposeful and efficient use of resources—manpower, materials and finances, in an organized manner, for achieving the predetermined objectives.

Components

- Planning: Determining what is to be done
- Organization: Setting up the framework and making it possible for groups to do work
- Communication: For motivating the people to do work
- Monitoring: Supervision of work to ensure satisfactory progress.

Management Methods and Techniques

- These are based on two principles:
  i. Behavioral sciences.
  ii. Quantitative methods.

Management Methods Based on Behavioral Sciences

a. Organizational management
  - It deals with designing the organization structure such that it meets the health needs and demands of the people by utilizing all the resources at disposal and prevents wastage of resources
  - This organizational structure should be periodically reviewed and changed depending upon the changing concepts, problems and technology.

  Significance
  - An effective organization ensures efficient delivery of health services.

b. Personnel management
  - It involves skillful use of human resources by proper method of selection, training, placement and motivation of the persons followed by division of responsibility and work load, incentives for better work, opportunities for promotion and professional advancement, etc.

  Significance
  - Personnel management is the fundamental principle behind the concept of health team.

c. Communication
  - Better communication among the members of the health team, public and government ensures efficient working of the organization and prompt healthcare delivery
  - Barriers in communication may cause decrease in quality of work by delay in regular reporting and notification, delays in compilation of statistics, delay in release of supplies and salaries, delays in institution of prompt remedial measures.

  Significance
  - Lack of communication especially between the government and health delivery organization is one of the major problems in health management in India.

  Health information systems
  - Information is must for day-to-day healthcare management and can come from both formal and informal sources
  - The information obtained is collected, classified, stored or transmitted, retrieved, transformed and displayed for monitoring and evaluating a health program.

  Significance
  - Providing right information to the right person in right time helps to take right decision ensuring better results.

d. Management by objectives (MBO)
  - It is a process wherein the superior and subordinate manager identifies the members of an organization and they together identify common goals and define responsibility of each member and finally assess the contribution of each member
  - The health team can also be grouped into subunits for the administrative convenience
  - These subunits then plan their activities accordingly.

  Steps
  - Setting the goals of the organization
  - Identification of different units and subunits
  - Subordinate goals are set for each unit at departmental level, section level, unit or individual level
  - The units then formulate a plan of action, taking into consideration the targets and resources
  - A periodic feedback system is established to understand if there is any problem and whether objectives need modifications
  - An appraisal of the performance is done at the end of the program by seniors
  - Subordinates with poor performance is penalized and similarly one with outstanding performance is rewarded.

Advantages	*Disadvantages*
▪ Since objectives are divided into each unit or individual, everyone knows their duties enabling better management ▪ Each person can take independent decision for doing their work ▪ The participation of subordinates in decision making helps improve efficiency resulting in better outcome ▪ As every individual is given a target, he can take corrective measures if he feels his performance is less	▪ Priority is given to short-term objectives, not so much for long-term or qualitative objectives ▪ It makes organization rigid ▪ Unrealistic and unattainable goals demoralizes the implementers ▪ The success depends upon the feedback system ▪ As objectives are divided, overcommitment leads to rivalry over use of company resources

Management Methods Based on Quantitative Methods[Q]

a. Cost benefit analysis
   - In cost benefit analysis, the amount of money spent for intervention is calculated followed by measurement of output of intervention in monetary units[Q]
   - The course of action that gives the highest monetary returns for the lowest investment is regarded the best one[Q]
   - But in the health fields, the benefits cannot be expressed in monetary terms, however attempt can be made to translate the outcome in terms like morbidity and mortality prevented by considering the direct and indirect cost
   - Direct costs saved are cost of drugs, hospitalization, investigations, etc.
   - Indirect costs are saving of loss of wages, etc.

   Approaches
   - Human capital approach
   - Willingness to pay approach.

   Disadvantages
   - At times, it is difficult to convert indirect benefits into monetary benefits
   - Some interventions have collateral benefits like provision of clean water not only prevents typhoid but also other waterborne diseases which leads to confusion in calculation of monetary units
   - The lead time or the interval between the application of the intervention and the benefit is often too long causing difficulties in converting the benefits into monetary units
   - Sometimes during allocation of budget for two program, one program being more important but availability of resources is limited, under such circumstances, money may be allotted to one program only and here the loss of benefit due to rejecting other program is not considered.

b. Cost-effective analysis
   - It is similar to cost benefit analysis except benefits are expressed in terms of results achieved[Q]
   - It measures the degree of attainment of predetermined objectives and targets

Types	*Procedure*	*Applications*
i. Fixed cost approach – Analysis is in terms of effectiveness for unit cost – Example: Number of deaths averted per lakh rupees ii. Fixed effectiveness approach – Analysis in terms of cost per unit of effectiveness – Example: Cost of averting one death	▪ Define the objectives of the program ▪ Identify the possible ways to achieve objectives ▪ Calculate the cost of each method and effectiveness of each method ▪ Implement the best method selected out all possibilities	▪ Identification of best option out of all health interventions ▪ Identification of choice of technology, choice of strategy, etc. ▪ Identification of better healthcare delivery system ▪ Identification of best component of program ▪ Identification of resources for better program

   Advantages
   - Here the benefits are not expressed in terms of monetary units but **expressed in terms of** natural units[Q] like number of lives saved, number of disabilities averted, etc.

   Significance
   - It is an expression of the desired effects of a program, service, institution or support activity in reducing health problem
   - Quality adjusted life year is the most comprehensive indicator of CEA[Q].

c. Cost accounting
   - It is the method of calculation of cost of a health program[Q] or any health intervention.

Methods	*Applications*
i. Input method – Here, the inputs can either capital investment in form of one time purchase of articles or recurring costs ii. Function or activity method – Here the cost is calculated by the money spent on activities such as training, management, supervision, evaluation, monitoring, transport, etc.	▪ It is a preliminary step in cost-benefit and cost-effective analysis ▪ Creates awareness about the financial aspects of the program ▪ Comparing cost of different programs ▪ Calculation and comparing the cost of different components of the program ▪ Identification and monitoring of costly component of a program ▪ Helps in making cost projections

d. Cost minimization analysis
   - Comparison of costs of different interventions that are assumed to provide equivalent benefits.
e. Cost utility analysis
   - Comparison of costs and benefit of health technologies that impact both quality and quantity of life
   - It measures health benefits such as healthy years, QALY, DALY
   - It is a multidimensional
   - Quality adjusted life year is most widely used to measure benefits in cost utility analysis
f. Input and output analysis
   - It is a management technique involving two components:
     - Input: Refers to all resources of the program like manpower, money, material and time
     - Output: Refers to the benefits derived from the interventions like number of lives saved, etc.

Steps	*Advantages*	*Disadvantages*
▪ Estimate the inputs required for interventions ▪ Calculate the output in terms of cost-effectiveness analysis ▪ Express the analysis in a tabular format	▪ It helps to calculate the required input for desired output or expect the output with known input ▪ Relatively easy	▪ Output measurement is difficult, sometimes even impossible

g. Model
   - Model or simulation study is a basic concept of management science and is a symbolic representation of idealized system and an abstraction of reality
   - A model incorporates different courses of action for a program thus it aids to understand how the factors in a situation affect each other and indicates probable results and outcome of each course of action.

Advantages	*Disadvantages*
▪ It enables to predict the outcome by a known mix of interventions ▪ It also provides view of effect of course of action on the system	▪ The assumptions about results are made on the basis of stability of variables which is impractical

h. System analysis
   - It a management tool for finding the cost effectiveness of a course of action

Objectives	*Steps*
▪ Help the decision makers to choose an appropriate course of action and find cost-effective alternative[Q]	▪ Identification of problem ▪ Investigation of problem ▪ Searching for objectives ▪ Finding alternative solutions ▪ Evaluation of alternatives for cost effectiveness ▪ Re-examination of objectives if necessary ▪ Identification of most cost-effective alternative

i. Network analysis
   - A network is graphic plan of all events and activities to be completed in order to reach an end objective[Q].

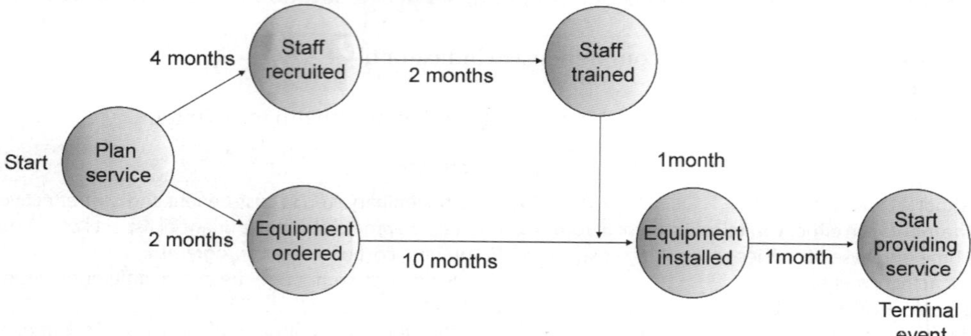

Fig. 1: Network analysis flowchart

Types

PERT (Program Evaluation and Review Technique)[Q]	*CPM (Critical Path Method)*
▪ It is a management technique enabling more detailed planning and more comprehensive supervision ▪ It can be best simplified by the example of a housewife who plans a meal so that each item in the menu is completed at the same time Features ▪ Construct an arrow diagram which represents the logical sequence in which the event must take place ▪ Such diagram permits calculating time for each activity and identify critical activities Advantages ▪ Provides a basic discipline by which all concerned in a project can know what is expected from them ▪ Minimize delays or crises in the implementation of the plan ▪ Allows better communication between the various levels of management ▪ Identifies potential problems ▪ Furnishes continuous, timely progress report ▪ Aids in planning, scheduling and monitoring the project Significance ▪ PERT is a useful management technique applicable to a great variety of projects and forms a solid foundation upon which an evaluation and checking system is built	▪ Critical path is the longest path of a network[Q] ▪ Here the emphasis mainly on the activities ▪ It is generally applied to projects that are repetitive in nature ▪ Here the cost considerations are important Significance ▪ Any delay in activity along critical path will result in delay of the entire project[Q]

Significance
– Network analysis brings about greater discipline in planning.

j. Planning=Programming-Budgeting system
– It is a system designed to help the decision makers to allocate resources to an organization for most effective use in order to achieve desired objectives in cost effective manner
– It calls for grouping of activities into programs.

Features
– It emphasizes the need for clearly defined objectives
– It searches for alternatives based on cost benefit implications
– Future cost implications are worked out for various alternatives
– It needs well established information system.

k. Work sampling
– It is a systematic observation and recording of activities of one or more individuals carried out at random intervals[Q]
– It provides quantitative measurements of various activities performed and time required for the same
– It helps in judging the efficiency of current staff and appropriateness of his job description and training
– It helps in standardizing the methods of performing job and determining the required manpower for the organization.

l. Decision making
– It involves taking decisions about development of resources, optimum work load for medical and paramedical workers, strategies for providing healthcare, etc.
– It is done at the level where best decisions can be made and made only after obtaining complete data.

7. Functions of World Health Organization (WHO).

Refer Question No. 5 June 2009 (RS2) Paper II.

8. Prevention of genetic disorders.

- Genetic disorders are disorders due to chromosomal abnormalities or any defect in genes.

Prevention of Genetic Disorders

A. Health promotive measures
  a. Eugenic measures
    - Eugenics is a science which aims to improve the genetic endowment of human population (Sir Francis Galton[Q])
    - It is study of hereditary improvement of human race by controlled selective breeding[Q] (Genetic manipulation)

Types

Negative eugenics[Q]	*Positive eugenics*[Q]
▪ Negative eugenics aims to reduce the frequency of hereditary disease and disability in the community to as low as possible ▪ It is the improvement in the population by killing the weak, defective and those with undesirable characteristics ▪ This practice of eliminating the weaker section of society was practiced by the Hitler in Germany who subjected millions Jews to concentration camps ▪ Another way by which negative eugenics can be practiced is prevention of procreation by sterilization of the people with harmful traits, abortion or other methods of family planning ▪ However in spite of eugenic sterilization, new cases of hereditary diseases will continue to arise partly because of fresh mutations and partly because of marital alliances between hidden carriers of recessive defects	▪ Positive eugenics aims to improve the genetic composition of the population by encouraging the carriers of desirable genotypes to assume the burden of parenthood ▪ However its application has very limited because ▪ Majority of socially valuable traits like intelligence, etc. though partially determined biologically are not inherited in such a simple way and have a complex multifactorial determination both genetic and environmental ▪ We cannot determine which we transmit to our children

Disadvantages
- Absence of agreement about the ascertainment of desirable characteristics
- Selective breeding as envisaged in eugenics reduces the genetic diversity and limits the capacity of the population to adopt to changing environment.

Applications
- Sterilization of person with harmful trait
- Prenatal diagnosis and abortion in the event of diagnosing harmful genetic disorder in fetus
- Artificial inseminations
- In vitro fertilization and embryo transfer
- Gene cloning.

b. Euthenics
- It is the manipulation of the immediate environment of the man because environment has an influence on the genetic development[Q] by enabling the genes to express them readily [Environmental manipulation]
- Manipulation means altering external factors such as education and the controllable environment, including the prevention and removal of contagious diseases, education regarding employment, home economics, sanitation and housing
- Greek: "euthenein" meaning thrive or flourish
- Euthenics is distinguished from eugenics primarily in that eugenics is concerned with improvement of human species through manipulation of genetic inheritance whereas euthenics is concerned with uninheritable improvements in human beings at a particular time and place, though this can have genetic consequences.

Significance
- Euthenics improves the genetic endowment of the human race.

c. Genetic counseling
- Genetic counseling is a process of offering advice to individuals to improve the genetic constitution at the level of individual family.

Types

	Prospective genetic counseling	*Retrospective genetic counseling*
	▪ Allows for true prevention of genetic disorder	▪ Most common genetic counseling offered today
Indications	▪ Individuals or couples who are at genetic risk	▪ Couples reporting voluntarily after birth of affected children
Timings	▪ Before the individual develops symptoms or couples produce their first child	▪ After birth of affected child

Contd...

Contd...

	Prospective genetic counseling	*Retrospective genetic counseling*
Content	▪ Avoiding marriages amongst heterozygote carriers identified by genetic screening procedures ▪ Education about MTPs in married couples with unfavorable prenatal diagnosis	▪ Probable risks associated with future pregnancies ▪ Facilities available for prenatal diagnosis and termination of suspected pregnancies ▪ Use of contraception or sterilizing techniques depending upon the attitudes and cultural environment of couples involved
Remarks	▪ Advantages ▪ Prevents birth of child with genetic disorders like thalassemia, sickle cell anemia, G6PD deficiency	

Significance

- Genetic counseling is the most immediate and practical solution genetics can render in healthcare.

d. Other measures
   - Prevention of consanguineous marriages because when blood relatives marry each other there is increased risk of expression of recessive trait in offspring thus preventing diseases like albinism, phenylketonuria, alkaptonuria
   - Avoiding late marriages can prevent certain chromosomal abnormalities like Trisomy 21.

B. Specific protection
   - Protection of individuals and communities against mutagens like X-rays, ionizing radiations, mutogenic chemicals
   - Protection of gonads in individuals undergoing X-rays examination
   - Avoiding X-ray examination in pregnant women
   - Immunization of pregnant mothers against rubella
   - Immunization of Rh–ve mothers with anti-D globulin to prevent erythroblastosis fetalis.

C. Early diagnosis and treatment
   a. Detection of genetic carriers
      - Healthy genetic carriers of many genetic disorders especially inborn errors of metabolism can be identified and such individuals should be counseled.

   b. Prenatal diagnosis
      - Prenatal diagnosis is an early detection technique employed in secondary prevention of genetic disorders.

Indications

Indications	*Methods*
▪ Advanced maternal age ▪ Previous child with chromosome aberration ▪ Intrauterine growth delay	▪ Cytogenetics (amniocentesis, chorionic villus sampling)
▪ Biochemical disorders	▪ Protein assay ▪ DNA diagnosis
▪ Congenital anomaly	▪ Sonography ▪ Fetoscopy
▪ Screening for neural tube defects and trisomy	▪ Maternal serum alpha fetoprotein and chorionic gonadotropin

Methods

i. Ultrasonography
   - It helps in visualizing fetal malformations, fetal growth abnormalities
   - It also helps in monitoring invasive prenatal diagnostic techniques like amniocentesis, chorionic villi sampling

ii. Amniocentesis
   - It is transabdominal aspiration of amniotic fluid from uterus for biochemical tests, culture of fetal cells and karyotyping
   - It is performed preferably between 14–16 weeks of gestation[Q].

   Indications[Q]

   - A mother aged 35 years or more (high-risk of Down's syndrome)

- Mother with a child with Down's syndrome or other chromosomal anomalies
- Parents with known chromosomal translocation
- Parents with a child with a metabolic defect detectable by amniocentesis
- Family history of sex-linked genetic disorder where sex determination is warranted.

Investigations
- Biochemical tests helps detect neural tube defects, anencephaly and spina bifida by elevation of serum alpha fetoprotein
- Culture of fetal cells detects inborn errors of metabolism
- Karyotyping detects chromosomal aberrations (Down's syndrome, Trisomy 18).

iii. Chorionic villi sampling
- It is done to obtain fetal trophoblastic tissue to study fetal DNA and enzymes found in amniocytes
- It also helps detect biochemical and structural anomalies.

c. Neonatal screening
- Neonate is subjected to battery of examination procedures to detect genetic disorders as follows:

❖ Clinical examination	Congenital dislocation of hip, congenital hypothyroidism
❖ Biochemical tests	Phenylketonuria, G6PD deficiency
❖ Hb electrophoresis	Sickle cell anemia, thalassemia
❖ Immunoreactive trypsin measurement	Cystic fibrosi

d. General population genetic screening
- This identifies individuals at risk of developing hereditary disorders before appearance of any symptoms by analyzing DNA.

Significance
- Genetic disorders though rare, are important health concerns and can be prevented if appropriate preventive strategy is used.

9. Write salient features of National Mental Health Program.

- National Mental Health Program was initiated by Government of India in 1982[Q] envisaged with integration of mental healthcare with general healthcare and welfare.

Aims	*Objectives*
▪ Prevention and treatment of mental and neurological disorders and their associated disabilities ▪ Use of mental health technology to improve general health services ▪ Application of mental health principles in total national development to improve quality of life	▪ To ensure availability and accessibility of minimum mental healthcare for all particularly to most vulnerable sections of population ▪ To encourage mental health knowledge and skills in general healthcare and social development ▪ To promote community participation in mental health service development and to stimulate self-help in community

Infrastructure

Mental hospitals	*Tertiary care institutions*	*Supportive organizations*
▪ State owned hospitals or private hospitals ▪ Provide custodial care rather than therapeutic care	▪ Institutions are involved with treatment, research and training ▪ National Institute of Mental Health and Neurosciences (NIMHANS), Bengaluru ▪ Central institute of Psychiatry, Ranchi ▪ Institute of Human Behavior and Allied Sciences, New Delhi	▪ Central Mental Health Authority and National Human Rights Commission which monitor implementation of Mental Health Act and functioning of state owned mental health hospitals respectively

Implementation

- National Mental Health Program is implemented through District Mental Health Program
- Its main objective is to provide basic mental health services to the community and to integrate these with other health services.

Revised Scheme 2

Activities under District Mental Health Program

- Training of mental health team at the identified nodal institutions
- Increase awareness about mental health problems
- Provide service for early detection and treatment of mental illnesses in the community (OPD/Indoor and follow up)
- Provide valuable data and experience at the level of community at the state and center for future planning and improvement in service and research
- Strengthening and modernization of mental hospitals.

Strategies (10th Five Year Program)

a. Integration into primary healthcare	▪ Expansion of District Mental Health Program (DMHP) to 100 districts all over country ▪ Integration of mental healthcare service with existing general health services ▪ Empowerment of Primary Health Care (PHC) doctor to offer care to mentally-ill persons at PHC ▪ Utilization of infrastructure such as village health guides and health workers for early detection and follow up services
b. Establishment and strengthening of infrastructure	▪ Establishment of tertiary care institutions for treatment of mental disorders ▪ Strengthening and modernization of existing mental hospitals to make treatment acceptable to the patients ▪ Upgradation of psychiatry wings in general hospitals/ medical colleges to enhance better training opportunities
c. Training	▪ Research and training in mental health for improving service delivery ▪ Training mental health teams at nodal institutions in state ▪ Training of trainers from states at NIMHANS
d. Health education	▪ IEC activities to improve public awareness and facilitate community participation ▪ Increasing awareness of mental health problems in community ▪ Eradicating stigmatization of mentally-ill patients and protecting their rights
e. Rehabilitation services	▪ Providing rehabilitation services for chronically disabled mental patients ▪ Providing counseling for alcoholics, drug addicts, delinquents

Targets Achieved

- Number of districts that have successfully implemented DMHP—542
- Improvement in service care in mental hospitals
- Lowering of stigma attached to mental illnesses
- Increased awareness of mental disorders.

Significance

- Major hindrance to proper and effective implementation of National Mental Health Program is lack of infrastructure, deficient manpower, attitude of society towards mental illness however now NGOs have joined hands in this program to help in community-based care of mentally-ill
- However, there is still a need for integrating mental health components in national level programs like ICDS, education system, and use of traditional systems like yoga, meditation, so that the mental health promotive activities become part of program.

10. Community Health Center.

Refer Question No. 2 December 2007 (RS2) Paper II.

11. How do you measure the burden of coronary heart disease in the community?

- Coronary heart disease or ischemic heart disease is impairment of heart function due to inadequate blood flow to heart compared to its needs due to obstructive changes in coronary circulation.

Measuring Disease Burden

a. Proportional mortality ratio	▪ It is proportion of all death attributed to coronary heart disease ▪ It is simplest measure
b. CHD incidence rate	▪ It is sum of fatal and nonfatal attack rates ▪ Accurate measurement is difficult because manifestations vary in different individuals ▪ However mortality rates can serve as crude incidence rate
c. Prevalence rate	▪ It can be estimated from cross sectional surveys using ECG for incidence of infarction and history of prolonged chest pain
d. Age-specific death rates	▪ It suggests true increase in incidence
e. Case fatality rate	▪ It is proportion of attacks that are fatal within 28 days of onset
f. Loss of life expectancy	▪ It is based on calculation of average gain in life expectancy following complete elimination of all cardiovascular deaths if other mortality rates remain unchanged
g. Measurement of risk factor level	▪ Includes measurements of levels of cigarette smoking, blood pressure, alcohol consumption and serum cholesterol
h. Medical care	▪ Measures levels of medical care in community

Significance

- Coronary heart disease has emerged as a major noncommunicable disease in recent decade.

12. Emergency contraception.

- Emergency contraception are contraceptive measures that if taken after sex, may prevent pregnancy
- Also called morning after or postcoital contraception
- However, these methods does not guarantee to prevent pregnancy.

Mechanism	*Indications*
▪ Acts by stopping ovulation or by interfering with implantation of ovum	▪ Unprotected intercourse ▪ Rape, sexual assault, incest ▪ Failure of contraceptive method such as rupture of condom, displacement of IUD, missing 2 or more OC pills ▪ Premature ejaculation in couple practicing coitus interruptus

Methods

- Oral contraceptive pills[Q] (Yuzpe and Lancee method[Q]—WHO)
  - Preparation of choice as it is less likely to cause adverse effects

  Regimens
  - Combined OC pills
    - Pills with 30 μg estrogen: Current recommendation
      - 4 pills immediately followed by 4 pills 12 hours later
    - Pills with 50 μg estrogen: Standard method
      - 2 pills immediately followed by 2 pills after 12 hours
    - Pills with 200 μg estrogen
      - 1 pill immediately followed by 1 pill 12 hours later
    - Mini pills (0.75 mg progestin only pills)
      - 1 pill immediately followed by 1 pill 12 hours later
    - High does estrogen
    - 5 mg estrogen OD for 5 days.

  Timing
  - Recommended within 48–72 hours of an unprotected intercourse
  - Sooner it is initiated, more effective the contraception and beyond 72 hours, the efficacy is reduced
  - A pregnancy test should be carried out if the period is >3 days late.

Side effects
- Nausea
  - Intrauterine cantraceptive device (IUCD) (Copper T^Q^)
- Copper IUCDs within a period of 3–5 days^Q^
- It is more effective than oral contraceptive pills
- It is more than 99% effective^Q^
  - Antiprogesterone (RU-486^Q^)
- Mifepristone (Ru – 486) 600 mg to be taken within 27th day of cycle irrespective of duration and number of intercourse.

Significance

- This method is a lance chance, secondary method of contraception to prevent an unplanned pregnancy and can save the lady from agony and embarrassment of resorting to illegal abortion.

SHORT ANSWERS

13. Describe rash in measles.

- Measles is an acute highly infectious disease characterized by fever and catarrhal symptoms of upper respiratory tract followed by a typical rash.

Rash in measles

- In measles, rash appears in 2nd stage (exanthematous or eruptive stage)
- It follows fever and catarrhal symptoms, appearing on 4th day of fever.

Features	*Progression*
▪ Rashes are pink (or dull red), velvety and maculopapular ▪ They remain discrete but often become confluent and blotchy ▪ They completely disappear and do not leave behind any permanent pock marks	▪ It first appears behind ear on 4th day after fever, then on forehead, face and down the trunk slowly taking 2–3 days to progress to hands and lower extremities ▪ Rashes begin to disappear from 5th or 6th day in same order as they appeared ▪ Lesions disappear completely from face but on trunk they leave behind brownish discoloration which may persist for about 6–8 weeks

Significance

- Rashes of measles are so typical of disease that word "Measles" is derived from word "maseles" meaning spots.

14. Planning–programming–budgeting system.

Refer Question No. 6 December 2011 (RS2) Paper II.

15. Enumerate Mendel's laws of inheritance.

- Laws of inheritance were derived by Gregor Johann Mendel, an Austrian monk conducting hybridization experiments in garden peas
- They are also called Mendel's Principles of Heredity or Mendelian inheritance.

Laws of Inheritance

Law of Segregation (The "First Law")	*Law of Independent Assortment (The "Second Law")*
▪ The Law of Segregation states that every individual possesses a pair of alleles (assuming diploidy) for any particular trait and that each parent passes a randomly selected copy (allele) of only one of these to its offspring. The offspring then receives its own pair of alleles for that trait. Whichever of the two alleles in the offspring is dominant determines how the offspring expresses that trait	▪ The Law of Independent Assortment, also known as "Inheritance Law", states that separate genes for separate traits are passed independently of one another from parents to offspring. That is, the biological selection of a particular gene in the gene pair for one trait to be passed to the offspring has nothing to do with the selection of the gene for any other trait

Contd...

Contd...

Law of Segregation (The "First Law")	*Law of Independent Assortment (The "Second Law")*
▪ More precisely, the law states that when any individual produces gametes, the copies of a gene separate so that each gamete receives only one copy (allele)	▪ More precisely, the law states that alleles of different genes assort independently of one another during gamete formation

Significance

- Mendel's law of inheritance have become core of classical genetics.

16. Prevention of neonatal tetanus.

Refer Question No. 12 June 2013 (RS2) Paper II.

17. Central Government Health Scheme.

- Central Government Health Scheme is a Health scheme introduced in 1954
- It is based on principle of cooperative effort by the employee and employer, to mutual advantage of both
- Previously called Contributory Health Service Scheme.

Objectives	*Beneficiaries*	*Facilities*
▪ To provide comprehensive medical care to Central Government employees	▪ Employees of Central Government, retired Central Government servants, employees of autonomous organizations, windows receiving family pension, Members of Parliament, e.g. Governers and retired Judges	▪ Out-patient care through a network of dispensaries ▪ Specialist consultation ▪ Antental, natal and postnatal services ▪ Pediatric services including immunization ▪ Laboratory and X-ray investigations ▪ Supply of necessary drugs ▪ Supply of optical and dental aids at reasonable rate ▪ Emergency treatment ▪ Hospitalization facilities at government and recognized private hospitals ▪ Domiciliary visits ▪ Family welfare services

Significance

- Central Government Health Scheme is a well organized health insurance scheme providing reasonable medical care and essential preventive and promotive health services to a large group of wage earner in India.

18. Disaster mitigation.

Refer Question No. 15 December 2009 (RS2) Paper II.

19. Secondary prevention of rheumatic heart disease.

Refer Question No. 11 December 2016 (RS2) Paper II.

20. Enumerate objectives of school health program.

Refer Question No. 4 December 2013 (RS2) Paper II.

21. Social security available for elderly population.

Refer Question No. 2 December 2009 (RS2) Paper I.

22. Indications for medical termination of pregnancy.

- Medical Termination of Pregnancy is governed by the MTP act 34 of 1971[Q] which came into force from 1st Jan. 1972
- This Act was subsequently amended in 2002 and then came to be known as The Medical Termination of Pregnancy Amendment Act, 2002 (No. 64 of 2002)
- This act has made certain provisions for legal medical termination of pregnancy.

Indication[Q] of the Medical Termination of Pregnancy

a. Therapeutic[Q]	▪ When the continuation of pregnancy endangers the life of women or may cause severe injury to her physical or mental health
b. Eugenic[Q]	▪ When there is risk of the child being born with serious physical or mental abnormality. This may occur – If a pregnant woman suffers from German measles, smallpox or chickenpox, viral hepatitis, toxoplasmosis or any severe viral infection during the first trimester – If a pregnant woman is treated with teratogenic drugs like thalidomide, cortisone or if she consumes hallucinogens or antidepressants ▪ If a mother is treated with X-rays or radioisotopes during pregnancy ▪ Insanity of the parents
c. Humanitarian	▪ When pregnancy has resulted out of a rape
d. Social[Q]	▪ When pregnancy is due to failure of contraceptive method ▪ When socioeconomic environment can injure the mother's health

Provisions

A. District Level Committee
- The Act Enables Establishment of District Level Committee to oversee implementation of the Act and also to award and renew licenses to the recognized MTP centers
- The committee would compose of One member of the district level Committee shall be the Gynecologist/Surgeon/Anesthetist and other members from the local medical profession, nongovernmental organization, and Panchayati Raj Institution of the District. Provided that one of the members of the committee shall be a woman
- The tenure of the committee shall be for two calendar years and the tenure of the nongovernment members shall not be more than two terms

B. Qualification and experience of the doctor[Q]

For termination up to 20 weeks for gestation	*For termination up to 12 weeks of gestation*
• A medical practitioner registered with State Medical Council immediately before the commencement of the act, should posses experience in the practice of obstetrics and gynecology for a period not less than 3 years • A medical practitioner who has been registered in a State Medical Register and who holds a post-graduate degree or diploma in obstetrics and gynecology, the experience or training gained during the course of such degree or diploma	• A medical practitioner registered with State Medical Council – If he has completed six months of internship in obstetrics and gynecology or – Unless the following facilities are provided therein, if he had experience at any hospital for a period of not less than one year in the practice of obstetrics and gynecology – If he has assisted a registered medical practitioner in the performance of twenty-five cases of medical termination of pregnancy[Q] of which at least five have been performed independently, in a hospital established or maintained or a training institute approved for this purpose by the government

C. Recognized center[Q]
- The recognized centers where MTP can be done should obtain license from District Level Committee which would inspect the place before approving the place
- No place shall be approved
  - Unless the Government is satisfied that termination of pregnancies may be done therein under safe and hygienic conditions; and
  - Unless the following facilities are provided therein, namely

For Termination up to 12 weeks of gestation	*For Termination up to 20 weeks of gestation*[Q]
• A gynecology examination/labor table, resuscitation and sterilization equipment, drugs and parental fluid, back up facilities for treatment of shock and facilities for transportation	• An operation table and instruments for performing abdominal or gynaecological surgery • Anaesthetic equipment, resuscitation equipment and sterilization equipment • Drugs and parental fluids for emergency use, notified by the Government of India from time to time

- The certificate of approval issued by the committee shall be conspicuously displayed at the place to be easily visible to persons visiting the place
- Government run hospitals are also the centers

D. Consent
- According to the act, the consent of woman is necessary to perform the MTP
- Consent of the husband is not necessary
- Abortion cannot be performed on the request of the husband if the woman herself is not willing
- In case of minor or lunatic a written consent from the guardian is required[Q]

E. Documents required
- The documentary proof of age of the women is not required. Statement of the woman of being over 18 years of age is accepted
- Even in cases of rape, the statement of the woman that she was raped is enough. It is not necessary to lodge a complaint in the police station

F. Length of pregnancy
- As per the act, all the indications of the MTP are applicable only upto 20 weeks of pregnancy[Q]
- If the period of pregnancy is below 12 weeks, it can be terminated on the opinion of single doctor[Q]
- If the period of pregnancy is above 12 weeks then two doctors must concur that there is an indication[Q]. Once the opinion is formed, the termination can be done by any one of the doctors
- However in emergency pregnancy can be terminated by a single doctor even without required training, without consulting a second doctor in an private hospital

Significance

- Medical Termination of Pregnancy Act has liberalized abortion in India thus has contributed to reduction of maternal mortality which used be caused due to criminal abortions.

MBBS PHASE III EXAMINATION

JUNE 2012

(Revised Scheme 2)

PAPER I

LONG ESSAYS

1. Define malnutrition. Describe the causes and clinical features of severe forms of malnutrition. How will you prevent malnutrition in children?

- Malnutrition is a pathological state resulting from a relative or absolute deficiency or excess of one or more essential nutrients.

For severe form of malnutrition (Protein Energy Malnutrition)

Refer Question No. 1 December 2012 (RS2) Paper I.

2. What is pneumoconiosis? What are the factors that influence causation of pneumoconiosis? What measures are taken to prevent it?

- Pneumoconioses or lung diseases are a group of lung diseases occurring out of the specific occupation, caused by inhalation of insoluble dust,[Q] over a prolonged period of exposure.

Pathology	*Clinical features*	*Treatment*
▪ Characterized by fibrosis of lung parenchyma followed by its complications ▪ Once established, it is usually progressive, permanent, pulmonary pathology	▪ Characterized by persistent cough, progressive breathlessness, gradually cripples the person by reducing the working capacity due to fibrosis of the lungs followed by the features of complications such as tuberculosis, emphysema, chronic obstructive pulmonary disease (COPD), pulmonary hypertension, cor pulmonale and even carcinoma in some cases	▪ No treatment or cure ▪ Prevention is the only intervention

Factors Influencing Pneumoconioses

a. Concentration of dust in air	▪ Higher the concentration, greater the health hazards ▪ Permissible limit is 200 μg/m^3 of air
b. Composition of dust	▪ More complicated the composition of the dust, greater the health hazard
c. Size of the dust particles (most important determining factor)	▪ Smaller the size of the dust particle, greater the tissue reaction (see particle size table below) ▪ Particles of size more than 0.1 μ and less than 5 μ is called respirable dust and is responsible for pneumoconiosis[Q]

Particle size	*Behaviour*
>10 μ	Settle down on the ground and become soil dust
<10 μ	Remain suspended in air
5–10 μ	Caught in upper respiratory passage
3–5 μ	Caught in mid respiratory passage
0.5–3 μ[Q]	Reach alveoli to lodge in respiratory tract[Q] and cause tissue reaction in form of fibrosis (most dangerous[Q])
<0.1 μ	Harmless because of Brownian movements they exhibit and they are absorbed

Contd...

Contd...

d. Duration of exposure	▪ Longer the duration of exposure to the dust, greater the health hazard ▪ Nearly 10–15 years of exposure is necessary for the development of tissue reaction
e. Individual susceptibility	▪ Better the health and nutritional status, lesser the chances of development of pneumoconiosis early

Common Pneumoconioses

Dust	*Disease*	*Industries*
a. Inorganic		
i. Silica	Silicosis	Sand stone industry, stone quarrying and dressing, granite industry, pottery and ceramic industry, gold, silver mica and steel industry
ii. Asbestos	Asbestosis	Asbestos cement factory, fireproof textiles, brake lining gaskets
iii. Iron	Siderosis	Iron ores and mines, iron and steel industries
iv. Coal dust[Q]	Anthrocosis[Q]	Coal mines
v. Aluminum	Aluminosis	Aluminum industries
vi. Berrylium	Berylliosis	Berrillum mining, manufacture of alloys
vii. Stone	Lithosis	Stone industries
b. Organic dust		
i. Cotton dust[Q]	Byssinosis[Q]	Textile industry[Q] (spinners[Q])
ii. Sugar cane dust[Q]	Bagassosis[Q]	Cane sugar factories, paper and cardboard industry
iii. Tobacco dust	Tabacosis	Tobacco factories
iv. Mouldy hay[Q]	Farmer's lung[Q]	Agricultural industry

Prevention and Control of Pneumoconioses

a. Health promotion	
i. Preplacement examination	▪ Consists of thorough examination of the individual before giving the job which includes not only thorough physical examinations but also routine investigations including X-ray of the chest
ii. Health education	▪ Employees at a risk of pneumoconioses are educated about the hazards of dust inhalation over long period ▪ They are also educated about the hazards of smoking as a precipitating factor and prevention of those hazards
iii. Provision of healthy physical environment	▪ Improvement in the sanitation such as cleanliness, adequate ventilation and good house-keeping (wet mopping of floors and walls) are mandatory
iv. Control of dust	▪ Prevention of formation of dust at the point of origin by water sprays or oil or steam, e.g. wet drilling of rock ▪ Prevention of escape of dust into the atmosphere by special enclosures or cabinets or hood for the machinery at the point of origin of dust and a with exhaust ventilation to draw into the hood and conveyed through ducts into collecting units ▪ Keeping moisture content below 20% and spraying 2% propionic acid (fungicide) controls bagassosis[Q] ▪ Use of safer type of asbestos like chrysolite (white form) and amosite (brown form) reduces hazards of asbestosis ▪ Removal of dust by special ventilatory arrangements
b. Specific protection	▪ Workers should protect themselves using face-masks, respirators and gas masks
c. Early diagnosis and treatment	▪ Periodic examination including X-ray of chest, so that the cases of respiratory diseases can be detected early and removed from the offending occupation and are given some other job ▪ If detected before the formation of fibrosis of the lungs and changed the job, resolution of the lungs can occur, except in asbestosis and anthracosis
d. Disability limitation	▪ Consists of limiting the further disability of the worker by detecting even the slightest degree of disability and immediately assigning some other suitable job
e. Rehabilitation	▪ Required for those workers, who have become handicapped due to the development of fibrosis of the lungs ▪ They require physical, psychological, social and vocational rehabilitation

Significance

- With industrialization, incidences of pneumoconioses are on rise and can become a major occupational health problem if preventive measures are not taken.

SHORT ESSAYS

3. Explain briefly dimensions of health.

Refer Question No. 3 December 2013 (RS2) Paper I.

4. Disability rates.

Refer Question No. 1 June 2008 (RS2) Paper I.

5. Sentinel surveillance.

- Sentinel surveillance is system of identifying the missing cases[Q] and thereby supplementing the notified cases[Q]
- Sentinel surveillance is used to supplement the routine reporting system.

Objective	*Procedure*	*Advantages*
▪ To know the disease prevalence in total population[Q]	▪ Here the interested and competent physicians (or institutions) in selected areas to enrolled as sentinel sites ▪ These sentinel sites regularly, timely and completely report the case of disease in their areas ▪ Over a period of time, they are developed into a notification system for providing more detailed information ▪ Under National AIDS control program wherein STD clinic, ANC clinic serves as sentinel sites[Q] to monitor trend ▪ Example: In AIDS, Malaria, Dengue, UIP	▪ Minimized reporting biases ▪ Simplified feedback information

Significance

- Sentinel surveillance provide more valuable and detailed information compared to traditional notification system
- It is a method of secondary prevention
- If properly implemented, it is less costly than developing and maintaining an ongoing notification system.

6. Difference between epidemiology and clinical medicine.

Points of difference	*Epidemiology*	*Clinical medicine*
a. Unit of study	Population or population at risk	Case or cases
b. Study of	Disease pattern in entire population	Disease pattern in an individual patient
c. Primary concern	Both sick and healthy (case and control respectively)	Only sick
d. Seeks	Source of infection, mode of spread or an etiological agent in order to determine future trend and recommend specific control measures	Diagnosis of diseases from which prognosis is derived and specific treatment is prescribed
e. Case finding	Active, i.e. going out to community to find sick or experience suspected causal factor in question	Passive, i.e. patient comes to doctor
f. Presentation of data	Conceptual and presented in form of tables and graphs	Factual and based on laboratory reports or post-mortem reports

Significance

- Though epidemiology and clinical medicine appears to be antagonistic but they are both closely related, coexistent and mutually helpful.

7. Uses of epidemiology.

- Epidemiology is the study of the distribution and determinants of health-related states or events in specified populations, and the applications of this study to the control of health problems.

Uses of Epidemiology

a. To study historically the rise and fall of disease in the population	▪ Health and disease pattern in a community is never constant and are fluctuating both over short and long periods of time ▪ Epidemiology provides a means to study disease profiles and time trends in human population ▪ By a study of these trends, useful projections into the future can be made and identification of emerging health problems and their correlates
b. Community diagnosis	▪ One of the uses of epidemiology is community diagnosis ▪ It generally refers to the identification and quantification of health problems in a community in terms of mortality and morbidity rates and ratios, and identification of their correlates for the purpose of defining those individuals or groups at risk or those in need of health care ▪ This helps to lay down priorities in disease control and prevention ▪ Quantification of morbidity and mortality serve as a benchmark for the evaluation of health services at a later date. ▪ Quantification of health problems becomes source of new knowledge about disease distribution, causation and prevention ▪ Epidemiology therefore has been described as a diagnostic tool of community medicine
c. Planning and evaluation	▪ Epidemiologic information about the distribution of health problems over time and place provides the fundamental basis for planning and developing the needed health services and for assessing the impact of these services on the people's problems ▪ Evaluation is an equally important concern of epidemiology ▪ The development of randomized controlled trial has made it possible to evaluate treatment modalities on a firm scientific basis
d. Evaluation of individual's risks and chances	▪ Besides the incidence rate and specific rates which are measures of absolute risk, the one can calculate relative risk and attributable risk for a factor related to or believed to be a cause of the disease
e. Syndrome identification	▪ Medical syndromes are identified by observing frequently associated findings in individual patients ▪ Epidemiological investigations can be used to define and refine syndromes
f. Completing the natural history of disease	▪ By studying disease patterns in the community in relation to agent, host and environmental factors the gaps in the natural history of disease can be filled up ▪ Epidemiological investigations have yielded a large amount of data on risk factors in relation to chronic disease
g. Searching for causes and risk factors	▪ By relating disease to interpopulation differences and other attributes of the population or cohorts examined, causes of disease can be identified ▪ The concept of "risk factors" gave renewed impetus to epidemiological research

8. Prevention of food adulteration Act (PFA Act).

Refer Question No. 11 December 2007 (RS2) Paper II.

9. Occupational cancer.

Refer Question No. 8 December 2007 (RS2) Paper I.

10. Barriers of communication and their prevention.

Refer Question No. 5 June 2010 (RS2) Paper I.

11. Biological transmission of diseases.

Refer Question No. 1 June 2009 (RS2) Paper I.

12. Herd immunity and its importance.

- Herd immunity is the level of resistance of a community or group of people to a particular disease.

- It concerns the freedom from infection individuals within a herd by sole virtue of the influence of the herd structure on transmission among individuals
- It provides an immunological barrier to the spread of disease in the human herd
- Herd structure is not constant[Q].

Determinants of herd immunity	*Changes in the herd immunity*
a. Age, sex and racial structure of the population b. Previous exposure of the herd to the disease concerned c. Stability of the herd with reference to emigrants and migrants[Q] d. Environmental factors conducive to the transmission of infection Example, water, supply, vectors, sanitation, etc. e. Artificial immunity in the individuals in the herd	▪ Herd immunity can increase due to: – Selective migration of susceptible persons – Death of susceptibles – Artificial acquisition of immunity by susceptibles – Subclinical infection in the herd ▪ Herd immunity can decrease due to: – Selective immigration of susceptibles – New birth

Significance

- If herd immunity is very high, the occurrence of disease will be very low
- If high level of herd immunity is maintained the disease eradication can be obtained as in case of polio, diphtheria
- However tetanus does not have herd immunity[Q].

SHORT ANSWERS

13. Modes of intervention.

Refer Question No. 1 December 2007 (RS2) Paper I.

14. Germ theory of disease.

- Germ theory is a theory of disease causation
- It was Proposed by Louis Pasteur[Q]
- Germ theory quotes that disease is caused by germs or microbiological agents like bacteria, etc.
- It gained momentum during 19th century and early 20th century with demonstration of bacteria in air by Louis Pasteur, causative agent of anthrax is bacteria by Robert Koch and then successful discoveries of many microbes like *Gonococcus*, typhoid bacilli, pneumococci, etc.
- This concept laid emphasis on one-to-one relationship between the causal agent and the disease.

Limitation

- Germ theory could not explain the reason for disease occurrence in only a few individuals after exposure to the causative agent and why some did not manifest disease even if they harbored the pathogen.

Significance

- Germ theory though took only one sided view of disease causation, it shifted the focus of epidemiologist from age old concept and provided a firm base for further research in scientific reason of disease causation.

15. Symposium.

Refer Question No. 2 June 2009 (RS2) Paper I.

16. Odds ratio.

Refer Question No. 1 June 2014 (RS2) Paper I.

17. Hazards of radiation.

Refer Question No. 8 December 2010 (RS2) Paper I.

18. Balanced diet.

Refer Question No. 4 June 2013 (RS2) Paper I.

19. Acculturation.

- Acculturation means culture contact^{Q} and diffusion of culture between individuals of different types of culture
- In simplified version, it is the process by which the cultural traits invented in one society are diffused or spread directly or indirectly to other societies
- Direct diffusion occurs when persons or groups have actual physical contact and indirect is without physical contact through media, commerce, etc.

Factors influencing acculturation (Channels of Acculturation)	*Barriers of acculturation*
▪ Conquest ▪ Prestige of diffused culture and its people ▪ Migration ▪ Industrialization ▪ Need of some new element to meet a crisis ▪ Education ▪ Propagation of religion ▪ Trade and commerce	▪ Resistance to cultural changes – Mores and taboos – Sense of superiority – General cultural inertia ▪ Adaptability of the recipients of the new culture ▪ Physical isolation

Role (Effects) of Acculturation

- Acculturation plays a very important role in development of a community
- It was due to acculturation that cultural traits from ancient civilization like Indus valley civilization, Greek civilization, Egyptian civilization, Roman civilization have spread to other areas of the world
- After renaissance, the center for would culture shifted to Great Britain, France and other European countries which spread to other countries through colonization
- Currently, USA has become the center of world culture and we Indians are borrowing their culture, good or bad through direct or indirect ways
- Indians have gone global, English has become a universal language.

Good effects of acculturation	*Bad effects of acculturation*
▪ Changes in food habits ▪ Introduction of scientific medicine ▪ Increased literacy ▪ Introduction of new ideas, concepts, ethics, etc.	▪ Smoking, alcohol consumption ▪ Drug abuse ▪ Junk food ▪ Sedentary lifestyle

Significance

- Acculturation is always very important for growth of a community or culture but cultural borrowing, i.e. borrowing ideas which would help the community is far better.

20. Break point chlorination.

Refer Question No. 9 December 2016 (RS2) Paper I.

21. Food fortification and food enrichment.

- Food fortification and food enrichment are two process to provide essential nutrients to required by the human body.

Food Fortification V/s Food Enrichment

Points of comparison	*Food fortification*	*Food enrichment*
▪ Definition	Addition of nutrients beyond that food originally contained	Addition of nutrients to replace that were lost during processing
▪ Example	Iodized salt	Vitamin B12 enriched refined flour

Ref:

Academy of Nutrition and Dietetics. "Enriched, Fortified: What's the Difference?" Accessed on February 12, 2008 http://www.eatright.org/cps/rde/xchg/SID-5303FFEA-D13B3A75/ada/hs.xsl/home_8388_ENU_HTML.htm.

22. Types of ventilation.

- Ventilation means replacement of vitiated (stagnant, warm and moist) air with controlled inflow of air in regards to temperature, humidity and purity in order to provide comfortable environment without risk of infection.

Types of Ventilation (Based upon Motive, which Originates them)

Natural ventilation	*Artificial ventilation (Mechanical)*
i. Perflation and aspiration of wind - Perflation means blowing of air through room when doors and windows are open - It is natural movement of air - When doors and windows face each other, it is called cross ventilation - During its movement, air in front dries it thus lessening pressure around it and causing surrounding air to move towards it by aspiration ii. Temperature difference - Air moves from area of high density to low density - Normally, outer cooler air is of higher density which rushes in through every opening whereas inside air is of lower density moves up - Temperature difference between outer and inner air determines velocity of incoming air until temperature difference is nullified - This is basis of natural ventilation - In tropics, reverse process takes place whereas in cold countries fires are used to room to keep inside air warm iii. Diffusion of gases - Diffusion is passing of air through smallest opening or spaces such as cracks and crevices - Very slow process and very small - Of little value as a ventilation mechanism	i. Vacuum system (exhaust system[Q] or extraction system) - In this system, foul, vitiated air is extracted or exhausted to outside using exhaust fans, operated electrically creating a vacuum which is filled in by sucking in of fresh air from outside - Usually fixed higher up in wall or roof because vitiated air is warmer and moves up - Air entry can be regulated by adjusting fan speed *Application* - As means of ventilation in large halls, auditorium, cinema halls - To remove dust, fumes and other contaminants in kitchen, industries ii. Plenum system[Q] (propeller system) - Here, fresh air is pushed or propelled or blown into room by centrifugal fans[Q] or high pressure fans - It creates positive pressure and displaces vitiated air - Air is delivered through ducts at desired points *Application* - To supply air in air conditioned buildings and factories iii. Balanced system - It employs combination of both exhaust system and plenum system of ventilation *Application* - Used in large halls with extensive sitting capacity and in air conditioning system iv. Air conditioning[Q] - Air conditioner is an equipment which conditions or controls external air with reference to physical and chemical conditions like cleaning, adjusting temperature and humidity to make it most comfortable and them letting it into room at a measured rate and volume of flow without producing draught and exhausted through ducts - Air is filtered when drawn into an air conditioner system from room - Excess humidity is removed and air is circulated back into room after heating or cooling it, to bring room temperature to required comfort zone - If temperature difference between outside air and air conditioned room is very large, to prevent sudden exposure to high or low temperature, transition rooms are provided *Applications* - Air conditioners are extensively used in operations theaters, hospitals, hotels, offices, homes, cinema halls, transport vehicles, etc.

Standards of ventilation	
a. Cubic space	• Recommended standard of fresh air supply is 3000 cubic feet of fresh air should be provided per hour per person (200 cubic feet for child) • This is required amount of air so that a person entering a room from outside should not perceive any smell or stuffiness **Calculation** • Amount of fresh air delivered per hour to an occupied room can be calculated as follows: d = e/p where • d = amount of fresh air to be delivered to a room • e = CO_2 exhaled per hour per person (about 0.6 cubic feet per person per hour) • p = limit of respiratory CO_2 per cubic feet of air beyond which one feels stuffiness (0.0002 cubic feet per cubic feet)

Contd...

Contd...

	Therefore d= 0.6/0.0002 = 3000 cubic feet of air per person per hour **Significance** • This standard proposed by De Chaumont uses CO_2 as indicator, however is no longer used
b. Air change	• Recommended air changes in living rooms is 2–3 per hour[Q] whereas in work rooms and assemblies 4–6 per hour • However, it depends upon size of room, i.e. for example, for a person in a 100 cubic feet, to receive 3000 cubic feet of air per hour, air should change 30 times in an hour whereas for a person in a 1000 cubic feet room, requires only 3 air changes • If air is changed more frequently, i.e. more than 6 times per hour, it produces draught which should be avoided **Calculations** • Number of air changes per hour is calculated by dividing total hourly air supply to room by cubic capacity of room
c. Floor area	• Recommended standard of ventilation is 50–100 square feet per person[Q] in a standard house which should be 150 square feet in general hospital and 200 square feet in infectious disease hospitals • Floor space below 50 square feet results in overcrowding favouring spread of droplet infection **Significance** • Floor area is an important standard of ventilation and more significant than cubic feet considering heights over 10–12 feet are ineffective from ventilation point of view

Significance

- Natural ventilation is cheapest method of ventilation but is subject to atmospheric conditions therefore mechanical ventilations are preferred nowadays as they supply consistent ventilation under all conditions.

MBBS PHASE III EXAMINATION

JUNE 2012

(Revised Scheme 2)

PAPER II

LONG ESSAYS

1. Describe the epidemiology, clinical features, prevention and control of measles in a community.

Refer Question No. 1 December 2010 (RS2) Paper II.

2. Describe the causes of maternal mortality in India. Suggest preventive and control measures for reduction of MMR.

- Maternal mortality or maternal death is defined as the death of a woman while pregnant[Q] or within 42 days of termination of pregnancy[Q] irrespective of the duration and site of pregnancy from any cause related to or aggravated by the pregnancy[Q] or its management but not from accidental or incidental causes
- Thus, MMR measures risk of women dying from puerperal causes.

Calculation

- Maternal mortality ratio is calculated as:

$$\text{MMR} = \frac{\text{Total No. of female death due to complications of pregnancy childbirth or within 42 days of delivery from puerperal causes in an area during a given year}}{\text{Total No. of live births in the same area during the same year}^{Q}} \times 100{,}000^{Q}$$

- MMR is expressed per 100,000 live births[Q] (earlier it was expressed per 1000 live births but yielded fractions so denominator was increased to make it more sensible)
- In India, it is estimated by RHIME[Q] (Representative, re-sampled, routine household interview of mortality, with medical evaluation) which is an enhanced form of verbal autopsy[Q].

Current Status

- Current MMR in India is 174 per 100,000 live births (World Bank 2015)
- Millennium development goal is to reduce maternal mortality to 105 by 2015.

Causes of Maternal Mortality

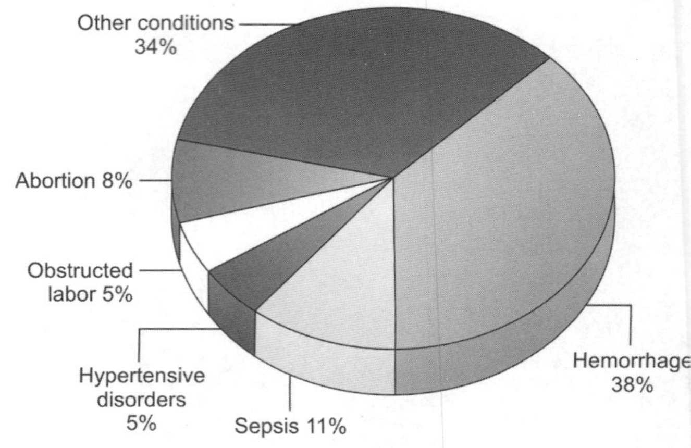

Fig. 1: Maternal mortality—medical causes

Medical causes				*Social causes (predisposing factors)*
Obstetric causes			*Nonobstetric causes*	
Antenatal	*Intranatal*	*Postpartum*		
▪ Toxemias of pregnancy ▪ Antenatal hemorrhage[Q] ▪ Placenta previa ▪ Abruptio placentae ▪ Multiple pregnancies ▪ Incomplete abortion followed by bleeding ▪ Ectopic pregnancy ▪ Criminal abortion[Q]	▪ Rupture of uterus ▪ Prolonged labour ▪ Obstructed labour (5%) ▪ Anesthetic shock during cesarean section ▪ Amniotic fluid embolism	▪ Puerperal sepsis[Q] (11%) ▪ Postpartum hemorrhage[Q] (MC– 38%) ▪ Thrombophlebitis	▪ Anemia[Q] ▪ Associated cardiac, renal, hepatic, metabolic or infectious diseases ▪ Malignancy ▪ Accidents	▪ Age at child birth (MC at 20–24 years) ▪ Parity ▪ Too close pregnancies ▪ Family size ▪ Malnutrition[Q] ▪ Poverty ▪ Illiteracy ▪ Ignorance and prejudices ▪ Lack of maternal services[Q] ▪ Shortage of health manpower ▪ Delivery by untrained dais ▪ Poor environmental sanitation ▪ Poor communication and transport facilities ▪ Social customs

Measures for Reduction of Maternal Mortality (Prevention and Control)

a. Efficient antenatal check-up	▪ Early recognition and registration of pregnancy ▪ Regular antenatal check-ups but at least 3 ▪ Antenatal investigations ▪ Antenatal advice including warning signals ▪ Dietary supplementation including treatment of anemia with iron and folic acid tablets ▪ Prevention of complications like eclampsia, malpresentation ▪ Treatment of medical conditions like hypertension, diabetes, tuberculosis ▪ Tetanus immunization ▪ Risk approach and primary healthcare for mothers with high-risk pregnancy
b. Efficient intranatal care	▪ Provision of safe delivery by trained person observing 5 cleans. ▪ Identification of danger signals and prompt attention ▪ Prevention of complications like ruptured uterus ▪ Training of local dais and female health workers ▪ Institutional deliveries for women with bad obstetric history and risk factors ▪ Establishment of first referral units for emergency obstetric care
c. Efficient postnatal care	▪ Regular postnatal check-ups and postnatal advice ▪ Infection and hemorrhage prevention during puerperium
d. Family welfare services	▪ Counseling about family planning services ▪ Family planning promotion to control family size preferably to one child ▪ Advice regarding spacing of about 3 years between two pregnancies
e. Health education	▪ About nutrition, drugs, exercise, habits, personal hygiene, about taking treatment of illness, etc. ▪ Attack on social and cultural taboos
f. Other services	▪ Encouraging female literacy ▪ Socioeconomic development of the community through active involvement of community ▪ Identification of every maternal death and searching for its cause

Significance

- Maternal mortality rate is a ratio[Q], not a rate
- Maternal mortality is a sentinel event to assess the quality of healthcare system.

SHORT ESSAYS

3. Describe the epidemiology and prevention of accidents.

Refer Question No. 2 June 2016 (RS2) Paper II.

4. What are the principles and elements of primary healthcare?

Definition

- "Primary healthcare is essential healthcare made universally accessible to individuals and acceptable to them through their full participation and at a cost the community and country can afford[Q]"
- The concept of primary healthcare was proposed by WHO[Q] and came into existence in 1978[Q] following an International Conference at Alma Ata[Q] (Erstwhile USSR)
- It is equally valid for all countries and has been accepted by all countries inclusive India
- It is the integral part of the India's health system.

Elements or Components of Primary Healthcare (Alma-Ata Declaration, 1978)[Q]

- E: Education concerning prevailing health problems and methods of preventing and controlling them[Q]
- L: Locally endemic diseases—Prevention and control
- E: Essential drugs
- M: Maternal and child healthcare including family planning[Q]
- E: EPI (immunization) against vaccine preventable diseases
- N: Nutrition and promotion of food supply
- T: Treatment of common diseases and injuries
- S: Safe water supply and basic sanitation[Q].

Principles[Q] or Determinants of Primary Healthcare

a. Equitable distribution[Q]
   - It means that the health services must be shared equally by all people irrespective of their ability to pay all (rich or poor, urban or rural) must have access to the health services
   - This principle is based on the fact that at present the healthcare services are concentrated in the towns and cities to the rich and curative oriented
   - On the other hand, the needy and vulnerable groups of population like the poor rural and the urban slums are neglected and who deserve the service the most
   - Primary healthcare aims to redress this imbalance by shifting the center of gravity of the healthcare system from cities to the rural areas and bring these services as near people's homes are possible.

b. Community participation[Q]
   - Involvement of individuals, families and communities in promotion of their own health and welfare is an essential ingredient of primary healthcare
   - This is based upon the fact that achieving universal coverage of primary healthcare is not possible without the involvement of the local community
   - Community involvement should be in the planning, implementation and maintenance of health services
   - Even the maximum reliance should be on the local resources such as man power, money and materials
   - It promotes social awareness and self-reliance of the community
   - It increases the community acceptance of the primary healthcare programs and reduces the distance between the provider and the consumer of the service
   - Examples of community participation are village health guides and trained dais who are selected from the local community and trained locally to deliver primary healthcare to the community they belong
   - They provide primary healthcare in way that is acceptable to the society by overcoming the cultural and communication barrier
   - They are the front line workers of the healthcare delivery system and have become essential feature of primary healthcare in India.

   Advantages
   - It is a cost-effective method of providing health services
   - People begin to view health more objectively, so they are more likely to accept the care
   - There will be greater commitment of the people resulting in the success of healthcare services
   - Health awareness becomes an integral part of village life
   - Health workers get greater support for their activities
   - People become more self-reliant in taking care of their health

- Healthcare services become more relevant to the health needs of the people
- There is less dependence on the government
- Quality of the healthcare improves.

Significance

- Community participation is aimed at placing the health of the people in their hands which contributes to their development and in turn the development of community.

c. Intersectoral coordination[Q]
- The Declaration of Alma—Ata states that the primary healthcare involves in addition to the health sector, all related sectors and aspects of national and community development in particular agriculture, animal husbandry, food industry, education, housing, public works, communications and other sectors[Q].

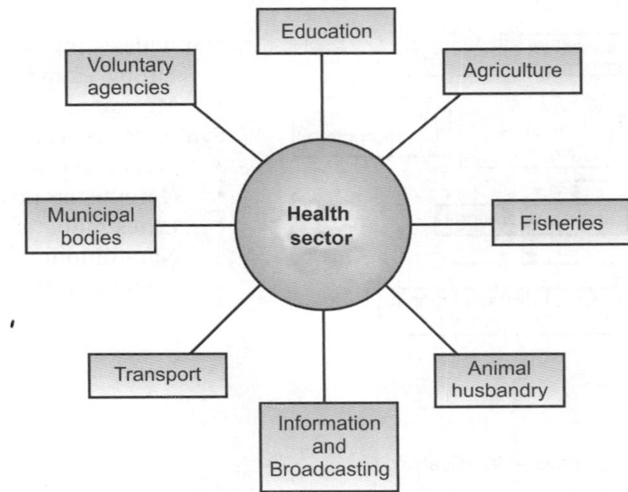

Fig. 2: Intersectoral coordination

- However, planning with other sectors is an important element of intersectoral coordination to avoid unnecessary duplication of activities
- But this requires a lot of political will because it demands administrative system review, resource reallocation and a suitable legislation
- Coordination committees set up to overlook this will make policies and implement in planned manner, so as to avoid duplication of the activities.

d. Appropriate technology[Q]
- Appropriate technology is that technology which is scientifically sound, adaptable to local needs and acceptable to those who apply it and those for whom it is used and that can be maintained by the people themselves in keeping with the principle of self-reliance with the resources, the community and country can afford[Q].

Elements	*Examples*
▪ Scientifically sound ▪ Effective and simple to use ▪ Acceptable to those who apply ▪ Acceptable to those who use ▪ In tune with local culture ▪ Capable of further development ▪ Based on self-reliance ▪ Easily understood by people and health volunteers ▪ Easily affordable to community	▪ Oral rehydration solution ▪ Immunization program ▪ Nutritional supplementation program ▪ DOTS ▪ Distribution of disposable delivery kits to domiciliary midwifery services ▪ Distribution of iron and folic acid tablets ▪ Family welfare services ▪ Biogas plant for cooking, heating and lighting

Significance

- Appropriate technology is a cheap and acceptable method of providing healthcare to the people
- Effective use of appropriate technology helps in bridging the urban-rural, rich-poor gap existing in the health sector
- Even the most vulnerable and weak sections will gain advantage from the use of appropriate technology suited to local needs.

Significance of Primary Healthcare

- Primary healthcare starts with the people themselves and has been described as "Health by the people, placing people's health in people's hands[Q]"
- Hallmark of primary healthcare are affordability, acceptability, accessibility and availability.

5. What are the different types of hormonal contraceptives? Write a note on mode of action, contraindications and complications of combined oral contraceptive pills.

- Hormonal contraceptive methods are the contraceptives containing gonadal steroids, i.e. synthetic estrogens and/ or synthetic progestogens.

Classification

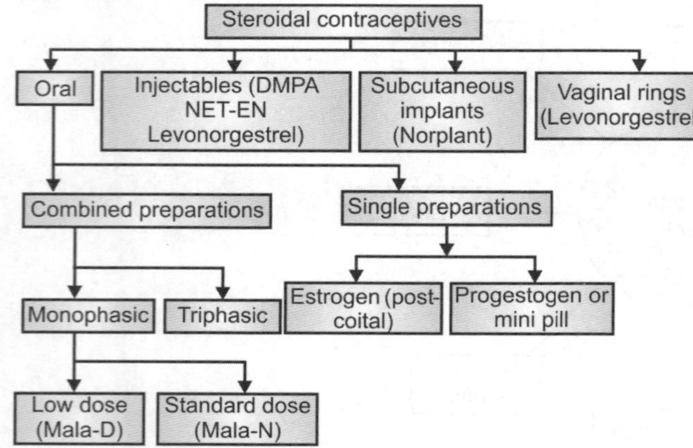

Fig. 3: Hormonal contraceptives—classification

Synthetic estrogens used:
- Ethinyl estradiol
- Mestranal

Synthetic progestogens used:
- Mederoxyprogesterone acetate[Q]
- Norethisterone acetate[Q]
- Lynestrenol[Q]
- Norethinodrel[Q]
- Levonorgestrel[Q]

Types

A. Combined oral contraceptive pills
   - They are so called because each pill has got a combination of estrogen and progestogen to be safe and effective.

Types

	Mala-N (Standard dose pill)	*Mala-D*
▪ Contents	▪ 30 μg of ethenyl estradiol[Q] ▪ 1000 μg of noresthisterone acetate[Q]	▪ 30 μg of ethenyl estradiol[Q] ▪ 500 μg of D-norgestrol[Q]
▪ Cost	▪ Provided free of cost under RCH program	▪ Provided at subsidized rate of 5 rupees

Mechanism of action

- Estrogen mainly inhibits ovulation and progestogen mainly causes the atrophy of endometrium and makes the cervical mucus thick, viscid and impenetrable to sperms, thereby preventing the pregnancy.

Formulations

<table>
<tr><th>Monophasic pills</th><th>Biphasic pills</th><th>Triphasic pills</th></tr>
<tr><td>▪ These pills deliver same amount of estrogen and progestin every day
Commercial preparations
▪ Containing 21 active (hormonal) pills
▪ Containing 28 pills (21 active + 7 placebos, i.e. reminder pills of different color is to make the women to have a continuity in taking the pills)</td><td>▪ These pills deliver same amount of estrogen every day</td><td>▪ Based upon the concept of administration of the pill of varying strengths of estrogen and progesterone in three phases, so that the regimen parallels more closely the normal hormonal cycle of the menstruating woman
Commercial preparation
▪ Triquilar
Contents
<table><tr><th>Ethynyl estradiol</th><th>Lenonorgestrel</th><th>Days</th></tr><tr><td>30 μg</td><td>50 μg</td><td>6</td></tr><tr><td>40 μg</td><td>75 μg</td><td>5</td></tr><tr><td>30 μg</td><td>125</td><td>10</td></tr></table></td></tr>
</table>

Precautions

- The woman is instructed to swallow one pill daily, preferably at bedtime, starting from the 5th day of the menstrual cycle, daily one, for 21 days, in the direction of the arrow over the packet, followed by a break of 7 days in case of 21 pill packet or continue one placebo daily in case of 28 pills packets, during which the woman will have menstruation
- The bleeding occurs within 2–3 days after the last hormonal pill and when bleeding occurs, it is considered as the first day of the next cycle
- The bleeding is called withdrawal bleeding because bleeding is not like normal menstruation but an episode of uterine bleeding from an incompletely formed endometrium caused by the withdrawal of the exogenous hormones
- Further the quantity lost is half of that occurring in the natural menstruation, thus, it is an anovular menstruation
- Whether bleeding occurs or not, she is instructed to start the next packet of the pills the very next day of the previous 28 pill packet or from the 5th day of the cycle in case of 21 pill packet
- Usually, she will have her cycles at the end of second course/packet
- She must not wait for more than 7 days between cycles of 21 pill packets
- She must continue to take packets after packets, as long as she does not desire pregnancy
- Pills should be taken every day to be most effective and if not taken correctly there will be risk pregnancy
- Missing the pills or starting new packet late are the most common mistakes and in such case.

Missed 1 pill	*Missed 2 pills or more in first 14 pills*	*Missed 2 pills or more in the 3rd row*	*Missed any pill in the 4th row*
Take missed pill as soon as she remembers and take the rest as usual	Take one pill as soon as she remembers and the rest as usual and meanwhile must also use another contraceptive method such as condoms or spermicides for 7 days or avoid sex for 1 week	Take the pill as soon as she remembers and take the rest as usual meanwhile she must also use another method such as condoms for 7 days or avoid sex for 1 week and she should start a new pack the next day after the completion of 3rd row and throw the last row of this pack away	Throw the missed pill away and take the rest as usual and start a new packet as usual on the next day thus forgetting to take placebos, she is still protected from pregnancy

Effectiveness	*Failure rate*
Low dose combined, either monophasic or triphasic, oral pills are very effective when used correctly and consistently	One pregnancies per 100 WYE

Contraindications

Absolute	*Relative (Requires medical surveillance)*
▪ Women beyond 35 years of age ▪ Women with hypertension or history of thromboembolism or cardiovascular diseases[Q] ▪ Cancer of breast and genitals ▪ Liver diseases[Q] ▪ Bleeding disorders ▪ History of thromboembolism ▪ Undiagnosed abnormal uterine bleeding ▪ Congenital hyperlipidemia[Q]	▪ Pregnancy ▪ Lactation[Q] ▪ Epilepsy[Q] ▪ Migraine ▪ Mild hypertension ▪ Chronic renal disease[Q] ▪ Diabetes mellitus ▪ Gallbladder disease ▪ Amenorrhoea ▪ History of frequent bleeding

Merits	*Demerits (Adverse effects/complications)*	*Noncontraceptive benefits of OCP[Q]*
▪ Highly effective ▪ Easy to use ▪ Nothing to do at the time of sex play unlike in barrier methods ▪ Increased sexual enjoyment because of no worry about pregnancy ▪ Can be used at any age during reproductive age preferably by newly wed to postpone for the first issue[Q] ▪ Can be used as long as she does not want pregnancy ▪ Reversible, i.e. fertility returns after stopping the pills ▪ Can be used as an emergency contraceptive after unprotected sex	▪ Nausea (common during first 2–3 months) ▪ Spotting or bleeding between menstrual periods especially if she forgets to take pills regularly ▪ Mild headache and migraine ▪ Breast tenderness ▪ Slight weight gain (due to water retention) ▪ Suppresses the quality and quantity of the breast-milk if she is lactating mother (because of estrogen content)	▪ Regularization of irregular menstrual cycle especially Stein-Leventhal syndrome (PCOD) ▪ Reduced incidence or improvement in – Dysmenorrhea – Anemia – Acne – Hirsutism – Ectopic pregnancy – Benign breast disease – Endometrial cancer

Contd...

Contd...

▪ Periods become regular, painless and fewer days of bleeding with minimal cramps[Q] ▪ Relieves premenstrual tension and acne ▪ Prevents anemia and malnutrition by preventing pregnancy ▪ Helps in preventing – Ectopic pregnancy – Ovarian cyst[Q] – Endometrial cancer[Q] – PID[Q] – Cancers of ovary and breast[Q] ▪ Safe for almost all women of any age whether or not they have had children ▪ Can be started any it is reasonably certain a woman is not pregnant	▪ May cause mood changes including depression, loss of libido ▪ Very rarely can cause cardiovascular effects such as hypertension, myocardial infarction, cerebral thrombosis and thrombosis in the deep veins of the legs especially among women with hypertension, aged above 35 years, and heavy smokers[Q] ▪ Does not protect against STDs including AIDS ▪ Worsens diabetic condition calling for more insulin[Q]	– Ovarian cysts – Ovarian cancer – Colorectal cancer – Pelvic inflammatory disease – Osteopenia and osteoporosis

B. Progestin only pills (Mini pill or Micro pill)[Q]
- These contain very small amounts of only one kind of hormone i.e. progestin[Q] (one half to one tenth of progestin percent in oral contraceptives) and they do not contain estrogen
- They are available in pack of 28 or 35 pills, all of the same color and there are no placebos
- This is a good choice for breastfeeding women who want an oral contraceptive

Mechanism of action
- Progestin thickens the cervical mucus, making it difficult for sperms to pass through
- It induces a thin, unfavorable, atrophic endometrium
- It also stops ovulation in about 50% of cases
- It does not work by disrupting the existing pregnancy

Indications
- The women can start at any time after child birth or miscarriage and no need to wait for the menstrual periods to return
- If periods have returned in a lactating woman, she can start POP at any time it is reasonably certain that she is not pregnant
- The first day of the bleeding is the best time to start if periods have returned
- She should take one pill every day[Q], preferably at the same time because delay by few hours increases the risk of pregnancy and missing 2 or more pills, greatly increases the risk
- When she finishes one packet, she should take the first pill from the next packet on the very next day and there is no wait between packets[Q]

Missed Pills	***Effectiveness***	***Failure rate***
• If she forgets to take one or more pills, she should take 1 as soon as she remembers and then keep taking one pill each day as usual • If more than 3 hours late taking a pill by a woman who is not breastfeeding or who is breastfeeding but her menses have returned should also use condoms or spermicide or else avoid sex for 2 days • She should take the missed pill as soon as she can	• Progestin only pill is very effective, much more than combined oral contraceptive because breastfeeding itself provides protection against pregnancy	• 1 pregnancy per 100 WYE

Merits	***Demerits***
• Good choice for a lactating mother, because it does not suppress lactation[Q] • Free from the side effects of estrogen • May help prevent benign breast disease, pelvic inflammatory disease, endometrial and ovarian cancer • May lengthen period of lactational amenorrhea • Can be used in women in whom combined oral contraceptive is contraindicated like women with hypertension, lactation, smoking, thromboembolic disorder and in women who cannot tolerate combined pills	• Irregularities in bleeding such as irregular periods, intermenstrual bleeding, spotting, etc. in nonlactating women • Headache and breast tenderness (less frequently) • To be taken daily at the same time because delay by even a few hours increases the risk of pregnancy • Does not prevent ectopic pregnancy • Prolonged infertility

C. Post coital pills (Emergency oral contraception)
- They are often called morning after conception pills because they can prevent pregnancy
- It should be taken within 48 to 72 hours of unprotected intercourse.
- This method should not be used in place of family planning methods

Mechanism of action
- They act by stopping ovulation or by interfering with implantation of the ovum

Indications
- Unprotected intercourse
- Rape, sexual assault, incest
- Failure of contraceptive method such as rupture of condom, displacement of IUD, missing 2 or more mini pills
- Premature ejaculation among couples practicing coitus interruptus

Methods

a. High dose estrogens
   - Diethylstilbestrol (DES) 50 μg a day for 5 days
   - Ethinyl estradiol 50 μg a day for 5 days
   - Estradiol benzoate 12.5 mg combined with oestradiol phenylpropionate 10.0 mg
   - Failure rate is less than 1%

b. Estrogen—progesterone combination
   - This method consisting of consuming either 8 low dose combined oral contraceptive pills (Mala-D) (4 as soon as possible followed by another 4 after 12 hours) or 4 standard dose combined pills (Mala-N) (2 pills followed by another 2-pills after 12 hours)
   - It is based on fact that combination of 100 mg of estrogen and 1 mg of progestogen, in a single dose renders the endometrium out of phase
   - Failure rate is 0.2 to 2.0%.

Merits	*Demerits*
• Simple • Safe • Cheap • Readily available	• Due to high doses of estrogen • Ineffective, if the implantation of ovum has already occurred

c. Danazol
   - It is a progestogen only with antigonadotrophic activity
   - It prevents implantation by making unfavourable endometrium

   Dose
   - 2 doses of 400 mg each at 12 hours interval

d. Mifepristone
   - It is antiprogesterone
   - It prevents ovulation when given in early proliferative phase and hinders the development of endometrium if given in the luteal phase, i.e. within 72 hours of unprotected sex

   Dose
   - 600 mg stat

e. Mechanical method
   - This consists of insertion of copper IUD within 3 to 5 days of unprotected intercourse
   - It prevents implantation due to endometrial changes and also possibly it has embryotoxic effect by copper ions
   - This is particularly useful when hormonal pills are contraindicated

Merits	*Demerits*
• Provides contraceptive protection for few more years • More effective than hormonal method	• Contraindicated in women who are at risk of STD because of rape

D. Injectable contraceptives (Depot formulations or slow release formulations)
   – These are the formulations containing only synthetic progesterone (and not estrogen) which is released slowly over a long period of time, thus providing long lasting hormonal contraceptive activity

Formulations

DMPA[Q] (Depot Medroxy Progesterone Acetate)	*NET-EN (Norethisterone Enanthate)*
• It is a microcrystalline suspension, to be given deep intramuscularly, once in 3 months[Q], each dose containing 150 mg of progestin (synthetic progesterone) and is less painful • Commercial preparation • Depo-Provera, Megestron	• It is an oily solution, to be given deep intramuscularly, once in 2 months, each dose containing 200 mg of synthetic progesterone • It is more painful • This disappears more rapidly from the circulation compared to DMPA, so it is given more frequently • Commercial preparation • Noristerat

Mechanism of action
– These synthetic progestogens inhibit ovulation by inhibiting the secretion of gonadotropins
– They also thicken the cervical mucus thereby forming a barrier to sperms[Q]
– They also induce a thin endometrium, less suitable for implantation

Time of administration
– These can be administered to women of any age, whether they have children or not
– It can be given at any time in the menstrual cycle, provided it is reasonably certain that she is not pregnant
– However, they are usually given during the first five days of menstrual period, to rule out the possibility of pregnancy
– For a lactating mother these injections are given as early as 6 weeks after childbirth and do not wait for periods to return
– It can also be given after abortion, within 7 days

Precautions	*Failure rate*	*Contraindications*
• Not to massage the site of injection, so that it is absorbed slowly • To take the injection once in 3 months if DMPA is given or once in 2 months if NET-EN is given • To come back on the due date for the next injection • That she will have her cycles once in 2–3 months, depending upon the type of injection • She should come back even if she is late • She should also come back if she develops side effects, such as heavy bleeding	• 0.3 pregnancies per 100 WYE	• Pregnancy • Early postpartum period • Suspected malignancy • PID • Bleeding disorders

Merits	*Demerits*
• Very safe, effective, convenient and reversible • Long-term pregnancy prevention (2–3 months) • Does not interfere with sex • Does not interfere with lactation • Quality and quantity of milk is not affected • Does not contain estrogen • Can be used by women of any age in the reproductive period, including nulliparous women • Helps prevent ectopic pregnancies, endometrial cancer and uterine fibroids • May help prevent ovarian cancer, iron deficiency anemia, and decrease the frequency of seizures among epileptic women	• Menstrual cycles become irregular, once in 2–3 months, depending upon the type • Changes in the menstrual bleeding are also likely such as varying from light spotting to heavy bleeding • May cause weight gain of 1–2 kg per year • Delayed return of fertility by 4–6 months or even longer • Injection to be taken regularly, every 2–3 months, depending upon the type • May cause headache, breast tenderness, mood changes and loss of libido

E. Subcutaneous implants (norplant implants)
   - This system consists of a set of 6 small, silicon rubber soft capsules, about the size of a small match-stick, each containing 35 μg of synthetic progestogen (Levonorgestrel), which when implanted subcutaneously, release the hormone slowly over a long period of time, providing contraceptive effect for at least 5 years

Insertion

- The capsules are inserted subcutaneously, by a small incision under local anesthesia in the upper arm of the woman using a template
- After all the capsules are inserted, the incision is closed with an adhesive bandage as stitches are not necessary
- Once inserted, they start functioning within 24 hours
- Removal is also by minor surgery, whenever pregnancy is desired

Mechanism of action

- These synthetic progestogens inhibit ovulation by inhibiting the secretion of gonadotropins
- They also thicken the cervical mucus thereby forming a barrier to sperms
- They also induce a thin endometrium, less suitable for implantation

Effectiveness	*Failure rate*
Contraception is provided for about 5 years	1–6 pregnancies per 100 WYE

Merits	*Demerits*
• Very safe, effective, convenient and reversible • Long-term pregnancy prevention (2–3 months) • Does not interfere with sex • Does not interfere with lactation • Quality and quantity of milk is not affected • Does not contain estrogen • Can be used by women of any age in the reproductive period, including nulliparous women • Helps prevent ectopic pregnancies, endometrial cancer and uterine fibroids • May help prevent ovarian cancer, iron deficiency anemia, and decrease the frequency of seizures among epileptic women	• Menstrual cycles become irregular, once in 2 to 3 months, depending upon the type • Changes in the menstrual bleeding are also likely such as varying from light spotting to heavy bleeding • May cause weight gain of 1 to 2 kg per year • Delayed return of fertility by 4–6 months or even longer • Injection to be taken regularly, every 2–3 months, depending upon the type • May cause headache, breast tenderness, mood changes and loss of libido

Significance

- Hormonal contraceptive is a classical example of exploitation of knowledge of body physiology for regulation of bodily functions
- They are most widely used contraceptive methods by females.

6. Briefly explain the modes of transmission of Hepatitis B infection.

Refer Question No. 1 December 2014 (RS2) Paper II.

7. Mention the steps involved in eradication of poliomyelitis.

Refer Question No. 1 June 2014 (RS2) Paper II.

8. What are the measures for control of sexually transmitted diseases?

- Sexually transmitted diseases are a group of communicable diseases that are transmitted predominantly by sexual contact.

Prevention and Control of STDs

Objectives

- To interrupt the transmission of sexually acquired infections
- To prevent the development of diseases, complications and sequelae
- To reduce the risk of HIV infection.

A. Primary prevention

Aim

– Reducing incidence of disease by preventing the acquisition of infection and disease through (i) Safer sexual behavior and (ii) Use of condoms for penetrative sexual acts.

Components

a. Health education
- Health education is an integral part of STD control program
- Principle aim is to help individual alter their behavior in an effort to avoid risk of getting infected
- Target groups include general public, patients, priority groups, community leaders, etc.
- It can be carried out through lectures, multimedia, flip charts, group or individual discussions and in mass media through articles in the periodicals/journals/newspapers read by general population
- Specific messages related to STD may include:
  - Abstinence is only way to completely prevent STI
  - Avoid sex with many different partners
  - Practice safe sex (e.g. using condoms)
  - Information that symptoms and signs may not be noticed, particularly in women, until complications appear
  - Description of recognizable signs and symptoms
  - A list of places where STD advice may be obtained (i.e. basic healthcare services) and, where available, categorical STD clinics and voluntary counseling centers.

B. Secondary prevention

Aim

– Reducing prevalence by shortening the duration of disease, thus minimizing the probability of complications or sequelae.

Components

a. Early detection and treatment
- Case detection

Screening	*Contact tracing*[Q]	*Cluster Testing*[Q]
▪ Screening is testing of apparently healthy volunteers from general population for early detection of disease ▪ High priority is given to special or high-risk groups like pregnant mothers, blood donors, sex workers, truck drivers, etc.	▪ Contact tracing is technique by which sexual partners of diagnosed patients are identified, located, investigated and treated ▪ It is one of the best method for controlling spread of infection ▪ It is relatively expensive in areas with low prevalence ▪ Key to success is patient himself who must disclose all sexual contact voluntarily	▪ Patients are asked to name other persons of either sex who move in same socio-sexual environment who are then screened

b. Effective STD care
- Adequate treatment of patients and their contacts is the mainstay of STD control

Objectives
- To make a correct diagnosis
- To provide effective treatment
- To reduce/prevent future risk—taking behavior
- To advise on treatment compliance
- To promote and provide condoms
- To ensure sexual partners are notified and appropriately treated.

Strategy
- Provide the comprehensive case management that includes diagnosis, curative treatment, reduction of risk - taking behavior and the treatment of sexual partners.

Case holding and treatment	*Epidemiological treatment*	*Syndromic management of STD*
▪ Most patient of STDs have tendency to disappear or drop out before treatment is complete therefore holding patient to ensure complete and adequate treatment is key to effective management	▪ Also called as contact treatment ▪ Consists of administration of full therapeutic dose of treatment to person recently exposed to STD while awaiting laboratory results	▪ Syndromic management refers to the approach of treating STI symptoms and signs based on the organisms most commonly responsible for such syndrome

c. Personal prophylaxis

Contraceptives	*Vaccines*
▪ Used of mechanical barriers is one of the easy and best method of preventing STD transmission ▪ When used along with spermicide, increases their efficiency ▪ However lack of motivation, acceptability and convenience limits their use	▪ Not many STDs are vaccines preventable except Hepatitis B

d. Notification of sexual partners
   - Known patients are encouraged to notify about their sexual partners even when no clinical signs of infection are evident because breaking the cycle of infection is a critical part of STI prevention
   - This is known as 'contact tracing'.

Approaches for contact tracing (WHO)

Patient referral	*Provider referral*
▪ Patient is given responsibility, after adequate health education and counseling, to contact sexual partners and ask them to present for treatment	▪ Patient is asked to provide names and addresses of sexual partners so that members of health staff can contact partners ▪ It is a costly exercise and will usually not be successful if it is perceived to threaten patient confidentiality

C. Support components
   a. Access to services
      - Provision of accessible, acceptable and effective services is important for control of STIs
      - It is recommended that routine STI services be integrated into primary healthcare whereas in urban settings specialized clinics can help specific high-risk groups such as sex workers and their clients, migrant workers, truckers, etc.
      - Establishment of STD clinic is staring point of STD control
      - STDs clinics should be established where all consultation, investigations and treatment, contact tracing and all other relevant services are available
      - Provision for laboratory services for providing correct aetiological diagnosis, contact tracing, morbidity surveillance and detection of microbial resistance.
   b. Training of healthcare providers
      - This includes
         - On- the- job training
         - Training within basic courses
         - Post-basic courses utilizing venereology expertise concentrated in those specialized clinics selected as referral/reference centers

- Training of trainers so that health workers are encouraged to train their colleagues (cascade principle)
- Distribution of national guidelines in a form that can be understood and used without special additional training

c. Healthy diversions
   - This includes provision of alternative healthy diversions, incentives and facilities for education and betterment in careers and providing a healthy psychological atmosphere through indoor and outdoor recreation, organized games, educational and recreational outings, amateur dramas and concerts

d. Social welfare measures
   - STDs are social problems with medial aspects thus warrant social therapy too
   - It includes rehabilitation of prostitutes, marriage counseling, etc.

Significance

- Control of sexually transmitted diseases is an important tool in reduction of risk HIV infection thus it serves dual purpose
- It is now considered that key to success of STD control program is integration of its essential elements into primary healthcare services
- Syndromic management of STDs has emergence as an important strategy in control of STDs as it is simple, feasible, economical and quite suited for Indian setup.

9. Cancer registries.

- Cancer registration is a secondary prevention measure for cancer control
- A uniform minimum data should be registered as per WHO handbook for Standardized Cancer Registers.

Types

	Hospital-based registries	*Population-based registries*
	▪ It includes all in-patient or out-patients treated by a particular institution	▪ It covers complete cancer situation in a geographic area with a population of 2–7 million
▪ Advantage	▪ Important in evaluation of diagnostic and treatment programs	▪ Provides incidence rate ▪ Useful tool for initiating epidemiological enquiries into causes of cancer, surveillance of time trends and planning and evaluation of operational activities in cancer control
▪ Disadvantage	▪ Limited use in epidemiological studies because of selected population under study	▪ Too large population to cover

Significance

- Cancer registries provides a base for assessing the magnitude of the problem and for planning necessary services.

10. Describe the job responsibilities of health worker female.

Refer Question No. 10 December 2007 (RS2) Paper II.

11. Describe the case finding tool for diagnosis of tuberculosis under Revised National Tuberculosis Central Program (RNTCP). Add a note on reasons for the false positivity and false negativity.

Refer Question No. 1 December 2009 (RS2) Paper II.

12. Describe the salient epidemiological features of dengue syndrome.

- Dengue is an acute, febrile, self-limiting infections disease.

Epidemiology

Agent factors	
a. Agent	▪ Engue is caused by dengue virus, a group B arbovirus, family of flaviviridae ▪ It presents four serotypes, namely, dengue type 1, 2, 3 and 4 and each one is infection to man[Q] ▪ Infection with one of these serotypes does not provide cross-protective immunity ▪ Infection with dengue viruses produce a spectrum of clinical illness ranging from a nonspecific viral syndrome to severe and fatal hemorrhagic disease
b. Reservoir of infection	▪ Man is the only known reservoir[Q], along with *Aedes* mosquito
c. Vector	▪ *Aedes aegypti* a domestic mosquito is the common and most effective vector ▪ Others are *A. albopictus*, *A. polynesiensis* and *A. scutellaris* which are less efficient
d. Mode of transmission	▪ *Aedes* mosquito female bites human during day[Q] and after feeding on an infected individuals blood, can transmit the infection immediately by a change of host when the blood meal is interrupted or after an incubation period where the virus multiples in salivary gland of the mosquito
e. Incubation period	▪ 3–14 days usually 5–7 days
Host factors	
a. Age and sex	▪ All age groups are equally affected ▪ No sex difference was found ▪ The disease is usually mild in children than in adults
b. Resistance	▪ Artificial or naturally acquired infection results in long lasting immunity
c. High-risk factors	▪ More severe disease and complications seen in: – Infants and elderly – Obesity – Pregnancy – Peptic ulcer disease – Menstruating women or abnormal bleeding – Haemolytic disease—G-6PD, thalassemia and hemoglobinopathies – Congenital heart disease; – Chronic diseases—Diabetes mellitus, hypertension, asthma, ischemic heart disease, chronic renal failure, liver cirrhosis – Patients on steroid or nonsteraidal anti-inflammatory drug (NSAID) treatment
Environmental factors	
a. Climate	▪ Tropical climate is more favorable for the spread of the disease ▪ Rainy season is conducive to *Aedes* breeding due to water collection in earthen vessels, flower pots, coconut shells, etc. hence maximum incidence is seen during August to October
b. Others	▪ Growing urbanization, poor house conditions, overcrowding and inadequate sanitation

WHO Classification

DF/DHF	*Symptoms/signs*	*Laboratory findings*
DF	▪ Fever with two or more of following: – Headache – Retro-orbital pain – Myalgia – Arthralgia – Rash – Hemorrhagic manifestations – No evidence of plasma leakage	▪ Leukopenia (WBC <5000 cells/mm^3) ▪ Thrombocytopenia (platelet count <150,000 cells/mm^3) ▪ Rising hematocrit (5–10%)
DHF I	▪ Above criteria for DF and hemorrhagic manifestation plus positive tourniquet test, evidence of plasma leakage	▪ Thrombocytopenia (Platelet count <100,000/mm^3) ▪ Hematorcit rise 20% or more

Contd...

Contd...

DF/DHF	Symptoms/signs	Laboratory findings
DHF II	▪ Above signs and symptoms plus some evidence of spontaneous bleeding in skin or other organs (black tarry stools, epistaxis, bleeding from gums, etc.) and abdominal pain	▪ Thrombocytopenia (Platelet count <100,000/mm^3) ▪ Hematorcit rise 20% or more
DHF III Dengue shock syndrome	▪ Above signs and symptoms plus circulating failure (weak rapid pulse, pulse pressure ≤ 20 mm Hg or high diastolic pressure, hypotension with the presence of cold clammy skin and restlessness)	▪ Thrombocytopenia (Platelet count <100,000/mm^3) ▪ Hematorcit rise more than 20%
DHF IV Dengue shock syndrome	▪ Signs as grade III plus profound shock with undetectable blood pressure or pulse	▪ Thrombocytopenia (Platelet count <100,000/mm^3) ▪ Hematorcit rise more than 20%

Clinical Criteria (As per National Guidelines)

Dengue fever	An acute febrile illness of 2–7 days duration with two or more of the following manifestations: Headache, retro-orbital pain, myalgia, arthralgia, rash, hemorrhagic manifestations
Dengue hemorrhagic fever (DHF)	a. A case with clinical criteria of dengue Fever plus b. Hemorrhagic tendencies evidenced by one or more of the following: – Positive tourniquet test – Petechiae, ecchymoses or purpura – Bleeding from mucosa, gastrointestinal tract, injection sites or other sites plus c. Thrombocytopenia (<100 000 cells per cumm) plus d. Evidence of plasma leakage due to increased vascular permeability, manifested by one or more of the following: – A rise in average hematocrit for age and sex ~ 20% – A more than 20% drop in hematocrit following volume replacement treatment compared to baseline – Signs of plasma leakage (pleural effusion, ascites, hypoproteinemia)
Dengue shock syndrome (DSS)	All the above criteria for DHF with evidence of circulatory failure manifested by rapid and weak pulse and narrow pulse pressure (–5.20% mm Hg) or hypotension for age, cold and clammy skin and restlessness

Treatment of Dengue

Dengue fever	Dengue hemorrhagic fever	Dengue shock syndrome
▪ Rest ▪ Fluids – Volume of fluid needed is similar to the treatment of diarrhea with mild-to-moderate isotonic dehydration – Liberal fluids intake including home available fluids like rice water, kanji, fruit juices, plain water or ORS solution are recommended for patient with excessive sweating, nausea, vomiting or diarrhea to prevent dehydration – If hydration level falls, IV fluids are given with monitoring of serial hematocrits, BP and urine output ▪ For fever – Give paracetamol with >6 hour interval (Avoid aspirin and NSAIDs) – Tepid sponging ▪ Monitoring – Continuous monitoring of blood pressure, hematocrit, platelet count and level of consciousness – Monitoring must be continued after defervescence	▪ Regular assessment by serial hematocrit levels or urine output ▪ Lookout for danger signs likes rise in hematocrit of ≥20% or single hematocrit value >40%, platelets count of ≥50,000/mm^3 and spontaneous hemorrhage	▪ Volume replacement—Most important treatment measure ▪ Immediate administration of IV fluids to expand plasma volume ▪ Close observation with good nursing care is imperative ▪ Blood transfusion—In case with significant hemorrhage ▪ Fresh frozen plasma or concentrated platelet transfusion—When DIC causes massive bleeding

Treatment Guidelines

Flowchart 1: Volume replacement algorithm for patients with moderate dengue fever (DHF grades I and II)

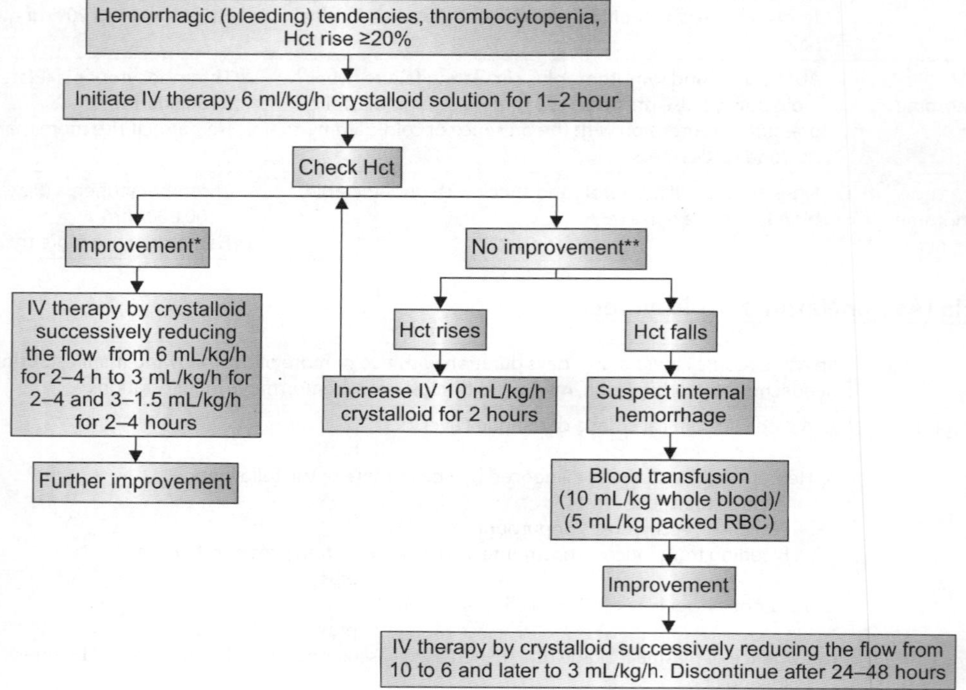

Note:
*Improvement: Hct falls, pulse rate and blood pressure stable, urine output rises

Abbreviation: Hct, hematocrit

Flowchart 2: Volume replacement alogorithm for patients with severe dengue fever (DHF grade III)

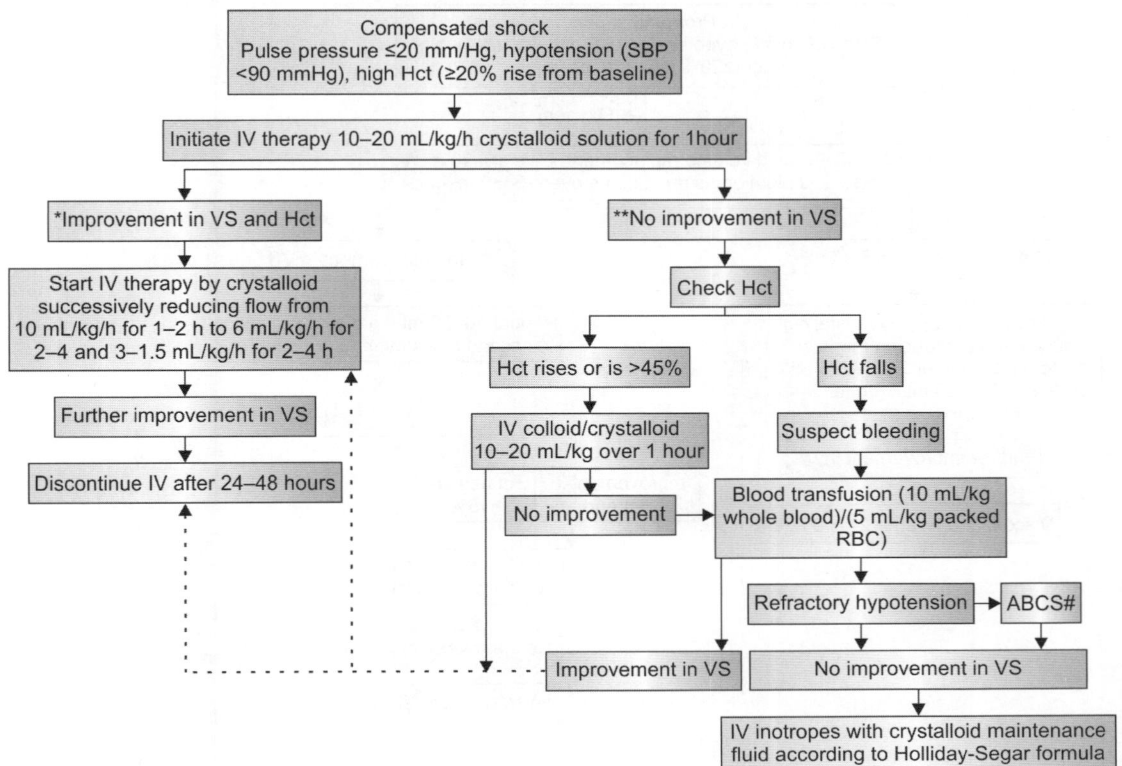

Crystalloid: Normal saline, Ringer's lactate
Colloid: Dextran 40/degraded gelatin polymer (polygeline)
#ABCS= Acidosis, bleeding, calcium (Na^{++} and k^{+}), sugar
Notes:
* Improvement: Hct falls, pulse rate and blood pressure stable, urine output rises
**No improvement: Hct or pulse rate rises, pulse pressure falls below 20 mm Hg, urine output falls
- Unstable vital signs: Urine output falls, signs of shock
- In cases of acidosis, hyperosmolar or Ringer's lactate solution should not be used
- Serial platelet and Hct determination: Drop in platelets and rise in Hct are essential for early diagnosis of DHF
- Cases of DHF should be observed every hour for vital signs and urine output.

Flowchart 3: Volume replacement algorithm for patients with severe dengue fever [DHF IV (DSS)]

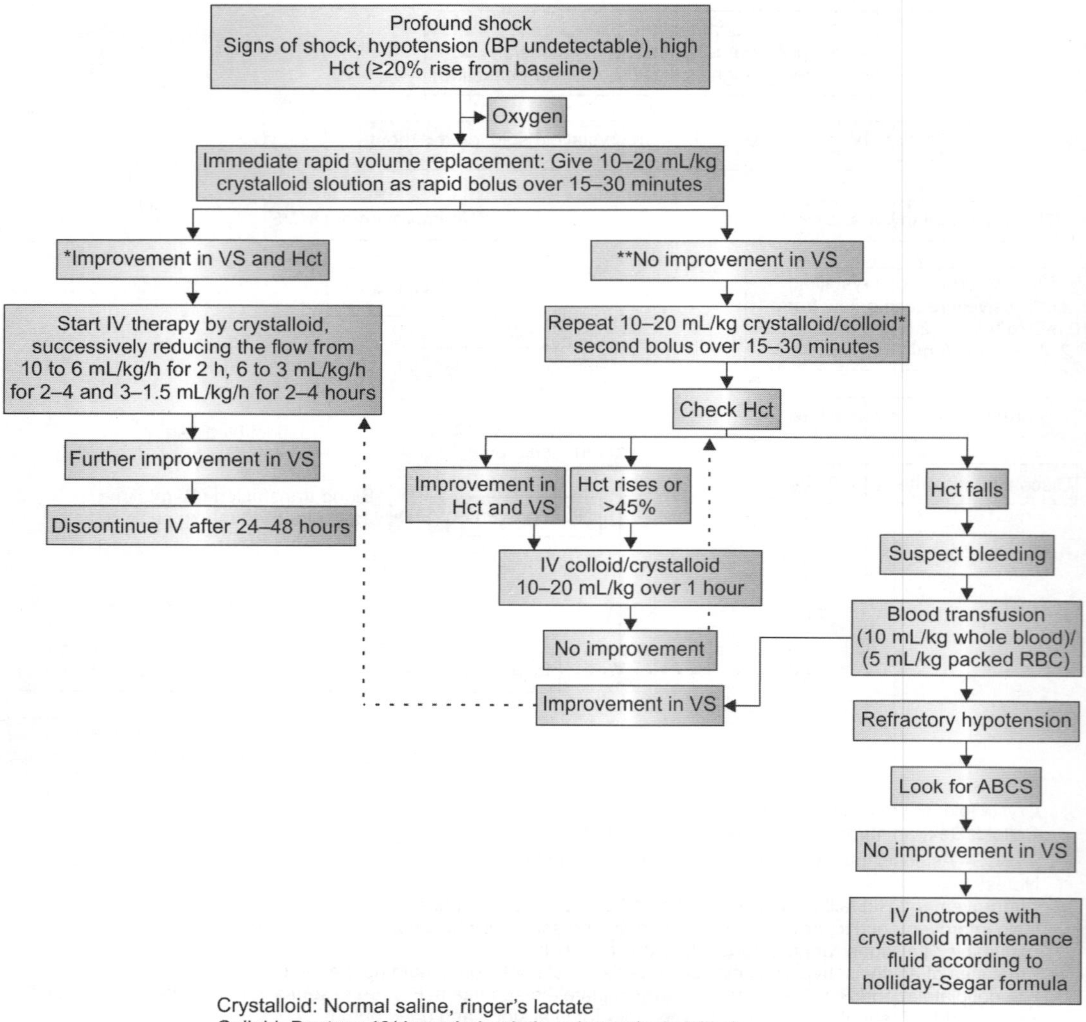

Profound shock
Signs of shock, hypotension (BP undetectable), high Hct (≥20% rise from baseline)

→ Oxygen

Immediate rapid volume replacement: Give 10–20 mL/kg crystalloid sloution as rapid bolus over 15–30 minutes

*Improvement in VS and Hct

Start IV therapy by crystalloid, successively reducing the flow from 10 to 6 mL/kg/h for 2 h, 6 to 3 mL/kg/h for 2–4 and 3–1.5 mL/kg/h for 2–4 hours

Further improvement in VS

Discontinue IV after 24–48 hours

**No improvement in VS

Repeat 10–20 mL/kg crystalloid/colloid* second bolus over 15–30 minutes

Check Hct

Improvement in Hct and VS

Hct rises or >45%

IV colloid/crystalloid 10–20 mL/kg over 1 hour

No improvement

Improvement in VS

Hct falls

Suspect bleeding

Blood transfusion (10 mL/kg whole blood)/ (5 mL/kg packed RBC)

Refractory hypotension

Look for ABCS

No improvement in VS

IV inotropes with crystalloid maintenance fluid according to holliday-Segar formula

Crystalloid: Normal saline, ringer's lactate
Colloid: Dextran 40/degraded gelatin polymer (polydeline)
ABC = Acidosis, bleeding, calcium (Na^{++} and K^{+}), sugar

Notes:

* Improvement: Hct falls, pulse rate and blood pressure stable, urine output rises

** No improvement: Hct or pulse rate rises, pulse pressure falls below 20 mm Hg, urine output falls

- Unstable vital signs: Urine output falls, signs of shock
- In cases of acidosis, hyperosmolar or Ringer's lactate solution should not be used
- Serial platelet and Hct determinations: Drop in platelets and rise in Hct are essential for early diagnosis of DHF
- Cases of DHF should be observed every hour for vital signs and urine output.

Prevention and Control Measures

A. Primary prevention

a. Health promotion (vector control)

- Disease is endemic in areas where mosquito breeding is common, so control of *Aedes* mosquito is the main step of controlling dengue

i. Anti-larval measures

- The environment should be cleaned up and got rid of water holding containers such as discarded tins, empty pots, broken bottles, coconut shells, etc.

- Spraying of mineral oils (diseal, kerosene, etc.) on the water once a week can also kill larvae by cutting off their air supply and specific toxic action
- Spraying of synthetic insecticides like Fenthion, Abate, Malathion, Chlorpyrifos is very effective.

ii. Anti-adult measures
- Residual sprays using DDT, malathion, propoxur, gamma—HCH
- Space sprays using pyrethrum.

iii. Protection from mosquito bites
- Use of mosquito nets
- Screening of building with copper or bronze gauze
- Use of skin repellents containing deet, indalone, dimethyl phthalate, etc.

b. Specific protection (vaccination)
- At present, there is no vaccine for dengue however clinical trials of live attenuated vaccine is underway.

B. Secondary prevention

a. Early diagnosis and treatment
- Early diagnostic of dengue cases and their treatment can render the man noninfective to mosquito thus breaking the transmission cycle
- The diagnosis is done by clinically and other lab investigations
- Treatment is symptomatic, and supportive, bed rest, and antipyretics
- Oral rehydration is required in dehydrated cases.

SHORT ANSWERS

13. What is exclusive breastfeeding? Enumerate the advantages.

- Exclusive breastfeeding means feeding the infant with mother's milk only and no other drinks like honey, water, glucose water, gripe water, juices, vitamin drops, animal milk, powdered milk or food that are given to newborn.
- The concept of exclusive breastfeeding was first introduced in 1979 jointly by WHO and UNICEF which was later adopted as global goal for optimum MCH and nutrition.

Average Duration

- About first 6 months[Q].

Advantages

- It protects the child from infections especially diarrheal diseases as the child is not exposed to external foods
- It helps in better development of the body
- Exclusive breastfeeding offer natural contraceptive benefit in just delivered mothers
- It promotes quick and early involution of uterus and reduces postpartum bleeding.

Significance

- Exclusive breastfeeding is very important strategy to reduce infant mortality rate as it protects the infant from infections

14. What is a blocked flea?

- Blocked flea is a rat flea with fully blocked proventriculus so that no food can pass through, leaving the stomach empty and leading flea to starvation.

Mechanism

- A rat flea can ingest upto 5 cu. mm of blood ingesting about 5,000 plague bacilli along with it
- These bacilli multiply enormously in gut of rat flea blocking proventriculus
- Such flea due inability to obtain blood meal, faces starvation and eventually death thus it makes frantic efforts to bite and suck blood over and over again
- In doing so, it inoculates plague bacilli into bite wound each time it bites.

Significance

- A blocked flea is an efficient transmitter of plague and a partially blocked flea is more dangerous than a completely blocked flea as it can live longer.

15. Mass drug administration for filariasis.

Refer Question No. 11 June 2011 (RS2) Paper II.

16. What is network analysis?

Refer Question No. 6 December 2011 (RS2) Paper II.

17. Treatment for leprosy.

Refer Question No. 5 December 2008 (RS2) Paper II.

18. Case definition used for diagnosis of AIDS.

Refer Question No. 10 June 2015 (RS2) Paper I.

19. What is Chandler's index?

Refer Question No. 4 December 2016 (RS2) Paper II.

20. What is rule of halves in hypertension?

Refer Question No. 12 December 2008 (RS2) Paper II.

21. What are the uses of growth chart?

Refer Question No. 22 December 2009 (RS2) Paper II.

22. Juvenile delinquency.

Refer Question No. 10 December 2012 (RS2) Paper I.

MBBS PHASE III EXAMINATION

DECEMBER 2012

(Revised Scheme 2)

PAPER I

LONG ESSAYS

1. Enumerate the nutritional problems in public health. Describe in detail protein-energy malnutrition with respect to its symptoms and preventive measures.

- In developing country like India where poverty is rampant, nutritional problems are quite common.

Nutritional Problems in Public Health

i. Low birth weight
ii. Protein-energy malnutrition
iii. Xerophthalmia (vitamin A deficiency[Q])
iv. Nutritional anemia (iron deficiency[Q])
v. Iodine deficiency disorders
vi. Endemic flourosis
vii. Lathyrism.

Protein-energy Malnutrition

- Protein-energy malnutrition (PEM) is a range of pathological conditions arising from coincidental lack in varying proportions of protein and calories, occurring most frequently in infants and young children and commonly associated with infections (WHO).

Epidemiology

a. Agent factors	▪ Protein-energy malnutrition is due to deficiency of energy and proteins in diet ▪ This deficiency may be marginal and precipitated by secondary factors like diarrhea, respiratory infections, worm infestations, malaria, etc.
b. Host factors	
i. Age	▪ Kwashiorkor is common in children between 1–3 years ▪ Marasmus is common in under fives
ii. Sex	▪ More common in female child due to traditional negligence
iii. Weaning	▪ Marasmus is common with prolonged breastfeeding without introduction of weaning ▪ Kwashiorkor is associated with early weaning due to variety of reasons

Contd...

Contd...

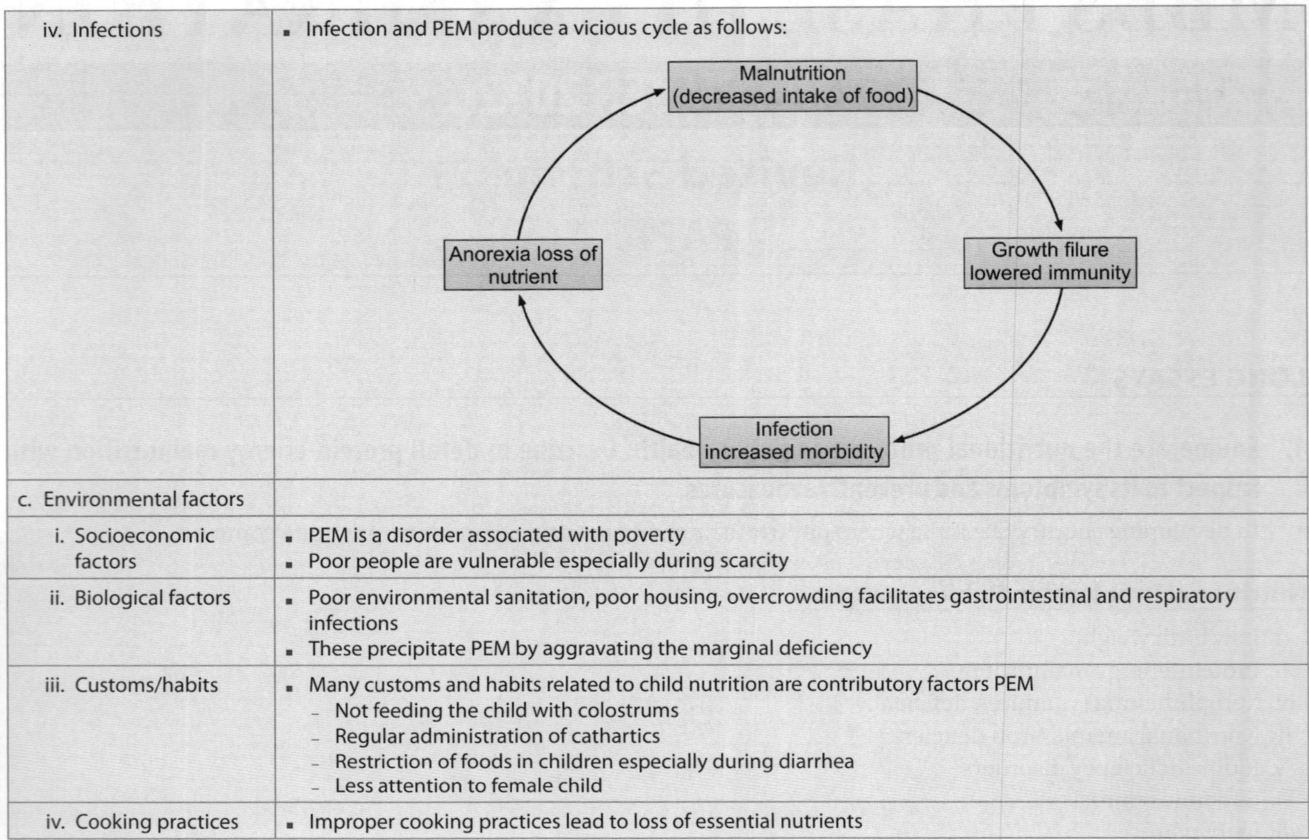

iv. Infections	▪ Infection and PEM produce a vicious cycle as follows: Malnutrition (decreased intake of food) → Growth filure lowered immunity → Infection increased morbidity → Anorexia loss of nutrient → Malnutrition (decreased intake of food)
c. Environmental factors	
i. Socioeconomic factors	▪ PEM is a disorder associated with poverty ▪ Poor people are vulnerable especially during scarcity
ii. Biological factors	▪ Poor environmental sanitation, poor housing, overcrowding facilitates gastrointestinal and respiratory infections ▪ These precipitate PEM by aggravating the marginal deficiency
iii. Customs/habits	▪ Many customs and habits related to child nutrition are contributory factors PEM – Not feeding the child with colostrums – Regular administration of cathartics – Restriction of foods in children especially during diarrhea – Less attention to female child
iv. Cooking practices	▪ Improper cooking practices lead to loss of essential nutrients

Classification

a. Clinical classification
   - Kwashiorkor
   - Marasmus

b. Anthropometric classification
   - It is based on the weight for age which is calculated as follows:

$$\text{Weight for age (\%)} = \frac{\text{Weight of the child}}{\text{Weight of a normal child of same age}} \times 100$$

i. Gomez's classification
   - Based on weight retardation[Q]
   - Child is compared with normal child of same age for his weight
   - Normal reference child is 50th percentile of Boston standards[Q]
   - Has prognostic value for hospitalized patients[Q]

Grade	*Weight for age*[Q]
Normal	90–110%
Grade I (mild malnutrition)[Q]	76–90%[Q]
Grade II (moderate malnutrition)	61–75%
Grade III (severe malnutrition)	≤60%

ii. Indian academy of pediatrics (IAP) classification—Adopted as ICMR guildlines[Q]

Grade	*Weight for age*
Normal	> 80%
Grade I (mild malnutrition)	71–80%
Grade II (moderate malnutrition)	61–70%
Grade III (severe malnutrition)[Q]	51–60%[Q]
Grade IV (very severe malnutrition)	≤50%

and alphabet K post-fixed in presence of edema.

iii. Welcome's classification

Condition	*Weight for age*
Kwashiorkor[Q]	60–80% with edema[Q]
Undernutrition	60–80% without edema
Marasusmus	<60% without edema
Marasmic kwashiorkor	<60% with edema

iv. Jelliffe's classification

Grade	*Weight for age*
Grade I	81–90%
Grade II	71–80%
Grade III	61–70%
Grade IV	≤60%

v. Waterlow's classification

Nutritional status	*% of height for age (stunting)—Index of duration*[Q]	*% of weight for height (wasting)—Index of severity*[Q]
Normal	>95	>90
Mildly impaired	94-87.5	90–80
Moderately impaired	87.4-80	80–70
Severely impaired	<80	<70

Clinical Forms/Types

Marasmus	*Kwashiorkor*	*Marasmic-kwashiorkor*
▪ PEM from severe deficiency of both dietary energy and proteins ▪ Characterized by muscle wasting with normal serum protein levels	▪ PEM due to diet very low in proteins ▪ Characterized by edema with decreased serum albumin levels	▪ PEM with features of both marasmus and kwashirokor, i.e. muscle wasting and edema

Clinical Features

Features	*Marasmus*	*Kwashiorkor*
a. Age group	▪ Common in children aged <5 years	▪ Commonly seen in children aged 2–5 years
b. Growth	▪ Mild retarded growth (child is grossly emaciated, and underweight) ▪ Depleted of subcutaneous fats with muscle	▪ Server retardation in growth and development ▪ Child is not emaciated rather looks blown up due to edema
c. Muscles	▪ Muscle wasting (characteristic)	▪ Weak and atrophic
d. Fat	▪ Severe loss of subcutaneous fat	▪ Fat often retained but not firm

Contd...

Contd...

Features	*Marasmus*	*Kwashiorkor*
e. Behavior (mental changes)	▪ Very hungry and cries continuously	▪ Apathy and anorexia (early manifestations) ▪ Child is less lively and refuses to eat
f. Appetite	▪ Usually good	▪ Poor
g. Diarrhea and vomiting	▪ Frequent small dark green mucous stools of "hunger diarrhea" (aggravates disease further) ▪ Vomiting more common	▪ Diarrhea almost always present and becomes chronic and remittent
h. Skin and mucus membranes	▪ Skin is thin, attached to bone, flaccid and wrinkled ▪ Bony prominences are marked ▪ Mucous membranes of mouth are usually reddish	▪ Skin lesions although not always present are very characteristic, patches of hyperpigmentation, exfoliation, desquamation and ulceration are seen in skin of legs, buttocks and perineum (flaky paint dermatosis) ▪ Unlike marasmus, some subcutaneous fats are present
i. Edema	▪ Absent	▪ Pitting edema (main clinical characteristic for diagnosis) ▪ Soft and painless, usually first affects legs and then spreads to upper extremities and face
j. Hairs and facies	▪ Hairs usually thin and lusterless ▪ Easily pluckable hairs ▪ Typical face of marasmic child compared to "little monkey" or Wisened Old Man look	▪ Hairs usually dry and thin ▪ Black hairs become brown or reddish yellow and sometimes even white ▪ Depigmented hairs alternate with more pigmented hairs (Flag sign) ▪ "Moon facies"
k. Hepatic enlargement	▪ None	▪ Sometimes, due to accumulation of fat
l. Weight for height	▪ Very low	▪ Low but may be masked by edema
m. Biochemical findings	▪ Serum albumin almost normal (2–3 g/dL) ▪ Blood urea level normal ▪ Serum cortisol increased ▪ Fasting glucose reduced ▪ Plasma/amino acid ratio—normal ▪ Serum K^+ normal	▪ Serum albumin markedly reduced (0.5–2 g/dL) ▪ Blood urea level reduced ▪ Serum cortisol normal or decreased ▪ Fasting glucose reduced ▪ Plasma/amino acid ratio elevated ▪ Serum K^+ decreased

Prevention and Control

a. Primordial prevention	▪ To prevent emergence of risk factors, the mothers with poor socioeconomic background are discourage to conceive more than 2 children or the mothers are educated about breastfeeding nutrition of self and the child, increasing demand of the child with age and growth, etc.
b. Primary prevention (WHO expert committee)	
i. Health promotion	▪ Measures directed to pregnant and lactating women like education, food supplement ▪ Promotion of correct breastfeeding practices ▪ Frequent feeds to a growing child ▪ Development of low cost weaning food ▪ Improving family diet ▪ Nutrition education ▪ Home economics to improve living condition and purchasing power ▪ Family planning and spacing of birth ▪ Family environment
ii. Specific protection	▪ Giving protein and energy rich diet to child possibly containing milk, eggs, fresh fruits ▪ Immunization ▪ Food fortification
c. Secondary prevention	▪ Periodic surveillance ▪ Early diagnosis of any lag in growth ▪ Early diagnosis and treatment of infections and diarrhea ▪ Development of programs for early rehydration of children with diarrhea ▪ Development of supplementary feeding programs during epidemics ▪ Deworming of heavily infested children
d. Tertiary prevention	▪ Nutritional rehabilitation services ▪ Hospital treatment ▪ Follow-up care

Significance

- PEM is the commonest and most common nutritional problem in under 5 age group[Q] requires all the available resources and man power to prevent but not without the involvement of mother.

2. Explain the levels of prevention and its mode of intervention with suitable examples.

Refer Question No. 1 December 2007 (RS2) Paper I.

SHORT ESSAYS

3. Epidemic curve.

Refer Question No. 4 December 2016 (RS2) Paper I.

4. Employees State Insurance Act, 1948.

Employees State Insurance Act, 1948 (ESI Act)[Q]

- ESI Act was passed in 1949[Q] and subsequently amended in 1975, 1984, 1989 and 2010
- ESI Act is an important measure of social security and health insurance in India
- It provides for certain cash and medical benefits to industrial employees in cases of sickness, maternity and employment injury thereby removing the economic and physical fear.

Scope

- The act extends to whole of India (except North Eastern states and UTs) and applies to all establishment employing ten or more persons in the preceding 12 months, irrespective whether it runs with power or without power[Q]
- Prior to amendments it covered power using factories employing less than 20 employees[Q] and factories employing more than 20 employees where power is not used[Q]
- The establishments coming under purview of this act are:
  - Hotels and restaurants[Q]
  - Cinemas and theaters[Q]
  - Road transport establishments
  - Newspaper establishments[Q]
  - Shops
  - Education institutions
  - Medical hospitals
- It covers all employees—manual, clerical, supervisory and technical getting up to ₹15,000 per month[Q]
- It can be extended to any other agricultural or commercial establishment
- However, it does not include defence establishment[Q], mines and railways.

Administration

- Administration of ESI scheme is entrusted to ESI Corporation, an autonomous body
- It consists of:
  - Chairman—The Union Labor Minister
  - Vice-chairmen—Secretary to Government of India, Ministry of Labor
  - Five representatives from central government
  - One representative from each state government
  - One representative form all union territories
  - Five representatives of employees
  - Five representatives of employers
  - Two representatives from medical profession
  - Three members of parliament
- A standing committee of 16 members is constituted among these to act as an executive body for administration of the scheme. This body meets four times a year.

- This committee is headed by chief executive officer who is the Director General of Corporation and he is assisted by four principal officers namely Insurance Commissioner, Medical Commissioner, Financial Commissioner and Actuary
- Medical benefit council is headed by the Director General of Health Services, Government of India, assisted by the Medical Commissioner and it advices the organization on medical relief
- ESI Corporation has 21 state wise regional officers and 15 subregional offices
- There are also inspecting officers throughout the country to inspect factories and for checking insecurability of employees and correct payment of contributions.

Finance

- Scheme is run by contributions by employees and employers and grants from central and state governments as follows:

Employee[Q]	1.75% of his wages[Q]	Employees getting daily wages below ₹ 100 (₹ 2600/month) are exempted
Employer[Q]	4.75% of employee's wages[Q]	
State Government[Q]	1/8th of total medical cost[Q]	
ESI Corp	7/8th of total medical cost	
Central Government[Q]	2/3rd of administrative expenditure	

Benefits to Employees

- ESI scheme provides following benefits to the employees:
  - i. Medical benefit[Q]
  - ii. Sickness benefit[Q]
  - iii. Maternity benefit[Q]
  - iv. Disablement benefit
  - v. Dependent benefit[Q]
  - vi. Dependent benefit
  - vii. Funeral benefit[Q]
  - viii. Rehabilitation benefit[Q]

A. Medical benefit
- It consists of full medical care including hospitalization, free of cost to the insured person in case of sickness, employment injury and maternity
- This benefit is provided in kind and not in cash.

Types (of medical care)

a. Full[Q]	▪ Includes hospitalization, free of cost not only to the insured person but also the members of the family in case of sickness, employment injury and maternity ▪ Services comprise – Out-patient care – Supply of drugs and dressings – Specialist medical and surgical services – Pathological and radiological investigations – Domiciliary services – Antenatal, natal and postnatal services – Immunization – Family planning – Emergency service – Ambulance – Health education – In-patient treatment ▪ If specialized treatment is necessary the employees are sent outside the state for treatment at the expense of ESI corporation ▪ Full medical care including hospitalization is being given at 116 centers only
b. Restricted	▪ Consists of only out-patient care
c. Expanded	▪ Consists of full medical care short of hospitalization

Medical care delivery

Direct pattern	*Indirection pattern (panel system)*
▪ Medical care is provided through service dispensaries of ESI corporation established with full time medical and paramedical personnel in areas having a concentration of 1,000 or more employee's family units ▪ On an average, a doctor need to attend about 80 cases per day in OPD and one home visit a day ▪ Part time dispensaries are established in area with less than 750 employee's family units ▪ Mobile dispensaries are established if the employee's are scattered over a long distance	▪ Medical care is provided through registered medical practitioners designated as Insurance medical practitioners ▪ They are paid remuneration quarterly according to the number of family units attached to them (maximum 750 family units per practitioner)

Miscellaneous medical facilities

- Free supply of artificial limbs, spectacles, hearing aids, hand driven cycles, walking calipers, surgical boots, dentures, spinal braces, etc. to patient who are incapacitated due to employment injury
- Preventive inoculations
- Free contraceptives and cash incentives for undergoing sterilization
- Training in yoga exercise.

B. Sickness benefits
- Consists of periodical cash payment to an insured person in case of sickness when he/she is unable to attend to work, provided his sickness is duly certified by an Insurance Medical Officer or Insurance Medical Practitioner
- Insured person is protected from dismissal or discharge from service by the employers during the period of sickness
- To become eligible for sickness benefit, one should have paid contribution for not less than 28 days during corresponding contribution period
- A factory can be held to pay excessive sickness benefit if sickness results from lack of sanitary conditions or improper maintenance of sanitary conditions.

Types

a. Ordinary sickness benefit
   - Benefit is payable for a maximum period of 91 days[Q] in any continuous period of 365 days. This benefit covers only short-term illnesses
   - However the person receiving sickness benefit is required to remain under medical treatment provided under the act.

b. Extended sickness benefit
   - In certain long-term diseases a person is entitled to extended sickness benefit in addition to 91 days and the benefit is payable up to 309 days[Q] provided the insured person has put in 2 years of continuous service
   - 34 diseases entitled for extended sickness benefit are:

i. Infectious diseases	Tuberculosis[Q], leprosy[q], chronic empyema, AIDS
ii. Neoplasm	Malignant diseases
iii. Endocrine, nutritional and metabolic disorders	Diabetes with complications like retinopathy, nephropathy and diabetic foot[Q]
iv. Disorders of CNS	Monoplegia, hemiplegia, paraplegia, hemiparesis, intracranial space occupying lesions, spinal cord compression, Parkinson's disease, neuromuscular dystrophy, immature cataract, detachment of retina, glaucoma
v. Diseases of CVS	Coronary artery disease, congestive heart failure[Q], cardiac valvular diseases with failure, cardiomyopathies, heart disease with surgical interventions
vi. Disorders of RS	Bronchiectasis, interstitial lung disease, COPD with cor pulmonale
vii. Diseases of liver	Cirrhosis of liver with ascites
viii. Orthopedic diseases	Dislocation of vertebra or prolapsed of intervertebral disc, nonunion or delayed union of fracture, post-traumatic surgical amputation of lower extremity, compound fracture with chronic osteomyelitis
ix. Psychosis[Q]	Schizophrenia, depression, dementia, depressive psychosis
x. Others	More than 20% burns with infections/complications, chronic renal failure, Reynaud's disease or Burger's disease

Amount

- Cash is paid at rate of 50% of the average daily wages[Q].

c. Enhanced sickness benefit
  - Full average daily wage for duration up to 7 days in case of vasectomy and up to 14 days in case of tubectomy.

C. Maternity benefits
- Benefit payable in cash to an insured woman for confinement/miscarriage or sickness arising out of pregnancy/ confinement or premature birth of child or miscarriage.

Duration of benefit

- Confinement	12 weeks[Q] (6 weeks before and 6 weeks after delivery)
- Sickness due to pregnancy	30 days
- Miscarriage and premature birth	6 weeks

Amount

- Benefit is allowed at about full wages.

D. Disablement benefit
- In event of temporary or permanent disablement due to employment injury is entitled to cash payment besides free medical treatment.
- Also includes disablement arising from accident occurring to an employee while commuting to and from office to residence and vice versa for duty, provided there is nexus between the circumstances and employment.

Amount

- Temporary disablement benefit	72% of wages as long as the temporary disablement lasts[Q]
- Total permanent disablement	72% of wages as life long pension
- Partial permanent disablement	Part of 72% of wages as life long pension

E. Dependent's benefit
- In case of death as a result of employment injury, the dependants of an insured person are eligible for periodical payments
- An eligible son or daughter is entitled to dependent's benefit up to age of 25 without any proof of education
- Benefit is withdrawn if the daughter marries early
- Widow gets the benefit life long or until she get remarried.

Amount

- Pension at rate of 40% more than the standard benefit rate is paid periodically to widow and children in accordance to prescribed share
- Minimum benefit to the dependent is Rs. 14 per day.

F. Funeral benefit
- An immediate cash payment payable on the death of an insured person irrespective of cause of death to the eldest surviving member of the family towards the expenses on his funeral.

Amount

- Amount is not exceeding Rs. 10000.

G. Rehabilitation benefit
- On monthly payment of Rs. 10 the insured person and his family members continue to get medical treatment after permanent disablement or retirement.

Benefits to employers[Q]

- Exemption from the applicability of Workman's Compensation Act, 1923
- Exemption from Maternity Benefit Act, 1961[Q]
- Exemption from payment of medical allowance to employees and their dependants or arranging for their medical care[Q]
- Rebate under IT Act on contribution deposited in the ESI account[Q]
- Healthy work force.

Significance

- Employee State Insurance Scheme is so named for following reasons
  - Employees because it is meant for the employees
  - State because the government or state takes the responsibility of intervening and providing remedial measures in event of worker meets with a crisis
  - Insurance because the workers have to pay a small percentage of their wages as premium.

5. Bias in case control studies.

Refer Question No. 6 June 2014 (RS2) Paper I.

6. How can genetic disorders be prevented in a community?

Refer Question No. 8 December 2011 (RS2) Paper II.

7. Write briefly the methods of purification of water at household level.

Refer Question No. 2 December 2013 (RS2) Paper I.

8. Describe Iceberg phenomenon of diseases with suitable examples.

Refer Question No. 3 June 2010 (RS2) Paper I.

9. Write briefly about effects of urbanization on health.

- Urbanization is phenomenon of population migration from the rural area to cities or urban areas.
- An urban area is one with:
  - Population more than 5,000
  - More than 75% of male population working in nonagricultural occupation
  - Population density of atleast 400/km^2.

Causes of Urbanization

- Employment opportunities
- Attraction of living conditions
- Educational, health, transport, entertainment and other facilities.

Health Effects of Rapid Urbanization

a. Physical or environmental effects	
i. Housing or living	▪ Because of migration of the population for the sake of employment in industries, slums will come up like mushrooms ▪ There will be poor standard of living, overcrowding, lack of sanitation, improper drainage system, etc. all predisposing for prevalence of communicable diseases often resulting in epidemics
ii. Environmental pollution	▪ Consists of air pollution, water pollution and soil pollution because of discharge and emission of industrial waste, dust, smoke, fumes, etc.
iii. Vector problems	▪ Collections of water in and around the industries and residential areas become the potential breeding places for the mosquitoes
b. Psychological effects	▪ Due to migration of the population, altered living conditions and food, failure of adjustment, etc. leads to mental illness, behavioral disorders, neurosis, psychoses, etc.
c. Social effects	▪ These are alcoholism, drug abuse, gambling, prostitution, divorces, broken homes, antisocial activities like theft, murder, rape, juvenile delinquency and such other crimes
d. Miscellaneous effects	▪ A nuisance to the people by noise, smoke and smell ▪ Particular health hazard due to particular industry ▪ Accidents, both industrial and vehicular ▪ Malnutrition, sexually transmitted diseases, etc.

Significance

- Urbanization has caused a social crisis in rural areas and health and demographic crisis in urban areas.

10. What is juvenile delinquency? Add a note on its causes and preventive measures.

- Juvenile delinquency is the unacceptable behavior which includes all deviations from normal youthful behavicr by a child below age of 18 years
- The incidence is highest amongst children aged above 15 years and is about 4–5 times more in boys than opposite sex.

Examples

- Crimes, disobedience to parents, deserting the homes, mixing with immoral people or indulging in antisocial activities like stealing, lying, gambling, burglary, cruelty, sexual offences, destructiveness, etc.

Causes

Biological causes	*Social causes*	*Others causes*
▪ Hereditary defects, feeble mindedness, physical defects and glandular imbalance are certain biological causes of juvenile delinquency ▪ Children with XYY karyotype (supermales) also exhibit such behavior	▪ Children living in broken homes like death parents, separation of parents, step mother show criminal tendencies ▪ Disturbed home conditions like poverty, alcoholism, parental neglect, ignorance about child care, too many children, etc. also predispose to juvenile delinquency	▪ Influence of cinema, television, immoral friends, etc..

Prevention

a. Improvement of family life	▪ Parents should be prepared for parenthood ▪ There should be appreciation of the child's need and they should be aptly met ▪ A family should well adjust to prevent delinquency
b. Schooling	▪ Schools play an important role in instilling discipline in children ▪ In schools, the teacher student relationship should be cordial ▪ Teachers should try to detect any early signs of delinquency and institute remedial measures
c. Social welfare program	▪ Reaction facilities, parent counselling, child guidance, education facilities and adequate general health services

Significance

- With increasing modernization and urbanization, the incidences of juvenile delinquency is on rise and need to curbed before it engulf the future of the nation.

11. Explain the barriers of communication in health education.

Refer Question No. 5 June 2010 (RS2) Paper I.

12. Prevention of vitamin A deficiency disorders.

- Vitamin A is fat-soluble vitamin occurring in 2 forms, retinol (animal sources) and β carotene (vegetable sources).

Vitamin A Deficiency

Etiology	*Predisposing factors*
• Inadequate supply of vitamin A • Defective absorption from gut due to gastrointestinal disorders	• Low socio-economic status • Poor nourishment or nutritional disorders like PEM • Recurrent infections like measles[Q], diarrhea[Q]

Clinical Features (Grouped Under Ocular and Extra-ocular Manifestations)

A. Ocular manifestations
   - Ocular manifestations of vitamin A deficiency is termed xerophthalmia[Q] (WHO and USAID committee)
   - Xerophthalmia (Xerosis = dryness)
   - Most common in children aged 1–3 years

WHO classification

XN	Night blindness (Nyctalopia)
X1A	Conjunctival xerosis
X1B	Bitot's spots
X2	Corneal xerosis
X3A	Corneal ulceration/keratomalacia affecting <1/3rd of corneal surface
X3B	Corneal ulceration/keratomalacia affecting >1/3rd of corneal surface
XS	Corneal scar due to xerophthalmia
XF	Xerophthalmic fundus

Features

a. XN (Night blindness[Q])
  - Earliest symptom[Q] in children
  - Sometimes termed chicken eyes
  - Means inability of child to see in dim light due to failure of dark adaptation because of decreased synthesis of rhodopsin in retina

b. X1A (Conjunctival xerosis)—1st clinical sign[Q]
  - One or more patches of dry, lusterless, nonwettable conjunctiva
  - Described as 'emerging like sand banks at receding tide' when child ceases to cry
  - Patches almost always involve inter-palpebral area of temporal quadrant and often nasal quadrant also
  - Almost always bilateral and is epithelial xerosis[Q]
  - Entire bulbar conjunctiva affected in advanced cases
  - Associated with conjunctival thickening, wrinkling and pigmentation

c. X1B (Bitot's spots[Q])—characteristic of vitamin A deficiency
  - Raised, silvery white, foamy, triangular patch of keratinized epithelium situated on bulbar conjunctiva in interpalpebral area
  - Base of triangle is at limbus and apex towards the outer canthus
  - Superficial and raised above conjunctiva
  - Usually bilateral and temporal and less frequently nasal
  - Extension of xerotic process and represent areas of sqaumous metaplasia
  - In young children they indicate vitamin A deficiency whereas in adults they are often inactive sequelae of earlier disease

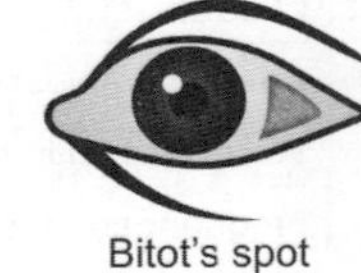
Bitot's spot

d. X2 (Corneal xerosis)—serious manifestation of vitamin A deficiency
  - Punctate keratopathy (begins in lower nasal quadrant)
  - Followed by haziness and/or granular pebbly dryness
  - Lusterless cornea

e. X3 (Corneal ulceration/keratomalacia[Q])—Grave medical emergency
  - Occurs in late stages due to colliquative necrosis
  - Circular and sharply demarcated small ulcers (1–3 mm) with steep margins surrounded by xerotic cornea occurs peripherally
  - Large ulcers and necrotic area extend centrally or involve entire cornea
  - Ulceration beings slightly inferior and nasal aspect
  - Stromal defects not treated immediately results in blindness

f. XS (Corneal scars)
  - Due to healing of stromal defects
  - Of various densities and sizes
  - May or may not cover papillary area

g. XF (Xerophthalmic fundus)
  - Typical seed like raised whitish lesions scattered uniformly over the part of fundus at the level of optic disk

B. Extraocular manifestations
  - Retardation of growth
  - Follicular hyperkeratosis (phrynoderma)
  - Anorexia
  - Increased incidence of respiratory and GIT infections
  - Urinary calculi

Prevention of Vitamin A Deficiency Disorders

- To combat nutritional vitamin A deficiency, Government of India initiated National Vitamin A Prophylaxis Program in 1970 to cover preschool children aged up to 5 years
- Currently the program is an integral component of RCH program which is now a part of NRHM.

Objectives

- Promoting consumption of vitamin A rich foods by pregnant and lactating women and by children under five years of age and appropriate breastfeeding

- Administration of massive dose of vitamin A up to five years (1st dose of 1lac IU at 9 months with measles vaccination followed by doses of 2 lac IU every 6 months up to 5 years)
- One dose of vitamin A to all children suffering from measles if they have not received it in previous month
- One additional dose of vitamin A to all cases of severe malnutrition
- All children sick with xerophthalmia to be treated at health facilities.

Strategy

a. Short-term action: Vitamin A prophylaxis
   - Vitamin A prophylaxis is a short-term action plan of under the National Program.

   Strategy
   - Here the strategy is to administer large doses of vitamin A (retinol palmitate) orally, in recommended doses to vulnerable groups on a period periodic basis
   - The vitamin A is supplied free of cost through PHCs as flavored syrup in 100 mL bottle with a concentration of 100,000 IU per mL[Q]
   - The bottle is supplied with a 2 mL capacity spoon[Q] thus providing 200,000 IU per spoonful[Q]
   - The bottle once opened should be used within 6–8 weeks.

   Recommended dosage vitamin A prophylaxis

Vulnerable group	*Oral dose*	*Timing*
Newborn	50,000 IU (27.5 mg[Q])	At birth[Q]
Children <1 year	100,000 IU (55 mg)	Once every 4–6 months[Q]
Children >1 year	200,000 IU (110 mg)	Once every 4–6 months[Q]
Women of child bearing age group	300,000 IU (165 mg)	Within one month of giving birth
Pregnant and lactating mothers	5,000 IU (2.75 mg)	Everyday
	20,000 IU (11 mg)	Once every week

   Vitamin A prophylaxis schedule (New guidelines—November 2006)—Under National Immunisation Schedule

Dose no.	*Age of the child*	*Dose*	*Remarks*
1	9 months	100,000 IU	Along with measles vaccine
2	1½ years	200,000 IU[Q]	With booster doses of DPT and OPV
3	2 years	200,000 IU	Nil
4	2½ years	200,000 IU	Nil
5	3 years[Q]	200,000 IU[Q]	Nil
6	3½ years	200,000 IU	Nil
7	4 years	200,000 IU	Nil
8	4½ years	200,000 IU	Nil
9	5 years	200,000 IU	Nil
	Total	**17,00,000 IU[Q]**	

   * Old guidelines had only 5 doses till age of 3 years thus total of 9 lakh IU

   - This is also known as immunization against xerophthalmia

   Merits
   - This is a flexible, short-term action plan with good results
   - This can be organized quickly and with minimum of infrastructure
   - Reduces incidence of keratomalacia by 80%.

b. Medium-term action
   - Fortification of certain food with vitamin A.

Revised Scheme 2

c. Long-term action
   - Promotion of consumption of green leafy vegetables
   - Promotion of breastfeeding for as long as possible
   - Improvement in environmental health
   - Immunization against measles
   - Prompt treatment of diarrheal diseases
   - Social and health education.

Significance

- Vitamin A deficiency is one the most common cause of preventable blindness and most common cause of blindness in children hence proper and timely institution of preventive measures can reduce prevalence of nutritional blindness in community.

SHORT ANSWERS

13. Physical quality of life index (PQLI).

Refer Question No. 16 December 2007 (RS2) Paper I.

14. Explain briefly the occupational hazards of agricultural workers.

Refer Question No. 5 June 2009 (RS2) Paper I.

15. Attributable risk.

Refer Question No. 1 December 2016 (RS2) Paper I.

16. What are the uses of screening?

Refer Question No. 1 December 2010 (RS2) Paper I.

17. What is blinding in randomized controlled trials?

Refer Question No. 1 December 2015 (RS2) Paper I.

18. Disability limitation.

Refer Question No. 1 December 2007 (RS2) Paper I.

19. Explain in brief about group discussion.

Refer Question No. 2 June 2009 (RS2) Paper I.

20. Endemic ascites.

- Endemic ascites is a toxicity produced due toxin found in food.

Cause

- It is produced due to pyrrolizidine alkaloid[Q], a heaptotoxin found in the weed Jhunjhunia seeds (crotalaria)[Q] which contaminates the millet *Panicum miliare* (locally known as *Gondhali*)
- It is endemic in Sargiya District of Madhya Pradesh affecting both sexes and all age groups except infants.

Clinical Features

- It manifests as sudden onset ascites and jaundice with overall mortality of 40%.

Prevention and Control

- Education of people.
- Deweeding of Jhunjhunia plants
- Removing seeds of Jhunjhunia at household level as its seeds are considerably smaller than those of the millet.

21. Medical social worker.

- Medico-social worker is a paramedical person qualified in sociology with training in health education and is attached to health institution, doing both medical and social work.

Activities

a. Assisting doctor in making a social diagnosis and treatment of the disease
   - Medico-social worker provides information to the doctor about the patient's social background, about the living conditions, socioeconomic status, nature of occupation, type of family, habits, family interactions, emotional overtones, occupational circumstance, etc. which has influence on the development of the disease and has an impact on the minds of the patient.

b. Providing health education, care and motivation to the patient
   - Medico-social worker provides information to the patient about the causation of the disease, its consequences, mode of transmission and how it can be controlled and cured
   - They remove the doubts and misconception about the disease and its treatment
   - They motivate the patient to take treatment correctly, completely and regularly
   - They help the patient in matters of social adjustment and social rehabilitation thus helps the patient to develop dignity and self confidence.

c. Providing health education and support to the family
   - Medico-social worker educates the family about the nursing the patient, showing sympathy, and extending cooperation towards him to promote speedy recovery
   - They provide emotional support for stress management
   - They arrange for financial assistance to the family from social welfare agencies for treatment of the patient.

d. Providing health education and promoting health of the community
   - Medico-social worker gives health education to the community by organizing film shows, video presentations, etc.
   - They motivate people for family planning
   - They participate in contact tracing and cluster testing of STDs and motivates them to undergo clinical examination and treatment
   - They take part in organization of health camps, cataract camps, tubectomy camps, immunization, etc.

Significance

- Medico-social worker acts as a link between the health institution or doctor and the community and between the community and social welfare agencies.

22. Registration of vital events.

Refer Question No. 21 June 2014 (RS2) Paper I.

MBBS PHASE III EXAMINATION

DECEMBER 2012

(Revised Scheme 2)

PAPER II

LONG ESSAYS

1. Describe the epidemiological determinants, prevention and control measures of plague.

- Plague is one of the oldest diseases known to man
- Also called as black sickness, Mahamari or the great death
- It is an acute, communicable disease, primarily a zoonotic disease that exists in nature between small mammals, usually wild rodents, and the fleas that they harbor.

Epidemiological Determinants

a. Agent factors	
i. Agent	▪ Etiological agent is *Yersinia pestis*[Q] ▪ Gram –ve, non-motile, non-spore forming, cocco bacillus ▪ Has safety pin appearance and exhibits bipolar staining with Wayson's stains[Q]
ii. Reservoir of infection	▪ Both rats and humans are reservoirs ▪ Wild rodents are natural reservoirs of infection and are responsible for maintenance and spread of disease ▪ In India, wild rodent *Tatera indica*[Q] is considered as main reservoir
iii. Source of infection	▪ Infected rodents ▪ Infected rat flea ▪ Cases of pneumonic plague
iv. Infective material	▪ Respiratory droplets (pneumonic plague) ▪ Pus (bubonic plague)
v. Incubation period	▪ 2–8 days in bubonic and septicemic plague ▪ 1–3 days in pneumonic plague
b. Host factors	
i. Age and sex	▪ Occur among people of all ages and of both sexes
ii. Immunity	▪ No natural immunity ▪ Immunity after recovery lasts for short period
iii. Human activities	▪ Commonly occurs in individuals employed in grazing, cultivation, harvesting, deforestation or hunting which offer numerous chances of flea-man contact
iv. Movement of people	▪ Often possible for a person to get a disease in a place where plague is not suspected at all due to fast and rapid transport means
c. Environmental factors	
i. Season	▪ In North India, plague season starts from September to May whereas in South India, there is not such seasonal variation
ii. Temperature and humidity	▪ Environment with temperature of 30°C and relative humidity of >60% is favorable for spread of plague as this environmental conditions favor growth of bacilli in vector and survival of vector
iii. Rainfall	▪ Heavy rainfall tends to flood rat burrows and control plague
iv. Natural calamities	▪ Natural disasters like earthquake, floods, war, etc. predispose to epidemics of plague

Contd...

Contd...

v. Urban and rural areas	▪ Plague has occurred in many towns due to unfavorable ecological conditions and lack of efficient flea vectors
vi. Housing conditions	▪ Poor housing conditions favor breeding of rats
d. Vectors	▪ Plague is most commonly transmitted to humans through bite of infected fleas ▪ Both sexes of rat flea transmit the disease[Q] ▪ Major flea vectors include – *Xenopsylla cheopis*[Q] (oriental rat flea[Q]; nearly worldwide in moderate climates)—most common and most efficient vector – *Xenopsylla brasiliensis* (Africa, India, South America) – *Xenopsylla astia* (Indonesia and Southeast Asia) – Pulex irritans (human flea) may be responsible for human-to-human transmission of plague *Features* ▪ These vectors are blood sucking ectoparasites which thrive on blood of rats and reside among their hairs ▪ When rat dies of plague, parasite leaves host to search for other vector and may bite human accidently ▪ A flea ingests about 0.5 cu mm of blood containing about 5,000 plague bacilli, which multiply in proventriculus of gut and after these bacilli reach optimum number, flea becomes infective (thus flea acts as amplifier vector) ▪ Time required for flea to become infective from its infection is called extrinsic incubation period which is about 10 days ▪ Once flea become infective, it remains infective for rest of its life and an infected flea may live up to 1 year ▪ Infective flea transmits infection by regurgitation of bacilli into bloodstream of humans during bite of flea
e. Mode of transmission	▪ Commonest mode of transmission of plague is by bite of infective blocked flea from wild rodent to periodomestic rodents and to domestic rodents and humans ▪ Humans can be directly infected from wild rodents when they enter forests ▪ In pneumonic plague, infection can be transmitted from man to man by droplet infection ▪ Infection can also be transmitted by droplets from cats which eat dead rats and develop pneumonic plague ▪ Contact transmission is possible from handing infected animals or infected material like pus from buboes ▪ Percutaneous transmission is possible following scratching over dried faces of rat fleas ▪ Aerosol transmission is also possible by inhalation of infected dust from burrows of rodents

Prevention and Control

A. Elimination or control of reservoirs
   a. Control of human reservoirs
      i. Early diagnosis
         - Death of rats (rat falls) provide warning signals of imminent outbreak
         - Community diagnosis can be made by large number of people suffering from fever and buboes (large painful enlargement of lymph nodes)
         - Diagnosis needs to confirmed by bacteriological examination.
      ii. Notification
         - Occurrence of cases is notified to concerned authorities as early as possible to institute control measures.
      iii. Isolation
         - All cases of pneumonic plague are isolated for at least for 5 days of chemotherapy.
      iv. Concurrent disinfection
         - Using 5% cresol, patient's sputum, discharges and personal belongings are disinfected
         - Dead bodies should be handled with aseptic precautions.
      v. Chemotherapy
         - Started immediately without waiting for confirmation
         - Drug of choice
            ❖ Streptomycin[Q] 30 mg/kg IM for 7–10 days
            ❖ Tetracycline 500 mg QID for 10 days
         - Alternatives
            ❖ Sulphonamides
            ❖ Streptomycin 30 mg/kg IM for 7–10 days (risk of complications due to release of endotoxin from massive destruction of plague bacilli)
            ❖ Chloramphenicol (in plague meningitis as it crosses blood-brain barrier).

b. Elimination of animal reservoirs (of domestic rodents and fleas)
   i. Trapping of rats
      - Done by using poisonous baits containing arsenic, warfarin or zinc oxide
   ii. Fumigation
      - A very effective method.

Agents used	*Method*	*Remarks*
▪ Cyanogas (commonly used) ▪ Sulfur dioxide	▪ Using a cyanogas pump, calcium cyanide powder is pumped into rat burrows and closed with mud ▪ On coming into contact with moisture, calcium cyanide releases hydrocyanic acid which is lethal on inhalation	*Advantages* ▪ Also destroys rat fleas *Disadvantages* ▪ Short lasting effect, hence has to repeated frequently ▪ Rats living in roofs not controlled ▪ Risk to person employed

   iii. Pesticides

Agents used	*Method*	*Remarks*
▪ 10% DDT (not effective) ▪ 3% BHC ▪ 2% carbaryl ▪ 5% malathion ▪ 1.5% dieldrein ▪ 2% aldrin *Dose* ▪ 2–3 g of pesticide for each sq meter of surface requiring treatment	▪ Before spraying, all foodstuffs and eating and cooking vessels should be removed ▪ Spraying should cover entire floor area, bottoms of all walls up to 3 feet above floor level, back of doors, roofing of thatched houses, crevices of walls, rat runs, clothing, bedding, cats, dogs and other pets ▪ Rat burrows should be insufflated with pesticide dust using dust blower	*Area covered* ▪ Up to radius of 5 miles around each infected locality *Advantages* ▪ Also controls rat fleas ▪ Residual effect lasting for 3–6 months

   iv. Long-term measures
      - Improvement of general sanitation
      - Improvement of housing and quality of life.

B. Breaking channel of transmission
   – Vectors (rat fleas) can be controlled by cyanogas fumigation and insufflations of rat burrows with pesticides—most effective method of breaking chain of transmission[Q]
   – Droplet spread of infection can be prevented by concurrent disinfection of patients sputum in 5–10% cresol.

C. Protection of susceptible
   – Susceptible include family contacts, medical and nursing staff attending patients
   – They are advised to wear gowns, gloves and masks.
   a. Chemoprophylaxis
      - Drug of choice is tetracycline[Q] 500 mg QID for a week
      - Alternative is Sulphonamides 3–5 g daily for a week.
   b. Immunoprophylaxis (vaccination).

   Plague vaccine
   - Plague vaccine available is developed by Haffkine and modified by Sokhey

Type	▪ Formalin-killed vaccine			
Constituents	▪ 2,000 million killed *Yersinia pestis* bacilli per mL			
Dose		*First dose*	*Second dose*	*Booster dose*
	▪ Adult male	1.0 mL	1.5 mL	1.0 mL
	▪ Adult female	0.75 mL	1.0 mL	0.75 mL
	▪ 1–4 years	0.2 mL	0.4 mL	0.2 mL
	▪ 5–10 years	0.3 mL	0.6 mL	0.3 mL
	▪ 11–16 years	0.4 mL	0.8 mL	0.4 mL

Route of administration	▪ Subcutaneous
Schedule	▪ Primary immunization – 2 doses 1–2 week apart ▪ Booster doses – Every 6 months (starting 6 months after 2nd dose of primary immunization) in high-risk group like geologist, biologists and anthropologists
Immunity	▪ Starts 5–7days after inoculation and lasts for about 6 months
Indications	▪ Endemic areas ▪ Suspicion of epidemic (1 single dose of double the routine dose at least 1 week before) ▪ Travellers to hyperendemic areas (50% protective)
Contraindications	▪ Pregnant mothers (potential risk of fetal damage and abortions) ▪ Infants below 6 months[Q] (protected by maternal antibodies) ▪ Plague epidemic (useless)
Reactions	▪ Pain, tenderness, headache (appear within few hours and subside in 1–2 days)

Significance

- WHO recommends that plague vaccine in all circumstance is only for prevention, not for control of human plague.

c. Surveillance of susceptible areas
   - Surveillance is necessary in areas with history of past infection or foci of natural plague
   - It should cover all aspects of rodents and human plague.

d. Health education
   - People in susceptible areas should be educated about
     - ❖ Sanitation in and around house
     - ❖ Not to keep food grains in open containers
     - ❖ Not to sleep on floors
     - ❖ Not to go into forested areas
     - ❖ Notification of appropriate authorities about rat falls.

Significance

- Plague has been known as a dreaded killer from times immemorial
- Plague is a notifiable disease under International Health Regulations but is no more a quarantinable disease
- A medical practitioner should consider plague as an differential diagnosis in any case of fever with lymphadenopathy or when multiple pneumonia cases occur in a community.

Revised Scheme 2

2. Discuss Revised National Tuberculosis Control Program.

- Revised National Tuberculosis Control Program (RNTCP) was launched by Government of India in 1993 as a pilot project and expanded in 1997 and is now covers the entire country since 24th March 2006.
- Its basic goal is to decrease incidence of tuberculosis to such a low level that it is no longer a major public health problem[Q].

Objectives

- Detection of at least 70% of estimated cases through quality sputum microscopy[Q]
- Achievement of at least 85% cure rate among newly detected sputum smear positive infectious case[Q].

Goal to be achieved by 2007 (as per 10th five year plan)

• Coverage under RNTCP	1070 million
• Number of patients examined	4.07 million
• Total number of patients on DOTS	1.00 million
• New sputum smear patients put on treatment	0.40 million
• Cure rate of new sputum smear positive patients	>85%

Organizational Setup

National level	*Ministry of Health and Family Welfare*	*Secretary*
State level	State Tuberculosis Office	State Tuberculosis Officer
	State Tuberculosis Training and Demonstration Center	Director
District level	District Tuberculosis Center	District Tuberculosis Officer
Subdistrict level	Primary Health Center	Medical Officer
	Tuberculosis Health Unit	Senior Treatment Supervisor and Senior TB Laboratory Supervisor
	Microscopy Center	Specially Trained Technician
Village level		DOTS Agent

Laboratory Network

- To provide appropriate, available, affordable and accessible diagnostic services for TB suspects and cases, a nationwide network of RNTCP quality assured designated sputum smear microscopy laboratories have been set up
- Tuberculosis unit has both radiological and microbiological facility[Q].

Setup

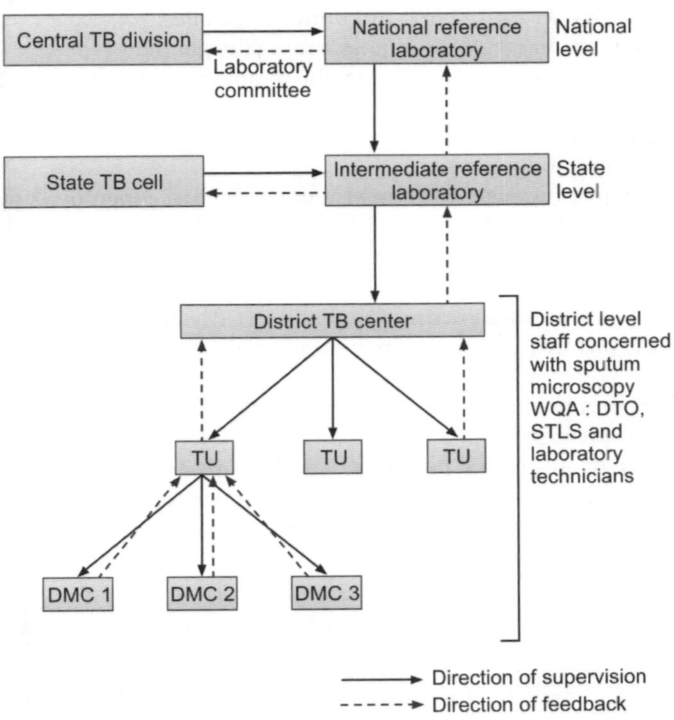

Fig. 1: Setup of RNTCP

Activities

- Carry out sputum microscopy with external quality assessment
- Drug resistance surveillance.

Strategies

- Directly observed treatment short course chemotherapy (DOTS)
- Involvement of NGOs
- IEC activities and improved operational research.

a. Directly observed treatment short course chemotherapy (DOTS)[Q]
   - DOTS or direct observed therapy supervised is a new strategy for the treatment of tuberculosis under Revised National Tuberculosis Program (RNTCP)
   - It is a community-based tuberculosis treatment and case strategy which combines the benefits of supervised treatment and community-based support and care
   - DOTS is a KEY strategy of revised national tuberculosis program.

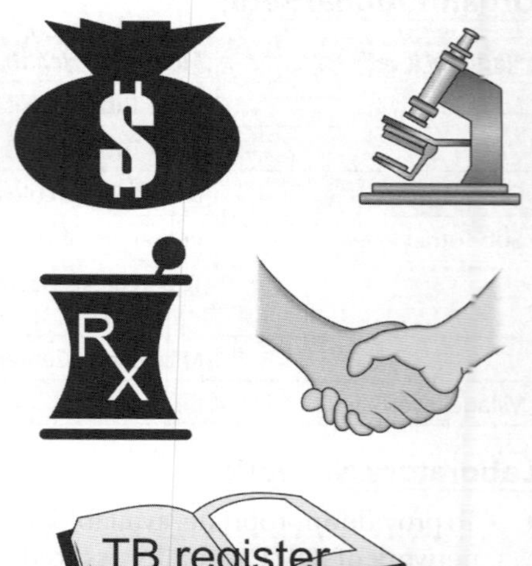

Fig. 2: Components of DOTS

Components[Q]
- Political and administrative commitment
- Good quality diagnosis by microscopy
- Adequate supply of quality drugs
- Directly observed treatment
- Systematic monitoring and accountability.

i. Political and administrative commitment
   - The political commitment for the control of tuberculosis is evident from the fact that the Government of India obtained a loan of US $ 142 millions from World Bank in 1997 for implementation of RNTCP
   - It celebrates World TB day on 24th March by conducting rallies, especially by cured patients to create awareness among the people
   - Mass media campaigns are launched to educate the people regarding the DOTS.

ii. Quality diagnosis by microscopy
   - Under RNTCP, sputum microscopy is the case finding tool
   - The case finding is passive and not active[Q]
   - Here the patient visiting a physician with persistent productive cough of >2 week duration with or without hemoptysis is suspected to be TB patient and TB has to ruled out by the physician by screening them with 2 sputum smear examinations[Q] by a specially trained technician in the designated RNTCP microscopy centers

Principle
- **2 sputum smear examinations is a must[Q]** under RNTCP because with one sample of sputum, the chances of detecting smear positive is 80%, with two samples 93%.

Procedure
- The early morning sample is taken because the secretions build up in the airways overnight and chances of detecting bacilli are more
- Since is difficult for an out-patient to provide 2 early morning specimens, spot-morning-spot samples are collected, i.e. a sample of sputum is collected on the spot when the patient attends the out-patient department and is then given a cup to collect the sputum of next day morning
- Smears are examined by the ZN staining[Q].

Grading of smears

If slide has	*Result*	*Grading*	*No of fields examined*
>10 AFB per field	Positive	+++	20
1–10 AFB per field	Positive	++	50
10–99 AFB per 10 fields	Positive	+	100
1–9 AFB per 10 fields	Positive	Scanty	100
0 AFB in 100 fields	Negative	—	100

Advantages
- Not only confirms the diagnosis but also helps in assessing the prognosis
- More objective and reliable than X-ray of chest and is 98% specific than X-ray
- Helps to categorize the patient by distinguishing between smear +ve and smear –ve patients (for patient to be +ve there should be at least 10,000 bacilli/mL of sputum[Q])
- Facilitates provision of appropriate treatment.

iii. Adequate supply of drugs
   - Under RNTCP, the entire course of drugs supplied free of cost, and patient is ensured about it before beginning the treatment, thus ensuring regular supply without interruption
   - The drugs are supplied as patientwise boxes, colored red, blue and green for category I, II and III respectively, containing full course of treatment
   - Each box has 2 chambers, the smaller containing drugs of intensive phase and the larger containing drugs of continuation phase
   - The drugs are packed in blister packs and for the intensive phase, each blister pack contains one day's medication and for the continuation phase each blister pack contains one week's supply of medication
   - The combipack for extension of intensive phase are supplied separately
   - Children and adolescents often fall into category III because they rarely cough up sputum and almost always smear negative.

iv. Directly observed treatment (DOT)
   - It envisages the direct observation or watching of the patient swallowing every dose of anti-TB drugs, all at a time, preferably in empty stomach in the intensive phase and only the first dose of the week during the continuation phase, by the treatment observer or health worker known as DOTS agents.
   - DOTS agents are, accessible and acceptable to the patients and accountable to the health system, such as teachers, anganwadi-workers, social-workers, ex-patients, members of NGOs, etc.
   - They are paid an honourarium of ₹ 150/- per patient completing the treatment
   - Family members are not made DOTS agents because they are not effective DOTS agents
   - The DOTS supervises the daily consumption of tablet during the intensive phase and the consumption of medicine in the continuation phase is also checked by return of multiblister combipack, when the patient comes to collect medicine for the next week
   - In this program, alternate day treatment is used.

   Advantages
   - DOT ensures 95% relapse free cure rate and also prevents MDR
   - It also builds a human bond between the health-care provider and the patient
   - Cost-effective strategy effective in controlling TB on mass basis
   - Internationally accepted.

v. Systematic monitoring and accountability
   - RNTCP ensures systematic monitoring, supervision and accountability at every level
   - Each level must do its part to ensure cure of the patient and to break the chain of its transmission
   - Therefore, at subdistrict level tuberculosis units (TU) are set up for the exclusive purpose of supervision and monitoring of TB control activities
   - It has both radiological and microbiological diagnosis facility[Q].

Tuberculosis Unit
- A TB unit covers a population of about 5 lakhs[Q] (2.5 lakh in hilly and tribal areas)
- It is staffed by a senior treatment supervisor and a senior TB laboratory supervisor
- A designated medical officer supervises the work in a TU
- A TU will have one microscopy center for every 100,000 population[Q] (50,000 in tribal, desert, remote and hilly regions) referred to as the designated microscopy center (DMC).

Activities
- Maintaining TB register containing information on diagnosis and treatment of every patient
- Ensure effective diagnosis by microscopy and treatment by directly observed treatment
- Complete quarterly reports on diagnosis, sputum conversion, treatment outcome and program management
- Recheck all +ve slides and 10% of –ve slides.

Advantages
- DOTS has reduced incidence and prevalence of tuberculosis
- It produces cure rates form 85% to 95%
- It prevents tuberculosis bacilli from spreading to others
- It alleviates poverty, saving of working days and lives, reduces the duration of illness

- It prolongs the survival of HIV infected tuberculosis patients
- It prevents treatment failure and reduces deaths due to multidrug-resistant tuberculosis and spread of multidrug-resistant tuberculosis
- It strengthens health services and confidence among the health workers about the curability of tuberculosis and multidrug-resistant tuberculosis.

Significance
- DOTS is a community based, supervised, anti-TB treatment care strategy which ensures that the patient takes right drugs, in right dose, at right interval for the right duration
- DOTS involve provision of basic, essential, utilitarian service starting by the people, of the people and for the people.

b. Involvement of NGOs
- NGOs are involved to inform, educate and communicate with the population
- They also motivate the patients to seek treatment and complete the course
- They can also be involved as DOT agents
- It is a novel feature of RNTCP[Q].

c. IEC activities
- These comprise of dissemination of information about tuberculosis through mass media, street plays, role play, etc.
- It tries to clear the misconception among the general public about the disease and informs that the disease is curable.

RNTCP—Phase II

- Phase II of RNTCP is a step forward in tuberculosis control to achieve TB related Millennium Development Goals.

Goals	*Strategy*	*Activities*
▪ Aims ▪ Increase access to services to hard to reach areas like tribal or hilly areas ▪ Targets ▪ Case detection rate of 70% ▪ Cure rate of 85%	▪ Provision of additional TB unit and DMCs in tribal/difficult areas ▪ Provision of TBHVs in urban areas ▪ Compensation for transportation of patient and attendant in tribal areas ▪ Higher rate of salary to contractual staff posted in tribal areas ▪ Enhanced vehicle maintenance and travel allowance in tribal areas ▪ Studies to document utilization by marginalized groups	▪ Consolidation, maintenance and further improvement of achievements of phase I ▪ Strengthen intersectoral collaboration, involve medical colleges and conduct need-based focused and people centric information, education and communication activities ▪ Scaling up state level intermediate referral laboratories ▪ Implementation of DOTS-Plus for multidrug-resistant TB

Guidelines

a. Tuberculosis suspect
   - Any person with cough 2 weeks or more

b. Number of specimen required for diagnosis of smear-positive pulmonary tuberculosis
   - Two
     - Spot sputum specimen (day 1)
     - Morning after sputum specimen (day 2).

c. Diagnosis of tuberculosis
   - None sputum positive: Doubtful
   - One sputum positive: Sputum positive pulmonary tuberculosis
   - Two sputum positive: Sputum positive pulmonary tuberculosis.

d. Management of clients
   i. None sputum positive
      - Give antibiotics for 10–14 days
        - ❖ Cough relieved: Nontuberculosis person
        - ❖ Cough persists: REPEAT two sputum smear examination
      - Chest X-ray
        - ❖ Findings suggestive of TB: Sputum negative tuberculosis: Start ATT
        - ❖ Nonfindings suggestive of TB: Nontuberculosis person

ii. One sputum positive
   - Start ATT
iii. Two sputum positive
   - Start ATT

Achievements

- Since implantation of RNTCP, because of DOTS and TB surveillance, the case detection rate is improved to 79% and DOTS cure rate is about 88% (2011).

SHORT ESSAYS

3. Describe "ASHA"s role and responsibilities under National Rural Health Mission.

Refer Question No. 2 June 2014 (RS2) Paper II.

4. Malarial indices.

- Malarial indices are parameters used for measurement of malaria (malariometry)
- It is necessary to routinely assess certain parameters to evaluate the success of surveillance activity.

Malarial Indices

- Malaria in an area can be measured by prevalence and incidence of malaria (Epidemiological parameters) and vector indices (entamological parameters).

a. Prevalence rate of malaria
   – These were routinely employed in pre-eradication era
   i. Child spleen rate
      - It is the percentage of children between 2–10 years showing splenic enlargement
      - Adults were excluded because in adults splenomegaly may occur due to reasons other than malaria.

      Application
      - Spleen rate is used for measuring endemicity of malaria in a community[Q]
      - Depending upon spleen rate, country was classified into following areas
        - Hypoendemic (<10%)
        - Mesoendemic (11–50%)
        - Hyperendemic (51–75%)
        - Holoendemic (>75%)

      Significance
      - Spleen rate is best indicator for malaria prevalence[Q] in a community.
   ii. Average enlarged spleen
      - It is a refined indicator, denoting average size of enlarged spleen
   iii. Child parasite rate
      - It is the percentage of children between 2–10 years positive for malarial parasite in their blood smears
   iv. Parasite density index
      - It is average number of malarial parasite per cu mm of blood estimated from all positive slides.

      Significance
      - It indicates average degree of parasitemia in a sample of well-defined group of population.
   v. Infant parasite rate
      - It is the percentage of infants positive for malarial parasite in their blood smears.

      Significance
      - Most sensitive indictor[Q] because it indicates active transmission of malaria in community
      - An area with zero infant parasite rate for 3 consecutive years, suggests absence of malaria transmission even in presence of anophenline mosquito (Anophelism without malaria).

vi. Proportional case rate
   - It is the number of cases diagnosed as clinical malaria for every 100 patients attending hospitals
   - It is a crude indicator because cases are not related to their time and place of distribution.

b. Incidence rates of malaria
   - These indices are used currently
   i. Annual parasite incidence[Q] (API)
   - It is the number of new confirmed cases of malaria occurring in an area during a given year and confirmed by blood-smear examination and is expressed per 1,000 population
   - It is based on intensive active and passive surveillance and cases confirmed by blood examination.

Calculations

$$API = \frac{\text{Confirmed cases during a given year}}{\text{Total population under surveillance}} \times 1000$$

Application
- For spray operations under modified plan of action, endemic areas in country were classified into following areas[Q]
  - Areas with API <2 : Regular insecticide spray
  - Areas with API >2 : Focal insecticide spray

Significance
- API is a sophisticated measure of malaria incidence in a community[Q]
- It depends upon annual blood collection and examination rates and sufficient number of blood slides must be systematically obtained and examined for malaria parasite to work out accurately annual parasite incidence.

ii. Annual blood examination rate[Q] (ABER)
   - It is the percentage of population examined for peripheral blood smear during a given year
   - If it is done monthly, it is called monthly blood examination rate (MBER).

Calculations

$$ABER = \frac{\text{Number of slides examined in a year}}{\text{Total population}} \times 100$$

Application
- MBER can be used to analyze trend of fever rate in community by comparing data from previous years or previous months of same year.

Significance
- ABER is an index of operational efficiency[Q]
- WHO recommends examination of slides equal to at least 1% of population however under modified plan of action for malaria control, slides equal to at least 10% of population should be examined monthly.

iii. Slide positivity rate[Q] (SPR)
   - It is the percentage of slides found positive for malarial parasites, irrespective of type of species.

Calculation

$$SPR = \frac{\text{Total no. of blood smear positive for MP}}{\text{Total no. of blood smears examined}} \times 100$$

Application
- SPR provides information about trends of malaria transmission by comparing data with previous years

Significance
- This gives information about parasite load in community

iv. Slide falciparum rate[Q] (SFR)
   - It is the percentage of slides found positive for *Plasmodium falciparum* parasites.

Calculation

$$SFR = \frac{\text{Total No. of blood smears +ve for } P.\ falciparum}{\text{Total no. of blood smears examined}} \times 100$$

Application

- SFR provides information about trends of malaria transmission by comparing data with previous years.

Significance

- SFR pinpoints areas of *P. falciparum* preponderance and indicates necessity for intensification of control measures on priority basis.

v. *Plasmodium falciparum* percentage (PF%)

- It is the percentage of positive blood smears positive for *P. falciparum*

Calculation

$$PF\% = \frac{\text{Total No. of blood smears +ve for } P.\ falciparum}{\text{Total no. of blood smears +ve for MP}} \times 100$$

Significance

- This gives information about incidence of falciparum malaria in relation to total case load of malaria

vi. Annual falciparum incidence[Q] (AFI)

- It is the confirmed new cases of falciparum malaria per 1,000 population during a given year.

Significance

- It is special parameter for *Plasmodium falciparum*

c. Vector indices (Entomological parameters)

i. Adult vector density (Mosquito density)

- It is the number of mosquitoes per man hour catch

ii. Human blood index

- It is the percentage of female aneopheline mosquito containing human blood in their stomach
- It indicates degree of anthrophilism.

iii. Sporozoite rate

- It is the percentage of female anopheline mosquitoes containing sporozoites in their salivary glands.

iv. Biting density (man biting rate)

- It is the average incidence of anopheline bites per day per person
- It is determined by catching mosquitoes by using humans as bait.

v. Inoculation rate

- It is the product of biting density and sporozoite rate.

Significance

- The malarial indices used to measure load of malaria in population are still from pre-eradication era, though malaria control policy has changed. These parameters are mostly parasitological in nature and unlikely to reveal true epidemiological picture
- Hence it is essential for malaria eradication that focus shifts on true epidemiological parameters and case detection machinery is fully supervised and made more efficient.

5. What is role of mass drug administration in controlling lymphatic filariasis?

Refer Question No. 11 June 2011 (RS2) Paper II.

6. Write briefly about the elements of primary health care.

Refer Question No. 4 June 2012 (RS2) Paper II.

7. Describe the services provided by UNICEF.

Refer Question No. 8 June 2010 (RS2) Paper II.

8. What is disaster preparedness?

- Disaster preparedness is a program of long-term development activities whose goals are to strengthen the overall capacity and capability of a country to manage efficiently all types of disasters. It should bring about an orderly transition from relief through recovery and back to sustained development.

- Phase of disaster preparedness is the predisaster phase of disaster management.

Objectives	*Components*
▪ To ensure that appropriate systems, procedures and resources are in place to provide prompt effective assistance to disaster victims thus facilitating relief measures and rehabilitation of services	▪ Evaluation, from past experiences about risk involving the region ▪ Location of disaster prone areas ▪ Adaptation of a standard operating procedure ▪ Organizing of communication, information and warning systems ▪ Ensuring coordination and response mechanism ▪ Development of public education program ▪ Coordination with news media ▪ National and international relations ▪ Organization of disaster simulation exercises that test response mechanism ▪ Training of health workers, social workers and members of NGOs ▪ Keeping stocks of food, drugs and other essential commodities

Significance

- Disaster preparedness is an ongoing multisectorial activity and forms an integral part of disaster management
- It should be active and energetic.

9. Define perinatal mortality rate. Enumerate the various causes of perinatal mortality in India.

Refer Question No. 2 December 2011 (RS2) Paper II.

10. What are the risk factors for hypertension? Discuss briefly its preventive measures.

- Hypertension is a chronic life style disorder, characterized by an increase in the arterial blood pressure of the individual
- It has gained importance due to its etiological role in coronary heart disease, stroke and other vascular complications.

Risk Factors

Nonmodifiable risk factors	
a. Age	▪ Prevalence of blood pressure rises with age in both sexes and the rise is greater in those with higher initial blood pressure ▪ Probably this represents an accumulation of environmental influences and the effects of genetically programd senescence in body systems
b. Sex	▪ Early in life there is little evidence of a difference in blood pressure between the sexes ▪ However, at adolescence, men display a higher average level ▪ This difference is most evident in young and middle aged adults ▪ Late in life the difference narrows and the pattern may even be reversed ▪ Post-menopausal changes in women may be the contributory factor for this change
c. Genetic factors	▪ There is considerable evidence that blood pressure levels are determined in part by genetic factors, and that the inheritance is polygenic ▪ The blood pressure values of monozygotic twins are usually more strongly correlated than those of zygotic twins ▪ Children of normotensive parents have 3% possibility of developing hypertension, whereas children of hypertensive parents have 45% possibility of developing hypertension
d. Ethnicity	▪ Black communities have higher blood pressure levels than other ethnic groups
Modifiable risk factors	
a. Obesity	▪ The greater the weight gain, the greater the risk of high blood pressure ▪ When people with high blood pressure lose weight, their blood pressure generally decreases ▪ Central obesity (increased waist to hip ratio) has positive correlation with high blood pressure in several populations

Contd...

Contd...

b. Diet	
i. Salt intake	▪ High salt intake of 7–8 g per day increases blood pressure proportionately ▪ Low sodium intake has been found to lower the blood pressure ▪ Potassium antagonises the biological effects of sodium, and thereby reduces blood pressure ▪ Potassium supplements have been found to lower blood pressure of mild-to-moderate hypertensives ▪ Other cations such as calcium, cadmium and magnesium have also been suggested as of importance in reducing blood pressure levels
ii. Saturated fat	▪ Saturated fat raises blood pressure as well as serum cholesterol
iii. Dietary fiber	▪ Risk of hypertension is inversely related to the consumption of dietary fiber ▪ Most fibers reduce plasma total and LDL cholesterol
iv. Alcohol	▪ High alcohol intake is associated with an increased risk of high blood pressure ▪ Alcohol consumption raises systolic pressure more than the diastolic
c. Heart rate	▪ Heart rate of the hypertensive group is invariably higher reflecting a resetting of sympathetic activity at a higher level
d. Physical activity	▪ Physical activity by reducing body weight may have an indirect effect on blood pressure
e. Stress	▪ Psychosocial factors operate through mental processes, consciously or unconsciously, to produce hypertension
f. Socioeconomic status	▪ In developed countries higher prevalence of hypertension have been noted in upper socioeconomic groups but in fast developing countries higher levels of blood pressure have been noted in lower socioeconomic groups also
g. Other factors	▪ There is an inverse relation between hypertension and levels of education, income and occupation ▪ Oral contraception, because of the estrogen component in combined preparations predispose to hypertension ▪ Other factors such as noise, vibration, temperature and humidity might play a role

Prevention (WHO)

A. Primary prevention (primordial prevention)

- Primary prevention includes all measures to reduce incidence of disease in a population by reducing risk of onset.

Objectives

- To modify or eliminate risk factors.

Strategies

a. Population strategy

- Directed at whole population based on fact that even small reduction in average blood pressure of population reduces incidence of hypertension to an large extent.

Objectives

- ❖ To shift community distribution of blood pressure towards lower levels or biological normality.

Components

i. Dietary modifications

- Reduce average consumption of salt <5 g/day[Q]
- Moderate fat intake
- Prudent diet
- Discourage consumption of alcohol
- Restrict energy needs only to body requirements
- DASH (dietary approach to stop hypertension) diet
  - ❖ Avoid saturated fat
  - ❖ Include mono-unsaturated fatty acids like olive oils
  - ❖ Include poly unsaturated fatty acids like sunflower, fish, cottonseed oils
  - ❖ Include fresh fruits and vegetables daily, specially potassium rich fruits like banana, oranges and vegetables like carrot, spinach, mushrooms beans, etc.
  - ❖ Include nuts, seeds or legumes
  - ❖ Choose whole grain over white flour
  - ❖ Choose moderate amount of protein, preferably fish or poultry.

ii. Weight reduction[Q]
- By diet control and promotion of physical activities
- Maintain normal body mass index (BMI <25).

iii. Exercise promotion[Q]
- Regular exercise reduces body weight, blood lipids and blood pressure.

iv. Behavioral changes
- Modify personal lifestyle, reduce stress, practice yoga or meditation
- Abstain from alcohol and smoking.

v. Health education
- Educate the people about risk factors and preventive measures for control of hypertension.

vi. Self care[Q]
- Patient is taught self care by taking his own blood pressure and keeping a log of it.

b. High-risk strategy
- Constitutes specific protection
- Aimed at prevention of attainment of blood pressure where treatment has to be started
- Directed at high-risk cases
- Done by regular recording of blood pressure in high-risk cases, i.e.
  - Obese people
  - Individuals above 50 years
  - Alcoholics
  - Diabetics
  - Sedentary workers
  - Pregnant woman
  - Individual with strong family history.
- These individuals are trained in self care, i.e. regular monitoring of blood pressure with follow up.

B. Secondary prevention

Objective
- To detect and control high blood pressure in affected individuals.

Strategies

a. Early case detection
- Achieved through screening of high-risk groups and followed by regular care
- Difficult considering fact that high blood pressure causes symptoms very late due to organic damage.

b. Treatment
- Aimed at reducing and maintaining blood pressure below 140/90
- Done through administration of antihypertensive drugs
- Also targeted towards other risk factors like smoking and raised blood cholesterol levels.

c. Patient compliance
- Patient compliance determines success of secondary prevention as treatment of hypertension must be continued life long
- This is obtained through health education directed to patients, families and community.

C. Tertiary prevention

a. Disability limitation
- Treat the patient intensively to limit the development of disease.

b. Rehabilitation
- Patients with handicap due to hypertension like hemiplegia (following stroke) or blindness (following retinopathy) are rehabilitated accordingly.

Significance

- Hypertension is most common cardiovascular disorder[Q] and an important life style disorder and an important risk factor for the cardiovascular deaths.
- Primordial prevention is best method of prevention, however, even secondary prevention has shown reduction in incidence of stroke and other complications due to it.

11. Classify hormonal contraceptives. Write briefly about their adverse effects.

Refer Question No. 5 June 2012 (RS2) Paper II.

12. Discuss the specific health protection given to the antenatal cases.

Refer Question No. 9 December 2010 (RS2) Paper II.

SHORT ANSWERS

13. Oral polio vaccine.

- Oral polio vaccine (OPV) or Sabin's polio vaccine is a live attenuated vaccine used for active immunization against poliomyelitis
- It was describe by Sabin in 1957

Nature	▪ Live attenuated virus vaccine of all the three types of polio viruses (trivalent vaccine) and is liquid
Composition	▪ Each dose of 2 drops contains 3 lakh $TCID_{50}$ of type 1 virus, 1 lakh $TCID_{50}$ of type 2 virus and 3 lakh $TCID_{50}$ of type 3 virus[Q] grown primary monkey kidney or human diploid cell cultures
Storage	a. Heat stabilized vaccine – 4°C – Vaccine remains potent for 4 years if cold chain is maintained and 1 month at room temperature b. Non-stabilized vaccine – -20°C in a deep freeze – Can also be kept in freezer compartment of refrigerator temporarily during immunization drive if deep freeze is not available
Dose	▪ 2 drops
Mode of administration	▪ Orally by the dropper ▪ Tilt the head of the child backwards and force the mouth open by gently squeezing the cheeks or pinching the nose ▪ Drops are dropped onto the tongue ▪ Mothers are advised not to administer hot liquids, food, breast milk half an hour prior to and after vaccination
Schedule	▪ Zero dose — At birth along with BCG ▪ First dose — At 6 weeks ▪ Second dose — At 10 weeks ▪ Third dose — At 14 weeks ▪ Booster dose — 18 months and 4–5 years
Immunity	▪ On administration, the live vaccine strain infect intestinal epithelial cells and multiply in the Peyer's patches resulting in viremia ▪ This leads to production of circulating antibodies which prevent dissemination of virus to the CNS thus prevents paralytic polio ▪ Intestinal infection stimulates production of IgA secretory antibodies[Q] thus preventing subsequent infection of the alimentary tract with wild strains of the polio virus ▪ 3 doses of OPV offer 85% protection, 4 doses confer 90% and 5 doses confer 95% immunity[Q] ▪ Multiple doses induce higher and lifelong immunity, both systemic and local
Indications	▪ For active immunization of infants against polio
Contraindications (Nil under National Pulse Polio Program)	▪ Acute febrile illness ▪ Diarrheal diseases (OPV is given but not counted) ▪ Leukemia and malignancy ▪ Immunosuprresive or steroid therapy
Adverse effects	▪ Mutation of type 3 virus[Q] in the intestine resulting in vaccine associated paralytic poliomyelitis[Q] ▪ Rare affecting 1 in millions and more so in adults
Advantages	▪ Easy to administer, painless ▪ Does not require highly trained staff ▪ Induces both local and systemic immunity ▪ Quick production of large quantity of antibodies even at single dose providing substantial immunity

	▪ Provides herd immunity as follows: – Vaccine virus is excreted in feces thus contaminating the water which when consumed by other children may infect them thus immunizing them too ▪ Useful in controlling epidemics ▪ Relatively inexpensive ▪ Easy to manufacture
Disadvantages	▪ Instability of vaccine at high ambient temperature ▪ Frequent vaccine failure even with fully potent vaccine ▪ Very small residual neurovirulence in OPV

Significance

- Oral polio vaccine was the sole reason for eradication of the polio from the India
- Under Mission IndraDhanush, Government of India is making a phased transition from OPV to IPV.

14. Mention the uses of growth chart.

Refer Question No. 22 December 2009 (RS2) Paper II.

15. What is couple protection rate?

- Couple protection rate the percentage of eligible couples effectively protected against childbirth by one or the other approved methods of contraception[Q], i.e. condom, OC pills, IUDs and sterilization
- Under RCH-II goal for CPR is set at >65%
- The current CPR is 46% (2000) whereas the target fixed for 2000 AD was 60%[Q]
- By attaining CPR 60%, it is almost equivalent to cut off almost all third or higher order of births, leaving 2 or less than 2 children per couple[Q], so that it is possible to achieve Net Reproduction Rate of 1[Q].

$$\text{CPR} = \frac{\text{Total no. of eligible couple protected by any 4 approved method}}{\text{Total no. of eligible couples in community}} \times 100$$

Significance

- This indicates the prevalence of contraceptive practice in the community[Q].

16. Congenital rubella.

Refer Question No. 3 June 2011 (RS2) Paper II.

17. Post-exposure prophylaxis of rabies.

Refer Question No. 2 December 2008 (RS2) Paper II.

18. Epidemiological basis for eradication of smallpox.

- Global eradication of smallpox is the most brilliant accomplishment and a historical milestone in history of medicine which was possible due to specific epidemiological features of smallpox
- WHO declared global eradication of smallpox on 8th May 1980 (In India , April 1977).

Epidemiological Basis for Smallpox Eradication

- No known animal reservoir
- Absence of subclinical cases
- No long-term carrier of virus
- No transmission of infection by individuals with subclinical infection
- Absence of second attacks
- Life long immunity after recovery from disease
- Comparatively easy recognition of disease (even by a non-medical person) because of appearance of characteristic rash on visible parts of body

- Availability of potent, heat stable, freeze dried vaccine with easy administration and conferring life long protection
- Successful cooperation from public
- Cooperation from international health agencies and all the countries.

Significance

- Smallpox is the first disease to be eradicated globally and has laid a foundation of eradication of other similar diseases like polio.

19. Mention the objectives of postpartal care. What are the complications which may arise during postpartal period?

- Care of the mother and the newborn after delivery is known as postnatal care.

Objectives	*Timing*
▪ To prevent complications of postpartal period ▪ To provide care for rapid restoration of mother to optimum health ▪ To check adequacy of breastfeeding ▪ To provide family planning services ▪ To provide basic health education to mother and family	▪ **Minimum recommended postnatal visits[Q] - 3** – 1st visit: <3 days – 2nd visit: 1 week – 3rd visit: 8 weeks

Components

A. To prevent complications of the postpartal period
   – Certain complications which arise during postpartal period should be diagnosed early and dealt promptly.

i. Puerperal sepsis	▪ Infection of the genital tract within 3 weeks of delivery characterized by fever, raised pulse rate, foul smelling lochia, pain and tenderness is lower abdomen, etc. ▪ Can be prevented by attention to asepsis before and after delivery
ii. Thrombophlebitis	▪ Infection of the leg veins frequently associated with varicose vein characterized by tenderness, paleness and swelling of leg
iii. Secondary haemorrhage	▪ Bleeding per vaginum anytime 6 hours after delivery to the end of perpeurium due to retained placenta or membranes
iv. Others	▪ Urinary tract infection and mastitis, etc.

B. To provide case for rapid restoration of the mother to optimum health
   – Care is provided to mother to recuperate physically psychologically and socially from her experience of delivery.

a. Physical	
i. Postnatal examination	▪ Soon after delivery, health check up is done twice a day during first 3 days and subsequently once a day till the umbilical cord drops off ▪ At each of these examination, temperature, pulse and respiration is checked, breast is examined, normal involution of uterus is checked, lochia is examined for any abnormality, urine and bowel is checked and advice is given on perineal toilet including care of stitches ▪ At the end of 6 weeks, involution of uterus is checked ▪ Thereafter once a month examination is done for first 6 months and thereafter once in 2 or 3 months till the end of 1 year ▪ In rural areas, if so many visits are difficult, then at least 3–6 postnatal visits are must
ii. Anemia	▪ Routine hemoglobin estimation is done during postnatal visits and in cases of anemia, it should be treated
iii. Nutrition	▪ Nutrition of mother should be adequately met because a malnourished mother secretes as much milk and a well nourished mother but poor in quality and at the cost of mother's health
iv. Postnatal exercises	▪ Postnatal exercises are necessary to bring the stretched abdominal and pelvic muscles back to normal ▪ Normal house-hold duties are resumed gradually
b. Psychological	▪ Common psychological problems encountered after birth are fear, timidity and insecurity which can be eliminated by proper instructions and support and companionship of her husband
c. Social	▪ Mother should be encouraged to raise the child in a wholesome family atmosphere developing her own methods

C. To check adequacy of breastfeeding
   - Breast milk is the main source of nourishment in the 1st year of life and in societies this may be for 1½ year or longer
   - Mothers can secrete as much as 400–600 mL of milk per day during 1st year[Q]
   - Mothers are advised to breastfed the exclusively for 4–5 months followed by supplementary food rich in proteins and other nutrients from age of 4–5 months introduced gradually in small amounts (Weaning)
   - Mothers should be discouraged from bottle feeding the child as they are nutritionally poor and bacteriologically dangerous.

D. Family planning
   - During postnatal visits, mothers are motivated to adopt a suitable contraceptive method for spacing the next birth or for limiting the size of family
   - In suitable candidates, postpartum sterilization is recommended on the 2nd day after delivery
   - In postpartum period, lactation offers some protection against conception and there fore can not be relied upon, their fire
   - During the first 6 months, UD and nonhormonal contraceptive are ideal choices and hormonal contraceptives are avoided as they suppress lactation
   - However injection of medroxy-progesterone acetate after delivery is successful contraceptive as it does not suppress lactation but because of its side effects its use is limited to multiparae at ages over 35 years or those who have completed their families.

E. To provide basic health education to mother/family
   - In postnatal period mother and her family is educated in regards to:
     - Hygiene—personal and environmental
     - Feeding for mother and infant
     - Pregnancy spacing
     - Importance of health check up
     - Birth registration.

20. Recommendations of Shrivastav Committee.

Refer Question No. 6 June 2010 (RS2) Paper II.

21. Screening for breast cancer.

Refer Question No. 11 June 2013 (RS2) Paper II.

22. Effect of urbanization on health.

Refer Question No. 9 December 2012 (RS2) Paper I.

MBBS PHASE III EXAMINATION

JUNE 2013

(Revised Scheme 2)

PAPER I

LONG ESSAYS

1. What are the sources and functions of iodine? Enumerate the spectrum of conditions under iodine deficiency disorders. Discuss about the components of Iodine deficiency disorders control program.

- Iodine is an essential trace element which is necessary for synthesis of thyroid hormones, namely triiodothyronine and thyroxine which regulate normal metabolism, growth and development.

Sources	*Daily requirement (<1 teaspoon over lifetime)–WHO/UNICEF*	*Distribution*	*Functions*
▪ Iodine requirement of body is met by food (90%) and water (10%) ▪ Dependent upon the iodine content of soil therefore iodine deficiency is geographical in nature *Rich sources* ▪ Sea foods such as fish, shrimps, prawns, crab, oyster, lobster, etc./Cod liver oil/Vegetables grown on iodine rich soil *Common sources* ▪ Milk, cereals, pulses, fruits and vegetables *Regular sources* ▪ Iodized salt, iodized oil	Preschool children (0–59 months) ▪ 90 µg School children (6–12 years) ▪ 120 µg Adult (>12 years) ▪ 150[Q] µg Pregnancy and lactation ▪ 250[Q] µg	Total body content ▪ 50 mg Thyroid gland ▪ 15 mg	▪ Iodine is essential for synthesis of thyroid hormones in thyroid gland ▪ It is essential for growth and development of fetus, deficiency of which causes cretinism

Iodine Deficiency Disorders

- Iodine deficiency disorders are disorders produced due to deficiency of iodine.

Spectrum of Iodine Deficiency Disorders

Age group	*Iodine deficiency disorders*
▪ Neonate	Cretinism—mental deficiency, deaf mutism, spastic diplegia, squint, psychomotor defects, neonatal goiter, neonatal hypothyroidism, delayed motor milestone[Q], Intrauterine foetal deaths[Q]
▪ Child/adolescents	Goiter, juvenile hypothyroidism, dwarfism, cretinism, impaired mental functions, educational backwardness, personality problems
▪ Adults	Goiter, hypothyroidism, impaired mental functions, myxedema

Epidemiology

a. Agent factors	
i. Iodine deficiency	▪ Nutritional deficiency of iodine is the main cause of IDD ▪ Iodine is essential for synthesis of T_3 and T_4 hormones which regulate numerous important functions of body

ii. Goitrogens	▪ Goitrogens are goiter producing substances which prevent up take of iodine by thyroid gland ▪ Example: Cabbage, cauliflower, PAS, sulfonylureas, lithium, cobalt, etc.
b. Host factors	
i. Age	▪ Age commonly affected are school going children in endemic areas and women in age group of 20 – 30 in nonendemic areas ▪ Children of mothers with iodine deficiency also develop iodine deficiency (cretinism)
ii. Sex	▪ In endemic areas male—female ratio is almost same but in nonendemic areas, female preponderance is seen
c. Environmental factor	
i. Geographic region	▪ Iodine deficiency disorders are endemic in hilly regions like Himalayas
ii. Water pollution	▪ Water pollution has proved to be causative agent of endemic goiter in initial studies

Clinical Features (Health Hazards)

Goiter	*Primary hypothyroidism*	*Juvenile hypothyroidism*	*Cretinism*
▪ Goiter is nontoxic nonneoplastic enlargement of thyroid gland ▪ If it increases in size, it produces pressure symptoms like stridor, wheezing, dysphagia, hoarseness of voice	▪ Clinical feature include slow, slurred speech, puffiness around eyes, dry, scaly cold thickened skin, coarse brittle hair, non pitting edema of lower extremities, slow pulse rate, faint heart sound, pericardial effusion	▪ Characterized by delayed milestones, growth retardation delay in closing of fontenelle, delayed mental development, myopathy, protracted sexual infantilism	▪ Severe iodine deficiency which starts in utero ▪ Manifests as dwarfism, mental retardation and deafness[Q] ▪ Prevalence of cretinism indicates severity of iodine deficiency in an area

Prevention and Control

a. Primary prevention	
i. Specific protection	▪ It consists of provision of iodine in form of iodized salt or based iodine injection ▪ Through National Program for Prevention of IDD, Government of India mandates iodinization of common edible salt with potassium iodate or sodium iodate in level of 30 ppm at production level and 15 ppm at consumer level ▪ Other measure is intramuscular injection of 2 mL of iodized poppy seed oil which provides protection of 4 years[Q]
ii. Health promotion	▪ It targets awareness regarding cause of iodine deficiency disorder, use of iodized salt, etc. through health education
b. Monitoring	▪ It is the monitoring of level of iodine in iodized by means of examining iodine content of salts collected at various points ▪ Besides this iodine content of soil, water and various other foods is also recommended
c. Surveillance	▪ Surveillance for prevalence of endemic cretinism is a part of National Program for Prevention of IDD as prevalence of endemic cretinism is indicative of severity of iodine deficiency[Q]
d. Manpower training	▪ Health personnel at various levels should be trained into surveillance of iodine deficiency, collection and examination of iodized salt samples and water from endemic areas

Iodine Deficiency Disorder Control Program[1]

- Iodine deficiency disorder control program was formerly known as National Goiter Program (1962)
- However due to failure of National Goiter Control Program to contain incidence of goiter and realization of prevalence of goiter beyond goiter belt, it was changed to IDD control program in 1992 with nationwide approach rather than area specific.

Objectives and components	*Goals*
▪ To ensure production, supply and used of iodized salt in place of common salt (universal component) ▪ Surveys to assess the magnitude of Iodine deficiency disorders ▪ Resurveys after every 5 years to assess extent of iodine deficiency disorders and impact of iodized salt ▪ Laboratory monitoring of iodated salt and urinary iodine excretion ▪ Health education and publicity	▪ Reduce incidence of IDD in adults to <10% by 2010 ▪ Reduce prevalence of goiter in age group of 10–14 years <5% ▪ Reduce numbers of cretins born to zero by 2000

Strategies

a. Surveys (to assess iodine deficiency)
   - Surveys are carried out to assess magnitude of iodine deficiency disorders and resurveys are done every 5 years to assess extent of IDD and impact of iodized salt.

District IDD/Goiter surveys
   - Survey is carried out in children aged 6–12 years[Q]
   - 20 villages/wards or schools are selected from district by cluster sampling[Q]
   - Proportionate to size sampling
   - Sample of 90 children (45 boys and 45 girls) are selected from each cluster
   - Salt sample is collected from house of every 5th child selected
   - Every alternate child from the child selected for salt sample is tested for urinary iodine excretion
   - Every month, about 50 salt samples and 25 urinary iodide excretion samples are tested

Indicators for epidemiological assessment of iodine deficiency	*Epidemiological criteria for assessing severity of iodine deficiency disorders*
▪ Prevalence of goiter ▪ Prevalence of cretinism ▪ Prevalence of neonatal hypothyroidism (most sensitive indicator of environmental iodine deficiency) ▪ Urinary iodine excretion (recommended for surveillance) ▪ Determination of serum levels of T4 and TSH	▪ Total goiter rate—Grade I + Grade II ▪ Median urinary iodine excretion ▪ Thyroid volume (ultrasound) ▪ Salt iodine content

b. Use of iodized salt and fortify all edible salt (in phased manner by end of 8th plan as National policy)
   - 31 states and union territories have banned use of salt other than iodized salt
   - Salt are iodized with potassium iodide (KI)—called as iodized salt or potassium iodate (KIO_3)-called as iodated salt
   - Potassium iodate is preferred as it is very stable and has melting point of 530°C
   - Level of iodization in salt should contain minimum 30 ppm at production level and 15 ppm at consumer level[Q] (PFA Act, 1954).

c. Monitoring and surveillance
   - An essential component of IDD control program is regular monitoring the effect of iodized salt on prevalence of IDD.

Criteria for tracking progress towards IDD elimination (IDD elimination criteria[Q])

▪ Proportion of enlarged thyroid (6–12 years)	<5%
▪ Urinary Iodine excretion below 100 µg/L	<50%
▪ Urinary Iodine excretion below 50 µg/L	<20%
▪ Proportion of houses consuming adequately iodized salt	<90%

d. Manpower training
   - Efficient and trained manpower are core to success of any program
   - Personnel involved in IDD control program are trained at biochemistry division of National Institute of Communicable Diseases, Delhi

e. Health education and publicity
   - Under IDD control program, regular advertisements are given in Print media, TV, radio emphasizing benefits of use of iodized salt to general public in local language.

Infrastructure and Administrative Set-up

Institute	*Location*	*Staffing pattern*	*Functions*
▪ Central nutrition and Iodine deficiency disorders cell	New Delhi at Director General of Health Services	Deputy Assistant Director General (IDD) Technical assistant Junior investigator Field assistants and attendants Office staff	Responsible for nationwide implementation of program through intersectoral coordination, coordination between state IDD control cells, managing IEC activities, etc.

Contd...

Contd...

Institute	*Location*	*Staffing pattern*	*Functions*
▪ Iodine deficiency disorders control cell	Located at State or UT level to ensure effective implementation of program	▪ Technical officer (IDD) ▪ Statistical analyst ▪ LDC/typist	▪ Carries out periodic surveys regarding the prevalence of IDD ▪ Responsible for checking iodine levels in salt, distribution of iodized salt, creating demand for iodized salt, monitoring, manpower training and health education
▪ National reference laboratory (IDD monitoring laboratory)	Set-up at Biochemistry division of National Institute of Communicable Diseases, Delhi	Laboratory technician Laboratory assistance	Responsible for monitoring IDD and training manpower
▪ Regional IDD monitoring laboratory	At Hyderabad (South), Kolkata (East and NE), New Delhi (West) and Delhi (North)	Laboratory technician Laboratory assistance	Responsible for monitoring IDD and training manpower

Indicators to Monitor Success of IDD Control Program

Process indicators	*Impact indicators*	*Sustainability indicators*
Monitor and evaluate the salt iodization process	Assess based IDD status and to monitor and evaluate the impact of salt iodization on the target population	Assess successful elimination of iodine deficiency and to judge sustainability and maintenance of achievement achieved for decades to come
i. Salt iodine content at production site ii. Salt iodine content at point of packing iii. Salt iodine content at wholesale and retail levels iv. Salt iodine content at households	i. Urinary iodine levels[Q] – Principal impact indicator – Recommended once a salt iodization program has been initiated ii. Goiter assessment – By palpation and ultrasound to establish baseline severity of IDD iii. Neonatal thyroid stimulating hormone (TSH) levels – Helpful if hypothyroidism screening program pre-exists in country	i. Median urinary iodine levels in target population 100 µg/L ii. Level of iodization[Q] (30 ppm at production level and 15 ppm at consumer levels) iii. Total goiter rate <5%

Significance

- India is home to largest single goiter belt in world (Himalayan Goiter belt) covering about 2400 km and addition to this are other isolated goiter belts
- Iodine deficiency is one of the easiest deficiency to prevent with simple, cheap and appropriate technology like iodized salt
- Hence effective implementation of IDD control program can bring down the incidence and prevalence of iodine deficiency disorders in India
- 21st October is celebrated as Global Iodine Deficiency Disorders Day.

Ref: Tiwari BK; Revised Policy Guidelines on National Iodine Deficiency Disorders Control Program—Revised Edition October 2006, available as PDF at *http://nrhm.gov.in/nrhm-components/national-disease-control-programs-ndcps/iodine-deficiency-disorders.html* assessed on 22nd May 2014.

2. What is a randomized controlled trial? Outline the steps involved in conducting a RCT.

Refer Question No. 1 December 2015 (RS2) Paper I.

SHORT ESSAYS

3. What are the salient features of carriers? Classify the different types of carriers with examples.

Refer Question No. 1 June 2009 (RS2) Paper I.

4. What is balanced diet? Write briefly about the recommended dietary goals.

- A balanced diet is defined as one which contains a variety of foods in such quantities and proportions that the need for energy amino acids, vitamins, minerals, fats carbohydrates and other nutrients is adequately met for maintaining health, vitality and general well-being and also makes a small provision for extra nutrients to withstand short duration of leanness.

Prescribing a balanced diet	*Components of balanced diet*
▪ For constructing a balanced diet, following guidelines should be followed ▪ First and foremost, it should fulfill the daily requirement of protein, i.e. 15–20% of daily energy intake[Q] ▪ Next comes fat requirement which should be limited to 20–30% of daily energy intake[Q] ▪ Carbohydrates rich in natural fibers should constitute remaining food energy ▪ Requirements of micronutrients should also be met ▪ Pattern of food production climatic conditions of the region, economic capacity, religion, customs, taboos, tastes and habits of the person should also be borne in mind while prescribing a balanced diet	▪ For adult male weighing 60 kg and involved in moderate work Cereals 520 Pulses 50 Leafy vegetables 40 Other vegetables 70 Roots and tubes 60 Milk 200 Oil and fat 45 Sugar and jaggery 35

Dietary Goals

- Dietary goals are set of recommendations made by the WHO Expert Committee which forms the framework for formulating a balanced diet for an individual
- A diet satisfying these goals is called "Prudent diet".

Dietary Goals (WHO)

i. Dietary fat should be limited to approximately 20–30% of total daily intake[Q]
ii. Saturated fats should contribute no more than 10% of the total energy intake[Q]; unsaturated vegetable oils should be substituted for the remaining fat requirement (New Guidelines = <7%)
iii. Excessive consumption of refined carbohydrate rich in natural fiber should be taken
iv. Sources rich in energy such as fats and alcohols should be restricted
v. Salt intake should be reduced to an average of not more than 5 g per day[Q]
vi. Protein should account for approximately 15–20% of the daily intake
vii. Junk foods such colas, ketchups and other foods that supply empty calories should be restricted
viii. Total cholesterol intake through diet should not exceed 200 mg per day.

Significance

- Ultimate objective is achieve cholesterol/HDL ratio <3.5[Q]
- All countries should develop a National Nutrition and Food Policy setting out dietary goals for achievement
- These dietary goals should be adhered to while formulating a balanced diet
- However, these conditions may not be applicable for special groups like pregnancy, lactating mothers, medical disorders like diabetes.

5. What is health information system and what are its uses?

- Health information system is a mechanism for the collection, processing, analysis and transmission of information required for organizing and operating health services and also for research and training.

Objectives	*Requirements/Features (WHO)*	*Components*	*Sources*
▪ To provide reliable, relevant, up-to-date, adequate, timely and reasonably complete information for health managers at all levels ▪ To provide ability of sharing of technical and scientific information including bibliographical to all health personnel participating in health services of a country	▪ System should be population based ▪ System should avoid unnecessary agglomeration of data ▪ System should be problem orientated ▪ System should employ functional and operation terms like episodes of illness, treatment regimens, laboratory tests, etc.	▪ Demography and vital events ▪ Environmental health statistics ▪ Health status: mortality, morbidity, disability and quality of life	▪ Census ▪ Registration of vital events ▪ Sample registration system ▪ Notification of diseases

Contd...

Contd...

Objectives	*Requirements/Features (WHO)*	*Components*	*Sources*
▪ To provide data at periodic intervals which will show general performances of health services ▪ To assist planners in studying their current functioning and trends in demand and work load	▪ System should express information briefly and imaginatively in form of tables, charts or percentages ▪ System should make provision for the feedback of data	▪ Health resources: facilities, beds, manpower ▪ Utilization and non-utilisation of health services: indices of outcome of medical care ▪ Financial statistics related to the particular objective	▪ Hospital records ▪ Disease register ▪ Record linkage ▪ Epidemiological surveillance ▪ Other health service records ▪ Environmental health data ▪ Health manpower statistics ▪ Population surveys ▪ Other routine statistics related to health ▪ Non-quantifiable information

Uses[Q] (Application)

- To measure the health status of the people and to quantify their health problems and medical and health care needs
- For local, national and international comparisons of health status. For such comparisons the data need to be subjected to rigorous standardization and quality control
- For planning, administration and effective management of health services and programs
- For assessing whether health services are accomplishing their objectives in terms of their effectiveness and efficiency
- For assessing the attitudes and degree of satisfaction of the beneficiaries with the health system
- For research into particular problems of health and disease.

Significance

- Health information system is an integral part of national health system which is a basic tool of management and a key input for progress of society
- Unfortunately it is still difficult to get information where it matters the most, i.e. at community level and no country at present has such a thoughtfully constructed system of health information to provide data at community level.

6. Outline the steps involved in disinfection of a well.

- Wells constitute the main source of water supply in rural areas
- Since most of the wells are shallow wells, liable for contamination, need to be disinfected periodically more so during epidemics of acute gastroenteritis, cholera
- During such epidemics of water borne diseases, well are superchlorinated everyday, preferably twice a day, once in the early morning and once in the late afternoon in case of heavily used wells.

Disinfectants Used

- Bleaching powder.

Steps of well Chlorination

a. Finding the volume water in wells[Q]
 – It is done by using the formula

Circular well	*Rectangular well*
▪ Volume of well = $\pi r^2 h$ Where π = 3.14 r = radius of the well in meters h = height of the water column in meters ▪ Volume expressed in cu. meters 1 cu. mtr. In 1000 liters ▪ Therefore volume of water in mtr^3 X 1000 = X liters	▪ l x b x h x 1000 = X liters Where l = length of well in meters b = breadth of well in meters h = height of well in meters

b. Estimating the quantity of bleaching powder required[Q]
   - It is done using Horrock's apparatus[Q] which estimates chlorine demand of water[Q]

   Harrock's apparatus

   Contents
   - 6 white cups, each of 200 mL capacity
   - 1 black cup with a white circular margin inside, near the brim
   - 2 metal spoons, each level spoonful holds 2 g of bl. powder
   - 7 glass stirring rods
   - 1 special pipette
   - 2 droppers
   - Starch iodide indicator[Q] (Produces blue color).

   Procedure

   i. Preparation of stock (standard) chlorine solution
      - Take one level spoonful (2 g) of bleaching powder in the black-cup and make into a thin paste by adding little water
      - Add more of water gradually with stirring till the level reaches the white circular mark
      - Stir well and allow to settle, so that calcium of the bleaching powder settles down
      - This is the stock chlorine solution.

   ii. Estimating chlorine demand
      - Fill all the six white cups with water from the well, to be tested up to a cm below the brim
      - With the help of the pipette add standard chlorine solution as follows one drop to first white cup, two drops to second cup, three drops to third cup, so on and six drops to sixth cup
      - Stir the water in each cup with separate stirrers for each cup
      - Wait for half an hour for the action of chlorine in the water (Chlorination)
      - Add three drops of Starch-iodide indicator[Q] (Starch -Cadmium/potassium-iodide) for all the six cups and stir again
      - Development of blue color indicates the presence of free residual chlorine
      - The intensity of the blue color is directly proportional to the quantity of free residual chlorine in the water
      - If blue color is not obtained even in 6th cup, then the first cup is considered as 7th cup and counted subsequently as 8th, 9th, 10th up and so on and the test is continued by adding chlorine solution, 7 drops, 8 drops, so on respectively to all the remaining cups and the first cup showing distinct blue color is noted.

   iii. Calculations
      - The cup number indicates the number of level spoonfuls of bleaching powder for disinfecting 455 liters of water, so as to give 0.5 ppm of free residual chlorine concentration
      - For X liters of water in the well, quantity of bleaching powder is estimated
      - For superchlorination, one extra spoon is added per 455 liters of water.

c. Preparation of chlorine solution
   - Take estimated amount of bleaching powder in a bucket and make into a thin paste by adding little water
   - Add more water till the bucket is three-fourths full
   - Stir well and allow to sediment for 1-minute so that lime settles down
   - Transfer the supernatant chlorine solution to another bucket and discard the chalk or lime and do not pour into the well, because it increases the hardness of well-water.

d. Delivery of chlorine solution
   - Lower the bucket containing chlorine solution into the well, below the surface of the water and agitate vertically and horizontally, so that chlorine solution mixes with the well water uniformly.

   Double pot method
   - It is advocated during epidemics to ensure a constant dose of chlorine to the well-water.

   Equipment
   - It consists of 2 cylindrical pots, one placed inside the other
   - The size of the cylinders being 30 cm height and 25 cm diameter for the outer pot and 28 cm height and 16 cms diameter for the inner pot.

- Both the pots have an opening on the side
- The outer pot has an opening of about 1cm diameter near the bottom and the inner pot has the opening near the brim.

Procedure

- A mixture of 2 kg of coarse sand and 1 kg of bleaching powder is put in the inner pot and moistened with water
- It is then put inside the outer pot
- The surface is then closed with a polythene foil
- The double pot is then lowered into the well by means of a rope, for about 1meter below the water surface, to prevent the damage caused by the buckets used by the public
- The water from the outer pot enters into the inner pot, mixes with bleaching powder mixture
- The chlorine solution comes out slowly over a long period of time, thus ensuring constant chlorination over a long period of about 15–20 days, for a well containing about 4500 liters of water, having a draw-off rate of about 400 litres per day
- After 15–20 days, it needs to be removed, emptied, refilled and replaced for further chlorination
- The other types of chlorine diffusers are pot diffuser and coconut shell diffuser.

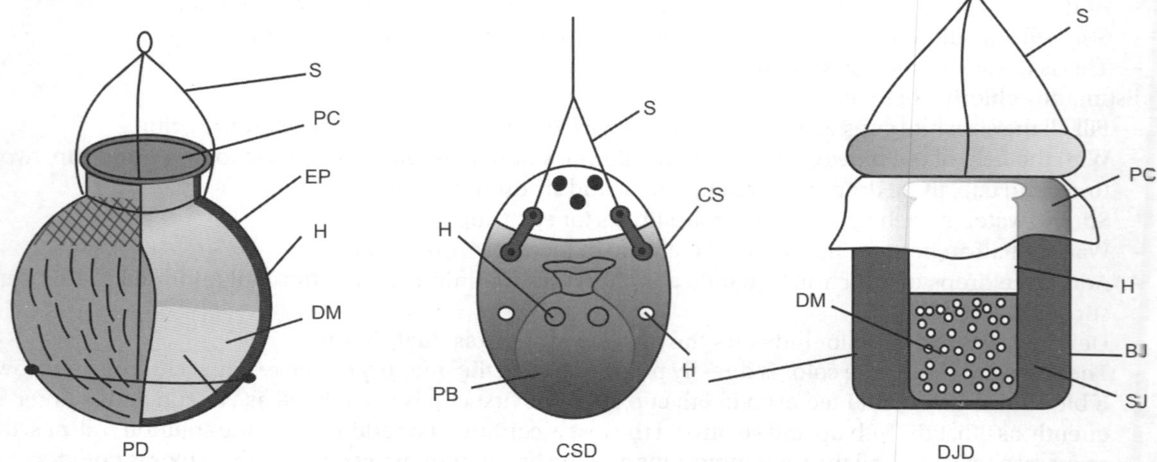

PD, pot diffuser; CSD, coconut shell diffuser; DJD, double jar diffuser; EP, earthenware pot; CS, coconut shell; BJ, big jar; SJ, small jar; H, hole; DM, disinfectant mixture; PB, polythene bag; PC, polythene cover; S, string

Fig. 1: Chlorine diffusers used during epidemics

e. Contact period
   - Allow contact period of one hour[Q] before the water is drawn for use.

f. Orthotoluidine test
   - It is done to verify whether water has been properly chlorinated or not[Q]
   - It free residual chlorine level is less than 0.5 ppm after contact period of one hour, the chlorination procedure should be repeated.

Significance

- Disinfection of well is the most basic procedure a doctor working in community needs to know as it goes a long way in preventing water borne diseases.

7. What are cross-sectional studies? Mention the advantages and limitations of this type of study design.

- Cross-sectional studies are a type of descriptive observational study conducted in population or a sample drawn from population over a very limited time span
- It is the simplest form of an observation study and is also called as prevalence studies
- This is a single examination of a cross-section of population wherein the exposure and the disease in a defined population is measured simultaneously.

Aims	*Steps*
▪ To find the disease pattern in the community to measure the disease burden ▪ To find the prevalence rate of diseases ▪ To formulate the etiological hypothesis ▪ To find the high-risk groups of various diseases ▪ To identify the risk factors or causes of various diseases	▪ Specify the aims of the study ▪ Define the study population ▪ Specify the problem to be studied ▪ Calculate the sample size depending upon the prevalence of problem under study ▪ Recruitment of sample by using appropriate sampling techniques ▪ Collection of information by using pretested questionnaire usually containing closed end type questions ▪ Analysis of collected data ▪ Formulation of hypothesis

Advantages	*Disadvantages (limitations)*
▪ Cross-sectional studies are simple and can be finished in short duration ▪ They are less costly than prospective study ▪ They are help to find out existence of both new and old cases of a disease (disease prevalence) ▪ They are more useful for chronic diseases ▪ They are usually starting point in prospective cohort studies ▪ They are useful for screening of diseases which are already existing in community ▪ They provide useful data for health care delivery systems like needs of the people, disease burden in the community, environmental data, nutritional data, etc. ▪ They allow formation of risk statements (though they may not be highly precise) ▪ They may help formulation of causal hypothesis by distribution patterns which can later be tested by analytical studies	▪ They give very less information about natural history of disease, time distribution of disease and incidence of disease ▪ They cannot be applied for short lived diseases like infections ▪ They do not provide direct estimates of risk factors ▪ They are prone to bias from selective survival ▪ Since exposure and disease are measured at same point of time, it is not possible to establish the temporality (time from exposure to development of disease) ▪ Concept of causativity (time sequence of disease) cannot be deduced from cross-sectional studies

Significance

- Cross-sectional studies are more advantageous than the case control studies
- They are useful for screening of population groups for undiagnosed diseases of public health importance.

8. Differentiate between monitoring and surveillance with examples.

Refer Question No. 7 June 2009 (RS2) Paper I.

9. What are the principles of health education?

Refer Question No. 2 December 2011 (RS2) Paper I.

10. What is neurolathyrism? Mention the causes, clinical features and interventions for control of the problem.

Refer Question No. 12 December 2009 (RS2) Paper I.

11. Write about the different methods of control of arthropods.

Refer Question No. 11 June 2010 (RS2) Paper I.

12. What are the functions of a family?

- Family is defined as a group of biologically related individuals living together and eating from a common kitchen.

Types	
a. Nuclear family (Elementary/Unitary family)	• Nuclear family is a type of family • Universal to all human societies *Characteristics* • It consists of married couple and their children till they are dependents[Q] • They occupy the same dwelling space • In a nuclear family, husband wife relationship is likely to be more intimate but the husband plays more dominant role • Another concept of nuclear family is new family which are families under 10 years of duration[Q] *Significance* • With rapid urbanization, nuclear family has become the norm even in developing countries
b. Joint or extended family	• Common in India, Africa, Far East and Middle East and more common in rural areas *Characteristics* • It consists of a number of married couples and their children who live together in the same household. All the men are related by blood and the woman of the household are their, wives, unmarried girls and widows of the family kinsmen • All the property is held in common. There is a common family purse to which all the family income goes and form which all the expenditures are met • All the authority is rested in the senior male member of the family who is the most dominant member and controls the internal and external affairs of the family. The senior female member by virtue of her being the wife of the male head shares his power so far the as the women of the family are concerned • Familial relations enjoy primary over martial relations • Merit of the joint family is based on the motto of 'union is strength' • Responsibilities are shared giving the family greater economic and social security • The old, helpless, unemployed and children are provided security socially and economically
c. Three generation family	• Fairly common in west *Characteristics* • Household where representative of three generations related to each other by direct descent live together • It usually occurs when young couples are unable to find separate housing accommodation and continue to live with their parents and have their own children

Functions

a. Residence
   - Family provides a clean and decent home to its members with cordial relations with each other providing safety and security
   - It is an identification and an address denoting an appropriate placement of the individual in the society
   - The homely comfort unwinds the tension of the hard working days and thus provides relaxation physically and mentally.

b. Division of labor
   - In a family, roles and functions performed by the members is well-distributed well-defined
   - Male members have sole duty to earn a living and support the family
   - Female members have total responsibility of running the household and case of children and elderly
   - However with modernization and urbanization, there is now greater sharing of responsibilities in a modern family.

c. Reproduction and bringing up of children
   - Very important function evident from the fact that a family originates after marriage
   - The biological urge of mating and procreation transforms the couple into parents, giving more meaning to life
   - In a family mother provides absolute care of the infant and children up to a certain age and father provides for education and food
   - Both parents together teach the child social customs and traditions.

d. Socialization
   - Family acts as a bridge between generation and between father and sons
   - It is the transfer point of civilization
   - By celebrating festivals and participating in social ceremonies and also by cultural and traditional practices, family helps to transmit cultural patterns and behaviors like eating cleanliness, dress, speech, language, behavior and attitudes from one generation to another.

e. Economic functions
   - Family handles issues like inheritance of the property and the ownership and or control of certain kinds of property like farm, shop or dwelling
   - The property is passes on from father to children in the family
   - All the income of the family is pooled and shared thus providing economic security to all the dependent members also in terms of food, clothes, shelter and other basic necessities of life.

f. Social care
   - Family provides social care by
     i. Giving status in a society to its members (Use of family names where it occurs)
     ii. Protecting its members from insult defamation, etc.
     iii. Regulating martial activities of its members
     iv. Regulating to a certain extent, political religious and general social activities
     v. Regulating sex relations through incest taboos
     vi. Education
   - Family is the temple of learning and the mother is the first teacher
   - Learning is far superior in the conducive atmosphere of love, care and personalized attention
   - The child learns the language, religion, morals, manners, habits and other elements of culture
   - The also learn traditional practices and religious beliefs
   - As they grow, they realize their rights, duties and responsibilities.

h. Emotional support
   - Family provides emotional support to its members at critical life events like failures, mishap, bereavement, loss, etc.
   - It provides support during pregnancy, child birth, marital conflicts, divorce, widowhood
   - It acts as buffer or shock absorber in the events of stress and strain.

i. Support
   - Family provides economic and social support to its members especially weaker individuals like elderly, handicapped individuals, children, widow, etc.

j. Bridging the generation gap
   - There is exchange of knowledge of culture from old to new generation while new generation brings in new modern concepts.

Significance

- Family is the basic component of a society and plays an important role in community medicine.
- It is the most powerful example of social cohesions[Q].

SHORT ANSWERS

13. Human development index.

Refer Question No. 3 December 2009 (RS2) Paper I.

14. Asbestosis.

- Asbestosis is a pneumoconiosis resulting from inhalation of asbestos dust over a long period of time
- Asbestos is fibrous, mineral silicate, i.e. silica combined with oxygen and other elements like calcium, magnesium, iron, sodium or aluminium
- Asbestosis does not usually appear until after 5–10 years of exposure[Q].

Types	*Industries using asbestos*
▪ Serpentine type or Chrysolite (white asbestos) (i.e. hydrated magnesium silicate) ▪ Amphibole type (hydrated silicate of iron, calcium and sodium)—most dangerous[Q] ▪ Crocidolite (or blue form)—more hazardous ▪ Amosite (or brown form)	▪ Manufacture of asbestos cement, sheets, pipes, gaskets, fire-proof textiles, etc. ▪ Mining, milling and in the manufacture of asbestos products

Pathology

i. Fibrosis	▪ There is fine, interstitial, diffuse fibrosis, around the terminal bronchioles, involving the walls of air spaces, tissue reaction being mainly due to mechanical irritation, usually in lower half of lungs ▪ Fibrosis is followed by bronchiectasis and emphysema ▪ X-ray chest shows "ground-glass" appearance of lower 2/3rd of the lungs and heart shows shaggy appearance without clear cut cardiac margins due to thickening of the pleura ▪ Sputum shows asbestos bodies, i.e. asbestos fibers coated with fibrin ▪ Pathology may progress even after cessation of exposure to asbestos dust
ii. Pleural calcification	▪ Pleura are thickened ▪ Calcified pleural plaques are seen, usually bilateral
iii. Neoplasms	▪ Common malignant lesion is bronchogenic carcinoma which is predisposed to by smoking ▪ Less common is malignant mesothelioma of pleura or peritoneum, often associated with effusion or ascites respectively
iv. Asbestos corns of skin	▪ This is due to local effect on the skin of the hands ▪ Spicules of asbestos penetrate the skin and result in corns and require excision

Prevention and Control

Refer Question No. 2 June 2012 (RS2) Paper I.

15. Predictive value of a screening test.

- Predictive value is an indicator of validity of a screening test
- It reflects diagnostic power of a screening test.

Depends Upon

- Sensitivity
- Specificity
- Disease prevalence (directly proportional to predictive value, i.e. more prevalent the disease, higher the predictive value).

Types

Predictive value of a positive test	*Predictive value of a negative test*
▪ It is the probability of an individual really having the disease, if the test result is positive, i.e. percentage of positives probably having the disease ▪ Mathematically, it is the ratio of true positives and the number of persons declared as having the disease by the screening test Predictive value of a positive test = $\frac{a}{a+b} \times 100$	▪ It is the probability of an individual really not having the disease, if the test result is negative, i.e. percentage of negatives probably not having the disease ▪ Mathematically it is the ratio of true negatives and the number of persons declared as not having the disease by the screening test Predictive value of a negative test = $\frac{d}{c+b} \times 100$

Significance

- A good screening test should also have high predictive value besides high sensitivity and specificity
- However, it is not a true indicator of validity of a screening test because it is affected by prevalence of the disease even if the sensitivity and specificity remain unchanged.

16. Differentiate between health education and propaganda.

Refer Question No. 11 December 2010 (RS2) Paper I.

17. Measures for the control of noise pollution.

Refer Question No. 4 December 2008 (RS2) Paper I.

18. What is sanitation barrier?

Refer Question No. 20 June 2008 (RS2) Paper I.

Revised Scheme 2

19. Acculturation.

Refer Question No. 19 June 2012 (RS2) Paper I.

20. Spot map.

- Spot map or geographic spot map is a pictorial depiction where the distribution of the disease frequency is represented in the form of dots or spots[Q], each dot representing an unit number of 10, 20, 30, etc. in the area map prepared
- Number of dots indicates the frequency in units, i.e. each dot (spot) marks one frequency.

Advantages

- These maps show at a glance areas of high/low frequency, the boundaries and patterns of disease distribution
- Deaths and disease can be marked separately by two different color dots.

Applications

a. Pictorial representation of disease frequency	Spot maps makes representation of disease frequency easy to see
b. Epidemiological studies	Spot maps helps in study of place of distribution, source or reservoir of infection and behavior of disease
c. Indentifying source of infection or common risk factor	If the map shows clustering of cases it may suggest a common source of infection or common risk factor
d. Monitoring a epidemics	These maps are prepared on weekly or monthly basis to help in monitoring changes in magnitude of epidemics over a period of time and also the direction of their spread
e. Study of inner and outer city disease frequency	Inner and outer city variations in disease frequency are well known and these variations are best studied with the aid of spot maps

21. What are nosocomial infections? Give examples.

- Nosocomial infection is an infection originating in a patient or others while in a hospital or other health care facility and manifesting either during hospital stay itself or after discharge
- It is cross infection occurring in the hospital and is also called as hospital acquired infection
- It denotes a new disease completely unrelated to patient's primary disorder, i.e. it was not present or incubating at the time of admission or residual of an infection acquired during a previous admission
- It also includes infections acquired in hospital but manifesting after discharge from hospital and also diseases occurring in a healthy staff of medical facility.

Examples

- Urinary tract infections
- Respiratory tract infections
- Infection of surgical wounds (postoperative infection)
- Hepatitis B.

Etiological agents	*Predisposing factors*	*Modes of transmission*
▪ Staphylococci (50%) ▪ Gram negative bacilli (45%)—*E. coli, Klebsiella, Proteus, Pseudomonas, Salmonella, Shigella,* etc. ▪ Others (5%)—viruses, protozoa, rickettssiae, fungi, etc.	▪ Failure to observe aseptic precautions ▪ Drug resistance among microorganisms ▪ Overcrowding in hospitals ▪ Poor environmental sanitation in hospitals ▪ Decreased resistance and increased susceptibility of vulnerable groups of patients	▪ By contact amongst patients themselves or contact with doctors ▪ By droplet infection ▪ By infected dust released while sweeping or bed making ▪ By fomites ▪ By parenteral or percutenous route (iatrogenic infections)

Prevention and Control

a. Elimination of sources and reservoirs	
i. Care of hospital staff	▪ Hospital staff suffering from any infectious disease should not be allowed to attend duties till complete recovery
ii. Care of the patients	▪ Admission of highly infectious cases in separate isolation wards only
iii. Treatment	▪ Prompt and specific treatment as early as possible to reduce infectivity
iv. Nursing care	▪ Barrier nursing—hospital staff acting as barrier to prevent cross infection by wearing gowns, gloves, masks while touching or examining certain infectious cases ▪ Task nursing—posting of nurses for specific tasks of patient, i.e. separate nurses for feeding, treatment, etc.
b. Breaking chain of disease transmission	▪ Disinfection of hands with soap and water or antiseptics soon after touching the patient suffering from contagious disease ▪ Isolation of highly infectious disease in isolation ward ▪ Concurrent disinfection of patient's discharges and fomites ▪ Avoiding overcrowding, adequate space, adequate lighting and adequate cross ventilation ▪ Vaccum cleaning of floor followed by wet mopping of floor preferably with phenyl ▪ Observing strict aseptic precautions and meticulous care and caution to prevent iatrogenic infections ▪ Safe and proper disposable of hospital waste ▪ Environmental engineering of hospital premises
c. Protection of susceptible host	▪ Highly susceptible patients should be isolated from others in special wards ▪ Protection of susceptible and hospital staff with vaccination like hepatitis B, tetanus, etc. ▪ Universal blood and body fluid precautions

Significance

- Prevalence of of nosocomial infection is estimated to be 25–40% in India and it is impossible to think in terms of eradication (though it is ideal) but infection rate of 1% is considered ideal.

22. What is pasteurization of milk? What are the tests used to check for the efficiency of pasteurization?

Refer Question No. 6 December 2009 (RS2) Paper I.

MBBS PHASE III EXAMINATION

JUNE 2013

(Revised Scheme 2)

PAPER II

LONG ESSAYS

1. Discuss epidemiology of malaria. Write briefly about its prevention and control.

- Malaria is a protozoal disease caused by infection with Plasmodium species of hemoparasites
- It is one disease that has taught health workers not to take any success lightly as it resurrected itself as a major health problem after being on verge of eradication.

Epidemiology

A. Agent factors
   a. Agent
      - In humans, malaria caused by 4 distinct species of the malaria parasite, namely
         - Plasmodium vivax (most common—70%)
         - *Plasmodium falciparum* (25–30%)
         - *Plasmodium malariae* (<1%)
         - *Plasmodium ovale* (very rare)
   b. Life cycle
      - Malarial parasite undergoes 2 cycles of development:
         - Asexual cycle in human (intermediate host)
         - Sexual cycle in mosquito (definitive host[Q])
            i. Asexual cycle
            It begins when an infected female anophelen mosquito bites a person and injects sporozoites
            Inside human host, *plasmodium* undergoes following phases of development

Hepatic phase	▪ Sporozoites disappear within an hour from peripheral circulation, most being destroyed by phagocytes, however, some reach the liver cells ▪ Depending upon species, sporozoites become hepatic schizonts in 1–2 weeks, which eventually burst releasing a shower of merozoites ▪ Number of merozoites produced from a single sporozoite varies considerably with infecting species (*P. falciparum* forms 40,000 merozoites whereas other species produce only 2,000 to 15,000 merozoites) ▪ Intrahepatic schizonts of plasmodia except falciparum do not burst all at the same time and remain dormant in the hepatocytes for considerable periods before they begin to grow and undergo pre-erythrocytic schizogony, thus liberating merozoites into blood causing relapses of these infections ▪ *P. vivax* and *P. ovale* may continue to relapse for 2 to 3 years and *P. malariae* may persist for 10 to 20 years or more ▪ *P. falciparum* does not exhibit this exo-erythrocytic phase ▪ Once the parasites enter the RBC, they do not reinvade the liver

Contd...

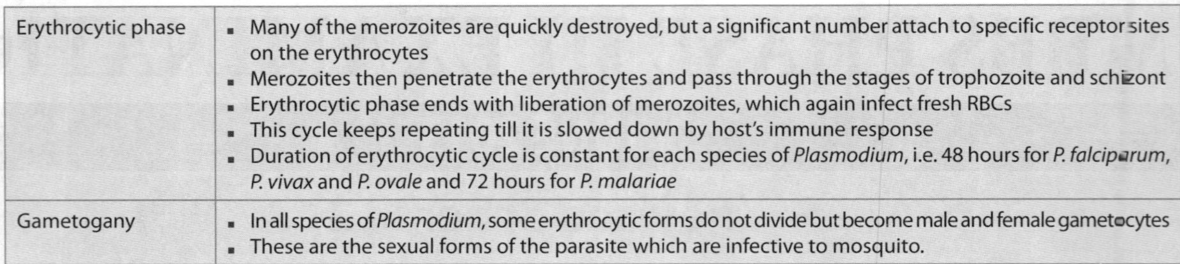

Erythrocytic phase	▪ Many of the merozoites are quickly destroyed, but a significant number attach to specific receptor sites on the erythrocytes ▪ Merozoites then penetrate the erythrocytes and pass through the stages of trophozoite and schizont ▪ Erythrocytic phase ends with liberation of merozoites, which again infect fresh RBCs ▪ This cycle keeps repeating till it is slowed down by host's immune response ▪ Duration of erythrocytic cycle is constant for each species of *Plasmodium*, i.e. 48 hours for *P. falciparum*, *P. vivax* and *P. ovale* and 72 hours for *P. malariae*
Gametogany	▪ In all species of *Plasmodium*, some erythrocytic forms do not divide but become male and female gametocytes ▪ These are the sexual forms of the parasite which are infective to mosquito.

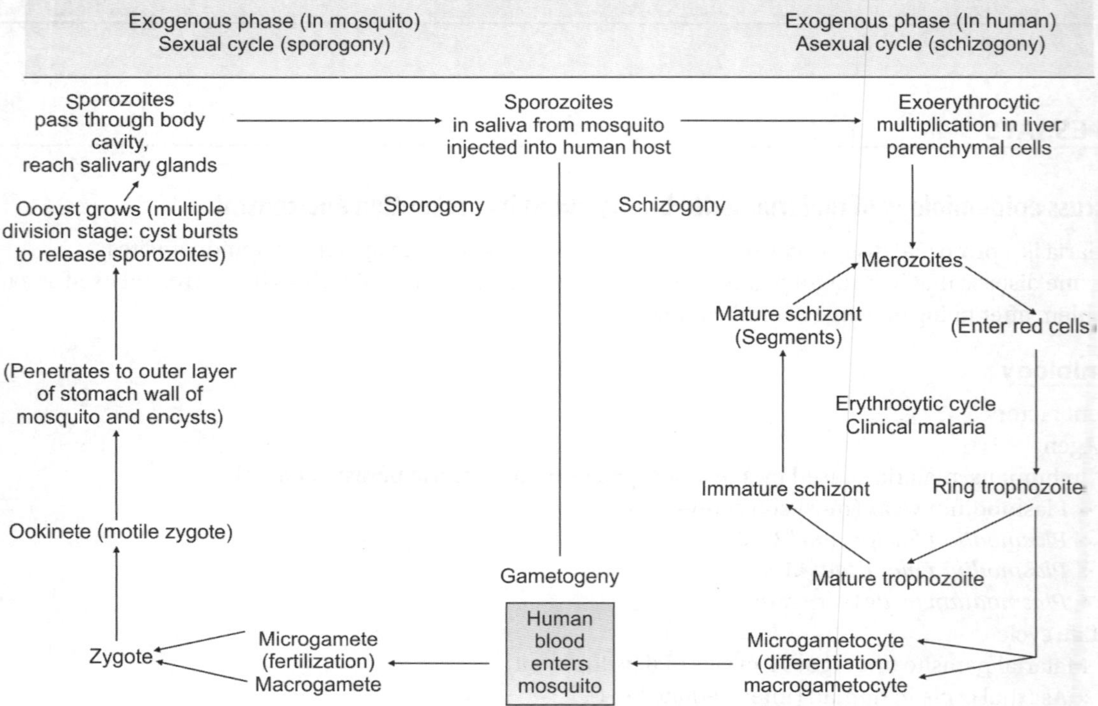

Fig. 1: Life cycle of *Plasmodium*

ii. Sexual cycle (sporogony)
- It begins when an anophelne mosquito ingests gametocytes while feeding on an infected person
- Gametocytes continue further development in the mosquito
- In stomach of mosquito 4–8 thread-like filaments called microgametes are developed by exflagellation of male gametocytes
- Female gametocyte undergoes a process of maturation and becomes a female gamete or macrogamete
- Microgametes are attracted towards the female gamete by chemotaxis, and one of the microgamete causes fertilization of the female gamete
- Resulting zygote is at first a motionless body, but within 18–24 hours, it becomes motile. This is known as Ookinete, which penetrates stomach wall of the mosquito and develops into an oocyst on the outer surface of the stomach
- Oocyst grows rapidly and develops within it numerous sporozoites, the infective form of parasite
- When mature, the oocyst bursts and liberates sporozoites into body cavity of mosquito
- Many sporozoites migrate to salivary glands of the mosquito, and the mosquito now becomes infective to man
- Time period required for development of parasite from gametocyte to sporozoite stage in the mosquito is called as extrinsic incubation period, which is about 10–20 days

- Extrinsic incubation period depends upon environmental conditions like atmospheric temperature and humidity.

c. Reservoir of infection
  - Human reservoir is one who harbors the sexual forms (gametocytes) of the parasite
  - A patient can be a carrier of several plasmodial species at the same time
  - Children are epidemiologically important reservoir than the adult because they are more likely to be gametocyte carriers than adults
  - For a person to serve as reservoir, he must harbor both sexes of mature, viable gametocyte in his blood in quantity sufficient density to infect mosquitoes
  - Only known animal reservoir is chimpanzees in tropical Africa, which may carry infection with *P. malariae*

d. Period of communicability
  - Malaria is communicable as long as mature, viable gametocytes exist in circulating blood in sufficient density to infect vector mosquitoes
  - In vivax infections, it is 4–5 days whereas in falciparum infections, it is 10–12 days period of maximum communicability is maximum in early stage of infection when gametocytes density may exceed 1,000/mm^3.

e. Relapses
  - Vivax and ovale malaria usually relapse more than 3 years after patient's first attack
  - It is derived from original, sporozoite-induced, liver schizonts which have lain latent long before bursting
  - Recurrences of falciparum malaria usually disappear within 1–2 years
  - *P. malariae* infection is known to persist for 40 years or more and causes prolonged low level, asymptomatic parasitemia
  - Relapses in *P. falciparum* and *P. malariae* infections is due to a chronic blood infection, i.e. erythrocytic schizogony persisting at a low level.

B. Host factors

a. Age	▪ No age is immune to malaria ▪ But newborns by virtue of presence of high concentration of fetal hemoglobin exhibit resistance to falciparum infection
b. Sex	▪ Females have less incidence of malaria because they are better clothed and live mostly indoor
c. Genetics (Race)	▪ Individuals with sickle cell trait manifest milder illness of falciparum ▪ People with duffy negative erythrocytes are resistant to vivax infection
d. Pregnancy	▪ Risk of malaria increases during pregnancy especially in primi para ▪ Causes intrauterine fetal death, premature labor and abortions
e. Socioeconomic development	▪ Prevalent in socioeconomic backward population
f. Housing	▪ Malaria is acquired mostly by insect bites within homes ▪ Ill-ventilated, ill-lighted houses are ideal indoor resting places for mosquitoes ▪ Site, type of construction, nature of walls, etc. influence selection of control measures
g. Population mobility	▪ Infected people amongst migrating population may import malaria parasites in their blood and reintroduce malaria into areas where malaria has been controlled or eliminated
h. Occupation	▪ Predominantly a rural disease and is closely related to agriculture practices
i. Human habits	▪ Man vector contact is influenced by habits such as sleeping out of doors, nomadism, refusal to accept spraying of houses, replastering of walls after spraying and not using measures of personal protection (e.g. bed nets)
j. Immunity	▪ Malaria epidemic is influenced by the immune status of the population which is acquired only after repeated exposure over several years ▪ Thus in endemic malarious areas, infants, young children, migrants and travellers from non-endemic areas suffer most from the disease ▪ Infants born of immune mothers are generally protected during the first 3–5 months by maternal IgG antibody whereas infants born of semi-immune mothers are only partially protected ▪ People living in endemic areas exposed continually to malaria develop considerable degree of resistance to clinical disease, but their partial immunity to malaria declines with time after they leave their endemic areas ▪ Active immunity is species—specific ▪ Both humoral and cellular factors play a role in this protection

C. Environmental factors

a. Season	▪ Seasonal disease with maximum prevalence seen in July to November
b. Temperature	▪ Optimum temperature for malarial parasite to develop is about 20–30°C
c. Humidity	▪ A relative humidity of 60% is necessary for mosquitoes to live their complete life span ▪ With rise in relative humidity, mosquitoes become more active and feed veraciously ▪ Fall in relative humidity, reduces the life span of mosquitoes
d. Rainfall	▪ Relationship between rainfall (total and its distribution) and mosquito breeding is fundamental importance ▪ Rain provides breeding opportunities to mosquitoes besides increasing their life span by increasing the relative humidity
e. Altitude	▪ Due to unfavorable climatic conditions, Anophelines mosquitoes are not found at altitudes above 2000 m
f. Drainage of sewage	

Vectors

- The vector of malarial parasite is female anopheline mosquito
- Out of about 45 species of anopheline mosquitoes in India, only a few are regarded as vectors of primary importance
- These include *An. culicifacies, An. fluuiatilis, An. stephensi, An. minimus, An. philippinensis, An. sundaicus* and *An. maculates*
- However, the most important vectors are *An. culicifacies*[Q] in rural areas and *An. stephensi*[Q] in urban areas.

Mode of Transmission

Vector transmission	*Direct transmission*	*Congenital malaria*
▪ Malaria is transmitted by bite of infected female anopheline mosquitoes having sporozoites in its salivary glands ▪ A single infected vector, during her life time, may infect several persons	▪ Malaria may be induced accidentally by hypodermic, intramuscular and intravenous injections of infected blood or plasma ▪ Blood transfusion poses a problem because parasites keep their infective activity during at least 14 days in blood bottles stored at–4°C	Congenital infection of the newborn from an infected mother may also occur, but it is comparatively rare

Incubation Period

- Usually not less than 10 days
- Varies with species of the parasite but on an average it is:
  - 12 (9–14) days for falciparum malaria
  - 14 (8–17) days for vivax malaria
  - 28 (18–40) days for quartan malaria
  - 17 (16–18) days for ovale malaria
- With some strains of *P. vivax*, it may be delayed for as long as 9 months.

Clinical Features

a. Febrile paroxysm
   - Primary manifestation is fever marked by paroxysms corresponding to the development of the parasites in the RBCs
   - Peaks of fever coincide with release into the blood stream of successive broods of merozites
   - Typical febrile paroxysm comprises three distinct stages, i.e. cold stage, hot stage and sweating stage, followed by an afebrile period in which the patient feels greately relieved

	Cold stage	*Hot stage*	*Sweating stage*
Features	▪ Onset is with lassitude, headache, nausea and chilly sensation followed in an hour or so by rigors ▪ Parasites demonstrable in blood	Feeling of burning hot and patient casts off his clothes	▪ Fever comes down with profuse sweating ▪ Feels relieved and often falls asleep
Temperature	Rises rapidly to 39–41°C	—	Drops rapidly to normal

Contd...

Contd...

Headache	Often severe and associated with vomiting	Intense but nausea commonly diminishes	—
Skin	Feels cold in early part this stage which later it becomes hot	Hot and dry to touch	Cool and moist
Pulse	Rapid and may be weak	Full and respiration rapid	Becomes slower
Duration	15–60 minutes	2–6 hours	2–4 hours

- This febrile paroxysms occur with definite intermittent periodicity repeating every third or fourth day depending upon the species of the parasite involved
- Classical 3 stages may not always be observed due to maturation of generations of parasite at different times
- Periods of latency may last several weeks or months
- In persons with poor immunity these paroxysms are associated with marked prostration.

b. Relapse
- Disease has a tendency to relapse and is characterized by enlargement of spleen and secondary anemia
- Febrile herpes is common in all malarial patients

Manifestations and Complications

Parasite	*Manifestations*	*Complications*
P. falciparum	▪ Primary fever in its first few days is usually irregular or even continuous and then the classical 48 hour periodicity becomes established or fever may continue to be irregular and the hot and cold stages ▪ Headache, nausea and vomiting usually more severe and greater tendency towards development of delirium, hemolytic jaundice and anemia ▪ Mortality is much greater than in other forms of malaria	Cerebral malaria, acute renal failure, liver damage, gastrointestinal symptoms, dehydration, collapse, anemia, blackwater fever
P. vivax	▪ Symptoms are same but are usually milder and more regularly divided into "hot" and "cold" stages	Anemia, splenomegaly, enlargement of liver, herpes, renal complications
P. ovale	▪ Milder than *P. vivax* and cease after a few paroxysms even if no treatment is given	
P. malariae	▪ Resemble those of *P. vivax* but the cycle is of 72 hours instead of 48 hours ▪ Tendency for long-term relapses to occur is marked	

Diagnosis

- Depends on demonstration of parasite in blood.

a. Microscopy
- Examination of blood films under microscope is useful in searching for and identification of malaria parasite
- Two types of blood films are prepared, thin film and thick film

Thick smear (sensitivity): Detects presence of malaria[Q]	*Thin smear (specificity): Identifies species*[Q]
▪ More reliable in searching for parasite, as large volume of blood is examined under each microscope field ▪ When scanty, parasite may be found about 20 times more rapidly in thick slide than in thin slide	▪ More valuable for identifying species of parasite as they are seen more clearly

- Stain used is JSB (Jaswant Singh Battacharaya) stain[Q]
- Recommended that both types of film be prepared on a single microscope glass slide

b. Malarial fluorescent antibody test
- Usually becomes positive 2 weeks or more after primary infection (by which time infection cures)

Advantages	*Disadvantages*
Greatest value in epidemiological studies and in determining whether a person has had malaria in past	A positive test is therefore, not necessarily an indication of current infection

c. Rapid diagnostic tests
   i. Dipstick tests (*P. falciparum* Histidine rich protein II – HRP II)
   - Used for rapid diagnosis of *Plasmodium falciparum*
   - Uses 2 antibodies specific for *Plasmodium falciparum* Histidine Rich Protein II Antigen[Q]
   - Is a antigen capture assay
   - Colloidal gold is used in the test card

Advantages	*Disadvantages*
▪ Latest, simple and rapid diagnostic technique ▪ Applied for evaluation of field trials and compare with microscopy ▪ Gives result in 3–5 minutes ▪ Specificity and negative predictive value is 99%	Not as effective when parasite level <100 parasite/ml of blood

d. Optimal test [Parasite specific lactic dehydrogenase (LDH dipstick test)]
   – Positive in *P. falciparum* and *P. vivax* parasitemia
   – Simple and rapid
   – Superior to HRP II[Q].

Prevention and Control

A. Elimination of reservoirs (i.e. control of parasites)
   a. Early diagnosis and treatment

Strategy

– First priority in malaria control is early diagnosis and prompt treatment of malaria cases to reduce morbidity and mortality as it is well within capability of existing primary health care system
– Under primary health care system, village health guides and multipurpose workers are fully trained to detect and treat cases of malaria at the community level with support from referral system, i.e. PHC and higher levels
– In addition, government has also established drug distribution centers and fever treatment depots manned by voluntary workers from community all across country in rural endemic areas to cope with malaria treatment
– As per new drug policy of 2013, all fever cases should be investigated for malaria either by microscopy or by rapid diagnostic test (RDT) and treat all positive cases
– Emphasis is on complete treatment in diagnosed cases of malaria rather than one single dose presumptive treatment to suspected case of malaria to avoid chloroquine resistance in *P. falciparum.*

   i. Case detection
   - All fever cases attending a PHC or hospital should be presumed to be of malaria and differential diagnosis should be clinical grounds.
   - 1 microscope per 30,000 population at PHCs in rural areas[Q] and for 50,000 population in urban areas
   - Diagnosis can be made by rapid diagnostic test
   - Diagnosis is aided by Link worker which caters to population of 2000[Q] in areas with high prevalence of *P. falciparum* who collects smears, and forward slides to PHCs
   - There is one fever treatment depot in every village.

   ii. Treatment
   - Extensive use of antimalarial drugs to prevent death and to reduce malaria morbidity are the declared objectives of the malaria program.

   a. Vivax malaria

Drug	*Duration*	*Day*	*Dose*	*Remarks*
Chloroquine	3 days	Day 1	10 mg/kg	
		Day 2	10 mg/kg	
		Day 3	5 mg/kg	
Primaquine	14 days		0.25 mg/kg	C/I in infants, pregnancy and G6PD def Taken after meals (not empty stomach)

b. Falciparum malaria
   i. In other states (other than North Eastern states)
      - Artemisine based combination therapy (ACT-SP)

Drug	Duration	Dose	Remarks
Artesunate	3 days	4 mg/kg	C/I in 1st trimester
Sulfadoxine	On day 1	25 mg/kg	C/I in children <5 months
Pyrimethamine	On day 1	1.25 mg/kg	
Primaquine	On day 2	0.75 mg/kg	

   ii. North-Eastern States
      - Artemether based combination therapy (ACT-AL)

Drug	Duration	Dose	Remarks
Artemether	3 days	80 mg BD	C/I in 1st trimester and children <5 kg
Lumefantrine	3 days	480 mg BD	
Primaquine	On day 2	0.75 mg/kg	

   iii. Uncomplicated Falciparum malaria in pregnancy
      - 1st trimester

Drug	Duration	Dose	Remarks
Quinine	7 days	10 mg/kg TDS	Should not be taken empty stomach

      - 2nd and 3rd trimester
         o ACT-SP in other states and ACT-AL in North-Eastern states

c. Mixed infections (*P. vivax* + *P. falciparum*)
   i. In other states (other than North Eastern states)
      - Artemisine based combination therapy (ACT-SP)

Drug	Duration	Dose
Artesunate	3 days	4 mg/kg
Sulfadoxine	1 day	25 mg/kg
Pyrimethamine	1 day	1.25 mg/kg
Primaquine	14 days	0.75 mg/kg

   ii. North-Eastern States
      - Artemether based combination therapy (ACT-AL)

Drug	Duration	Dose
Artemether	3 days	80 mg BD
Lumefantrine	3 days	480 mg BD
Primaquine	14 days	0.75 mg/kg

d. *Plasmodium* malariae
   - Treat as *P. falciparum*

e. *Plasmodium* ovale
   - Treat as *P. vivax*

f. Severe and complicated malaria

Initial parenteral treatment for 24–48 hours	*Oral treatment (following parenteral treatment)*	*Duration*	*Remarks*
Quinine 20 mg/kg (IV infusion at the rate of 5 mg/kg/hr OR IM divided doses) followed by 10 mg/kg 8 hourly (maintenance dose)	Quinine (10 mg/kg TDS) + Doxycycline (100 mg OD)	7 days	
	Quinine + Clindamycin	7 days	Pregnancy and children <8 years
Artemisin derivative Artemether—3.2 mg/kg IM at admission then 1.6 mg/kg/day Artesunate—2.4 mg/kg IV or IM at admission then at 12 hours and 24 hours, then OD Arteether—150 mg IM for 3 days	ACT-SP + Primaquine	3 days + On day 2	In other states
	ACT-AL + Primaquine	3 days + On day 2	In Northen Eastern states

iii. Chemoprophylaxis[Q]
- Though reliable, it can play a useful role in reducing the risk of infection
- Can be used for short-term (≤6 weeks) or for long-term (>6 weeks)
- Recommended regimes are:

Drug	*Dose*	*Start*
Chloroquine	300 mg (base) once a week on same day each week	1 week before travel
Chloroquine	100 mg (base) daily for 6 days per week	1 day before travel
Proguanil	200 mg OD	1 day before travel
Mefloquine	250 mg once a week on same day each week	2 weeks before travel
Doxycycline (for short-term only)	100 mg OD	1 day before travel

- It is usually recommended for travelers to areas or as a short-term measures for soldiers, police personnels or laborers serving in highly endemic areas
- It is also advocated for pregnant woman living in areas of high transmission to prevent low birth weight anemia
- Chemoprophylaxis should preferably begin a week before arrival[Q] in the malarious area and continued for at least 4 weeks or preferably 6 weeks after leaving[Q] the endemic area
- Chemoprophylaxis should be accompanied with personal protection and other methods of vector control.

B. Breaking the channel of transmission (control of vectors, i.e. anopheline mosquitoes)

a. Antilarval measures

i. Physical method (source reduction)
- Consists of reduction in the sites of mosquito breeding like drainage of filing, deepening or flushing, management of water level, changing salt content of water and intermittent irrigation, etc. are some of the classical methods of malaria control
- And if feasible, the major attention should be give to permanent reduction of sources by improvement of the environment.

ii. Chemical method
- Consists of application of larvicides over the breeding places
- Before applying larvicides, the breeding places should be cleared of scum and vegetations so as to maximize the efficiency
- Antilarval measures include oiling the collections of standing water or dusting them with paris green
- Application of temephos confers long effect with low toxicity
- However, larviciding must be repeated at frequent intervals making it a costly affair.

iii. Biological method
- Consists of using biocides such as using *Bacillus sphaericus* and *B. thuringensis*, which are effective against larvae of anopheline mosquitoes.

b. Antiadult measures
  i. Residual spraying
    - Spraying of indoor surfaces of houses with residual insecticides is still the most effective measure to kill the adult mosquito
    - It reduces the longevity of the vector to less than 10 days[Q]
    - Most commonly used insecticides are organophosphates—malathion and fenitrothion

Insecticide	*Vector resistance*	*No. of round*	*Dosage (g/m² surface)*
DDT	Sensitive to DDT	2	1.0 g
Malathion	Resistant to DDT	3	2.0 g
Pyrethrin	Resistant to DDT and malathion	2 (6 weeks apart)	0.25 g

Disadvantages
    - Spraying once applied may need to be continued for an indefinite period
  ii. Space spraying
    - Ultraflow-volume method of pesticide dispersion in form of fog or mist using special equipment by air or on ground
    - It reduce vector population quickly

Advantages
    - Effective and economical
  iii. Individual protection
    - Use of repellants, protective clothing, bed nets mosquito coils, screening of houses, etc. are some measures of individual protection of great value if properly employed
    - However, their cost is the major limiting factor.

C. Protection of susceptible
  a. Personal prophylaxis
    i. Insecticide treated bed nets
      - Use of insecticide treated bed nets resulted in significant decline in malaria incidence and API

Chemical used
      - Synthetic pyretheroids
      - Deltamethrine: 2.5% doasage of 25 mg/m^2
      - Cyfluthrine: 5% in dosage of 50 mg/m^2
      - Permethrin
      - Lambdacyhalothrin
      - Etofenprox
      - Cypermethrin.

Effectiveness of pyretheroids
      - 6–12 months (retreatment every 6 months)
      - Long lasting insecticidal mosquito nets use pyretheroids along with a chemical binder that allows nets to be washed >20 times allowing for use >3 years.

Quality of mosquito nets
      - Number of holes per square inch: >150
      - Diameter of each hole: <0.0475 inch.
    ii. Insect repellants
      - Chemicals that are rubbed on exposed parts of body to repel mosquitoes.

Chemical used
      - DEET (N, N-diethyl-m-toluamide)
      - Allethrine
      - Essential oil of lemon ecucalyptus
      - Icaridin (picaridin)
      - Nepetalactone (catnip oil)
      - Citronella oil

  - Permethrin
  - Soyabean oil
  - Neem oil.

b. Health education
  - The community at large has to be educated about the hazards of the disease, modes of transmission, importance of sanitation, cooperation in the night blood surveys, importance of taking complete treatment, use of mosquito nets and their cooperation in carrying out antimosquito measures.

c. Malaria vaccine
  - Even with significant progress in malaria vaccine development, valid candidate vaccines have been slow to enter clinical trial and an effective vaccine is thought to be at least 10 years away
  - Only promising vaccine is RTS, S/AS02 which has potential to prevent infection and/or ameliorate disease has been safely tested in adult volunteers with protection in 70% adults.

Significance

- In the absence of a vaccine, vector control is the only practical approach to malaria control
- The priorities and approaches for malaria control is based on epidemiological considerations, adverse effects on health, economy, technical feasibility, functional resources, human resources and community participation.

2. Define perinatal mortality rate. Describe the measures taken to reduce the same.

Refer Question No. 2 December 2011 (RS2) Paper II.

SHORT ESSAYS

3. Under-fives clinic.

Refer Question No. 2 December 2010 (RS2) Paper II.

4. Health problems of the elderly.

Refer Question No. 2 June 2009 (RS2) Paper II.

5. Vision 2020.

- Vision 2020 or the Right to Sight is a global initiative launched by WHO on 18th February 1999 to reduce avoidable (preventable and curable) blindness
- Government of India expressed its commitment by launching it on 14th October 2004.

Objective	*Goals*
▪ **To reduce avoidable (preventable and curable) blindness by 2020[Q]** by assisting member countries in developing sustainable system enabling them to eliminating avoidable blindness from major causes	▪ To reduce current projection of 75 million blind people to 25 million by 2020 ▪ To reduce prevalence of blindness in India to 0.5% by 2012 ▪ No childhood blindness needlessly after 2012 ▪ Provision of vision guardian for every 5000 population by 2020

Strategy

- Identification of target diseases like **cataract, refractive errors and low vision, onchocerciasis, childhood blindness, glaucoma, diabetic retinopathy[Q]**, trachoma and corneal blindness and their prevention and control

Global vision 2020 (**5 diseases[Q]**)	*Indian vision 2010* (**7 diseases[Q]**)
1. Cataract 2. Refractive errors and low vision 3. Childhood blindness 4. Trachoma 5. Onchocerciasis	1. Cataract 2. Refractive errors and low vision 3. Childhood blindness 4. Trachoma (Focal) 5. Glaucoma 6. Diabetic retinopathy 7. Corneal blindness

- Development of human resources by increasing the capacity and skill of ophthalmic personals
- Strengthening of existing eye care infrastructure
- Use of appropriate and affordable technology
- Mobilization of resources
- Development of 4 tier infrastructure and technology as follows:

Tier	*Situation*	*Center*	*Number*	*Services/Activities*
First	Primary level	Vision centers	20000	▪ Refractive and prescription of glasses ▪ Primary eye care ▪ School eye screening program ▪ Screening and referral services
Second	Secondary level	Service centers	2000	▪ Cataract surgery ▪ Other common eye surgeries ▪ Facilities for refraction ▪ Referral services
Third	Tertiary level	Training centers	200	▪ Tertiary eye care including corneal transplantation, glaucoma surgery, etc. ▪ Training and CME
Fourth	Tertiary level	Centers of excellence	20	▪ Professional leadership ▪ Strategy development ▪ CME ▪ Laying standards and quality assurance ▪ Research

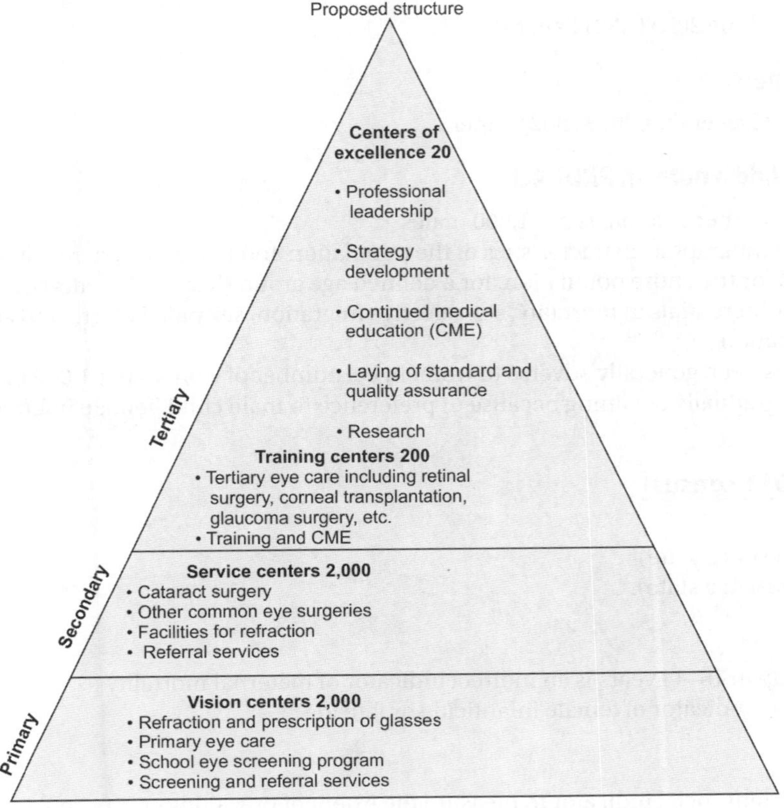

Fig. 2: Vision 2020—proposed infrastructure

Targets (Under 10th Five year Plan)

- Increase cataract surgery rate to 450 operations per one lakh population
- Improve visual outcome (>6/18) after cataract surgery in 80%
- Intraocular lens implantation in >80% of cataract surgery cases
- Development of 50 pediatric ophthalmology units in tertiary care hospitals
- Screen known diabetics for diabetic retinopathy
- Screen for glaucoma for those >35 years attending eye clinics
- Basic refraction services available in all districts
- 4000 vision centers manned by trained optometrist/refractionist/ophthalmic assistant
- Low vision centers at 590 centers of excellence/tertiary care
- 25 fully functional accrediated safe eye banks
- About 75% coverage for regular vitamin A supplementation (till 5 years of age).

Significance

- The Vision 2020 is a concept centered around the right issues, i.e. Recognition of sight as a fundamental human right.

6. Postexposure prophylaxis for rabies.

Refer Question No. 2 December 2008 (RS2) Paper II.

7. Mass drug administration against filariasis.

Refer Question No. 11 June 2011 (RS2) Paper II.

8. Functions of World Health Organization.

Refer Question No. 5 June 2009 (RS2) Paper II.

9. Disaster preparedness.

Refer Question No. 8 December 2012 (RS2) Paper I.

10. What is sex-ratio? Add a note on PNDT Act.

- Sex ratio is ratio of number of females per 1,000 males
- It is one the basic demographic characteristics of the population and it plays a vital role in study of any population
- It can be calculated for the entire population, for a defined age group (like 15–44 years) or at birth
- It is affected by sex differentials in mortality, sex selective migration, sex ratio at birth and at times sex differential in population enumeration
- Sex ratio in India has been generally adverse to women, i.e. number of woman per 1,000 males has always been less than 1,000 and it is gradually declining because of preference to male child, female infanticide, sex selective illegal abortions, etc.

Sex Ratio in India (2011 census)

- India—940
- Kerala—1084 (highest in a state)
- Haryana—877 (lowest in a state).

Applications

- Sex ratio of age group in 15–44 years is an indirect indicator of maternal mortality
- Sex ratio at birth is an indicator of female infanticide or feticide.

Significance

- Sex ratio is an important social indicator to measure the extent of prevailing equity between males and females in a society at a given point of time.

Preconception and Prenatal Diagnostic Techniques (Regulation and Prevention of Misuse) Act, 1994

- This act was passed by Parliament in 1994 and later amended in 2003
- It came into effect from January 1996.

Objectives

- To prevent misuse of modern prenatal diagnostic techniques particularly for selective abortion of female fetuses (To prevent female feticide).

Features

- It defines and prescribes prenatal diagnostic techniques
- It prohibits sex selection before and after conception
- It mandates registration of centers involved in prenatal diagnosis (genetic counseling centers, laboratories, USG centers, etc.)
- It imposes display of board specifying that sex determination is not done at this center
- It prohibits communication of sex of the fetus determined through any prenatal diagnostic technique through words/gesture/signs
- It requires consent of mother only
- It seeks to permit prenatal diagnostic techniques on a woman only in certain specified circumstances and in registered institutions.

Minimum Requirement for Performing Prenatal Diagnostic Technique

- Age of woman should be 35 years or more
- Should have undergone 2 or more spontaneous abortions or fetal loss
- Has been exposed to potentially teratogenic agents (drugs, radiations, infections or chemicals)
- Family history of mental retardation, genetic or chromosomal aberration in mother or father.

Records

- All records, charts, forms, consent letters and any other documents under this act has to be maintained for period of 2 years and if any criminal proceedings is instituted against any laboratory, the records should be preserved till final disposal of such proceedings.

Punishment

- Violation of any provision of this act is cognizable, non-bailable and compundable offence punishable with imprisonment up to 3 years and fine up to 10,000 and on subsequent occasions with imprisonment up to 5 years and fine up to 50,000
- If a registered medical practitioner is found to be involved in prenatal sex determination, in such case his name will be erased from the register of State Medical Council for a period of 2 years for first offence and permanently for subsequent offences.

Significance

- PNDT Act is a classical example of intercoordination between various ministries of Government of India to reduce fetal feticide.

11. Cancer screening in India.

- Early detection and prompt treatment of early cancer and precancerous condition provide the best possible protection against cancer
- Cancer screening is defined as search for unrecognized malignancy by means of rapidly applied tests.

Principle of Cancer Screening

- In many instances, malignant disease is preceded for a period of months or years by a premalignant lesion, removal of which prevents subsequent development of cancer
- Most cancers begin as localized lesions and if cured at this stage, high cure is obtained
- As much as 75% of cancers are accessible for screening.

Methods of Cancer Screening

Mass screening by comprehensive cancer detection examination	*Mass screening at single sites*[Q]	*Selective screening*
▪ A rapid clinical examination and examination of one or more body sites by the physician ▪ One of the important approaches for cancer screening	▪ Examination of single sites such as uterine **cervix**[Q], **breast**[Q]	▪ Examination of at risk people

Cancer Screening in Women

- Most common cancers seen in women are cervical cancer and breast cancer.

a. Screening for cancer cervix[Q]
   - Screening for a cancer cervix is very important aspect of prevention due to the following favorable facts
     - Cancer cervix is preceded by premalignant localized lesions such as cervical tear, chronic cervicitis, erosion, ectroprion
     - It has preinvasive stage, i.e. carcinoma in situ
     - The site is accessible unlike any other viscera
     - The lesion is localized for a fairly long time of about 8–10 years before it becomes invasive.

   Methods

   i. Pap smear or cervical smear examination for exfoliative cytology
      - Pap smear is very useful screening test in cancer cervix as it not only helps in detection of cases of cervical cancer but also prevents them from developing into invasive cancer
      - All women should have Pap test[Q] at the beginning of sexual activity and then every 3 years along with periodic pelvic examination
      - PAP smear is more useful but visual examination with acetic acid is more realistic
      - It should be directed at parous women of lower socioeconomic strata upwards of 35 years of age which are greatest risk of developing disease

   Disadvantages

Related to disease	*Related to test*	
	Response rate	*Sensitivity of PAP smear*
▪ Frequency with which the preinvasive phase progresses to invasive phase ▪ Frequency with which invasive cancer is preceded by abnormal smears	▪ It is least among women from poor socioeconomic status and also among illiterates	▪ PAP smear test has sensitivity of 89% and false negative is 20% and this sensitivity can be improved by taking the smear correctly and expert reporting

   ii. Colposcopic examination
      - The cervix is examined for change in color after application of Shill's iodine or acetic acid in high-risk women.
      - The change in color indicates cervical dysplasia which is even an earlier stage to carcinoma in situ.

b. Screening for cancer breast[Q]
   - Screening for breast cancer has a favorable effect on mortality from breast cancer

   Methods

   i. Breast self-examination by the patient (Breast self-examination)
      - All women should be encouraged to perform breast self-examination
      - Breast cancers are more frequently found by women themselves than by a physician during a routine examination
      - It is a useful adjuvant to early case detection

- Palpation is unreliable for large fatty breasts
- It forms the only feasible approach to wide population coverage.

ii. Palpation by a physician
- In high-risk groups cases or cases with lump in breast are examined by the physician.

iii. Thermography
- A safe method but not sensitive
- Can be employed in mass screening
- It has the advantage that the patient is not exposed to radiation.

iv. Mammography[Q]
- Most sensitive and specific tool[Q]
- Detects even small masses that may be missed on palpation
- Can be employed for selective screening.

Disadvantages
- Exposure to radiation (500 milliroentgen)
- Requirement of technical equipment of a high standard and radiologists with very considerable experience
- Biopsy from a suspicious lesion may end up in a false-positive.

c. Screening for endometrial cancer

Methods
i. Pap smear (not much useful)
ii. Ultrasonography[Q]
iii. Office endometrial washing[Q]
iv. Color flow imaging.

Cancer Screening in Both Sexes

a. Lung cancer
– It is doubtful whether disease satisfies criteria of suitability for screening.

Techniques
i. Chest radiography
ii. Mass radiography at six monthly interval is suggested for early diagnosis
iii. Sputum cytology

Significance

- Cancer screening is most important secondary prevention tool to prevent mortality and morbidity from cancer as most cancers are amenable to treatment when detected early.

12. Prevention of neonatal tetanus.

- Tetanus neonatorum or neonatal tetanus is form of generalized tetanus occurring in newborns
- Also called 8th day disease (because first symptom appears on 7th day)

Etiology	*Predisposing factor*	*Pathology*	*Clinical features*
Causative agent • Spores of *Clostridium tetani* Cause • Infection of umbilical cord stump due to lack of aseptic precautions while conducting the delivery	• Lack of maternal immunization with TT during pregnancy • Lack of hygiene environment during delivery • Lack of aseptic precautions while conducting delivery • Brutal habits of cutting the umbilical cord with rusted blade or knife, followed by application of cow dung to the umbilical cord to control bleeding • Use of dirty cloth to cover umbilical cord	• Spores on entry into body through umbilical stump, cause inflammatory process which provides favorable environment like presence of warmth and absence of oxygen for the spores to geminate into vegetative forms which later multiply and on autolysis producing exotoxins which enters the circulation, resulting in toxemia and ultimately lodge in the anterior horn cells of spinal cord and block inhibition of spinal reflexes	• Begins with poor suckling and excessive crying • Followed by trismus, difficulty in swallowing opisthotonus and tetano-spasms

Prevention and Control

- Training of dias or traditional birth attendants in conducting safe deliveries[Q]

- Providing disposable home delivery kits to pregnant mothers during antenatal checkups
- Provision of facilities for clean and safe deliveries in all PHCs and subcenters
- Ensuring essential newborn care with special reference to umbilical cord
- Education and practice of 5 clean practices[Q]
  - Five cleans is a strategy for elimination of neonatal tetanus wherein home deliveries are conducted under safe hygienic condition with more emphasis to aspesis
  - Local dais are taught these 5Cs during their training at PHCs and are provided a midwifery kit contains all essential equipments for practice of five cleans.

Components

Clean hands[Q] and fingernails	*Clean delivery surface[Q]*	*Clean cord cut[Q]*	*Clean cord tie*	*Clean cord stump*
Local dais should clean her hands before delivery with soap or antiseptic solution and use gloves through the delivery	Delivery should be conducted on a clean surface, preferably a clean plastic sheet or a disinfected bedsheet	Clean blade[Q] used to cut umbilical cord of newborn which should be preferably new or atleast sterilized	Clean thread used to tie cut umbilical cord should be new and sterilized	Stump of cut umbilical cord should be clean and practice of application of cow dung should be discouraged

Significance

- Introduction and regular practice of 5Cs by midwifes has improved maternal mortality and infant mortality rate significantly
- Sometimes these are also called 3 cleans, i.e. Clean delivery surface, Clean hand and Clean cord care (cut, tie and stump)
- Also suggested is seven cleans[Q] which includes 5Cs and clean water[q] and clean towel[q] for handwashing.

- Immunization
  - 100% coverage of expected mother with two doses of TT is very important for elimination of neonatal tetanus
  - Mother should be immunized with TT, first as early as possible during pregnancy and second at least a month later and at least 3 weeks before delivery if she is unimmunized[Q]. In immunized mothers, a single booster dose is sufficient[Q].
  - Infants born to the mothers who have not previously received 2—doses of TT can be protected by injection of antitoxin 750 IV, administered within 6 hours of birth.

Classification of Districts for Neonatal Tetanus Elimination

	Neonatal tetanus Incidence rate	*TT coverage to pregnant mothers*	*Attended deliveries*
High-risk districts	>1 per 1,000 live births	<70%	<50%
Control districts	<1 per 1,000 live births	>70%	>50%
Elimination districts[Q]	<0.1 per 1,000 live births[Q]	>90%	>75%

Significance

- Neonatal tetanus constitutes an important cause of preventable infant mortality in our country
- It carries very mortality and the case fatality rate is >90%
- It is easily preventable.

SHORT ANSWERS

13. *Aedes aegypti* index.

- *Aedes aegypti* index is an index of surveillance of *aedes* mosquito
- Also known as House index or Breteua index
- It is percentage of houses, in a defined area showing actual breeding of larvae of *Aedes aegypti* mosquitoes

$$\text{Aedes aegypti index} = \frac{\text{No. of houses showing actual breeding of larvae}}{\text{Total no. of houses in defined area}} \times 100$$

Revised Scheme 2

Normal Value

- Not more than 1.

Significance

- Aedes aegypti index is a WHO recommended index for surveillance of yellow fever, i.e. if this index become more than 1, then there is fear of outbreak of yellow fever
- It mandatory to ensure *Aedes aegypti* index around international airports and seaports to be maintained at zero in a 400 m perimeter[Q] (WHO International Health Regulations)
- This index can also be used to evaluate antilarval control measures.

14. Hardy -Weinberg law.

- Hardy-Weinberg law[Q] states that "in a large randomly breeding population, allelic frequencies will remain the same from generation to generation assuming that there is no mutation, gene migration, selection or genetic drift"
- Also called as Hardy-Weinberg principle
- This law was independently enunciated by Godfrey H Hardy, an English Mathematician and Wilhelm Weinberg, a German Physician in 1908
- It is a mathematical relationship that relates genotypes to allele frequencies which predicts how gene frequencies will be transmitted from generation to generation given a specific set of assumptions
- When a population meets all of the of the Hardy-Weinberg conditions, it is said to be in Hardy-Weinberg equilibrium (HWE).

Mathematical formula

- $p^2 + 2pq + q^2 = 1$
- Where 'p' and 'q' represent the frequencies of alleles and it is important to note that p added to q always equals one (100%).

Example

- The genes for height are represented as tall (TT), intermediate (Tt) and short (tt) and if they are to mate randomly, the several generations further will still have the same genes

Advantages	*Limitations*	*Application*	
		Is application only for[Q]	*Fails if applied to*[Q]
▪ Gives biologists a standard from which to measure changes in allele frequency in a population	▪ It assumes human population is static which never is the case	▪ Infinitely large populations ▪ Random mating populations ▪ Static populations	▪ Small populations ▪ Dynamic populations ▪ Non random mating ▪ Assortative mating ▪ Mutations ▪ Natural selection (mortality selection, fecundity selection) ▪ Gene flow ▪ Genetic drift ▪ Migration

Significance

- Hardy Weinberg law (Genetic equilibrium) forms the basic foundation and crucial unifying concept of population genetics, the entire principle is based on Mendelian genetics.

15. Contributions of Red Cross Society.

Refer Question No. 10 December 2013 (RS2) Paper II.

16. Triage.

- Triage is a different approach of medical treatment followed during disaster management where the number of casualties is very high and resources and medical supplies are limited.

Concept

- Triage consists of rapidly classifying the injured on the basis of the severity with prompt medical interventions and likelihood of their survival[Q]
- It does not follow regular "first come first serve" basis[Q]
- Highest priority is given to victims whose immediate or long-term prognosis can be dramatically affected by simple intensive care
- Low priority is given to those who are severely affected but even with treatment their survival is questionable.

International 4 Color Code System of Triage[Q]

Priority	Colors	Patient condition
a. Priority I (highest priority)	Red	Critically ill patients who need immediate medical/surgical treatment within 6 hours
b. Priority II (high)	Yellow	Moderately ill requiring resuscitation within 24 hours
c. Priority III (low)	Green	Ambulatory patients with minimum risk
d. Priority IV (least)	Black[Q]	Dead or moribund patients[Q]

Procedure

- Triage yields best results when carried out at disaster site[Q] and should be carried out at the disaster site[Q] in order to determine the transportation priority and admission to the hospital or treatment center where patients needs and priority will be reassessed.
- Triage sieve: Quick survey to separate the dead and the walking from the injured
- Triage sort: Remaining casualties are assessed and allocated to categories
- Tagging: Tagging of patient with identification, age, place of origin, triage category, diagnosis and initial treatment
- Training in triage should be done while training local health workers in disaster management
- Persons with minor or moderate injuries should be treated at the disaster site or their homes to void social dislocation where as seriously ill should be transported to hospital with specialized care.

Types of Triage

Simple triage	*Rapid triage*	*Reverse triage*
▪ Used in a scene of mass casualty, in order to sort patients into those who need critical attention and immediate transport to the hospital and those with less serious injuries ▪ This is required before transportation becomes available ▪ Categorization of patients based on the severity of their injuries can be aided with use of printed triage tags or color flagging	▪ START (Simple Triage And Rapid Treatment[Q]) is a simple triage system that can be performed by lightly trained lay or emergency personnel in emergencies ▪ It is not intended to supersede or instruct medical personal or techniques ▪ It may serve as an instructive example ▪ It has been field proven in mass casualty incidents such as train wrecks and bus accidents	▪ Here less wounded are treated in preference to more severely wounded in special situations ▪ A situation such as war where military setting may require solders to be returned to combat as quickly as possible ▪ Disaster situations where medical resources are limited in order to conserve resources for those likely to survive but requiring advanced medical care

Merits	*Demerits*
Triage is the only approach that can provide maximum benefits to the greatest number of injured in major disasters	It is an unethical practice

17. Rule of Halves.

Refer Question No. 12 December 2008 (RS2) Paper II.

18. Net reproduction rate.

- Net reproduction rate is a demographic indicator

- It is defined as the number of daughters a newborn girl will bear during her lifetime assuming fixed age specific fertility and mortality rates
- It is best index to assess recent fertility rate[Q]
- Net reproduction rate = ½ Total fertility rate (approximately)[Q].

Significance

- This is a measure of the extent to which mothers produce female infants who survive to replace them
- If NRR is 1, it means the female population is maintained exactly and population remains almost constant
- If NRR is less than 1, the population will decrease and vice versa if NRR is more than 1, the population will increase
- NRR of 1 can be achieved only if 60% of eligible couples practice one or the other method of family planning[Q] which is equivalent to attaining 2 child norm per couple[Q]
- Current level of NRR in India is 1.4[Q] which was to be reduced to 1 by 2006.

19. Incentives under National Family Welfare Program.

- National Family Welfare Program was launched in 1951 with the objective of "reducing the birth rate to the extent necessary to stabilize the population at a level consistent with the requirement of the National economy
- To increase the reach and acceptability of the contraceptive methods, it introduced cash incentives for the beneficiaries.

Incentives

a. For sterilization procedures[1]
   - ₹1,500 per case for vasectomy
   - ₹ 1000 per case for tubectomy in BPL/SC/ST cases
   - ₹ 650 per case for tubectomy for general category

Procedure	*Category*	*Individuals benefited*	*Incentive (₹)*
Vasectomy		Beneficiary	1100
		Motivator	200
		Surgeon	100
		Paramedical/Camp management	50
		Medicine	50
Tubectomy	BPL/SC/ST	Beneficiary	600
		Motivator	150
		Surgeon	75
		Paramedical/Camp management	50
		Anesthetist	25
		Medicine	100
	General	Beneficiary	250
		Motivator	150
		Surgeon	75
		Paramedical/Camp management	50
		Anesthetist	25
		Medicine	100

b. For institutional deliveries (government and accredited private institutions)[2,3]

Beneficiary	*Incentive (₹)*	*States*	*Categories*
Mother (up to 2 live births)	700 (rural)	High performing states (Andhra Pradesh, Gujarat, Haryana, Karnataka, Kerala, Maharashtra, Punjab, Tamil Nadu, West Bengal)	BPL, SC/ST and age ≥ 19 years
	600 (urban)		

Contd...

Contd...

	1,400 (rural)	Low performing states (Assam, Bihar, Madhya Pradesh, Odisha, Rajasthan, Uttar Pradesh, Uttaranchal, Chattisgarh, Jharkhand, Himachal Pradesh, and Jammu and Kashmir)	All pregnant women
	1,000 (urban)		
Cesarean delivery	1,500		
Travel allowance	250		
ASHA	600		

Significance

- Since introduction of cash incentives under Family Welfare Program, the number of permanent contraceptive procedures has increased thus indicating positive impact of the scheme.

Ref:

1. *http://pbhealth.gov.in/major12.htm* assessed on 23rd May 2014
2. Dongre A. Effect of monetary incentives on institutional deliveries: Evidence from the Janani Suraksha Yojna in India; A part of doctoral thesis available at *http://www.cdedse.org/ws2011/papers/Ambrish_Dongre_JSY.pdf* accessed on 23rd May 2014
3. Lahariya C. Cash Incentives for Institutional Delivery: Linking with Antenatal and Post Natal Care May Ensure 'Continuum of Care' in India. Indian J Community Med. 2009;34(1):15-8.

Revised Scheme 2

20. Enumerate the causes for maternal mortality in India.

Refer Question No. 2 June 2012 (RS2) Paper II.

21. Vaccine vial monitor.

- Vaccine vial monitor (VVM) is a heat sensitive chemical indicator label attached to the vaccine container by the vaccine manufacturer which records its cumulative heat exposure through a gradual change in its color
- It is a small, square-shaped, heat sensitive material placed on an outer circle of blue color printed on the label or on the vial cap in case of freeze dried vaccines
- The outer blue colored circle is used as reference to compare the color change in the central square of vaccine vial monitor.

Principle

- VVM is a label containing a heat sensitive material which is placed on a vaccine vial to register cumulative heat exposure over time
- Combined effects of time and temperature causes the central white square of vaccine vial monitor changes its color gradually from the light color at the starting point to darker with exposure to heat
- This darkening process is irreversible
- It indicates efficacy of cold chain[Q] (temperature maintenance)
- Main purpose is to ensure heat damaged vaccines are not administered.

Types	*Location*	*Vaccines with vaccine vial monitor*
▪ VVM2, VVM7, VVM14 and VVM30 ▪ The numbers indicate time in days that takes for the inner square to reach the discard point if vial is exposed to a constant temp of 37°C	a. On vaccine vial LABEL – Once opened, can be kept for subsequent sessions up to 28 days, regardless of formulation b. On location other than Label (cap, neck, etc.) – Once opened must be discarded at end of immunization schedule or within 6 hours of opening, regardless of formulation	▪ Oral polio vaccine ▪ Hepatitis B vaccine

Reading of Vaccine Vial Monitor

- Compare the darkness of inner square with that of outer circle
- If the inner square is lighter than the outer circle and the expiry date has not passed, the vaccine may be used
- If the inner circle matches the outer circle or even the darker the outer circle and if the expiry date has not passed, the vaccine is ineffective and must not be used[Q].

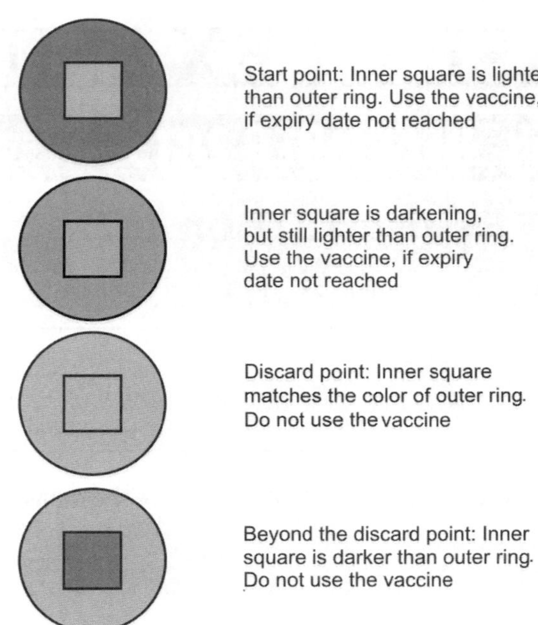

Fig. 3: Reading of vaccine vial monitor

WHO Grading (for OPV)

WHO grade	*Outer circle*	*Inner square*	*Inference*[Q]
Grade I	Blue	White	OPV can be used
Grade II	Blue	Light blue	OPV can be used
Grade III	Blue	Blue	OPV cannot be used
Grade IV	Blue	Purple/black	OPV cannot be used

- Thus OPV can be used up to Grade II[Q] whereas Grade III is discard point for OPV

Advantages	*Disadvantage*
▪ Vaccine vial monitor can help identify heat damaged vaccine ▪ Avoid unnecessary discarding of vaccine because of suspected heat exposure ▪ Can extend accessibility to vaccinations in remote areas beyond the reach of cold chain ▪ Can monitor the amount of vaccine discarded due to excessive heat exposure ▪ Can help identify cold chain problems	▪ Vaccine vial monitor does not directly measure the potency of the vaccine but gives information about the potency of the vaccine

Significance

- Use of vaccine vial monitor has become mandatory since 1998 thus ensuring quality assurance of the immunization program as it enables the health worker to ascertain whether the vaccine is potent[Q] or not
- It helps minimize vaccine wastage and helps health worker decide which vaccines to be used first (based on heat exposure rather than expiry dates).

22. Directly observed treatment (DOT).

Refer Question No. 2 December 2012 (RS2) Paper II.

MBBS PHASE III EXAMINATION

DECEMBER 2013

(Revised Scheme 2)

PAPER I

LONG ESSAYS

1. Discuss the epidemiology of protein-energy malnutrition. What are the measures taken for its prevention and control?

Refer Question No. 1 December 2012 (RS2) Paper I.

2. Define safe water. Enumerate the sources of water. What are the various methods of purification of water on small scale?

- Water is essence of life but not all water is safe for consumption
- Only safe and wholesome water is safest for human consumption
- If water does not meet the criteria of safe and wholesome water, it is considered to be contaminated or polluted.

Definition

- Safe and wholesome water[Q] is the water that is:
  - Free form pathogenic agents
  - Free from harmful chemical substances
  - Pleasant to taste, i.e. free for color and odor
  - Usable for domestic purpose.

Sources of Water

- Water source is any point in hydrological cycle which confirms two essential criteria
  - Quantity provided must be sufficient to meet present and future requirement
  - Quality of water must be acceptable.

Sources

Rain	Surface water	Ground water
	i. Impounding reservoirs ii. Rivers and streams iii. Tanks, ponds and lakes	i. Shallow wells ii. Deep wells iii. Springs

Purification at Small Scale (Domestic Level)

- Purification of water is of great importance in community medicine.
- The household or domestic purification of water can be done by single or combined use of any of the following method.

a. Boiling
  - Boiling is a satisfactory method of purifying water for household purposes
  - To be effective the water must be brought to a 'rolling boil' for 5–10 minutes because it kills all bacteria, spores, cysts and ova

– Water should be preferably stored in the same container in which water is boiled to avoid further contamination.

Advantages	*Disadvantages*
▪ It kills all bacteria, spores, cysts and ova ▪ It removes temporary hardness by driving of CO_2 and precipitating $CaCO_3$	▪ Taste of water is altered but this is harmless ▪ It offers no 'residual protection' against subsequent microbial contamination

b. Chemical disinfection

Chlorination

– The principle of chlorination is to ensure a free residual chlorine of 0.5 mg/L at the end of 1 hour of contact[Q]
– Disinfection action of chlorine is due to formation of hyochloric acid[Q]
– Most effective method water treatment in rural set-up[Q].

i. Bleaching powder	▪ Bleaching powder or chlorinated lime is a white amorphous powder with a pungent smell of chlorine ▪ Freshly made bleaching powder contains 33% available chlorine[Q] ▪ It is an unstable compound[Q] and rapidly loses its chlorine content on exposure to air, light and mixture ▪ But it retains its strength when mixed with excess of lime and is called stabilized bleach ▪ Therefore, it should be stored in cool, dark and dry place in a closed container and its chlorine content should be checked frequently
ii. Chlorine solution	▪ Prepared from the bleaching powder by mixing 4 kg of bleaching powder with 25% available chlorine is mixed with 20 liters of water to attain 5% solution of chlorine ▪ They are also liable to lose chlorine content on exposure to light or on prolonged storage. Therefore they should be kept in a dark, cool and dry place in a closed container
iii. High test hypochlorite	▪ High test hypochlorite (HTH) or perchloron is a calcium compound which contains 60–70% available chlorine ▪ More stable than bleaching powder and deteriorates much less on storage
iv. Chlorine tablets	▪ A chlorine tablets of 0.5g is sufficient quite good to disinfect 20 liters of water[Q] *Disadvantage* ▪ Tablets are costly
v. Iodine	▪ Used for emergency disinfection where 2 drops of 2% of ethanol soln. Of iodine suffice for 1 liter of clear water ▪ A contact time of 20–30 minutes is needed for effective disinfection *Advantages* ▪ Does not react with ammonia or organic compounds hence remain in its active molecular form over a wide range of pH values and water conditions and persists longer *Disadvantage* ▪ High cost ▪ Physiological activity of the iodine
vi. Potassium permanganate	▪ A powerful oxidizing agent *Advantage* ▪ Active against cholera vibrios

c. Filtration

– For small scale purifications filters such as Pasteur Chamberland filter, Berkefeld filter and Katadyn filters can be used
– The candle which is the essential part of the filter is made up of different material in different filters like porcelain in Chamberland type, kieselgurh or infusorial earth in Berkefeld filter, etc.
– In Katadyn filter, the surface is coated with a silver catalyst which kills the microorganism by its oligodynamic action.

Advantages	*Disadvantages*
▪ Cheap ▪ Removes bacteria	▪ Cannot remove viruses ▪ Only clean water should be used ▪ Requires periodic cleaning by scrubbing with hard brush under running water and boiling at least once a week

d. Ultraviolet radiation
   - Consists of direct exposure of film of water of about 1.5 cm thick to UV rays of 2538 Anstrom units (200–300 mm) emitted by mercury vapor quartz lamp
   - Thinner the water film, rapid the absorption of rays
   - Water should be free from turbidity.

Advantages	*Disadvantages*
▪ Destroys both vegetative and spore form of bacilli ▪ No residual effect ▪ Not harmful ▪ No taste or odor	▪ High cost of operation ▪ Regular maintenance ▪ Effectiveness diminished by color, turbidity and iron in water ▪ No rapid test for assessment

e. Reverse osmosis
   - Reverse osmosis is based on water reverse theory in nature.

Process

Stage	*Component*	*Significance*
▪ Stage 1	5μ sediment filter	Removes suspended impurities (sand, silt, dust and rust particles)
▪ Stage 2	Activated carbon block filter	Removes chemical impurities (chlorine, organic matters, colors and bleaches)
▪ Stage 3	Gag filter	Removes bad taste, color and odor causing harmful chemicals
▪ Stage 4	Reverse osmosis membrane (TF composite membrane with 0.0001 mm pore)	Removes dissolved salt, organics, bacteria, viruses, compound metals and minerals (allows only water molecules to pass through)
▪ Stage 5	Bacteriostatic silver impregnated activated carbon	Prevents growth of bacteria at point of use and removes color and odor

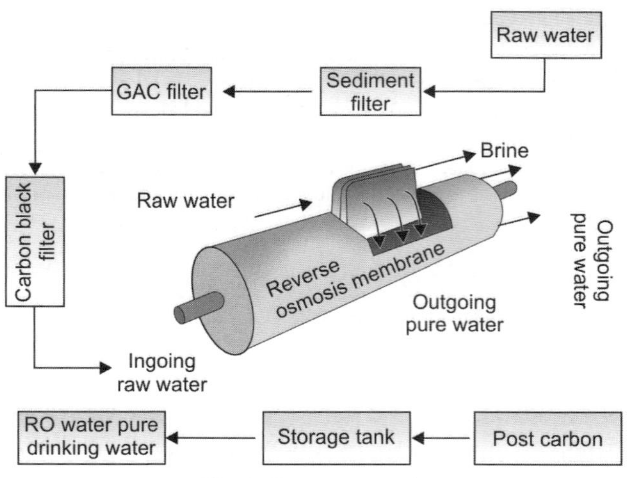

Fig. 1: Reverse osmosis

Advantages	*Disadvantages*
▪ Besides removing all pathogens, restores or improves natural taste of water	▪ Loss of naturally occurring minerals ▪ Slow process requiring long time to purify ▪ Wastage of water (for every 1 L of pure water, 4 L is wasted) ▪ Costly (initial investment high but becomes economical in long run) ▪ Regular maintenance

Significance

- Purification of water is very important aspect of environmental sanitation and every household should be well versed with method purification of water at domestic level for prevention of water-borne diseases.

SHORT ESSAYS

3. Define health. Enumerate the dimensions of health.

Most widely accepted definition of health given by World Health Organization in the preamble of its constitution is as follows:

- "Heath is a state of complete physical, mental and social well-being and not merely an absence of disease or infirmity."
- However, during 1997 Alma Ata conference, it has expanded to:
  - "Heath is a state of complete physical[Q], mental[Q] and social[Q] well-being and ability to lead socially and economically[Q] productive life and not merely an absence of disease or infirmity."

Dimensions of Health

- Health is a multidimensional entity
- These dimensions must contribute for positive health.

Dimension of Health

a. Physical dimension
  - The physical dimension of health implies the notion of "perfect functioning" of the body
  - It conceptualizes health biologically as a state in which every cell and every organ is functioning at optimum capacity and in perfect harmony with the rest of the body.

Signs of physical health	*Evaluation of physical health in an individual*	*Evaluation of physical health in a community*
▪ A good complexion ▪ A clean skin ▪ Bright eyes ▪ Lustrous hair ▪ A body well clothed with firm flesh, not too fat ▪ A sweet breath ▪ A good appetite ▪ Sound sleep ▪ Regular activity of bowels and bladder ▪ Smooth, easy, coordinated bodily movements ▪ All the organs of the body are of unexceptional size and function normally ▪ All the special senses are intact ▪ Resting pulse rate, blood pressure and exercise tolerance are within the normal range	▪ Self-assessment of overall health ▪ Inquiry into symptoms of ill health and risk factors ▪ Inquiry into medications ▪ Inquiry into levels of activity (e.g. number of days of restricted activity within a specified time, degree of fitness) ▪ Inquiry into use of medical services (e.g. the number of visits to a physician, number of hospitalizations) in the recent past ▪ Standardized questionnaires for cardiovascular diseases ▪ Standardized questionnaires for respiratory diseases ▪ Clinical examination ▪ Nutrition and dietary assessment ▪ Biochemical and laboratory investigations	▪ It is assessed by such indicators as death rate, infant mortality rate and expectation of life ▪ Ideally, each piece of information should be individually useful and when combined should permit a more complete health profile of individuals and communities

b. Mental dimension
  - Mental health is a state of balance between the individual and the surrounding world, a state of harmony between oneself and others, a coexistence between the realities of the self and that of other people and that of the environment
  - Thus mental health is not mere absence of mental illness but is the ability to respond to the many varied experiences of life with flexibility and a sense of purpose
  - Role of mental health can be understood by the fact that certain psychological factors can induce all kinds of illness, not simply mental ones like essential hypertension, peptic ulcer and bronchial asthma
  - Similarly some major mental illnesses such as depression and schizophrenia have a biological component

- The underlying inference is that there is a behavioral, psychological or biological dysfunction and that the disturbance in the mental equilibrium is not merely in the relationship between the individual and society.

Assessment of mental health in an individual	*Assessment of mental health in community*
▪ A mentally healthy person is free from internal conflicts; he is not at "war" with himself ▪ He is well-adjusted, i.e. he is able to get along well with others. He accepts criticism and is not easily upset ▪ He searches for identity ▪ He has a strong sense of self-esteem ▪ He knows himself: his needs, problems and goals (this is known as self-actualization) ▪ He has good self-control-balances rationality and emotionality ▪ He faces problems and tries to solve them intelligently, i.e. coping with stress and anxiety	▪ Assessment of mental health at the population level may be made by administering mental status questionnaires by trained interviewers ▪ The most commonly used questionnaires seek to determine the presence and extent of organic disease and of symptoms that could indicate psychiatric disorder; some personal assessment of mental well-being is also made

c. Social dimension
   - Social well-being is quantity and quality of an individual's interpersonal ties and the extent of involvement with the community
   - It implies harmony and integration within the individual, between each individual and other members of society and between individuals and the world in which they live
   - The social dimension of health includes the levels of social skills one possesses, social functioning and the ability to see oneself as a member of a larger society
   - In general, social health takes into account that every individual is part of a family and of wider community and focuses on social and economic conditions and well-being of the whole person in the context of his social network.

d. Spiritual dimension
   - Spiritual health refers to that part of the individual which reaches out and strives for meaning and purpose in life
   - It includes integrity, principles and ethics, the purpose in life, commitment to some higher being and belief in concepts.

e. Emotional dimension
   - A person is emotionally healthy when he does not lose temper or does not develop tension and possesses self-control.

f. Vocational dimension
   - An individual is healthy vocationally when he is capable of earning sufficiently to lead the life successfully
   - When work is fully adapted to human goals, capacities and limitations, work often play a role in promoting health, both physical and mental.

Others

- These include:
  - Philosophical dimension
  - Cultural dimension
  - Socioeconomic dimension
  - Environmental dimension
  - Nutritional dimension
  - Curative dimension
  - Preventive dimension.

Significance

- Dimensions of health symbolize a huge range of factors besides medical which contribute to attain a level of health that will permit individuals to lead a socially and economically productive life.

4. Integrated vector control.

Refer Question No. 11 June 2010 (RS2) Paper I.

5. Write the steps involved in a randomized controlled trial.

Refer Question No. 2 June 2013 (RS2) Paper I.

6. Stratified random sampling.

Refer Question No. 1 June 2016 (RS2) Paper I.

7. Cultural factors influencing health and disease.

Refer Question No. 12 December 2010 (RS2) Paper I.

8. Barriers in health communication.

Refer Question No. 5 June 2010 (RS2) Paper I.

9. What is web of causation? Explain with a suitable example.

- Web of causation is a concept of disease causation which considers all the predisposing factors like social, economic, cultural, genetic, and psychological factors
- This concept is ideally suited for the study of chronic diseases where the disease agent is often not known but outcome of interaction of multiple factors
- It shows that many risk factors interact with each other in disease causation but it does not imply that the disease cannot be controlled unless all the multiple causes or chains of causation or atleast a number of them appropriately controlled or removed
- Sometimes removal or elimination of just only one link or chain may be sufficient in pathogenic process.

Example

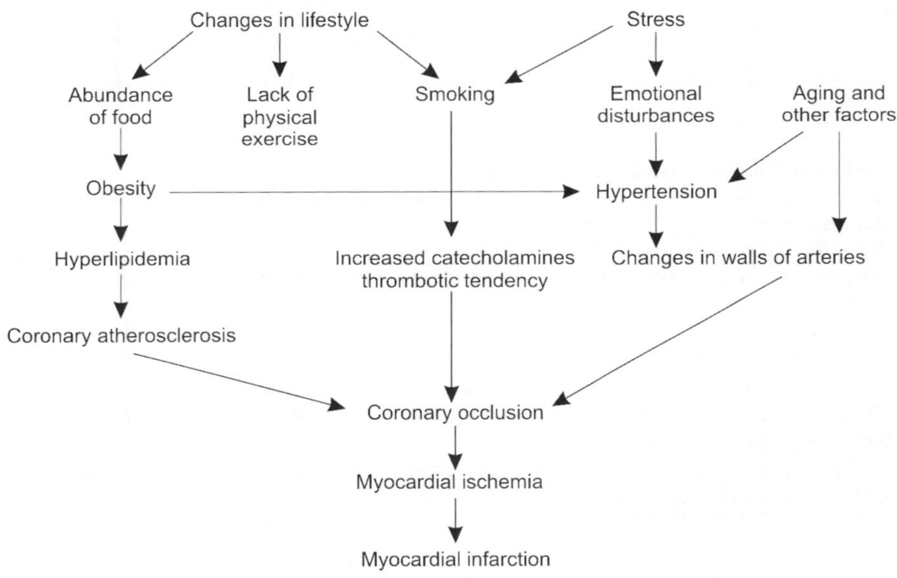

Fig. 2: Web of causation

Significance

- The concept on web of causation offers multiple approaches for the prevention and control of disease.

10. Disability indicators.

Refer Question No. 1 June 2008 (RS2) Paper I.

11. Epidemiology of silicosis.

- Silicosis is a pneumoconiosis caused by prolonged inhalation of dust containing free silica or silicon dioxide (SiO_2)

Industries

- Silica constitutes 1/4th of earth's crust and thus silicosis the most common industrial diseaseQ

- It is found in miners (of granite, sandstone, slate, coal, gold, tin and copper), quarry workers, tunnellers, sandblasters, grinders, ceramic workers, foundry workers, manufacturing of abrasives containing silica and peculiar to India in pencil, slate and agate grinding industry.
- About million workers in India are at risk of developing silicosis.

Epidemiology of Silicosis

Agent factors	
i. Chemical composition	• More complicated the composition of dust, greater the health hazard
ii. Size of particles	• Particles of 0.5–3 μm diameter are most dangerous
iii. Total dose	• Higher the dose of exposure, earlier the manifestation appear
iv. Duration of exposure	• Prolonged exposure leads to severe disease
Host factors	
i. Susceptibility of individuals	▪ Individuals with respiratory tract infections are more susceptible ▪ Better the health and nutritional status, lesser the chances of development of silicosis
ii.Occupation	▪ Seen in individuals employed in sand stone industry, stone quarrying and dressing, granite industry, pottery and ceramic industry and gold, silver, mica and steel industry
Environmental factors	
i. Poor ergonomics	If the industry does not employ methods to reduce silica dust, incidence of silicosis in its employees increases

Etiopathogenesis

Silicosis is caused prolonged inhalation of silicon dioxide or silica, often a few decades.

- The outcome depends upon the chemical composition of the dust, size of the particles total dose and duration of exposure and individual susceptibility.
- Incubation period varies from a few months up to 6 years of exposure.
- The pathogenetic mechanism of silicosis is as follows:
  - Silica particles between 0.5 μm and 5 μm size are taken up by the alveolar macrophages, which undergo necrosis. New macrophages engulf the debris and thus a repetitive cycle of phagocytosis and necrosis is set up.
  - Some silica laden macrophages are carried to the respiratory bronchioles, alveoli and in the interstitial tissue. Some of the silica dust is transported to the subpleural and interlobar lymphatics and into the regional lymph nodes. The cellular aggregates containing silica become associated with lymphoyctes, plasma cells, mast cells and fibroblasts.
  - Silica dust is fibrogenic. Crystlline form particularly quartz is more fibrogenic than non-crystalline form of silica.
  - Silica is cytotoxic and kills the macrophage which engulf it. The released silica dust activates viable macrophages leading to secretion of macrophage derived growth factors such as interleukin-1 that favor fibroblast proliferation and collagen synthesis.
  - Simultaneously, there is activation of T and B lymphocytes resulting in increased serum levels of immunoglobulins (IgG and IgM), antinuclear antibodies, rheumatoid factor and circulating immune complexes as well as proliferation of T cells.

DIAGNOSIS

Clinical Features

- Functional effects develop slowly and insidiously
- The manifestations can be divided into three stages:

First stage	*Second stage*	*Third stage*
There is mild dyspnea (dyspnea on exertion) which gradually increases. Clinical signs merge with little unproductive irritant cough and pain in chest. Working capacity is slightly affected	Marked dyspnea which impairs patient's ability to work and with clinical signs of bronchial breathing, dullness on percussion and scattered rhonchi. Total lung capacity is impaired due to development of obstructive or restrictive pattern of disease	Patient is totally incapacitated with signs of right heart failure

Investigations (Chest X-ray)

- Chest X-ray initially shows fine nodularity while later there are larger and coalescent nodules (Snow storm appearance)
- Radiological picture can be divided into four stages.

Latent stage	*Early stage*	*Late stage*	*Complicated stage*
Reticulation of lung fields due to thickening of perivascular and intercommunicating lymphatics	Nodules reach optimum size looking like "Lace", plus there is enlargement of hilar opacity. Silicotic nodules are 2–5 mm in diameter, homogenous in density and usually bilaterally symmetrical	Nodules coalescence giving "Snow storm appearance"	Large opacities with cavities indicating silico-tuberculosis

Treatment

- No effective treatment is available.

Complications

- Complications such as pulmonary tuberculosis (Silico-tuberculosis), rheumatoid arthritis (Caplan's syndrome) and cor pulmonale may occur.

Prevention and Control

- Silicosis can be controlled but fibrotic change cannot be reversed
- Measures for preventing silicosis are:

a. Health promotion	
i. Preplacement examination	▪ This consists of thorough examination of the individual before employing him in silica industry ▪ It should not only include thorough physical examination but also routine investigations including X-ray of the chest
ii. Health education	▪ Employees at the risk should be educated about the hazards of dust inhalation over long period ▪ They should be also educated about hazards of smoking as a precipitating factor and prevention of those hazards
iii. Provision of healthy physical environment	▪ Improvement of sanitation such as cleanliness, adequate ventilation, good house keeping like wet mopping of floors and walls are mandatory in industries
iv. Control of dust	▪ Prevention of formation of dust at the point of origin by water sprays, e.g. wet drilling of rocks ▪ Preventing escape of dust into atmosphere by special enclosures or cabinets or hoods for machinery at the point of origin of dust and such enclosures should be combined with exhaust ventilation so that the dust is drawn into the hood and conveyed through ducts into collecting units ▪ Arrangements to removal dust can also be made using special ventilatory mechanisms
b. Specific protection	▪ Workers should protect themselves by using face masks and other protective measures such as respirators and gas masks
c. Early diagnosis and treatment	▪ Workers should undergo periodic medical examination including chest X-ray so that the cases of silicosis can be detected early and removed from the job and transferred to some other job
d. Disability limitation	▪ Consists of limiting the further disability of the worker by detecting even the slightest degree of disability and immediately assigning some other suitable job
e. Rehabilitation	▪ Required to those workers who have become handicapped due to development of fibrosis of lungs. They require physical, psychological, social and vocational rehabilitation

Significance

- Silicosis is a notifiable disease under Factories Act, 1948 and Mines Act, 1952

Among occupational diseases, silicosis is the major cause of permanent disability and mortality.

12. Explain "specific protection" as an intervention in preventing a disease.

Refer Question No. 1 Jan. 2008 (RS2) Paper I.

SHORT ANSWERS

13. Physical quality of life index.

Refer Question No. 16 December 2007 (RS2) Paper I.

14. What do you mean by "de-professionalization of medicine"?

- De-professionalization of medicine means involvement of laymen in delivery of health care
- New cadre of health workers like community health workers, anganwadi workers, multipurpose workers, social workers, etc. are being considered and tried for providing health care to the community with relatively little training and support
- It is essential for providing primary health care.

Significance

- Though physician still holds unique position in health care in general however he can no longer restrict himself to his traditional role as detector of ailments, provider of treatment but is now also has become an educator, case finder, preventer, counsellor and an agent of social change.

15. What is "residual chlorine"?

Refer Question No. 5 June 2011 (RS2) Paper I.

16. What is euthenics?

Refer Question No. 8 December 2011 (RS2) Paper II.

17. Write briefly about odd's ratio.

Refer Question No. 1 June 2014 (RS2) Paper I.

18. Name any 4 criteria for a disease to be chosen for screening.

Refer Question No. 1 December 2010 (RS2) Paper I.

19. Mention the important duties of an anganwadi worker.

Refer Question No. 2 June 2010 (RS2) Paper II.

20. What is food adulteration? Give examples.

Refer Question No. 21 June 2010 (RS2) Paper I.

21. What are the health hazards due to overcrowding in a house?

- Overcrowding is the situation in which more people are living within a single dwelling than there is space for, so that movement is restricted, privacy secluded, hygiene impossible, rest and sleep difficult.

Standards

Persons per room		*Floor space*	
1 room	2 persons	100 sq feet or more[Q]	2 personsQ
2 rooms	3 persons	90–100 sq feet	1½ persons
3 rooms	5 persons	70–90 sq feet	½ person
4 rooms	7 persons	under 50 sq feet	Nil
5 or more	10 persons		

Health Hazard of Overcrowding (Role in Disease Transmission)

- Infectious diseases are more likely to spread rapidly in conditions of overcrowding

- There is increased risk of transmission of respiratory infections like tuberculosis, influenza, measles, whooping cough, common cold
- Due to proximity to each other, skin infections like scabies, impetigo, fungal infections, streptococcal and staphylococcal infection as likely to spread due to direct contact or fomites.

22. What are the diseases transmitted by aedes mosquitoes?

- Aedes mosquito is a group of mosquitoes

Habits	*Important species*	*Diseases caused*
▪ Widely distributed in India ▪ Most abundant during rainy season ▪ Breed in artificial collection of water in and around human dwellings	▪ Aedes aegypti ▪ Aeds vittatus ▪ Aedes albopictus	▪ Yellow fever (not in India) (first proved mosquito vector of viral disease) ▪ Dengue ▪ Dengue hemorrhagic fever ▪ Chikungunya fever ▪ Chikungunya hemorrhagic fever ▪ Rift valley fever ▪ Filariasis (not in India)

Significance

- Aedes mosquitoes occupy special importance in community medicine
- Aedes aegypti index is used as an important parameter for International Health Regulation at major ports.

MBBS PHASE III EXAMINATION

DECEMBER 2013

(Revised Scheme 2)

PAPER II

LONG ESSAYS

1. What are the epidemiological factors contributing to acute diarrheal diseases? Discuss briefly about its prevention and control measures.

- Acute diarrhea is defined as an attack of sudden onset of passage of loose, liquid or water stools which usually lasts 3–7 days but may last upto 10–14 days (WHO/UNICEF).

Epidemiological Factors

<table>
<tr><td>Agent factors</td><td></td></tr>
<tr><td>i. Etiological agents</td><td>
▪ In India, diarrhea is almost universally infectious in origin and a wide assortment of organism cause acute diarrhea
<table>
<tr><th colspan="3">Infectious</th><th rowspan="2">Non-infectious (20–30%)</th></tr>
<tr><th>Viruses</th><th>Bacteria</th><th>Others</th></tr>
<tr><td>▪ Rotavirus (15–25%)
▪ Astrovirus
▪ Adenoviruses
▪ Calciviruses
▪ Coronaviruses
▪ Norwalk group viruses</td><td>▪ Enterotoxigenic E. coli (10–20%)
▪ Campylobacter jejuni (10–15%)
▪ Shigella (5–15%)
▪ Salmonella (1–5%)
▪ Vibrio cholerae (5–10%)
▪ Vibrio parahaemolyticus
▪ Bacillus cereus
▪ Yersnia enterocolitica</td><td>▪ Cyptosporodium (5–15%)
▪ E. histolytica
▪ Giardia intestinalis
▪ Trichuriasis
▪ Intestinal species</td><td>▪ Kwashiorkor
▪ Sprue
▪ Celiac disease
▪ Pellagra</td></tr>
</table>
</td></tr>
<tr><td>ii. Reservoir of infection</td><td>▪ Man in principal reservoir for some enteric pathogens (E. coli, shigella, V. cholerae, Giardia lamblia, E. histolytica) whereas animal is important reservoir for some other enteric pathogens (Campylobacter jejuni, Salmonella, Y. enterocolitica)</td></tr>
<tr><td>Host factors</td><td></td></tr>
<tr><td>i. Age</td><td>▪ Diarrhea is most common in children especially between 6 months to 2 years
▪ Highest incidence is seen in age group of 6–11 months (when weaning occurs)
▪ Younger the age, faster the development of dehydration</td></tr>
<tr><td>ii. Sex</td><td>▪ Both sex are equally affected</td></tr>
<tr><td>iii. Coexisting conditions</td><td>▪ Diarrhea is more common in child with malnutrition
▪ Reduced gastric acidity, immunodeficiency can also predispose to diarrhea</td></tr>
<tr><td>iv. Socioeconomic factors</td><td>▪ Poverty, illiteracy, prematurity, lack of personal and domestic hygiene and incorrect feeding practices are contributory factors
▪ Malpractices in breastfeeding such as feeding prelacteal feeds, discarding colostrums, using feeding bottles, premature weaning play a significant role in infantile diarrhea</td></tr>
</table>

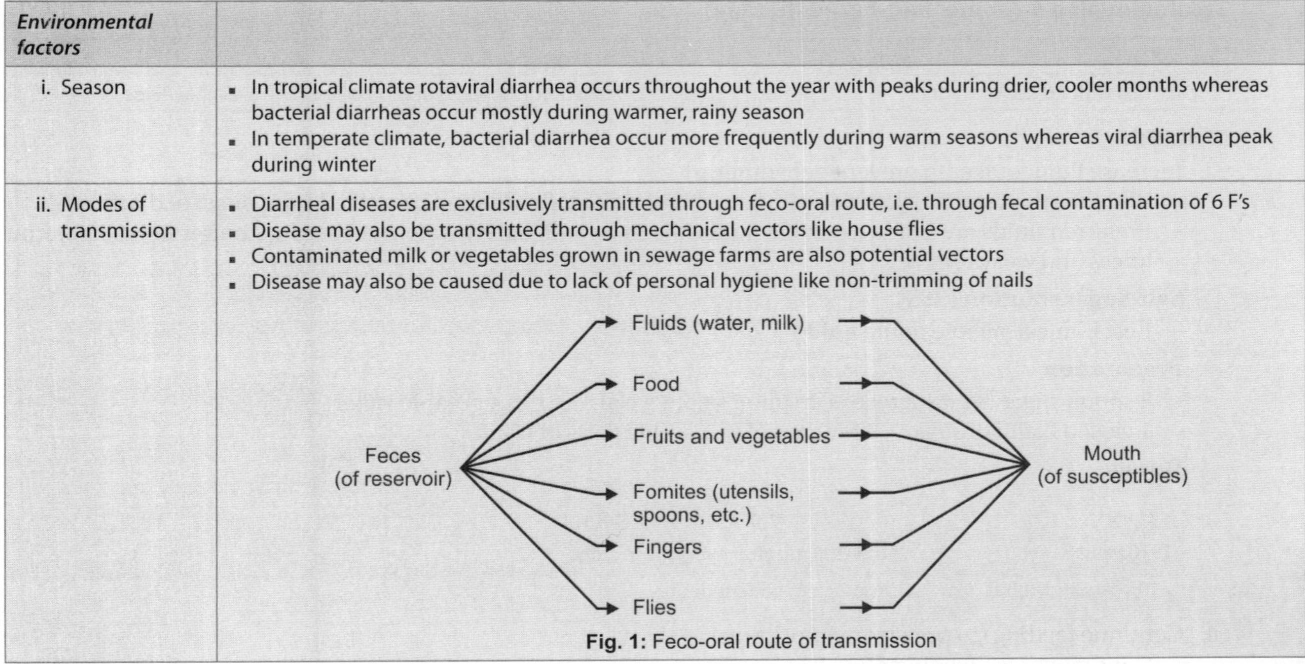

Environmental factors	
i. Season	▪ In tropical climate rotaviral diarrhea occurs throughout the year with peaks during drier, cooler months whereas bacterial diarrheas occur mostly during warmer, rainy season ▪ In temperate climate, bacterial diarrhea occur more frequently during warm seasons whereas viral diarrhea peak during winter
ii. Modes of transmission	▪ Diarrheal diseases are exclusively transmitted through feco-oral route, i.e. through fecal contamination of 6 F's ▪ Disease may also be transmitted through mechanical vectors like house flies ▪ Contaminated milk or vegetables grown in sewage farms are also potential vectors ▪ Disease may also be caused due to lack of personal hygiene like non-trimming of nails

Fig. 1: Feco-oral route of transmission

Assessment of a Child with Diarrhea

*Degree of dehydration**	*A*	*B*	*C*
Look for			
▪ General condition#	Well, alert	Restless, irritable#	Lethargic, floppy#, unconscious
▪ Eyes	Normal	Sunken	Deeply sunken and dry
▪ Tears on cry$	Present	Absent	Absent
▪ Tongue and mouth	Moist	Dry	Very dry
▪ Thirst#	Not thirsty (drinks normally)	Thirsty# (drinks eagerly)	Very thirsty# (drinks poorly or unable to drink)
Feel for			
▪ Skin pinch@	Goes back quickly within a second	Goes back slowly#, taking 1–2 seconds	Goes back very slowly#, taking more than 2 seconds
▪ Anterior fontenelle	Normal	Depressed	Very much depressed
Fluid deficit	<5% of body weight	5–10% of body weight	>10% of body weight
Diagnosis	No dehydration—Patient has no signs of dehydration	Some dehydration—Patient has 2 or more signs including atleast 1 key sign#	Severe dehydration—Patient has 2 or more signs including atleast 1 key sign#
Treatment	Plan A—With home available fluids to prevent dehydration	Plan B—With WHO recommended ORS solution to correct some dehydration	Plan C—With IV infusion urgently to correct severe dehydration and to prevent death

#KEY signs
*Always move from column C to column A for assessment and management
@Skin pinch is less useful in patients with malnutrition and obesity
$Tears on cry is a relevant only among infants and young children

Prevention and Control

A. Elimination of reservoir
   a. Prevention of dehydration (treatment plan A)

Treatment plan A (home fluid-based therapy)

Indications	*Objectives*
▪ Diarrhea with no dehydration	▪ Prevent further dehydration with home available fluids

Modalities

i. Increase fluid intake (to prevent dehydration)
- With diarrhea starts risk of dehydration, therefore oral fluids must be started from onset of diarrhea
- Preferred fluids are home available fluids like rice ganji, barely water, carrot soup, butter milk, lassi, fruit juices and weak tea

Salt-Sugar solution (SSS)
- Best home available home fluid

Preparation
- 8 spoon sugar (40 g sucrose) + 1 spoon salt (5 g NaCl) + 1 L of potable water
- 1 closed fistful of sugar + 3 pinches of salt + 1 big glass of water

Dosage

<2 years	50–100 mL after every loose stool
2–10 years	100–200 mL after every loose stool
>10 years and adults	As much as patient desires

ii. Continue feeding (to prevent malnutrition)
- Continue breastfeeding more frequently
- Give more soft cooked food if child is on solid food
- Give additional meals after episode of diarrhea

iii. Watch for signs of dehydration (to prevent acidosis, renal failure and death)
- Educate the mother to watch for signs of dehydration
- Instruct her to bring the child to doctor, if child does not improve even after 2 days or if he develops signs of dehydration.

b. Correction of some and severe dehydration (treatment plan B and C)

Treatment plan B

Indications	*Objectives*
▪ Some dehydration	▪ Correction of dehydration with WHO/UNICEF recommended formulations

Modalities

i. Oral rehydration therapy
- WHO recommended formulations (Reduced Osmolarity ORS—Low Na ORS[Q])

Composition (grams)		*Osmolar concentration (mmol/L)*	
Sodium chloride	2.6 g	Sodium	75 mmol/L
Trisodium citrate dehydrate	2.9 g	Potassium	20 mmol/L
Potassium chloride	1.5 g	Chloride	65 mmol/L
Glucose	13.5 g	Citrate	10 mmol/L
Potable water	1 L	Glucose	75 mmol/L
Total	20.5 g	Total	245 mmol/L

Dosage
- 50–100 mL/kg body weight per 4 hours

Age	<4 months	4-11 months	1–2 years	2–4 years	5–14 years	15 year
Weight in Kg	<5	5–8	8–11	11–16	16–30	>30
ORS in mL	200–400	400–600	600–800	800–1200	1200–2200	>2200
Local measure (glass)	1–2	2–3	3–4	4–6	6–11	12–20

Follow-up

- After 4 hours reassess child for degree of dehydration by moving from column C to column A
  * If there is improvement and no signs of dehydration → shift treatment to Plan A
  * If there is no improvement and some dehydration persists → continue Plan B
  * If there is severe dehydration → Shift treatment to Plan C.

Treatment plan C

Indications	*Objectives*
▪ Severe dehydration	▪ Urgent correction of dehydration with IV fluids

Modalities

i. Hospitalization and IV infusion
   - Child is immediately hospitalized
   - Fluid and electrolytes are replaced by intravenous infusion.

Fluids

Ringer lactate solution (Hartmann's solution for injection)	*Diarrhea treatment solution*
▪ Best IV fluid commercially available ▪ Supplies adequate concentration of sodium and potassium and lactate yields bicarbonate for correction of acidosis ▪ Used to correct dehydration due to acute diarrheas of all causes	▪ Ideal polyelectrolyte solution for intravenous infusion *Contents (per 1 lit)* ▪ NaCl: 4 g ▪ Na acetate: 6.5 g ▪ KCl: 1 g ▪ Glucose: 10 g

Dosage

Dosage	*30 mL/Kg*	*70 mL/kg*	*Total*
Infants	In 1 hour	In 5 hours	100 mL/kg in 6 hours
>1 year	In 30 minutes	In 150 mininutes	100 mL/kg in 3 hours

Follow-up

- Reassess child every 1 hour after stating IV infusion for signs of improvement (strong radial pulse, improved level of consciousness, improved ability to drink, skin turgor, passing of urine)
- Suspect renal failure, if patient does not pass urine within 3–4 hours and change over to mannitol drip till patient passes urine
- As general condition improves → change to Plan B

c. Maintenance of hydration
   - After correction of initial fluid and electrolyte deficit (indicated by reversal of signs of dehydration), hydration should be maintained using home-based fluids or ORS solutions till the patient is cured.

Principle

- Oral fluid intake should equal rate of continuing stool loss.

Dosage

	For children <10 years		*For children >10 years and adults*
Amount of diarrhea	Mild diarrhea (not more than 1 stool every 2 hours or longer or less than 5 mL stool/kg/hr)	Severe diarrhea (more than 1 stool every 2 hours or longer or more than 5 mL stool/kg/hr)	—
Amount of oral fluid	100 mL/kg body weight per day till diarrhea stops	Replace stool losses volume for volume, if not measurable give 10–15 mL/kg/hr	Provide as much as they like as thirst is adequate guide

d. Chemotherapy
   - Chemotherapy is indicated only when cause is known with fair degree of certainty
   - Antimicrobials have no role in viral diarrheas but they are essential to control bacterial and protozoal diarrheas
   - Antimicrobials do not shorten the duration of illness except cholera
   - Antimotility drugs should be avoided as they offer no specific protection but may prolong illness by giving time to bacteria to multiply in gut
   - Binding agents like pectin, kaolin, etc offer temporary psychological comfort by making stool more solid

e. Zinc supplementation
   - Zinc sulfate has shown to substantially reduce use of unwanted drugs, reduce infant mortality by 3-5% and also decrease further episodes of diarrhea following 2–3 months.

   Dosage (WHO/UNICEF)
   - It is given for 2 weeks as daily single dose of 20 mg for children above 6 months and 10 mg for children between 2–6 months

f. Restoration of nutritional status
   - Frequent breastfeeding or regular soft diet to older children helps to counter malnutritional effects of diarrhea

g. Treatment of associated features
   - Associated symptoms like fever, vomiting, abdominal pain are treated symptomatically

h. Notification
   - Cholera is a notifiable disease and any case of confirmed cholera needs to be reported to district health authorities

i. Isolation
   - Isolation is of little value in acute diarrheal diseases like cholera however cases and carriers should be isolated from drinking water sources

j. Surveillance
   - Maintaining records of all cases of diarrhea and their analysis helps to determine spread and pattern of disease outbreak
   - Pre-placement and periodic checkup of food handlers especially stool examination is also essential component of surveillance of diarrheal diseases.

B. Breaking chain of transmission

Sanitation	*Food hygiene*
▪ Provision of safe drinking water ▪ Sanitary disposal of excreta and sewage ▪ Hand washing after defecation, before eating or feeding infants ▪ Use of sanitary latrines to control vector-borne transmission ▪ Fly control ▪ Sanitary disposal of excreta and protection of food reduces vector borne transmission	▪ Proper care about food hygiene of children's food ▪ Use of safe water for cooking ▪ Food should be boiled and cooked properly ▪ It should be consumed when freshly cooked

C. Protection of susceptible

Health education (about)	*Specific protection*
▪ Mode of transmission of diarrheal diseases ▪ Diagnosis of dehydration at home ▪ Importance of ORS in treatment of diarrhea ▪ Use of sanitary latrines ▪ Washing of hands after defection to act as sanitary barrier ▪ Improvement in living conditions ▪ Sanitation in and around the house ▪ To maintain personal hygiene ▪ Correct weaning and feeding practices ▪ To use protected water for drinking and cooking purpose ▪ Disinfection of water on short scale, i.e. use of boiled and cooled water	▪ Immunization ▪ Regular measles immunization prevents post measles acute gastroenteritis ▪ Immunization against cholera during fear of outbreaks however it is of no use during epidemic ▪ Rota virus vaccines are also available ▪ Vitamin A prophylaxis ▪ Vitamin A prophylaxis for children below 3 years to prevent diarrhea by improving integrity of intestinal epithelium

Significance

- Diarrheal diseases are one of the major health problem faced by the community health worker but is easily preventable with proper health education and prompt treatment
- It is one disease where cost benefit ratio is better compared to others.

2. What are the millennium development goals (MDG's)? Critically analyse India's progress in achieving the goals with respect to maternal and child health.

- Millennium development goals are the goals set by the Millennium summit held in September 2000 at New York and attended by 189 countries.
- Baseline year of millennium development goal is 1990 and deadline year is 2015.

Goals

- To eradicate poverty and hunger
- To achieve universal primary education
- To promote gender equality and empower women
- To reduce child mortality
- To improve maternal health
- To combat HIV/AIDS, malaria and other communicable diseases
- To ensure environmental sustainability with an access to safe drinking water
- To develop a global partnership for development
- The charter prepared consists of 8 goals, 18 targets to achieve and 48 indicators to assess the efforts put in for achievement of these goals.

Important Health Related Millennium Development Goals in India

MDG	*Goals, targets and indicators*	*Year*	*India*
Goal 1	**Eradicate extreme poverty and hunger**		
Target 2	Halve between 1990 and 2015, the proportion of people who suffer from hunger		
Indicator 4	Prevalence of underweight children under 5 years of age	2014	29.4
Indicator 5	Proportion of population below minimum level of dietary energy consumption	2011	17.5
Goal 4	**Reduce child mortality**		
Target 5	Reduce by two-third between 1990 and 2015, the under five mortality rate		
Indicator 13	Under five mortality rate	2015	47.7
Indicator 14	Infant mortality rate	2015	38.0
Indicator 15	Proportion of 1 year old children immunized against measles	2015	83.0
Goal 5	**Improve maternal health**		
Target 6	Reduce by three quarters, between 1990 and 2015, the maternal mortality ratio		
Indicator 16	Maternal mortality ratio	2015	167
Indicator 17	Proportion of births attended by skilled health personnel	2010–2015	52
Target B			
	Contraceptive prevalence rate	2010–2015	55
	Adolescent birth rate	2013	31.5
	Antenatal care coverage (3 or more)	2006–2013	50
	Unmet needs for family planning	2006–2013	21.0
Goal 6	**Combat HIV/AIDS, malaria and other diseases**		
Target 7	Have halted by 2015 and begun to reverse the spread of HIV/AIDS		
Indicator 18	HIV prevalence among young people 15–24 years age group%	2012	0.1 (M) 0.1 (F)
	HIV prevalence among young people 15–49 years age group%	2012	0.1
Indicator 19	Condom use in high-risk population	2008–2012	32 (M) 17 (F)
Indicator 20	Ratio of children orphaned/non-orphaned in schools	2008–2012	72
Target 8	Have halted by 2015 and begun to reverse the incidence of malaria and other major diseases		
Indicator 21	Malaria death rate per 100,000 in children between 0–4 years Malaria death rate per 100,000 in all age groups Malaria incidence rate per 100,000	2008–12 2012 2012	8 2.3 1538

Contd...

Contd...

MDG	*Goals, targets and indicators*	*Year*	*India*
Indicator 22	Proportion (%) of population in malaria risk areas using insecticide treated bed nets Proportion (%) of population under age 5 with fever being treated with anti-malaria drugs	1990 1990	NA NA
Indicator 23	Tuberculosis death rate per 100,000 Tuberculosis prevalence rate per 100,000	2013 2013	19 211
Indicator 24	Proportion of smear positive pulmonary tuberculosis patients detected and put under DOTS	2012	64
	Proportion of smear positive pulmonary tuberculosis patients detected and cured under DOTS	2012	88
Goal 7	**Ensure environmental sustainability**		
Target 9	Integrate the principles of sustainable development into country policies and program and reverse the loss of environmental resources		
Indicator 29	Proportion of population using biomass fuels	2013	64
Target 10	Halve by 2015, the proportion of people without sustainable access to safe drinking water		
Indicator 30	Proportion of population with sustainable access by an improved water source	2011 2012	87 (F) 93 (U)
Target 11	By 2020 to have achieved a significant improvement in the lives of at least 100 million slum dwellers		
Indicator 31	Proportion of urban population with access to improved sanitation	2011	60
Goal 8	Develop global partnership for development		
Target 17	In cooperation with pharmaceutical companies, provide access to affordable, essential drugs in developing countries		
Indicator 46	Proportion of population with access to affordable essential drugs on a sustainable basis	1997	80

Health-related Goals[Q]

- 3 (i.e. 3, 4 and 6) out of 8 goals, 8 out of 18 targets and 18 out of 48 indicators are directly related to health.

Significance

- The areas of focus to improve the health are the communicable diseases, noncommunicable disease, nutrition and maternal and child health and these goals to be achieved not later than 2015[Q].

Analysis of Goals 4 and 5 in Regards to Maternal and Child Health

MDG	*Goals, targets and indicators*	*1990*	*2003–04*	*2007*	*2012–13*	*2015*
Goal 4	**Reduce child mortality**					
Target 5	Reduce by two-third between 1990 and 2015, the under five mortality rate (Target – 74.0)					
Indicator 13	Under five mortality rate	112.0	85.0	72.0	59.0	43.0
Indicator 14	Infant mortality rate	80.0	58.0	54.0	42.0	37.0
Indicator 15	Proportion of 1 year old children immunized against measles	32.7	56.0	--	--	87.0
Goal 5	**Improve maternal health**					
Target 6	Reduce by three-quarters, between 1990 and 2015, the maternal mortality ratio (Target–105)					
Indicator 16	Maternal mortality ratio	420	301	--	212	174
Indicator 17	Proportion of births attended by skilled health personnel	36	43	--	49	ε1 (2014)

- The above table clearly indicates the improvement in maternal and child health by fact that maternal and child mortality have reduced and proportion of birth conducted by skilled health professionals and vaccination cover against measles is improved
- Though we might have achieved the target 5 but we are very far from target 6.

Significance

- India is slowly but steadily moving towards achievement of millennium development goals by the deadline year 2015 all thanks to special focus on MCH services delivered to RCH program and NRHM.

Sustainable Development Goals

- Millennium development goals came to end of their term in December 2015, since 1st Jan 2016 they were replaced by 17 sustainable development goals
- It emphasises on development that meets the needs of the present without compromising the ability of future generations to meet their own needs
- It is unique in fact that it comprises of 5P's—People, Planet, Prosperity, Peace and Partnership
- It is designed to benefit all with basic motto of "Leaving no one behind"

Advantages	*Disadvantages*
SDGs call for action by all countries to promote prosperity while protecting the planet	It does not specifically mention that health is a human right

Health-related Goals

- Health is centrally placed within the 2030 agenda with one comprehensive Goal – SDG-3 "Ensure healthy lives and promote well-being of all ages"
- It includes 13 targets covering all major health priorities

	Goal and Targets	*Year*	*Indicator*
3.1	Reduce global MMR to <70 per 100,000 live births	2030	• MMR • Skilled delivery
3.2	Reduce under five mortality NMR - 12 per 1,000 live births U5 MR - 25 per 1,000 live births	2030	• NMR • U5 MR
3.3	End of epidemics of AIDS, TB, malaria and neglected tropical diseases and combat hepatitis, water borne diseases	2030	• % of new HIV infection • TB incidence • Malaria incidence • New Hep B infection per 100,000 population • Number of people requiring intervention against neglected tropical diseases
3.4	Reduce premature mortality by 1/3rd	2030	• Specific mortality rate (CVS disorder, cancer, diabetes, chronic RS disease) • Suicide mortality rate
3.5	Substance abuse – Prevention and treatment	—	• Coverage of treatment intervention • Per capita alcohol consumption
3.6	Reduce global deaths and injuries from RTA by half	2020	• Number of fatal RTA injuries within 30 days per 100,000 population
3.7	Universal access to sexual and reproductive health care services	2030	• Percentage of women in reproductive age group who have their needs for family planning satisfied • Adolescent birth rate
3.8	Universal health coverage		• Coverage of tracer interventions • Fraction of population protected against catastrophic/ impoverishing out-of-pocket health expenditure
3.9	Reduce number of deaths and illnesses from chemicals and pollution	2030	• Mortality rate due to household and ambient air pollution per lac population • Mortality rate due to chemicals, water and soil pollution

	Goal and targets	*Year*	*Indicator*
3.a	Implementation of WHO Framework Convention of Tobacco Control		• Age standardized prevalence of tobacco use in person aged >15
3.b	Support research and development in health care		• Proportion of population with aces to affordable medicine and vaccine • Total net official development assistance to medical research
3.c	Increase health financing and development of health workforce		• Health worker density and distribution per 10,000 population
3.d	Strengthen capacity of early warning, risk reduction and management of health risks		• Percentage of attributes of 13 core capacities been attained at specific point in time

Significance

- Along with the world, even India too adopted the SDGs and the priorities of SDGs are in convergence with the vision of the new Central Government which is a promising sign for the health sector
- Core principle of SDGs is end poverty and deprivation in all forms, leaving no one behind while making the development economically, socially and environmentally sustainable which is similar to policy of Central Government of "Sabka Sath Sabka Vikas".

SHORT ESSAYS

3. Specific protection for Japanese encephalitis.

Refer Question No. 6 December 2008 (RS2) Paper II.

4. School health program.

- School health is an important branch of community health which is an economical and powerful means of raising community health and more important future generations
- It was initiated in year 1960[Q]
- Renuka Roy School Health Committee (1961) laid the foundation for comprehensive school health program in India.

Objectives

- Promotion of position health
- Prevention of diseases
- Early diagnosis, treatment and follow-up defects
- Awakening health consciousness in children
- Provision of healthful environment
- Recognizing the child as a "change-agent" in the family.

Organization

- Health of the school child is the responsibility of the parents teachers, health administrate and the community and success or efficiency of school health services depends upon effective coordination between them
- The organizational set-up of school health service in Karnataka is as follows
- Most important functionary is school teacher[Q].

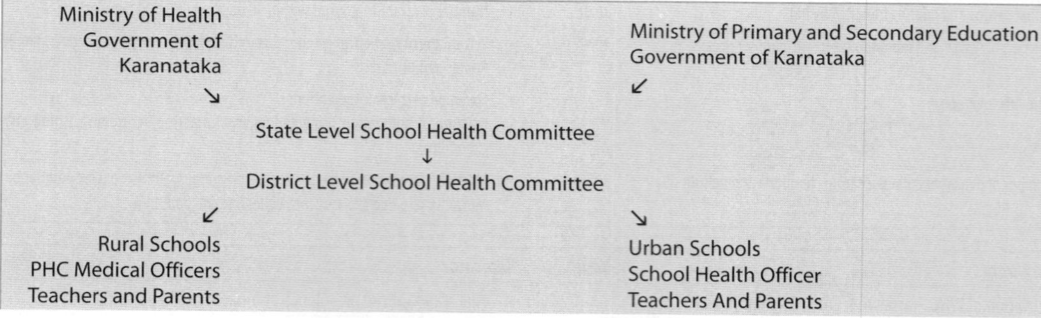

Health Problems of School Child

- A school health program should consider the health problems of school child
- The common health problems of a school child are:
  i. Malnutrition (123.5 per 1,000)
  ii. Infectious diseases
  iii. Intestinal parasites
  iv. Diseases of skin, eye and ear
  v. Dental defects like caries (180.3 per 1000)
  vi. Goiter (123.8 per 1,000)
- These problems will be addressed by the school health services.

Components (School health services)

a. Health appraisal of school children and school personnel
   i. Periodic medical examination of school children
      - A child should be examined at the time of entry into school and there after every 4 years
      - Under NHRM, school children are examined every 6 months[Q] (New Guidelines)
      - The initial examination should be thorough and detailed enough to include a careful history, physical examination, and tests for vision, speech and hearing
      - Laboratory examination of blood and urine should also be carried out
      - Special emphasis should be on diagnosis of any nutritional deficiency and any helminthic infestations.
      - A school teacher can assist this periodic medical examination by recording the medical history, quarterly recording the height and weight, annual testing of vision
      - He can also make understand the children the importance of medical appraisal thus preparing them for examination.
   ii. Periodic medical examination of school personnel
      - School personnel should be subjected to periodic medical examination as they are also part of school environment.
   iii. Daily morning inspection to children by teachers
      - Teacher is supposed to carry out daily morning inspection to detect any change in appearance or of the child such as:
         - Unusually flushed face
         - Any rash or spots
         - Symptoms of acute cold
         - Coughing or sneezing
         - Sore throat
         - Rigid neck
         - Nausea and vomiting
         - Red or watery eyes
         - Headache
         - Chills or fever
         - Listlessness or sleepiness
         - Disinclination to play
         - Diarrhea
         - Body pain
         - Dermatological conditions like scabies, ringworm
         - Pediculosis.
      - Such children should be referred to the school medical officer
      - For this function of school teacher, they should be trained adequately during teacher training courses and subsequently by short in service training courses.

b. Remedial measures and follow-up
   - Every medical examination should be followed by appropriate treatment and follow-up
   - For these purposes special clinic should be conducted at PHC in rural areas or at selected school or hospitals per 5000 students in urban with prior intimation to the concerned school regarding to date and time
   - These clinics should have doctors in all sphere with special emphasis on dental, eye and ENT doctors
   - There should be provision for beds as and when required in the referral hospitals for children.

c. Prevention of communicable diseases
   - A well-planned program should be conducted in school against the common communicable diseases
   - A record of all should be maintained as a part of the school health record and this record should accompany the student when the child migrates to another.

d. Provision of healthful school environment
   - A healthful school environment is necessary for the best emotional social and personal health of pupil
   - A school also serves as a demonstration center of good sanitation of community
   - The minimum standards for school environment and sanitation suggested in India

i. Location	▪ The school should normally be centrally situated with proper approached roads and at a fair distance from busy places and roads, cinema, houses, factories, railway tracks and markets ▪ School premise should be properly fenced and kept free from all hazards
ii. Site	▪ The school site should be on high land and not subjected to inundation or dampness and can be properly drained ▪ The prescribed land for a higher elementary school is 10 acres and for primary school 5 acres with additional 1 acre per 100 students ▪ A public park or playground should be made available to the students in urban congested areas
iii. Structure	▪ Nursery and secondary schools should be preferably single storied ▪ Exterior walls should have minimum thickness of 10 inches and should be heat resistant
iv. Classrooms	▪ A classroom should accommodate not more than 40 students[Q] and per capita space for students should be more than 10 sq. feet[Q] ▪ Every classroom should be attached to verandas
v. Furniture	▪ It is desired that every student should be provided single desks and chairs appropriate to the age of the child ▪ The desks should be of minus type[Q] and chairs should have proper back rests and facilities for desk work
vi. Door and windows	▪ The windows should be broad at level of 2 feet 6 inch from floor with bottom sill on opposing walls for cross ventilation ▪ The total door and window area should be at least 25% of floor area[Q] and ventilators should be more than 2% of floor area
vii. Color	▪ The classroom should be white and painted periodically
viii. Lighting	▪ Classrooms should have adequate natural light preferably from left but not from front
ix. Water supply	▪ There should be provision for continuous, safe and potable source of water to be distributed through taps
x. Eating facilities	▪ There should be clean hygienic place for eating or for midday meals ▪ Vendors other than those approved by the school authorities should be prohibited from school premises
xi. Lavatory	▪ A separate arrangement of privies and urinals should be for boys and girls with provision of at least one urinal per 60 students[Q] and 1 latrine per 100 students[Q]

e. Nutritional services
- The diet of school going children should contain all nutrients in proper proportions, adequate for maintenance of optimum health so that he can take full advantage of schooling
- An effort should be made to provide proteins, vitamin A and C, riboflavin, thiamine, calcium and iron
- The various schemes to combat nutritional deficiency as a part of school health program are:
  i. Midday school meal
    - Midday school meal program was started in 1962 on recommendations of School Health Committee[Q].

Objectives	*Principles*	*Model menu*
▪ Attract more children to school ▪ Prevent dropouts ▪ Combat malnutrition and improve health of school going children.	▪ An ideal midday meal should supply at least 1/3 of calorie requirement and ½ of protein requirement of the child[Q] ▪ It should be a supplement not a substitute to home diet, i.e. it should be provided at "no profit no loss" basis in school canteen to those cannot afford to bring their tiffin from home ▪ The menu should be such that it can be easily prepared in school without any complicated cooking process ▪ Use of locally available food should be encouraged ▪ Menu should be changed frequently to avoid monotony ▪ A child should receive 250 feeds per year	▪ Cereals and millets: 75 g ▪ Pulses: 30 g ▪ Oils/fats: 8 g ▪ Leafy vegetables: 30 g ▪ Non leafy vegetables: 30 g

  ii. Applied nutrition program
    - UNICEF is assisting the applied nutrition program in form of implement, seeds, manure and water supply equipments
    - If facilities are available, UNICEF provides assistance to develop school gardens to produce vegetable
  iii. Specific nutrients
    - Where ever feasible an attempt is done to provide specific nutrient responsible for nutritional deficiency

f. First aid and emergency care
- All teachers should receive adequate training during teacher training program or in-service training program regarding administration of first aid and emergency care in case such as:
  - Accidents leading to minor or serious injuries

- Gastroenteritis, colic, epileptic fits fainting, etc.
- A school should have a fully equipped first aid post.

g. Mental health
- Physical health and the learning process of a child is dependent on mental health
- Child is more prone for juvenile delinquency, maladjustment and drug addiction
- A school is most strategic place for shaping the child's and promoting mental health where school teacher has both positive and preventive role
- Every effort should be made to relieve the tedium of the classroom by planning school routine such that there is enough relaxation between periods of intense work
- In schools, no discrimination should be made amongst the students based on race, religion, casts, immunity intelligence family status, etc.
- There should be a vocational counselor and psychologist in schools for guiding the children to choose suitable career.

h. Dental health
- Children frequently suffer dental diseases especially dental caries and periodontal disease therefore there should be a provision for dental examination at least once a year
- Teachers should also teach dental hygiene to the students.

i. Eye health services
- School and amblyopia and detection and treatment of refractive errors, treatment of squint and amblyopia and detection and treatment of eye infections such as trachoma,
- Children at risk of developing xero-ophthalmia should be identified and they should be administered vitamin A.
- Under school eye screening program
  - Focus is on middle school (10-14 years age in 5th–8th std)
  - A single teacher examines 150 students[Q]
  - Children with visual acuity <6/9[Q] are referred to PHC.

j. Health education
- Besides academics a child should be taught about health to bring about desirable changes in health knowledge, in attitude and in practice
- Providing health education is the job of school teacher with assistance of teaching material and advice from health officer, public health nurse/health worker/health assistant
- Advantage of providing health education to children is that they take back the information to their parents and most important can pass it on to their children when they grow up
- Health education in school comprise

i. Personal hygiene	▪ School health education should be lively, practical and based on every day needs and interest such as hygiene of skin, hair, teeth and clothing ▪ Attention should be paid to posture of the child and such tendencies should be corrected at this stage only
ii. Environmental health	▪ Encourage young people to take part in health activities and keep their environment clean ▪ Take school children on visit to observe community health program and should be encourage to participate in them
iii. Family life	▪ Concerns with the development of health lives and healthy attitudes towards human reproduction

k. Education of handicapped children
- With cooperation of health, welfare, social and educational agencies, the handicapped children and his family is assisted so that the child will be able to reach their maximum potential to lead as normal a life as possible to become independent as possible and to become a productive and self-supporting member of society.

l. School health records (Swarna Aragya Chaitnya)
- A cumulative health record of each student should be maintained which should comprise.
  - Identifying data–name date of birth, parent's name and address, etc.
  - Post health history
  - Record of findings of physical examination and screening tests and record of services provides.
- These health records helps to have a cumulative information on the health aspects of school children in order to give continuing intelligent health supervision which is useful in analyzing and evaluating school heath programs and providing a useful link between the home school and the community.

5. Salient features of National Program for Control of Blindness.

Refer Question No. 2 December 2015 (RS2) Paper II.

6. Ring immunization.

- Ring vaccination is a process of administering vaccine only to the people who are in close contact with an isolated infected patient
- It is a process of isolation characterized by surrounding an infected patient or a non-immune person by a group of immune persons or vaccinated individuals.

Principle	*Procedure*	*Advantages*
▪ It prevents spread of highly infectious disease by surrounding the patient with a ring of immunization ▪ Idea is to form a buffer of immune people to prevent the spread disease in the event of an outbreak ▪ A film of vaccine virus prevents spread of wild or infective virus	▪ Ring immunization is done following a report of a vaccine preventable disease ▪ Usually the doses are given for a population of 5000 or 5 villages whichever is high ▪ However, there is no hard and fast criteria and can be modified as per the requirement	▪ Controls an outbreak of an epidemic ▪ Monitoring is made easy ▪ Can be used to protect nonimmunized children also

Example

- Measles
- Polio
  - Whenever a suspected case of polio is reported, all children below the age of 5 years (minimum 5,000 children) in he affected area covering an area of radius of 5 km are given extra dose of oral polio vaccine within 24–48 hours and extra dose is repeated to the same children after one month.

Significance

- Ring immunization can be compared to fire lines in forest used to prevent forest fires from spreading.

7. Strategies for measles elimination.

Refer Question No. 1 December 2010 (RS2) Paper II.

8. Down's syndrome.

- Down's syndrome or mangolism or trisomy 21 is a chromosomal disorder due to nondisjunction.

Karyotype	*Etiology*	*Pathogenesis*	*Clinical features*
▪ Trisomy 21	▪ Advanced maternal age	▪ During the first meiotic division the two chromosomes of a 21st instead of separating at anaphase, may both go to the same pole ▪ The resulting gamate then has 24 chromosomes instead of normal 23 ▪ At fertilization by this gamate the zygote will therefore have 47 chromosomes there being three identical chromosoms instead of one of the normal 21st pair	▪ The child has a broad face with obliquely placed palpebral fissures, epicanthus, a furrowed lower lip, mental retardation, hypotonia, a single line in palm (simian line) susceptible to infection and often have congenital heart disease ▪ They die young

For Preventive measures

Refer Question No. 8 December 2011 (RS2) Paper II.

9. Planning cycle.

Refer Question No. 8 June 2008 (RS2) Paper II.

10. Name important voluntary health agencies in India. Write briefly about any one of the agency.

- Voluntary health agency is an organization that is administered by an autonomous board which holds meetings, collects funds for its support chiefly from private sources and expends money, with or without paid workers in conducting a program directed primarily to furthering the public health by providing health services or health education or by advancing research or legislation or by a combination of these activities.

Voluntary Health Agencies in India[Q]

Objectives	*Activities*
a. Indian Red Cross Society (of India) – Established in 1920 by an Act of Indian Legislature	
– Improvement of health – Prevention of disease – Mitigation of suffering	▪ Provision of amenities to soldiers in time of war ▪ Organizing disaster relief service in times of flood, gamine, earthquake, etc. in the form of distribution of milk, medicines, clothes, blankets, etc. ▪ Maintaining blood banks and promoting blood donation for the benefit of those wounded in wars and disasters ▪ Development of maternity and child welfare services ▪ Maintaining the Red Cross Home in Bengaluru for disabled ex – serviceman ▪ Providing amenities like newspaper, periodicals, musical instruments and other comfort goods to patients in military hospitals ▪ Acting as an auxiliary of the country's health services
b. Tuberculosis Association of India[Q] – Organized during the year 1939 with its headquarters at New Delhi and branches in all the states of India	
	▪ Raising funds by conducting a TB seal campaign every year[Q] ▪ Training of doctors, health visitors and social workers in antituberculosis work[Q] ▪ Promotion of health education[Q] ▪ Promotion of consultation, research and conferences ▪ Publishing periodicals related to TB ▪ Operation of TB sanitoria at New Delhi, Kasuali, Mehrauli and Dharampur ▪ Management of New Delhi Tuberculosis Center
c. Family Planning Association of India[Q] – Established during 1949 with its headquarters at Mumbai and branches in all the states of India – It has two regional training centers at Hyderabad and Gwalior	
	▪ Provision of family welfare services, including MTP and sterilization through its clinics ▪ Conducts mobile camps in rural areas ▪ Conducts training programs for doctors, paramedical workers, volunteers and opinion builders in family planning areas ▪ Imparts education about population control, family planning, safe sex, prevention of STDs, etc. ▪ Organizes seminars, workshops and conferences ▪ Publishes quarterly journal related to family welfare ▪ Undertakes community development activities through its Parivar Pragati Pariyojna ▪ Provides financial assistance to other NGOs to undertake family welfare activities ▪ Provides answers to queries on family planning by correspondence or by personal interviews at its head quarters
d. Hind Kusht Nivaran Sangh – Founded in 1950, with its headquarters at New Delhi	
	▪ Provides financial assistance to leprosy homes and clinics ▪ Provides health education through publications and posters ▪ Provides training to medical workers and physiotherapists ▪ Encourages research and field investigations in leprosy ▪ Holds periodic All India Leprosy Workers Conferences ▪ Brings out "Leprosy in India", a quarterly journal
e. Voluntary Health Associations of India – A federation of organization in field of health and community development – First organization to popularize concept of Well Baby Clinic	
– Training of health trainers	▪ Develops and distributes health education material ▪ Brings out newsletters and journals devoted to health and community development ▪ Sets up stalls at exhibitions across India ▪ Imparts training to medical professionals, paramedical workers and other involved with health care delivery
f. Bharat Sevak Samaj – A non-political and non-official organization was formed in 1952 with its branches in all the states and districts	

Contd...

Contd...

Objectives	*Activities*
- To help people to achieve their health by their own actions and efforts	▪ Improvement in sanitation in the villages
g. Indian Council for Child Welfare[Q] - Established in 1952 with network of State and District councils all over the country	
- Development of children, physically, mentally, socially, morally and spiritually in a healthy and normal manner and in conditions of freedom and dignity	
h. Central Social Welfare Board - An autonomous body set-up by Government of India in August 1953 under the control of Ministry of Education	
	▪ Surveys needs and requirement of voluntary welfare organizations in the country ▪ Promotes the formation of social welfare organizations on voluntary basis ▪ Provides financial aid to deserving welfare organizations and institutions ▪ Initiated "Family and Child Welfare Services" in rural areas for welfare of women and children through various activities like mothercraft, social education, literacy classes, milk distribution, play centers, etc. ▪ Started a scheme for Industrial Cooperative to help the lower middle class women in urban areas to supplement their family income by doing paid work
i. Kasturba Memorial Fund - Fund of about ₹ 1 crore formed in 1944 in commemoration of Kasturba Gandhi	
	▪ Improve health of rural women through gram sevikas ▪ Utilization of the fund for various welfare projects
j. All India Women's Conference - Established in 1926 with branches all across the country	
- Welfare of women of India (the only voluntary health organization organized for the purpose)	▪ Runs MCH and family planning clinics, adult education centers to improve female literacy and milk distribution centers
k. All India Blind Relief Society - Established in 1946 for relief of the blind	
	▪ Conducts ophthalmic camps ▪ Works in coordination with other institutions and organization for the welfare of blind

Functions of Voluntary Health Agencies

a. Supplementing work of Government agencies	▪ Lending personal or by contributing funds for special equipment supplies or services, the voluntary health agencies strengthen the work of financial and statutory restricted government agencies
b. Pioneering	▪ Exploring ways and means of doing new things as in research is an area where voluntary health agencies can take initiative ▪ If an effort by voluntary health agency succeeds then the Government of India can step into take cover with considering of benefitting the large population ▪ Family planning program of India is an example, which was spearheaded by family planning association of Indian has evolved into a national policy
c. Education	▪ Voluntary health agencies can supplement the efforts of government agencies in regards to health education of masses
d. Demonstration	▪ By putting up demonstration and experimental projects the voluntary health agencies have advanced the cause of public health ▪ Demonstration of borehole latrine by the Rockefeller foundation has helped to solve the problem of hook worm in India to an extent

Contd...

Contd...

e. Guarding the work of Government agencies	▪ Voluntary health agencies can guide and criticize the work of governmental agencies
f. Advancing health legislation	▪ For the benefit of whole community the voluntary agencies can mobilize public opinion and advance legislation on health matters

Significance

- Voluntary health agencies are an important part of health care delivery system of any nation and they are true representative of health care delivery as their efforts are voluntary and selfless and directly to benefit the needy.

11. Prevention of diabetes mellitus.

Refer Question No. 1 June 2010 (RS2) Paper II.

12. Enumerate functions of multipurpose worker female.

Refer Question No. 10 December 2007 (RS2) Paper II.

SHORT ANSWERS

13. Cost effective analysis.

Refer Question No. 6 December 2011 (RS2) Paper II.

14. Body mass index.

Refer Question No. 4 June 2010 (RS2) Paper II.

15. Mention the elements of primary health care.

Refer Question No. 4 June 2012 (RS2) Paper II.

16. What is demographic gap?

Refer Question No. 15 June 2008 (RS2) Paper II.

17. Case definition for malaria.

- Malaria is vector-borne febrile disease caused by protozoal parasite *Plasmodium*, transmitted by bite of infected female anophelin mosquito.

Case Definitions[1]

Suspected case (Case that meets the clinical case definition)		*Confirmed case (Suspected case with laboratory confirmation)*
Uncomplicated malaria (clinical case definition)	*Severe malaria (clinical case definition)*	
▪ Fever or history of fever associated with symptoms such as nausea, vomiting and diarrhea, headache, back pain, chills, myalgia, where other infectious diseases have been excluded	▪ Fever and symptoms as for uncomplicated malaria but with associated signs such as disorientation, loss of consciousness, convulsions, severe anemia, jaundice, hemoglobinuria, spontaneous bleeding, pulmonary edema, shock	▪ Demonstration of malaria parasites in blood films by examining thick or thin smears or by rapid diagnostic kit for *P. falciparum* diagnosis

Ref:

1. www.the-ecentre.net/toolkit/Health/HTM-1(a).doc accessed on 28th May 2014.

18. What are cancer registries?

Refer Question No. 9 June 2012 (RS2) Paper II.

19. Recommendations of Bhore Committee.

- Bhore committee or the Health Survey and Development Committee was appointed under the chairman of Sir Joseph Bhore in October 1943[Q] to survey the then existing position, regarding the health conditions and health organization in the country and to make recommendations for the future development
- The committee submitted its 4 volume report in January 1946, putting forward a comprehensive proposal for the development of a National Program of health services for the country.

Observations

- The committee observed "if the nation's health is to be built, the health program should be developed on a foundation of preventive health work and that such activities should proceed side by side with those concerned with the treatment of patients".

Recommendations

- Integration of preventive and curative services at all administrative levels[Q]
- It visualized development of primary health center[Q] in two stages.

Short-term measures	*Long-term program (3 million plan)*
▪ Each primary health center in the rural area should cater to a population of 40,000[Q] supported by 3 subcenters and a secondary health center to serve as a supervisory, coordinating and referral institution ▪ The staff pattern of each PHC would be: Medical officers 2 Public health nurses 4 Nurse 1 Midwives 4 Trained dais 4 Sanitary inspectors 2 Health assistants 2 Pharmacist 1 Class IV employees 15	▪ Setting up primary health units with 75 bedded hospitals for each 10,000-20,000 population and secondary units with 650 bedded hospitals again regionalized around tertiary units (district hospital) with 2500 beds ▪ Major changes in medical education which includes 3 months training in preventive and social medicine to prepare "Social Physicians"[q]

Significance

- The Bhore Committee provided guidelines for national health planning in India through its concept of primary health center functioning as focal point for providing a package of comprehensive health care, comprising preventive, promotive and curative services.

20. Community health center.

Refer Question No. 2 December 2007 (RS2) Paper II.

21. Earthquake mitigation.

- Disaster mitigation involves measure designed either to prevent hazards or to lessen the likely effects of disaster.

Earthquake Mitigation Measures[1]

- Constitution of National core group for earthquake risk mitigation consisting of experts in earthquake engineering and administrators
- Drawing up a strategy and plan of action for mitigating impact of earthquakes
- Zoning of India in various seismic zones
- Laying down building construction norms for various seismic zones
- Evolving system for training of municipal engineers and masons
- Preparing plan for hospital preparedness
- Educating the general population in risk areas about safety drill and other protective measures.

Significance

- Earthquake is a natural disaster which can neither be predicted or prevented however institution of proper mitigation measures can help save lives and property.

Ref:

1. http://ndmindia.nic.in/Mitigation/index.htm accessed on 28th May 2014.

22. Advantages of intradermal rabies vaccine.

- Intradermal rabies vaccination with second generation anti-rabies vaccine was initiated in Thailand.

Vaccines used	*Sites used*
• Human diploid cell vaccine • Purified vero cell vaccine • Purified chick embryo vaccine • Purified duck embryo vaccine	• Abdominal wall (most common) • Deltoid • Suprascapularis • Thigh

Procedure

- The area for vaccination is divided into quadrants and a different site is used for each injection
- The injections are given deep subcutaneously
- To ensure proper administration a fold of skin is lifted between the thumb and other finger in the patients lying down or standing position and the vaccine is injected into the base of this fold using a fresh disposable with 1 mL syringe of 27 gauge needle
- The antigenic content of the rehydrated vaccine should be atleast 0.25 IU per 0.1 mL
- Production of papule indicates successful injection.

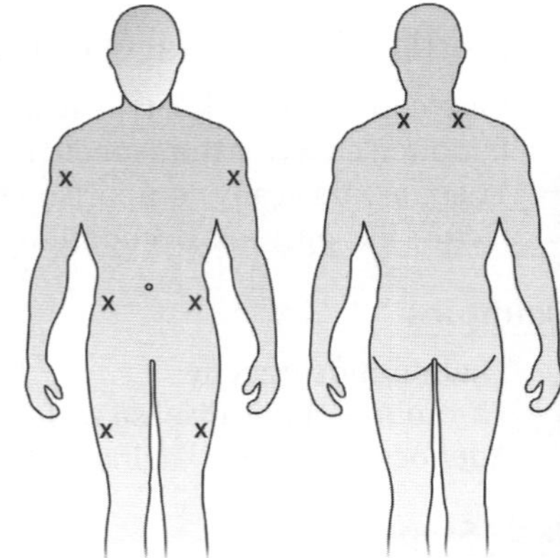

Fig. 2: Sites intradermal rabies vaccine

Regime: They are described by number of does on days 0, 3, 7, 14, 28 and 90.

Thai red cross regime	*Indian regime*	*WHO regime*
(2 – 2 – 2- 0 – 1 – 1)	(8 – 0 - 0 – 4 – 0 – 1)	(8 – 0 – 4 – 0 – 1 – 1)
Consists of two intradermal injections on days 0, 3 and 7 followed by an intradermal injection each on days 28 and 90	Consists of 8 intradermal injections on day 0 followed by 4 intradermal injection on day 14 and finally 1 injection on day 90	Consists of 8 intradermal injections on day 0 followed by 4 injection on day 7 and finally 1 injection each on 28th and 90th day

Advantages	*Disadvantages*
▪ Intradermal rabies vaccinations are effective showing adequate titres of rabies virus neutralizing antibodies in 80% patients as early as 7 days and all 100% on day 14 ▪ They lower the cost of vaccination	▪ Numerous injections ▪ Requires trained manpower ▪ Requires atleast 3 visits

MBBS PHASE III EXAMINATION

JUNE 2014

(Revised Scheme 2)

PAPER I

LONG ESSAYS

1. Describe the basic stages in a "case control study" with suitable examples.

- Case control study is a type of analytical epidemiology[Q]
- It is often called as retrospective study (from effect to cause[Q]) and is common first approach to test causal hypothesis
- These are basically comparison studies where cases and controls are compared with respect to know confounding factors like age, sex, occupation, social status, etc.

Examples

- Thalidomide tragedy
- Thromboembolic disease with use of oral contraceptives
- Adenocarcinoma of vagina with exposure of diethyl stilboestrol in fetal life.

Basic Steps

Four basic steps in conducting a case control study are:

a. Selection of cases and controls
b. Matching
c. Measurement of exposure
d. Analysis and interpretation

A. Selection of cases and controls
   - First step is to identify a suitable group of cases and a group of controls.
   i. Selection of cases

Definition of a case	*Sources of cases*
It involves two specifications a. Diagnostic criteria - Before study is started, the diagnostic criteria of the disease and the stage of disease if any to be included in study should be clearly specified - Once a diagnostic criteria is established, it should not be altered or changed during the period of study b. Eligibility criteria - A customary criterion is that only newly diagnosed cases within a specified period of time are eligible than old cases or cases in advanced stage of the disease	a. Hospitals - Often convenient - Drawn from a single or a network of hospitals admitted during a specified period of time - Entire case series or a random sample it is selected b. General population - All cases of study within a defined geographic area during a specified period of time are ascertained - Cases should be fairly representative of all cases in the community

ii. Selection of controls
   - Controls must be free from the disease under study
   - They must be similar to the cases as possible except for the absence of disease under study

- As a rule, a comparison group is identified before a study is done
- If the disease under study occurs in subclinical forms whose diagnosis is difficult then selection of controls may be difficult.

Source of controls	*Number of controls*
a. Hospital controls – Controls may be selected from the same hospital as the cases but with different illnesses other than the one under study – Ideally, the controls should have undergone the same diagnostic work ups as cases but have been found to be negative b. Relatives – Relative like spouses and siblings may also be used as control – However, sibling controls are unsuitable where genetic conditions are under study c. Neighborhood controls – Controls can also be drawn from people living in the same locality, working in the same place or studying in same school as cases d. General population – Individuals free from disease under study selected by random sample from a defined geographical areas form population control	▪ One control per case if many cases are available, large study is contemplated the cost of collecting a case and control is almost equal ▪ As many as 2, 3, or even 4 per case if study group is small say under 50 ▪ Selection of proper cases and controls is crucial for the interpretation of the results of a case control studies ▪ It is also desired to conduct more than one case control study preferably in different geographic area ▪ The validity of the study is increased, if the findings at two areas are consistent

B. Matching
- The controls may differ from the cases in number of factors such as age, sex, occupation, social status, etc.
- Matching is defined as the process by which we select controls in such a way that they are similar to cases with regard to certain pertinent selected variables which are known to influence the outcome of diseases and which if not adequately matched for comparability could distort or confound the results
- Comparability between cases and controls is very important as:
  - A confounding factor is defined as one which is associated both with exposure disease and is distributed unequally in study and control groups
  - While matching, suspected etiological factor or the variable under consideration should not be matched because its etiological role is eliminated.

Types

Group matching	*Pair matching*
▪ Assigning cases to subcategories based on their characteristics like age, occupation, etc. and then establishing appropriate controls	▪ It is finding a control for particular case as closely resembling as possible except for the disease under study ▪ Matching should not be overdone otherwise it becomes difficult to obtain controls and the odds ratio may be reduced

C. Measurement of exposure
- It is also important to define fix criteria for exposure
- Information about exposure should be obtained precisely in same manner in both the cases and controls
- It can be recorded by interviews, by questionnaires or by studying past records.

D. Analysis
- It is the final step to find out.
  i. Exposure rate among cases and controls to suspected factor.
  ii. Estimation of disease risk associated with exposure.

a. Exposure rates
- A case control study provides a direct estimation of the exposure rates to suspected factor in disease and non-disease groups

- In the following example exposure rate is calculated as follows:

	Cases	*Controls*
Exposure +ve	36 (a)	52 (b)
Exposure –ve	04 (c)	28 (d)
Total	**40**	**80**

Exposure rates

Cases $\frac{a}{a+c} = \frac{36}{40} = 90\%$

Controls $\frac{b}{b+d} = \frac{52}{80} = 65\%$

- Next step is to ascertain whether there is a statistical association between exposure status and occurrence of disease which is resolved by calculating the P value
- Particular test of significance depends upon the variables under investigation
- In case of discrete variables, results are presented as rates or proportions of those present or absent in the study in the control group and usual test of significance is standard error of difference between two proportions or chi-square test
- In case of continuous variables data have to be grouped and usual test of significance is standard error of difference between two means or the test
- $P < 0.05 \rightarrow$ statistically significant
- Smaller the P value greater the statistical significance or probability that the association is not due to chance alone
- However, statistical association does not imply causation.

b. Estimation of risk
- Estimation of disease risk associated with exposure is the second analytical step
- It is obtained by an index known as 'Relative risk' or (risk ratio) or odds ratio[Q].

Relative risk	*Odds ratio*
▪ Relative risk is the ratio between the incidence of disease among exposed and incidence among non–exposed[Q] $\text{Relative risk} = \frac{\text{Incidance among exposed}}{\text{Incidance among non-exposed}}$ $= \frac{a}{(a+b)} + \frac{c}{(c+d)} = \frac{36}{88} + \frac{4}{32}$ $= 0.4091/0.125$ $= 3.41$ ▪ A typical case control study does not provide incidence rates directly because there is no appropriate denominator or population at risk to calculate rates	▪ It is a measure of the strength of association between the risk factor and outcome[Q] ▪ It is closely related to relative risk and is key parameter in the analysis of case control studies[Q] ▪ It is based on three assumptions – Disease being investigated must be relatively rare – Cases must be representative of those with the disease – Control must be representative of those without the disease ▪ For the example cited above Odds ratio $= ad/bc$ $= 37 \times 28/52 \times 4$ $= 1008/2\text{–}8$ $= 4.85$ ▪ For example, people with exposure are 4.85 times at more risk for developing the disease

Advantages	*Disadvantages*
▪ Relatively easy to carry out ▪ Rapid and inexpensive compared to cohort study[Q] ▪ Requires comparatively few subjects[Q] ▪ Particularly suitable to investigate rare diseases or disease about which little is known[Q] ▪ No risk to the subject	▪ Problems of bias[Q] relies on memory or past records, accuracy of which is doubtful, validation of information obtained is difficult or sometimes impossible ▪ Selection of an appropriate control group may be difficult ▪ Incidence can not be measured[Q], only relative risk can be estimated[Q]

Contd...

Revised Scheme 2

Contd...

Advantages	Disadvantages
▪ Allows the study of several different etiological factors[Q] like effect of smoking, physical activity, diet in myocardial infarction ▪ Risk factors can be identified thus helps to formulate rational prevention and control program ▪ No attrition problems, because case control studies do not require follow up of individuals into the future ▪ Minimal ethical problems	▪ Not suited to the evaluation of therapy or prophylaxis of disease ▪ Another major concern is representiveness of cases and controls

Significance

- In recent years, case control study has emerged as a permanent method of epidemiological investigation.

2. Enumerate the vector-borne diseases and add a note on "prevention and control".

- Vector-borne diseases are diseases which require a vector (an arthropod or any living carrier) to transport the infectious agent to a susceptible host.

Vector-borne Diseases

Disease	*Vector*
▪ Malaria	▪ Anopheles (mosquito)
▪ Filariasis	▪ *Culex fatigans* (mosquito)
▪ Kala-azar	▪ *Phlebotomus argentipes* (sand fly)
▪ Japanese encephalities	▪ *Culicine vishnui* (mosquito)
▪ Chikungunya fever	▪ Aedes, Culex and Mansonia (mosquitoes)
▪ Epidemic typhus	▪ Louse
▪ Tick typhus	▪ Hard tick
▪ Q fever	▪ Soft tick
▪ Plague	▪ Rat flea
▪ Chagas disease	▪ Ruduviid bug
▪ Scrub typhus	▪ Trombiculid mite
▪ Guinea worm disease	▪ Cyclops
▪ Scabies	▪ Itch mite
▪ Sleeping sickness	▪ Tsetse fly

Prevention and Control

I. Primordial prevention
   a. Source reduction
      - Reduction in sources of vector breeding are the best method of preventing vector-borne diseases
      - Consist of elimination of nonessential water bodies which includes periodical emptying of domestic water container, sealing of water tanks, filling pot holes, puddles, burrow pits and canalizing drains so that water does not stagnate.
   b. Environmental modification
      - Government can undertake engineering activities to reduce breeding sources like leveling of lands, filling of depressions and making soakage pits.

II. Primary prevention (integrated vector control)
   – Primary modality of primary prevention is integrated vector control
   – Integrated vector control is the utilization of all appropriate technological and management techniques to bring about an effective degree of vector suppression in a cost-effective manner
   – It avoids the excessive use of any one method but tries to combine one or more methods whether they are directed towards only the larvae or adults or both, with a view to obtain maximum result with minimum inputs and also to prevent environmental pollution with toxic chemicals and development of resistance among vectors.

Measures

Offensive	*Defensive*	*Corrective*
▪ Comprises attacking arthropods and killing them using insecticides etc	▪ Comprise personal protective measures such as use of repellants, mosquito nets, etc	▪ Comprise modification of environment such that it become unfavorable for arthropods to lay eggs thus controlling vector population

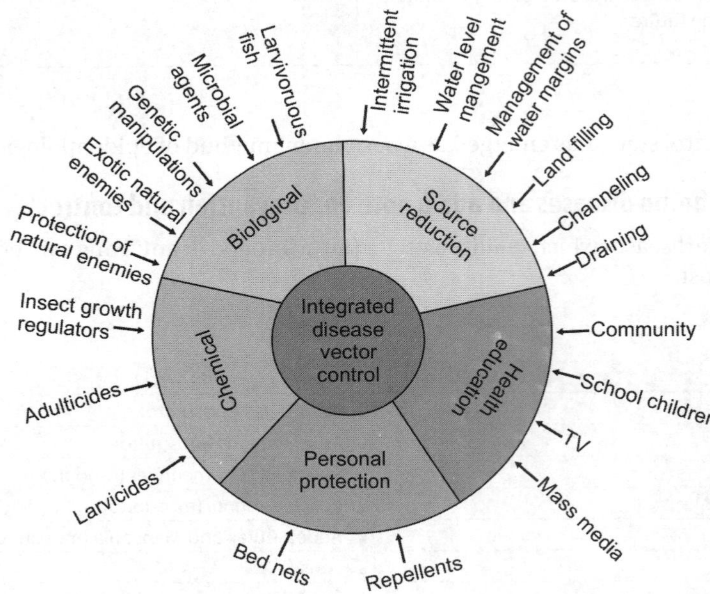

Fig. 1: Integrated management of vector—components

Components

A. Antilarval measures

- Antilarval measures are divided into three types

a. Environmental control

* This is also known as source reduction direction towards eliminating the mosquito breeding places.
* It comprises
  - ❖ Filling of low lying areas where water accumulation is possible (Anopheles)
  - ❖ Leveling or covering or drainage of cesspools ditches and sewers which are present near the houses (culex and anopheles)
  - ❖ Removal of water plants such as Pistia plants with herbicides (mansonia)
  - ❖ Clean up the environment and get rid of water holding containers such as empty pots coconut shells discarded tins, broken bottles, etc. (Aedes)
  - ❖ Weekly emptying of household water collections intermittent irrigation, cultivation of banana plants where water accumulates near the house
* Source reduction methods generally provide permanent results.

Significance

* Best approach to vector control[Q].

b. Chemical control

* Chemical control is the use of larvicides to kill the larvae
* These larvicides may act as stomach poisons when it is ingested by larva while feeding or as contact poison which penetrate the body wall or respiratory tract
* It is usually employed where source reduction is not feasible.

i. Mineral oils[Q]

- ❖ Diesel oils, fuel oils, kerosene when applied on water forms a thin film which cuts off the air to the larvae and pupae[Q] and cause death within 1–2 hours of application.

- The oil is applied at rate of 40–90 L per heater simply by dipping from a bucket or pouring from a water can
- However, mineral oil should be applied once in a week as the mosquito's life cycle is of 8 days.

ii. Paris green[Q]

- Paris green or copper acetoarsenite is an emerald green, micro crystalline powder containing more than 50% arsenious oxide
- It is a stomach poison[Q] and effective mainly against Anopheles[Q] which are surface feeders
- It is applied as 2% dust (prepared by mixing 2 kg Paris green in 98 kg diluents such as soapstone powder or slaked lime in a rotary mixer) in dose of 1 kg of actual Paris green per hectare of water surface.

iii. Synthetic insecticides

- These are organophosphorus compounds[Q] such as fenthion[Q], chlorpyrifos[Q], malathion, abate[Q], etc.
- Abate is a very effective larvicide at a concentration of 10 ppm
- Organochlorine compounds such as DDT, HCH are not recommended because of their long residual effect
- They applied in following doses

	Dose (g/hectare)	*Duration of action*
Chlorpyriphos[Q]	10–20	3–17 weeks
Fenthion[Q]	20–110	2–12 weeks
Malathion[Q]	220–1000	1–2 weeks
Temephos	60–110	2–4 weeks
Fenitrothion	100–1000	2–11 weeks
Abate	60–100	2–4 weeks

Advantages

- Mosquitoes are destroyed before they disperse to human populations
- Operations can be carried out in very short time
- Widely available
- Can be applied by hand.

Disadvantages

- Temporary control and costly repetitions
- Affection of other organisms
- Human toxicity.

c. Biological control

i. Bacteria (biocides)

- Certain bacteria are useful to kill the larva of mosquitoes which are
  - o *Bacillus sphaerizus*—500–5000 g/hour, acting for 1–2 weeks
  - o *Bacillus thiringiensis*—100–6000 g/hour, acting for 2–8 weeks

ii. Fishes

- A wide range of small fish feed readily on mosquito larvae and best known among them are *Gambusia affinis*[Q] and *Labister reticulatus*
- These fishes can be used in burrow pits, sewage, oxidation ponds, cisterns and farm ponds.

iii. Other biological agents

- *Notonectids*: Aquatic insects, feeding veraciously on larvae in ponds and rice fields
- *Hydra:* Coelenterates useful for mosquito predators
- *Flatworms:* Planaria feed on mosquito larvae
- *Fungi*: *Culicinomyces, Coelomomyces* are considerably effective against larvae
- *Nematodes: Ramanomermis culicivorax* and *R. iyengari* are under trial
- *Viruses*: *Polyhedrosis* viruses and indoviruses are under trial.

Advantages of biological control

* Does not cause chemical pollution.

B. Anti-adult measures

– Adult mosquitoes can be killed by:

a. Residual sprays[Q]
   - In this method a long-acting insecticides is sprayed on walls[Q] and other surfaces where mosquitoes rest
   - The commonly used insecticides are:

	Dosage (g/m^2)	*Duration of action*
Organochlorines		
▪ DDT[Q]	1–2[Q]	More than 6 months
▪ Lindane	0.2–0.5	3 or more months
Organophosphous		
▪ Malathion[Q]	1–2	1–3 months[Q]
▪ Fenitrothion	1–2	1–3 months
▪ Methyl pirimphos	1–2	2–3 months
Carbamates		
▪ Propoxus	1–2	2–3 months
▪ Bendiocarb	0.2–0.4	2–3 months
Pyrethroids		
▪ Permethrin	0.5	2–3 months
▪ Cypermethrin	0.5	4 or more months
▪ Deltamethrin	0.05	2–3 months

   - Good residual insecticide should:
     * Be toxic to target vector
     * Have long-lasting effect on a given surface
     * Be safe to human a dometic animals
     * Be acceptable to house owners
     * Be cost effective
     * Be stable during storage and transport
     * Not be irritant or repelient to targent insects to ensure that insects pick up a lethal dose
     * Mix well with water and be harmless to spraying instrument.

b. Space sprays
   - Space sprays are those where insecticidal formulations are sprayed into the atmosphere in the form of mist or fog to kill the insects which habitat outside the house
   - The principle is to fill space with a mist of small droplets that are picket up by the insects when they fly
   - Here a quick acting insecticide is usually used but residual insecticides such as malation[Q], fenitrothion are also used in form of ultra-low volume fogging[Q]
   - The mist may contain either organophosphorus compounds like malation, fenibrothion, diaginon, cypermethrin, etc. and the fog contains pyrethrum extract from pyrethrum flower[Q] which contains pyrethrin as active principle a nerve poison. It is a surface-acting insecticide which enters the mosquito through surface and used in dose of 10 z of spray solution per 1000 cu feet
   - The procedure carried out using a hand gun for domestic purpose or power sprayers or aerosol dispenser for large scale application.

Advantages	*Disadvantages*
▪ It has an immediate effect on adult population of insects and is therefore suitable for the control of disease outbreak ▪ It is less laborious for a single application ▪ Large areas can be treated fairly quickly ▪ Uses less insecticide per application ▪ Kills mosquitoes that does not rest in house	▪ Temporary effect ▪ High recurrent cost therefore unsuitable for multiple application ▪ Costly equipment and costly maintenance ▪ Need for specially trained staff ▪ May cause contamination of nontarget areas and organisms and air pollution ▪ Non acceptability due to pungent odor

c. Genetic control
  - Genetic control comprises methods like sterile male technique, cytoplasmic incompatibility, chromosomal translocation, sex distortion and gene replacement.

  Advantages
  - Cheaper and more efficient
  - No vector resistance.

d. Newer methods
  - Newer methods include methods such as insect growth regulators, chemosterilants, sex attractants and pheromones (a substance secreted by arthropod, received by another resulting in change in its behavior or developmental process).

C. Protection against bite

a. Mosquito nets
  - These offer protection against mosquito bites during sleep
  - The mosquito nets should be white to allow easy detection of mosquitoes
  - Net should be tucked under mattress to provide adequate protection
  - The size of the opening in the net should not exceed 0.0475 inch[Q] and number of holes per sq inch is usually 150[Q]

b. Insecticide impregnated bed nets
  - Mosquitoes can be made more effective by treating them with insecticides
  - These nets have efficacy of 6 months when not washed.

  Procedure

  i. Calculations
    * Surface area of net in $m^2 = 2 (a + b) + c$
      Where a = length × height
      b = height × width
      c = length × width
    * Quantity of insecticide needed (target dose of 25 mg/m^2)
      Quantity in grams = Surface area of net in $m^2 \times 0.025$
    * Volume of formulation required =

$$\text{Volume of formulation (mL)} = \frac{\text{Weight (Quantity in grams)}}{\text{\% formulation of insecticides}} \times 100$$

  ii. Commonly used insecticides
    * 2.5% delatmethrin
    * 5% cyfluthrin

  iii. Treatment
    * Using protective gloves, mix quantity of insecticide with cold water
    * Soak in net in water
    * Dry in net in shade (never in sunlight)
    * Discharge left over water into sewage drain or latrine but nerve near a water body used for drinking water source.

c. Screening
  - Screening of building with copper or bronze gauze having 16 meshes to inch is recommended
  - The diameter should not exceed 0.0475 inch
  - It is a costly but effective method.

d. Repellents[Q]
  - Diethyltolumide applied on skin[Q] remains active against culex mosquito for 18–20 hours
  - Indalone, dimethyl phthalate, dimethyl carbate, etc. are also effective.

D. Health education
  – Health education is an important component of integrated vector control
  – People should be educated regarding the breeding places and life cycles of common insects and should be taught to take domestic measures such as source reduction, personal protection, etc.

- People should be informed to cooperate in regards to other measures of vector control such as space sprays, residual sprays, etc.

Significance

- Integrated vector control has successfully tackled the following problems.
  - Technical problems like development of resistance to older insecticides
  - Financial problems like cost of newer insecticides
  - Environmental problems like environmental pollution by insecticides
  - Operational problems like lack of public cooperation for indoor spraying of insectides.

III. Secondary prevention
- Early diagnosis and treatment
  - Early diagnosis and treatment of the infected cases renders the case ineffective for vector to transmit the infection from the patient to new healthy individual.

Significance

- Vector-borne diseases form major bulk of disease load in a developing country thought they are easily preventable
- Many of these diseases like dengue, malaria are responsible for fatalities and rest are responsible for morbidity
- World Health Organization has prioritize this by initiating a global campaign to prevent vector-borne diseases in 2014 with WHO day theme being "*Small Bite – Big Threat*".

SHORT ESSAYS

3. Relationship between prevalence and incidence.

The relationship incidence and prevalence can be expressed as:

- Prevalence (P) = Incidence (I) × Mean duration (D)[Q] (In stable condition, i.e. 0 new cases)
- Thus it means that prevalence depends upon two factors, incidence and mean duration of illness
- That means decrease in incidence leads to decrease in prevalence
- Prevalence can be compared with a photograph, an instantaneous record and incidence with a film, a continuous record
- Prevalence is a ratio[Q]
- The relationship between incidence and prevalence can be best represented as:

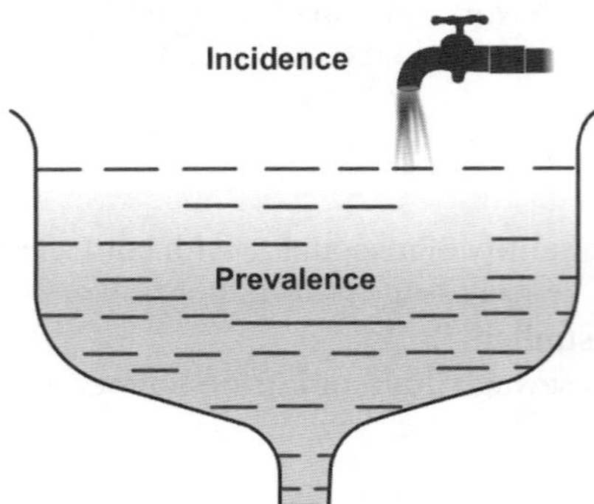

Fig. 2: Relationship between incidence and prevalence

4. Disease carriers.

Refer Question No. 1 June 2009 (RS2) Paper I.

5. Live vaccines.

- Live vaccines are preparations of microorganisms which have been attenuated by serial passage through tissue culture or chick embryo and have lost their capacity to induce full blown disease but retain their immunogenicity

- Attenuated organisms are organisms with reduced pathogenicity or virulence but retaining antigenicity or immunogenicity.

Mechanism of action	*Properties*	*Advantages (over killed vaccines)*	*Disadvantages (over killed vaccines)*
▪ Attenuated organism multiplies in host resulting in larger antigenic dose ▪ Have all major and minor antigenic components ▪ Engage certain tissues of the body (e.g. OPV engages intestinal mucosa) ▪ May be other mechanism like persistence of latent virus	▪ Immunization is generally achieved with a single dose (except OPV[Q]) ▪ Should not be administered to pregnant mothers, immunodeficient individuals ▪ 2 live vaccines can be administered simultaneously at different sites (or at an interval of 3 weeks) ▪ Mimics natural disease	▪ More potent ▪ Dose required is less ▪ Single dose sufficient ▪ Induces local immunity ▪ Produces durable immunity	▪ More incidences of adverse effects ▪ Contraindicated in pregnancy, immunosuppressive individuals ▪ Requires proper storage

Examples

Bacterial	*Viral*	*Rickettsial*
▪ BCG ▪ Typhoid ▪ Plague	▪ Sabin's oral polio vaccine ▪ 17 D (Yellow fever) ▪ Measles ▪ Rubella ▪ Mumps ▪ Influenza	▪ Epidemic typhus

Significance

- In any national programs, live vaccines are preferred over killed vaccine for the benefits they offer like single dosage and durable immunity however proper storage guidelines need to be followed.

6. Discuss the types of bias.

- Bias means a systematic error that is made unintentionally or unknowingly in the determination of the association between the exposure and disease[Q]
- It reflects some type of non-comparability between the study and control groups.

In case control studies	*In cohort and experimental studies*
Types	
a. Selection bias – Bias that occurs during selection of cases and control for the study i. Prevalence—incidence bias – Due to selective survival among prevalent cases. ii. Admission rate (Berkesonian) bias[Q] – Due to selective factors in admission to hospital and occurs commonly in hospital based studies iii. Wrong sample size – Due to insufficient sample size and most common type of preventable bias b. Ascertainment bias – Bias that occurs during measurement of exposure to the risk factors or during getting information about exposure to the risk factors i. Diagnostic bias – Due to disproportionately high performance of a diagnostic procedure on cases as compared to controls ii. Recall bias/Memory bias – Due to incorrect description of history by the controls when compared to cases	a. Assembly bias or selection bias – Due to · Refusal to participate in a study · Difference in the study of cohorts and control cohorts in the extent of disease · Presence of other diseases · Presence or absence of prior treatment b. Migration bias – Due to dropout of some participants in study due to death, recovery, side effects of treatment, etc. c. Measurement bias – Due to fault in measuring instruments

Contd...

Contd...

In case control studies	*In cohort and experimental studies*
Recommendations for minimizing bias	
▪ Cases should be limited to incident cases ▪ They should be homogenous in nature ▪ Definition of cases and control before study starts ▪ Strict criteria should be followed for inclusion and exclusion of cases in the study ▪ To prevent ascertainment bias, standardization procedure is advised ▪ At least two control groups should be selected, one hospital based and another community based ▪ Matching is advised to prevent confounders ▪ Analysis should be completed by a stratification and multivariate technique	▪ Restriction of study subjects to only those with narrow range of characteristics ▪ Matching of the patients in both the groups in terms of age, sex, stage of severity of disease, etc ▪ Stratification of the data ▪ Standardization of the data to be compared ▪ Multivariate adjustment to give equal weights to a number of variables ▪ Assuming the worst possible maldistribution of a unknown factor ▪ Randomization of groups so that each patient has equal chance of getting into the study

7. The food guide pyramid.

- A food guide pyramid is a pyramid shaped guide of healthy foods divided into sections to show the recommended intake for each food group.

History

- The first food pyramid was published by National Board of Health and Welfare of Sweden in 1974
- Most popular and widely used food pyramid was released by the United States Department of Agriculture in 1992, which was updated in 2005, and then replaced in 2011
- Over 25 other countries and organizations have also published food pyramids based on local dietary customs and available nutritional resources.

Principle

- The idea of food guide pyramid is based on principle of dividing daily diet into "basic foods" that were both cheap and nutritious, and "supplemental foods" that added nutrition missing from the basic foods.

Features

- The pyramid is divided into various sections as follows:

Level	*Composition*	*Nutrition*	*Servings*
Base	Foods that come from grains, i.e. cereals, breads, rice and pasta	Supply bulk of calories and fiber	6-11 servings
1st tier	Food that come from plants like vegetables and fruits	Vitamins, minerals and fibers	2–5 servings
2nd tier	Food that comes from animals like milk, yogurt and cheese, and meat, poultry, fish, eggs Beans and nuts	Protein, calcium, iron and zinc	2–3 servings
Apex	Food rich in fat, oils and sugar	Excess calories	Use sparingly

- Each section of pyramid represents added sugar or already present fat in food in form of symbols
- Food guide pyramid emphasises food from five major food groups shown in 3 lower sections of pyramid
- Each of these food groups provide some but not all of nutrients one needs
- Foods in one group cannot replace those in another
- No one food group is more important than other and for good health, one needs them all.

Advantages	*Disadvantages*
▪ Pyramid calls for eating a variety of foods to get the nutrient one needs and at the same time the right amount of calories to maintain or improve the weight ▪ Diagrammatic representation makes it ideal tool to explain importance of nutrition to illiterate population	▪ No provision or alternation for vegetarians ▪ Misconception about fatty foods as certain individuals may completely stop eating them

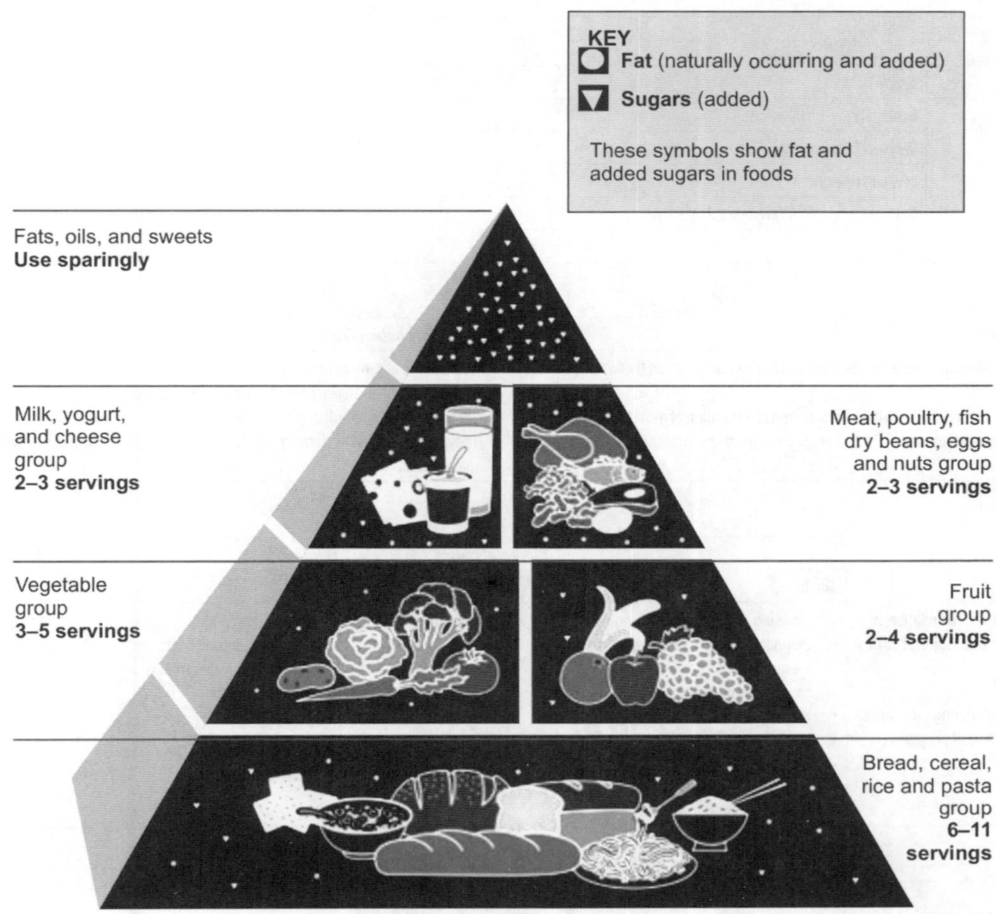

Fig. 3: Food guide pyramid

Other Forms of Dietary Representations

- The World Health Organization, in conjunction with the Food and Agriculture Organization, published guidelines that are represented as a table relating to objectives to prevent obesity, chronic diseases and dental caries
- New version of food pyramid released by USDA in 2011 is in form of a plate which is divided into four slightly different sized quadrants, with fruits and vegetables taking up half the space, and grains and protein making up the other half. The vegetables and grains portions are the largest of the four (My plate).

Significance

- The food pyramid is an outline of what to eat each day but it is not a rigid prescription but a general guide that lets you choose a healthful diet that is right for a person.

8. Low birth weight—prevention.

- Low birth weight is defined as a birth weight of less than 2.5 kg[Q] irrespective of gestational age[Q] (WHO), the measurement being taken preferably within the first hour of life[Q], before significant postnatal weight loss has occurred
- It includes both preterm (<37 weeks POG) and full-term (>37 weeks POG) babies
- Average birth weight in India is 2.8 kg (2.7–2.9 kg)
- Depending upon the population, the percentage of low birth weight is based on measurement of at least 500 babies[Q]

Grading

Birth weight	*Grade*
<1000 g	Extremely low birth weight
1000–2000 g	Very low birth weight
2000–2500 g	Low birth weight
2500–3500 g	Normal birth weight (average 2.7–2.9 kg)
>3500 g	Obese

Types

Preterm babies (30%)	*Small for date babies (70%)*
• Infants born after 28 completed weeks but before 37 weeks of gestation (between 196–259 days) • Their growth and development is within normal limits for duration of gestation • These babies easily catch up growth in 2–3 years given good neonatal care	• Infants born at term or preterm • Weigh less than 10th percentile for the gestational age • They are result of retarded intrauterine fetal growth • They have high risk of fatality and have more chances of getting infected or protein energy malnutrition

Etiology

Maternal causes		*Placental causes*	*Fetal causes*	*Risk factors (predisposing social factors)*
Medical	*Social*			
• Malnutrition (MC)—Liner relationship between maternal nutrition and birth weight • Severe anaemia • Heavy physical work during pregnancy • Hypertensive diseases of pregnancy • Malaria • Toxemia	• Smoking, addiction (smoking during pregnancy reduces birth weight by an average 170 g) • Low economic status • Short maternal stature • Very young age • High parity • Close birth spacing • Low education status	• Placental insufficiency • Placental abnormalities	• Fetal abnormalities • Acute intrauterine infections • Chromosomal abnormality • Multiple gestation	• Malnutrition • Infection • Unregulated fertility

Calculations

$$\text{(\%) Proportion of low birth weight babies} = \frac{\text{Live born babies with birth weight less than 2.5 kg}}{\text{Total number of live births}} \times 100$$

Status in India = 28% (2013)

Prevention and Control

Primary prevention	*Secondary prevention*
I.Direct intervention measures – Directed at identification of at risk pregnant women and providing efficient antenatal care with special attention to: a. Health promotion i. Prevention of malnutrition – By supplementary feeding[Q] – Fortification and enrichment of food – Nutritional education[Q] ii. Prevention of anemia – Distribution of iron and folic acid tablets during last trimester iii. Lifestyle change – Avoid strenuous exercise, smoking and alcohol b. Specific protection i. Control of infections – Early detection and treatment of infections which affect the fetal growth – Examples: Malaria, UTI, TORCH complex	I.Early diagnosis and treatment – Low birth weight babies require intensive neonatal care comprising of: i. Prevent hypothermia – Care of new born in incubator with function to adjust temperature, humidity and oxygen supply (incubatory care) with careful monitoring of O_2 supply – Bath is not given till baby gains 2500 g – Baby is wrapped in clean dry and warm cotton cloth covering entire body including head except face to prevent heat loss – If needed, bottles filled with warm water and covered with thin cloth are kept on either sides ii. Prevent malnutrition (Feeding) – As baby cannot suck, feeding is done often by nasal catheter preferably breast milk if available almost every alternate hour

Contd...

Contd...

ii. Controlling medical conditions – Early detection and treatment of hypertension, toxemias and diabetes II. Indirect interventions – Family planning – Deciding age at marriage (not earlier than 18 years) – Deciding age at the first child – Deciding number of children – Spacing between children[Q] (at least 3 years suggested) – Improvement of social measures such as literacy level, living conditions, quality of life – Avoiding workload during pregnancy – Improvement of availability of health services to women[Q]	iii. Prevention of infection – Infection is foremost cause of death in low birth weight babies, hence prevention of infection especially respiratory infection is very important to reduce infant mortality – Following precautions can be followed * Gentle handling, minimum handling * Handling with clean hands, no handling by sick person * Handling by minimum number of persons * Room must be warm, clean and dust free * Immunization should be given at right time * Prophylactic antibiotic to prevent septicemia * Task nursing (separate nursing for feeding and attending for soiling) * Barrier nursing to prevent cross infection * Expert nursing care **Duration** ▪ For a day or two for infants weighing between 2–2.5 kg ▪ Longer duration for infants weighing less than 2 kg till their weight reaches >2 kg

Significance

- Birth weight of an infant is the single most important determinant of its chance of survival, healthy growth and development[Q]
- Low birth weight is one of the most serious challenges in child health in both developed and developing countries and it amounts for ½ of perinatal and 1/3rd of all infant mortality
- Currently in India, 28% of infants born are low birth weight[Q]
- Low birth weight is single most important factor determining survival chance of child (survival chance is directly proportional to birth weight)
- Percentage of infants born with low birth weight closely reflects health status of mother during adolescence and pregnancy and also quality of antenatal care
- Multiplicity of causes of low birth weight makes it difficult to curtain the incidence of low birth weight but proper preventive measures can certainly bring it down
- 50% of incidence of low birth weight are preventable and attempt should be made to prevent them as low birth weight causes considerable suffering and wastage of human efforts, money but still recovery rate is very slow.

9. Occupational dermatitis.

- Occupational dermatitis is an occupational hazard.

Types of Dermatitis Producing Agents

Primary	*Sensitizing or allergic*
Cause dermatitis in workers exposed in sufficient concentration and for a long enough period of time	Occurs in small percentage of cases due to sensitization of skin

Epidemiology (Causes[Q])

a. Agent factors	*Physical*	*Chemical*	*Biological*	*Plant products*
	▪ Heat	▪ Acids	▪ Viruses	▪ Leaves
	▪ Cold	▪ Alkalis	▪ Bacteria	▪ Vegetables
	▪ Moisture	▪ Dyes	▪ Fungi	▪ Fruits

Contd...

June 2014 (Paper-I)

Contd...

	Physical	***Chemical***	***Biological***	***Plant products***
	▪ Friction	▪ Solvents	▪ Parasites	▪ Flowers
	▪ Pressure	▪ Grease		▪ Vegetable dust
	▪ X-rays and other rays	▪ Tar		
		▪ Chlorinated phenols		
b. Host factors				
i. Age	▪ More among young adults than older group of persons			
ii. Sex	▪ More among men than women because women take better care of their skin			
iii. Habits	▪ Alcoholism predisposes to dermatitis			
iv. Nature of skin	▪ Fair skin is more susceptible than dark skin			
v. Season	▪ Incidence is higher in summer than winter due to sprasity of clothes and excessive sweating			
vi. Person hygiene	▪ Lack of personal hygiene predisposes			
vii. Other skin lesions	▪ Presence of other skin lesions impairs resistance and predisposes			

Pathogenesis

- Primary dermatitis producing agents act:
  - By dissolving keratin
  - By dissolving fat
  - By dehydrating the tissue
  - By precipitating the proteins by oxidation or reduction
  - By keratogenic action.

Prevention and Control

a. Health promotion measures	
i. Preplacement examination	▪ Workers should be medically examined before employment and the ones with suspected or established dermatitis or ones with predisposition to skin disease should be rejected for the jobs involving skin hazard
ii. Health education	▪ All those who are at risk should be educated about maintenance of personal hygiene, frequent washing of hands, keeping machines clean, changing clothes everyday ▪ They must be educated about correct methods of handling irritant chemicals
b. Specification protection	
i. Protective clothing	▪ Provide adequate protection to the worker against direct contact with dermatitis producing agents by protective clothing, long leather gloves, aprons and boots ▪ Protective clothing should be washed frequently and kept in good order ▪ Barrier creams must be used regularly and correctly
ii. Personal hygiene	▪ Plentiful supply of warm water, soap and towel should be made available ▪ Workers should be educated and encouraged to use them
c. Early diagnosis and treatment	
i. Periodic inspection	▪ Conduct periodic medical checkup of all workers for early detection and treatment and if required transfer to a job not exposing him to risk
ii. Patch test	▪ Patch test is done to diagnose cases of allergic dermatitis
iii. Treatment	▪ Saline wash, potassium permanganate compresses, application of ointments and antibiotics

Significance

- Occupational dermatitis accounts for major share of all occupational diseases and its incidence is on rise due to industrialization and thus constitutes a major health problem in industrial areas.

10. Social security.

Refer Question No. 2 December 2009 (RS2) Paper I.

11. Types of mental illness.

- Mental and behavioral disorders are clinically significant conditions characterized by alteration in thinking, emotions or behavior associated with personal distress and/or impaired functioning.

Types of Mental Illness [International Classification of Diseases (ICD-10)]

Category	*Features*	*Examples*
a. Organic, including symptomatic mental disorders	Brain dysfunction is present. Disturbances of cognition, perception, mood and behavior	Includes dementia, delirium, mental disorders resulting from physical conditions, personality or behavioral disorders due to brain disease or injury
b. Mental and behavioral disorders due to psychoactive substance abuse	Disorders due to direct consequence of drug use and could not have occurred without consumption of drugs	Alcoholism, addiction to narcotics, sedatives
c. Schizophrenia, schizotypal and delusional disorders	Distortion of thinking, perception and mood that is not related to organic condition	Schizophrenia, schizotypal disorders, persistent delusional disorders, acute and transient psychotic disorders and schizoaffective disorders
d. Mood (affective) disorders	Disturbances of mood (affect) with other symptoms that are consistent with mood	Manic episodes, depressive disorders, bipolar affective disorders, recurrent depressive disorder and persistent affective disorder
e. Neurotic, stress related and somatoform disorders	Historically recognized as neurosis and have psychological causation	Phobic disorders, other anxiety disorders, obsessive compulsive disorder, stress and adjustment disorders, dissociative and conversion disorders and somatoform disorders
f. Behavioral syndromes and mental disorders associated with physiological disturbances and hormonal imbalance	Disorders with physiological and hormonal factors involved in causation	Eating disorders, psychogenic sleep disorders, sexual dysfunction, mental disorders associated with purperium
g. Disorders of adult personality and behavior	Expressions of individuals lifestyle and mode related to self and others Tends to be persistent	Personality disorders, enduring personality change, habit and impulse disorder, gender identify disorder and sexual preference disorder
h. Mental retardation	Arrested or incomplete development of mind manifested by impairment of skill commonly associated with intelligence	Mild, moderate, severe and profound grade of mental retardation
i. Disorders of psychological development	Begin at infancy or childhood and there is delay in development of functions related to nervous system	Speech disorders, specific developmental disorders, childhood autism
j. Behavioral and emotional disorders with onset usually occurring in childhood and adolescence	Onset in childhood and fluctuating course	Hyperkinetic disorders, conduct disorder, emotional disorder, tick disorder

Significance

- With rapid development and fast lifestyle, stressful life style has increased prevalence of mental illness so much so that WHO has dedicated 2001 world health day for mental health as "Mental Health: Stop Exclusion, Dare to Care"

12. Record linkage.

- Record linkage is the process of bringing together two or more records relating to the same entity (e.g. person, family, event, community, business, hospital, or geographical area), i.e. it refers to the task of finding entries that refer to the same entity in two or more files.

Applications

- It links morbidity and mortality data and provides information for studies of health care utilization and for descriptive epidemiology of disease as analyzed by characteristics of time, place, and event
- It can be used to improve data holdings, data collection, quality assessment, and the dissemination of information
- Data sources can be examined to eliminate duplicate records, to identify underreporting and missing cases (e.g. census population counts), to create person-oriented health statistics, and to generate disease registries and health surveillance systems. Some cancer registries link various data sources (e.g. hospital admissions, pathology and clinical reports, and death registrations) to generate their registries
- It is also used to create health indicators
- It can help in follow-up studies of cohorts or other groups to determine factors such as vital status, residential status, or health outcomes
- It can aid in developing recommendations about regulatory standards at the national and international levels.
- It is particularly suitable method of studying association between diseases as these association may have etiological significances.

Limitations

- Main problem with record linkage is the volume of data that can be accumulated, therefore in practice it is applied only on a limited scale like measurement of morbidity, family and genetic studies, etc.
- It is beyond reach of many developing countries.

Significance

- Record linkage is an important tool in creating data required for examining the health of the public and of the health-care system itself.

SHORT ANSWERS

13. Aims of epidemiology.

Refer Question No. 13 December 2011 (RS2) Paper I.

14. Odds ratio.

Refer Question No. 1 June 2014 (RS2) Paper I.

15. Iodized salt.

- The iodinization of salt is now the most widely used prophylactic public health measure against endemic goiter
- It consists of incorporation of sodium or potassium iodide to common edible salt.

Rationale for Choosing Salt

- It is consumed by all
- Added iodine does not change appearance or taste of salt
- Excess consumption of salt is not possible hence no risk of overdosage.

Composition	*Level of iodinization (according to Prevention of Food Adulteration Act)*	*Dose of iodide*
▪ Moisture content <6% by weight ▪ Sodium chloride >96% by weight	▪ Not less than 30 ppm at production point[Q] ▪ Not less than 15 ppm at consumer level[Q]	▪ 50 kg of potassium iodate (KIO_3) is added to 100,000 kg of salt ▪ This provides 50 ppm of potassium iodate equivalent to 30 ppm of iodine ▪ Since it is unstable, it comes down to 15 ppm of iodine at consumer level

Methods of Iodization

Dry mixing	*Mixing salt with potassium iodide*
▪ Spray mixing	Spraying aqueous solution of potassium iodate on salt and then mixing in a blender
▪ Submersion process	Mixing salt with a solution of potassium iodate in a tank and then drying

Health Benefits

- Iodized salt provides iodine which is very important in prevention of iodine deficiency disorders especially in endemic regions
- It promotes mental growth and development in children
- However, to have maximum benefit, iodized salt should be added to food after cooking.

Significance

- The iodized salt is most economical, convenient and effective means of mass prophylaxis of iodine deficiency disorders in endemic areas
- It is an example of food fortification.

16. Test to check the adequacy of pasteurization of milk.

Refer Question No. 6 December 2009 (RS2) Paper I.

17. Bar charts and its uses.

Refer Question No. 8 June 2017 (RS2) Paper I.

18. Difference between eugenic and euthenics.

Points of difference	*Eugenics*	*Euthenics*
a. Definition	Study of hereditary improvement of human race by controlled selective breeding	Manipulation of the immediate environment of the man because environment has an influence on the genetic development[Q] by enabling the genes to express them readily
b. Manipulations of	Genetic	Immediate environment
c. Inheritance of manipulation/ improvement	Yes	May be
d. Benefits	Entire population	Certain group of individuals
e. Effects on progeny	Prominent and visible	Negligible

19. Biological effects of radiation.

Refer Question No. 8 December 2010 (RS2) Paper I.

20. Passive smoking.

- Passive smoking is inhalation of environmental tobacco smoke, the smoke exhaled by someone else or emitted by the tip of a burning cigarette
- Also called as involuntary smoking or second hand smoking
- As a passive smoker, the nonsmoker breathes “sidestream” smoke from the burning tip of the cigarette and “mainstream” smoke that has been inhaled and then exhaled by the smoker.

Adverse Effects on Health

In children (most affected)	*In adults*	*In pregnancy*
▪ Pneumonia and bronchitis ▪ Coughing and wheezing ▪ Worsening of asthma ▪ Middle ear disease ▪ Stunted growth ▪ Allergies ▪ Possibly neurobehavioral impairment and cardiovascular disease in adulthood	▪ Increased risk of cancer in general, lung cancer (increase of 20–30%), breast cancer and brain tumors ▪ Predisposition to cardiac diseases (increase of 23%) ▪ Diseases of upper and lower respiratory tracts, exacerbation of asthma	▪ Increased risk of miscarriage ▪ Premature delivery ▪ Low birth weight ▪ Sudden infant death syndrome (SIDS)

Preventive Measures

a. Health education	▪ Educating smokers to about ill effects of passive smoking on their friends and family and couraging them to give up smoking especially when they have kids at home
b. Legislation	▪ To prevent individuals from passive smoking, Government of India has banned smoking in public places

Significance

- If smoking can be equated with suicide attempt then smokers should be held responsible for attempted homicide for passive smoking they cause.

Ref:

1. http://www.who.int/tobacco/en/atlas10.pdf accessed on 24th June 2014.
2. http://en.wikipedia.org/wiki/Passive_smoking accessed on 24th June 2014.

21. Vital events.

- Vital events are live births[Q], deaths[Q], fetal deaths, marriages, adoptions, legitimations, recognitions, annulments and legal separations[Q] (United Nations)
- These vital events are basis of various parameters/indices used to determine health status of a the population like birth rate, death rate, infant mortality rate, etc.
- The most common way of collecting information on these events is through civil registration system.

Significance

- Registration of vital events is foundation of vital statistics and helps calculate various indicators of health.

22. Mass media for health education—advantages and disadvantages.

Refer Question No. 2 June 2009 (RS2) Paper I.

MBBS PHASE III EXAMINATION

JUNE 2014

(Revised Scheme 2)

PAPER II

LONG ESSAYS

1. Describe in detail the strategies for polio eradication in India.

- Polio is next disease on list of WHO for global eradication as it has favorable epidemiological features.

Strategies for Eradication of Poliomyelitis[Q]

- Under National Polio Eradication Programs the strategies adopted for polio eradication are:

A. Sustain and maintain high level of routine immunization coverage of infants
   - For eradication of polio, it is essential to routinely immunize all children including newborns because unimmunized children maintain foci of infection
   - High level of immunization coverage reduces incidence of poliomyelitis to such a low level that it will set the stage for eradication of polio
   - It also important to contain the spread of wild polio strain.

   Strategy
   - Routine immunization of every child aged <1 year with at least 3 doses of oral poliovirus vaccine (OPV) at ages 6, 10 and 14 weeks.
   - Conduct pulse polio immunization days every year until polio is completely eradicated
   - Monitor OPV coverage in all districts at district level and below.

B. Pulse polio immunization
   - Pulse polio immunization is a program aimed at eradication of polio from the community
   - It is done by sudden, rhythmic, simultaneous and mass administration of OPV on two days 6–8 weeks apart to all children below the age of 5 years[Q] irrespective of their previous immunization status and therefore it is called pulse immunization
   - Was first introduced in 1995[Q]
   - Pulse polio immunization is over and above the routine immunization.

   Rationale
   - An epidemic of an infectious disease reaches a peak and declines rapidly because of the very high herd immunity consequent upon the epidemic spread of the causative agent
   - Soon after an epidemic the transmission may be interrupted and the agent will re-establish itself in the community only when sufficient numbers of susceptible children accumulate over a period of time
   - Pulse polio immunization is based on this principle
   - When a large proportion of susceptible children are vaccinated in a short period of time an epidemic is stimulated and the consequently resulting herd effect (i.e. decline in the incidence of a disease in unimmunized population because of break in transmission of the causative agent due to presence of larger proportion of immunized individuals[Q]
   - PPI replaces wild virus with vaccine virus from the community
   - For the diseases like polio which have inter epidemic intervals of more than one year. The pulse immunzation is carried out annually especially in winter months[Q] because
     - Virus has lowest transmission rate[Q]

- Efficiency of cold chain improves in winter[Q]
- 8 months preparation time can be obtained for next annual PPI[Q].

Activities or Components

a. National immunization days (NIDs)
   - National immunization days are defined as a day on which simultaneous administration of extra doses of oral polio vaccine to hundred percent of children under five years of age, irrespective of their previous immunization status is done in a single day[Q].

   Objectives[Q]
   - To curtail the transmission of wild polio virus by total elimination of the same as a part of Global Polio Eradication Strategy[Q].

   Strategy
   - Two rounds of NID are conducted in months of January and February, 6–8 weeks apart on Sundays in all zones of India
   - In addition, four additional rounds of NIDs will be conducted in June and July and in October and November in high-risk areas
   - The NIDs will be conducted on same dates throughout the country
   - A propaganda about the NID is made through posters, media, etc
   - A list of all children below the age of 5 years is made
   - It done through fixed post and house to house approach
   - In fixed post-approach, on the NID, booths are set up in all government hospitals private nursing homes, railway stations, bus stands, fairs, temples, etc. In villages, schools are also selected for polio booth. Therefore, this date is also termed booth activity day
   - This is followed by door-to-door campaign to ensure 100% coverage
   - All children below the age of 5 years who are immunized are marked by applying non removal ink on their index finger nail of right hand
   - Special efforts are taken for the high-risk area which are:
     - A district or ward where poliomyelitis cases has occurred in previous year
     - Areas with poor AFP surveillance
     - Urban slums
     - Remote and sparse populations
     - People living in areas not formally recognized by civil authorities
     - Mobile populations/tribes
     - Area of civil unrest.

b. Mop-up rounds
   - Immediately after the NID, review of the immunization done is taken up for 2-3 days in mop up rounds.
   - Here a house to house survey is done to find a unimmunized child and is immunized on the spot
   - In case, more than 5 unimmunized children are found in a locality, the polio immunization is repeated in the locality[Q].

c. Additional PPI rounds
   - In states where many cases of polio are reported, i.e. Uttar Pradesh, Bihar, etc. additional pulse polio immunization days are conducted.

Significance

- Pulse polio immunization program has seen drastic fall in incidence of poliomyelitis in the country except certain pockets of UP and Bihar thus signifying the success of this approach in Global Eradication of Poliomyelitis.

C. Acute flaccid paralysis surveillance
   - Acute flaccid paralysis surveillance is one of the strategies for the polio eradication.
   - It was introduced in 1997 when the incidence of poliomyelitis reduced drastically by 90%
   - It means detection, reporting and investigation of all cases of acute flaccid paralysis
   - Acute flaccid paralysis is sudden onset of flaccid paralysis (of lower motor neuron type) of limb of less than 4 weeks duration in child below 15 years[Q], with decreased or loss of tone and deep tendon reflexes and the limb is floppy or flaccid without sensory loss.

Objectives

To identify high-risk areas	*To monitor progress*	*To certify a country polio free*
▪ High-risk area – Is one where a case of poliomyelitis has been reported during the last one year or likely to occur and allows supplementary immunization to be focused – Is a one where surveillance system is poor – Is an urban area – Is an area with poor access to immunization services ▪ Is an area where specific group is not interested in vaccination	▪ The program manager determines whether the strategies are implemented effectively or not ▪ AFP rate in children below 15 years of age is an indicator of the sensitivity of the surveillance system	▪ It is done if there is no report of new case of poliomyelitis for 3 consecutive years inspite of adequate surveillance

Types

Routine surveillance	*Active surveillance*
▪ It consists of immediate reporting or notification of a case of AFP in children below 15 years of age, every month/week ▪ When no case is detected, reporting units should still send monthly/weekly report indicating zero cases which is called zero reporting ▪ Zero reporting ensures that surveillance activities are going on	▪ This is done by designated health person from the Department of Health who makes weekly visits to Department of Pediatrics and Neurology to enquire about new cases of AFP

Surveillance sensitivity

The surveillance sensitivity is measured by AFP rate as follows:

- The expected number of AFP cases in absence of poliomyelitis is 1 case per 100,000 children under 15 years.

$$\text{AFP rate} = \frac{\text{Reported number of AFP cases}}{\text{Expected number of AFP cases*}} \times 100$$

$$\text{Expected No. of APF cases} = \frac{\text{Estimated population under 15 years*}}{100{,}000} \times 1$$

*Estimated population under 15 years = Total population × 0.39

Components

a. AFP case classification
b. Line listing of the cases
c. Analysis of the data
d. Reporting of the findings

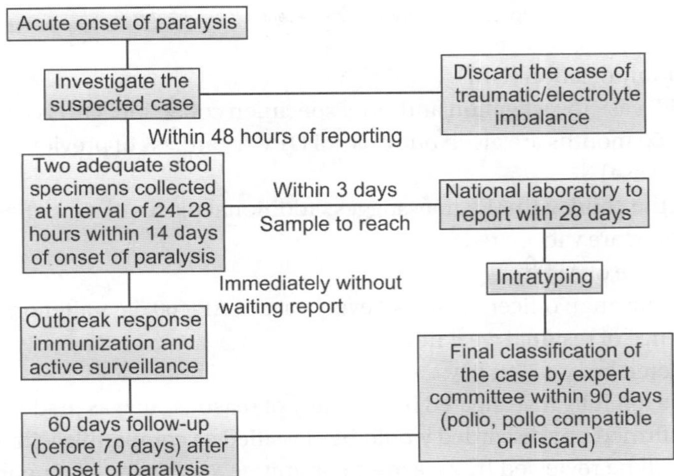

Fig. 1: AFP surveillance—process

a. AFP case classification
- Suspected AFP cases on detection should be reported to District Immunization Officer (DIO) by the quickest possible means for investigation to classify the case
- The concerned DIO should investigate the case within 48 hours and send a copy to state headquarter
- AFP cases are classified as polio or non-polio on the following scheme.

i. Active case search in community
   - A house to house active case search is conducted in the community where an AFP case resides or where an AFP cases visited during the incubation period for polio (4–25 days before onset of paralysis[Q]) to find the additional AFP cases that may have occurred
   - It is carried out along with outbreak response immunization
   - A search is conducted for any children <15 years who have had the onset of AFP within the preceding 60 days[Q]
   - All cases that are found are investigated immediately with collection of two stool specimen before administration of OPV.

ii. Adequate stool sample collection[Q]
   - From every case of AFP, stool samples are collected for diagnosis of poliomyelitis
   - Two stool specimens of adequate quantity (8–10 g) are collected at least 24 hours apart and within 14days of onset of paralysis[Q] (late cases up to 60 days)[Q] and sent to WHO accredited laboratory in clean container and good condition in reverse cold chain (2–8°C) for detection of polio virus.

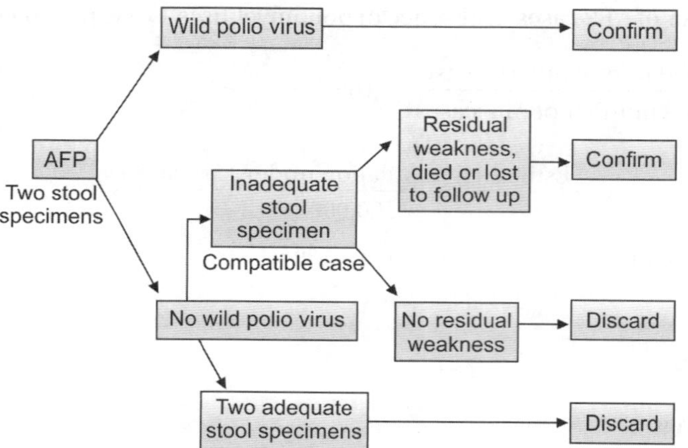

Fig. 2: AFP surveillance—case classification

iii. Outbreak response immunization (ORI)
   - Following the AFP case investigation and stool specimen collection, ORI is organized in the community
   - Children aged 0–59 months are given one dose of OPV regardless of previous immunization (in the villages or locality of AFP case)
   - Travel history of the child with AFP may suggest additional places of stay where ORI should be conducted
   - At least 500 children are vaccinated[Q]

iv. 60 day follow-up in a case of AFP[Q]
   - The district immunization officer must visit every case of AFP 60 days after onset of paralysis to confirm the presence or absence of residual weakness[Q]
   - Activity is completed before 70th day.
     * If AFP cases are not fully investigated for a variety of reasons such as inadequate stool specimen or could neither be confirmed nor discarded would be classified as compatible with poliomyelitis and such compatible cases will be reviewed by an expert committee, consisting of a neurologist, a pediatrician and a viriologist, who will then decide to confirm or discard the case.

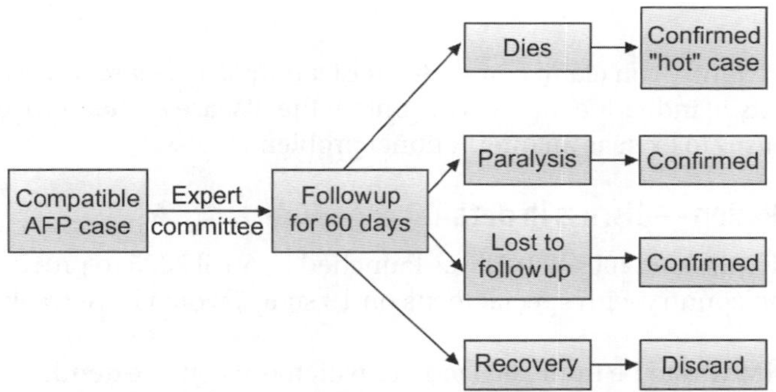

Fig. 3: AFP surveillance—compatible AFP cases

- Recovery from paralysis occurs in AFP cases other than polio and hence such cases are discarded.

b. Line listing of cases
   - This consists of reporting every case of AFP, by registering the case in prescribe proforma, which provides information such as name of the child, age, sex, address, immunization status, date of onset of paralysis, clinical findings, name of the reporting officer with contact details
   - Once a case is reported, active search is made to detect additional cases if any by house-to-house visits in that area.

   Advantage
   - Line listing helps in:
     - Avoiding duplication of case
     - Follow up of the cases
     - Helps to detect only fresh cases
     - Identification of high-risk areas
     - Implementation of containment measures.

   Significance
   - Acute flaccid paralysis surveillance is an important component of polio eradication program because polio virus has demonstrated ability to locate and infest pockets of susceptible person even in the countries with high level of vaccination coverage.
   - The immunization coverage may fail to reflect true levels of immunity in the general population.
   - Therefore, such high-risk areas or infected pockets will continue to serve as reservoir of infection and detection of the last reservoir or case of poliomyelitis is the greatest challenge which can be accomplished only with highly sensitive surveillance.

D. Mop-up immunization
   - Also called ring immunization or containment immunization or outbreak response.

   Objective
   - Contain polio outbreak in a limited jurisdiction and prevent spread of polio in community when poliovirus transmission has been reduced to well-defined and focal geographic areas.

   Strategy
   - On regular basis, door-to-door and child-to-child immunization is done in high-risk districts over period of days where wild polio virus is known or suspected to be still circulating to break the final chain of virus transmission
   - Consider every case of polio outbreak in an areas with >85% immunization coverage as an epidemic of polio and handle it on level of public health emergency
   - On confirmation of polio case in the jurisdiction of a PHC, medical officer should immediately take up administration of OPV to all children under five years living within 5 km radius from infected house or about 2000–3000 children in urban area irrespective of their immunization status
   - This should be done within 48 hours of reporting of acute flaccid paralysis and completed within a week
   - Second dose should be given after 1 month.

Significance

- In this era of jet travel, no country can claim complete eradication of a disease unless it is eradicated from the globe
- Hence it is the responsibility of individual nations to contain the disease in their jurisdiction and also step up efforts to eradicate it so that it ceases to exist as an international problem.

2. National Rural Health Mission—discuss in detail.

- The National Rural Health Mission (2005–2012) was launched in April 2005 to provide effective health-care to rural population throughout the country with special focus on 18 states, which have weak public health indicators and/or weak infrastructure
- The total duration of NRHM was to be from 2005 to 2012 which is recently extended up to 2017.

Principles	*Key components*	*Goals*
▪ Promote equity, access, efficiency, quality and accountability in public health system ▪ Enhance people-oriented and community-based approaches ▪ Decentralize and involve local bodies. ▪ Ensure public health focus ▪ Recognized value of traditional knowledge base of communities ▪ Promote new innovations, method and process development	▪ Provision of health activist in each village ▪ Village health plan to be prepared by village panchayat ▪ Strengthening of rural hospitals ▪ Integration of vertical health and family welfare programs at district level ▪ Strengthening delivery of primary health-care	▪ Reduction in infant mortality rate (imr) and maternal mortality ratio (MMR) ▪ Universal access to public health services such as women's health, child health, water, sanitation and hygiene, immunization, and nutrition ▪ Prevention and control of communicable and non-communicable diseases, including locally endemic diseases. ▪ Access to integrated comprehensive primary health-care ▪ Population stabilization, gender and demographic balance ▪ Revitalize local health traditions and mainstream AYUSH ▪ Promotion of healthy life styles

Targets

By 2015	▪ Filariasis elimination by 2015
By 2012	▪ IMR—to be reduced to 30/1,000 live births by 2012 ▪ Maternal mortality—to be reduced to 100/100,000 live births by 2012 ▪ TFR—to be reduced to 2.1 by 2012 ▪ Malaria mortality—50% reduction by 2010, additional 10% by 2012 ▪ Kala azar mortality reduction—100% by 2010 and sustaining elimination until 2012 ▪ Filaria/microfilaria reduction—80% by 2012 ▪ Dengue mortality reduction—50% by 2010 and sustaining at that level until 2012 ▪ Cataract operations—increasing to 46 lakh until 2012 ▪ 6,500 community health centers strengthened/established with 7 specialists and 9 staff nurses by 2012 ▪ 1,800 taluka/subdivisional hospitals and 600 district hospitals strengthened to provide quality health services by 2012
By 2010	▪ Filaria/microfilaria reduction—70% by 2010 ▪ All subcenters functional with two anms by 2010 ▪ All primary health centers with three staff nurses to provide 24 × 7 services by 2010
By 2008	▪ Over 5 lakh ASHAs, one for every 1,000 population/large habitation, in 18 special focus states and in tribal pockets of all states by 2008 ▪ Untied grants and annual maintenance grants to every SC, PHC, and CHC released regularly and utilized for local health action by 2008 ▪ All district health action plans completed by 2008
By 2009	▪ Mobile medical units for each district by 2009 ▪ Functional hospital development committees in all CHCs, subdivisional hospitals, and district hospitals by 2009
General (not time bound)	▪ Leprosy prevalence rate—reduce from 1.8 per 10,000 in 2005 to less that 1 per 10,000 thereafter ▪ Tuberculosis DOTS—maintain 85% cure rate through entire mission period and also sustain planned case detection rate ▪ Upgrading all health establishments in the districts to Indian Public Health Standards (IPHS) ▪ Increase utilization of first referral units from bed occupancy by referred cases of less than 20% to over 75%

Objectives

- Train and enhance the capacity of Panchayati Raj Institutions (PRIs) to own, control and manage public health services
- Preparation of health plan for each village through Village Health Committee of the Panchayat

- Strengthening subcenters through an untied fund to enable local planning and action
- Each subcenter will have an Untied Fund of ₹10,000 per annum which would be be deposited in a joint bank account of the ANM and Sarpanch and operated by the ANM, in consultation with Village Health Committee
- Provision of 24-hour service in 50% PHCs by addressing shortage of doctors, especially in high focus states, through mainstreaming AYUSH manpower
- Preparation and implementation of an intersectoral District Health Plan prepared by the District Health Mission, including drinking water, sanitation and hygiene and nutrition
- Integrating vertical Health and Family Welfare Programs at National, State, Block, and District levels.

Organization Structure

Level	*Organization*
Central	▪ Mission Steering Group (MSG) headed by Union Minister for Health and Family Welfare ▪ Empowered Program Committee (EPC) headed by the Union Secretary for Health and Family Wefare
State	▪ State Health Mission[Q] headed by Chief Minister of the State and State Health and Family Welfare Society to carry out functions of the mission ▪ Composition ▪ Chairperson: Chief Minister ▪ Co-Chairperson: Minister of Health and Family Welfare, State Government ▪ Convener: Principal Secretary/Secretary (Family Welfare) ▪ Nominated nonofficial members (5 to 8 members) such as health experts, representatives of medical associations, NGOs and Representatives of Development Partners ▪ Frequency of meetings ▪ At least once in every 6 months
District	▪ District Health Mission[Q] ▪ Composition ▪ Chairperson: Chairman, Zilla Parishad ▪ Co-Chairperson: District Collector ▪ Vice-Chairperson: CEO Zilla Parishad ▪ Mission Director: Chief Medical Officer
Village	▪ Village health, sanitation and nutrition committee ▪ Rogi Kalyan Samiti (for community management of hospitals)

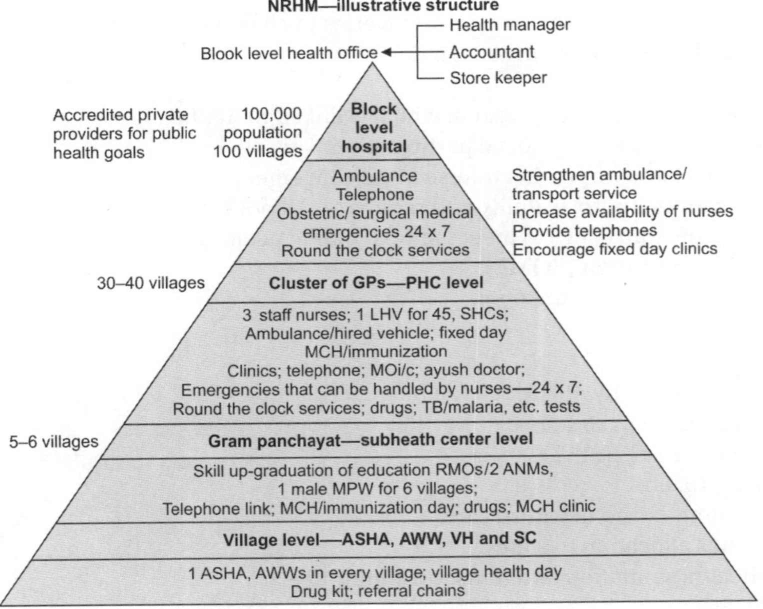

Fig. 4: NHRM—organization structure

Strategies

a. Train and enhance capacity of Panchayati Raj Institutions.
b. Decentralized village and district level health planning
   - Development of Village Health Plan for each village is a core strategy of NHRM. It is prepared by ASHA with help from Village Health Samiti of Panchayat
   - Similarly at district level, District Health Mission prepares Intersectoral District Health Plan including drinking water, sanitation, hygiene and nutrition
   - Village is lowest level at which health plans[Q] are formulated and district is core unit of planning, budgeting and implementation[Q].
c. Rogi Kalyan Samiti; a registered society comprising of community leaders who acts as trustees to manage affairs of the hospital and are responsible for upkeep of facilities and ensure provision of better care.
d. Promote access to improved health-care at household level by recruitment and training of accredited social health activist (ASHA)[Q].
e. Strengthening the public health service delivery system, particularly at village, primary and secondary level. by developing and implementing the Indian Public Health Standards
   - Strengthening of subcenters through united fund (10,000 per annum) and provision of multipurpose workers and ANMs
   - Strengthening of existing PHCs and CHCs to provide 24 hours service (in at least 50% PHCs), providing second doctor to PHCs
   - Developing CHCs as First Referral Units (FRUs) by providing special care in specialities of Medicine, Surgery, Obstetrics and Gynecology, and Pediatrics
   - Provision of 30–50 bedded CHCs per lakh population.
f. Mainstreaming of AYUSH (Indian Systems of Medicine).
g. Improved management capacity to organize health systems and services in public health.
h. Establishment of village health sanitation and nutrition committee.
i. Emphasizing evidence-based planning and implementation through strengthening capacities for data collection, assessment and review.
j. Formulating transparent policies for development of human resources.
k. Developing capacities for preventive health-care at all levels.
l. Strengthen of Janani Suraksha Yojana[Q], a safe motherhood initiative to promote institutional deliveries among poor women by cash incentives.
m. Janani Shishu Suraksha Karyakram providing free deliveries to all pregnant women.
n. National Mobile Medical Units Services in 333 districts.
o. National ambulance services.
p. Web-enabled Mother and Child Tracking system which is linked to Aadhar.
q. Prompting non-profit factor to increase social participation.
r. Promoting health behaviors and improving intersectoral convergence.
s. Regulation of private sector to improve equity and reduce out of pocket expenses.
t. Foster public private partnership (PPP) to meet national public health goals.
u. Re-orientation of medical education (ROME).
v. Raising health security/insurance for the poor.

New Initiatives

a. Home delivery of contraceptives by ASHA.
b. District level household survey in 26 states.
c. Promotion of menstrual hygiene in 152 districts.
d. Differential financial approach.
e. ASHA involvement in home-based newborn care.
f. Performance-based funds allocation to states.
g. Formation of village health, sanitation and nutrition committee.
h. Mainstreaming of AYUSH.

i. Rashtriya Bal Swasthya Karyakram (Feb 2013) for detection and management of 4D's—Defects at birth, Diseases, Deficiencies and Developmental delays.
j. Rashtriya Kishor Swasthya Karyakram (Jan 2014) to adolescent health-care.
k. Mother and child health wings of 30–100 beds in existing health-care infrastructure.
l. Free drugs and free diagnostic services.
m. National Iron + to supply weekly iron and folic acid supplementation in adolescents.
n. Delivery points for RMNCH+A services.
o. Universal health coverage.
p. Comprehensive primary health-care.
q. Kilkari—IVR based services delivering time sensitive audio messages to pregnant women and mothers of infants.

Functionary

- Accredited Social Health Activist (ASHA)
  - Accredited Social Health Activist (ASHA) is a cadre under National Rural Health Mission[Q], selected by the Village Health and Sanitation Committee of the Panchayat and is accountable to panchayat[Q]
  - She is not entitled to any pay and is a honorary volunteer[Q] receiving performance based compensation for promoting universal immunization, referral and escort services for RCH, construction of household toilets and other health-care delivery programs
  - She works under the overall guidance of District Health Mission and under direct guidance of anganwadi worker and auxillary nurse midwife
  - There is one ASHA for 1,000 population[Q] and in hilly and tribal areas it is one ASHA per habitation and is posted at village level[Q]

Selection criteria	*Training*
▪ ASHA must be a woman either married, widow or divorced ▪ She must the resident of the village ▪ Her age should be preferably 25–45 years ▪ She should have formal education up to 8th class[Q] ▪ She should have good communication skills and leadership qualities ▪ Preferably she should belong to disadvantaged population group to ensure better service that group	▪ ASHA will be trained in health promotion and treatment activities by the anganwadi worker and auxillary nurse midwife[Q] ▪ She would be provided with drug kit containing generic AYUSH and allopathic medicines form common ailments which would be replenished periodically by the anganwadi workder ▪ Government of India bears the cost of training, incentives and medical kits supplied to her

Duties assigned (role of ASHA)

- ASHA will create awareness and provide information to the community on determinants of health like nutrition, basic sanitation and hygiene, healthy living and working condition, information health services, and the need for timely utilization of health and family welfare services
- She will promote good health practices and provide a minimum package of curative care as appropriate and feasible and make timely referrals
- She will counsel women on birth preparedness, importance of safe delivery, breastfeeding and prevention of common infections including reproductive tract infection/sexually transmitted diseases[Q] and care of the young child
- She will mobilize and facilitate the community in accessing health and health-related services available at the anganwadi/subcenter/primary health center such as immunization, antenatal check-up, postnatal check-up, supplementary nutrition, sanitation and other services
- She will be a part of Janani Surakhsa Yojana and help reduce MMR[Q]
- She will develop a comprehensive village health plan[Q] with help from village health and sanitation committee of the panchayat
- She will arrange escort/accompany pregnant women and children requiring treatment[Q] to nearest medical facility
- She will provide primary medical care for minor ailments[Q] such as diarrhea, fevers, and first aid for minor injuries
- She will be a DOTS agent[Q]
- She will act as a depot holder for essential provisions like oral rehydration therapy, iron folic acid tablets, chloroquine, disposable delivery kits, oral pills and condoms, etc[Q].

- She will inform about the births and deaths in her village and any unusual health problems or disease outbreaks in the community to the sub-center/primary health center
- She will promote construction of household toilet under total sanitation campaign.

Monitoring and evaluation of ASHAs work

Process indicators	*Outcome indictors*	*Impact indicators*
▪ No. of ASHAs selected ▪ No. of ASHAs trained ▪ % of ASHAs attending review meeting after 1 year	▪ % of newborn weighed and families counseled ▪ % of deliveries with skilled assistance ▪ % of institutional deliveries ▪ % of JSY claims made by ASHA ▪ % of completed immunization in age group of 12–23 years ▪ % of unmet needs in BPL ▪ % of fever cases received chloroquine within 1 week in endemic areas	▪ Infant mortality rate[Q] ▪ Child malnutrition rates ▪ No. of cases of TB/leprosy detected compared to last year

Significance

- ASHA is an important functionary in the health-care delivery system acting as a bridge between ANM and village[Q] is an important link person between the community and the public health-care services[Q].

Significance

- Since independence, our country has created a vast public health infrastructure and has employed a large cadre of health-care providers yet, this vast infrastructure is able to cater to only 20% of the population, while 80% of health-care needs are still being provided by the private sector
- More than 70% of its population lives in rural areas, but only 20% of the total hospital beds are located there. Rural India is suffering from long-standing health-care problems and most of them are preventable and easily treatable
- National Rural Health Mission (NRHM) has been launched by Government of India to address these issues.

SHORT ESSAYS

3. Define sensitivity and specificity.

Refer Question No. 1 December 2010 (RS2) Paper I.

4. Pandemic influenza A—vaccine and treatment.

- Influenza pandemic occurs when there is an antigenic shift in influenza virus due to genetic reassortment or recombination of human virus with avian or animal virus in body of animal leading to a novel subtype virus for which humans have no immunity
- If such virus has sufficient gene from human influenza virus, then it can be readily transmitted from person to person resulting in pandemic.

Pandemic Influenza A

- Pandemic influenza A (H_1N_1) differs from seasonal influenza in its pathogenecity in regards to:
  - Majority of human population has little or no preexisting immunity to virus thus impact of infection has been in a wider age range
  - Virus can infect lower respiratory tract thus causing rapidly progressive pneumonia especially in children and young to middle aged adults.

Prevention

A. Elimination of reservoir
   a. Early diagnosis
      - Early diagnosis of cases of utmost importance as early symptoms are nonspecific

- Several rapid influenza diagnostic tests are commercially available
- Blood and stool cultures are vital investigations to diagnose cases.

b. Notification
- Notification of outbreak should be done wherever it is mandatory.

c. Isolation
- Cases need to be isolated from population for 7days after onset of illness or 24 hours after resolution of fever and respiratory symptoms whichever is longer.

d. Treatment
- Treatment of diagnosed cases is important to reduce the risk of transmission.

Drugs of choice	*Mechanism of action*	*Pharmaceutical actions*
▪ Oseltamivir and zanamivir (neuraminidase inhibitors)	▪ Prevent penetration of influenza virus into host cell thus prevent virus replication	▪ Shorten duration of fever, headache, cough, sore throat, general malaise and also reduce virus shedding

Dose

Oseltamivir		*Zanamivir*
Age/weight	Dose	2 inhalations (2 × 5 mg) BD for 5 days in children >5 years and adults
0–1 month	2 mg/kg BD for 5 days	
1–3 months	2.5 mg/kg BD for 5 days	
3-12 months	3 mg/kg BD for 5 days	
<15 kg	30 mg BD for 5 days	
15–23 kg	45 mg BD for 5 days	
24–40 kg	60 mg BD for 5 days	
>40 kg	75 mg BD for 5 days	

Treatment guidelines

- Treatment with oseltamivir should be initiated as early as possible in patient with severe or progressive clinical illness
  - It applies to all patient groups, including pregnant women and young children <2 years including neonates
  - Higher dose and longer duration of therapy with oseltamivir (up to 150 mg BD) can be given in patients not responding to standard regimen
  - Zanamivir should be used in case of inavailability, inability to use or resistance to oseltamivir
- Patients with higher risk of developing severe or complicated illness but presenting with uncomplicated illness should be treated as soon as possible following onset of illness
- Patients not considered to be at higher risk of developing severe or complicated illness, need not be treated with antivirals.

Significance

- Antiviral treatment should be started early following onset of symptoms but can be used at any stage of active disease when ongoing viral replication is anticipated and earlier treatment is associated with better outcomes.

B. Protections of susceptible

a. Immunization (Vaccination)

Indications (in order of priority—WHO)

- Health-care workers
- Pregnant women
- Individuals aged more than 6 months with one of the several chronic medical conditions
- Healthy young adults between age 15–49 years
- Healthy children
- Healthy adults between age 49–65 years
- Healthy adults aged more than 65 years.

Vaccines

i. Inactivated vaccine

* It is a split virion, inactivated, monovalent vaccine

<table>
<tr><td>Contents</td><td>▪ 15 μg of hemagglutinin per 0.5 mL of dose + thiomersal (vaccine preservative)</td></tr>
<tr><td>Storage</td><td>▪ 2–8°C (not to be frozen)</td></tr>
<tr><td>Indications</td><td>▪ During pandemic
▪ Along with seasonal influenza vaccination</td></tr>
<tr><td>Route of administration</td><td>▪ Intranmuscular (never gluteal)
▪ Children: Anterolateral aspect of thigh
▪ Adults: Deltoid</td></tr>
<tr><td>Immunity</td><td>▪ 14 days after vaccination
▪ Only systemic immunity, no local immunity
▪ No 100% immunity but only reduces risk of disease</td></tr>
<tr><td>Contraindications</td><td>▪ Children below 6 months
▪ Pregnant and lactating mothers</td></tr>
<tr><td>Dosage and schedule</td><td><table>
<tr><th>Age</th><th>Dose</th><th>Schedule</th></tr>
<tr><td>6–35 months</td><td>0.25 mL</td><td>2 doses, a month apart</td></tr>
<tr><td>3–9 years</td><td>0.5 mL</td><td>2 doses, a month apart</td></tr>
<tr><td>>9 years</td><td>0.5 mL</td><td>Single dose</td></tr>
</table></td></tr>
<tr><td>Adverse effects</td><td>▪ Local reaction—soreness, swelling and redness at injection site
▪ Fever, muscle or joint aches or headache—mild, lasting 1–2 days (frequent in children)
▪ Allergic reactions—hives, rapid swelling of deeper skin layers and tissues, asthma, hypersensitivity (rarely)</td></tr>
</table>

ii. Live attenuated vaccine

* It is a live attenuated, freeze dried

Route of administration	▪ Intranasal via nasal spray
Immunity	▪ Produces both systemic and local immunity in nose
Indications	▪ Children over 3 years of age ▪ Adults
Adverse effects	▪ Runny nose, nasal congestion, cough ▪ Sore throat, low grade fever, irritability and muscles aches and headaches (less frequently) ▪ Wheezing and vomiting (rarely in children)

b. Chemoprophylaxis

- Indicated in high-risk people such as children, elderly, close contacts and debilitated persons

<table>
<tr><th>Indications</th><th>Drug of choice</th><th>Dosage</th><th>Duration</th></tr>
<tr><td>▪ Health-care personnels
▪ Close contact of suspected or confirmed case</td><td>Oseltamivir</td><td><table>
<tr><th>Age/weight</th><th>Dose</th></tr>
<tr><td><3 months</td><td>Not recommended unless critical</td></tr>
<tr><td>3–5 months</td><td>20 mg OD</td></tr>
<tr><td>6–11 months</td><td>25 mg OD</td></tr>
<tr><td><15 kg</td><td>30 mg OD</td></tr>
<tr><td>15–23 kg</td><td>45 mg OD</td></tr>
<tr><td>24–40 kg</td><td>60 mg OD</td></tr>
<tr><td>>40 kg</td><td>75 mg OD</td></tr>
</table></td><td>10 days after last exposure</td></tr>
</table>

c. Personal protection
   - Appropriate infection control measures (standard and droplet precautions) should be followed
   - Strict adherence to hand hygiene with soap and water or alcohol based hand sanitizer
   - Cover mouth and nose with tissue or handkerchief when someone is coughing or sneezing.

d. Health education
   - Educate the community about modes of spread of disease, detection of early symptoms, personal protection measures via mass media
   - Conduct camps to diagnose inapparent cases in the community.

Significance

- Influenza pandemics show cyclic trends of 10–30 years
- Based on knowledge about past pandemics, the H_1N_1 virus is expected to continue to circulate as a seasonal virus for some years to come
- While level of concern is now greatly diminished, vigilance on part of national health authorities remain important because behavior of H_1N_1 virus as a seasonal virus cannot be reliably predicted.

5. Collection of sputum sample in tuberculosis.

- examination of sputum is the best criteria to diagnose tuberculosis according to WHO[Q].

Collection of Sputum in Tuberculosis

- Under RNTCP, sputum microscopy is the case finding tool
- Here the patient visiting a physician with persistent cough of 2 weeks duration is suspected to be TB patient and TB has to ruled out by the physician by screening them with 2 sputum smear examinations[Q] by a specially trained technician in the designated RNTCP microscopy centers.

Principle

- 2 sputum smear examinations is a must[Q] under RNTCP because with one sample of sputum, the chances of detecting smear positive is 80%, with two samples 93%.

Procedure

In adults	*In children*[1]
▪ The early morning sample is taken because the secretions build up in the airways overnight and chances of detecting bacilli are more	a. Sputum induction – Standard method of sputum collection in children – Sputum can be collected from even very young children by inducing cough and sputum production with nebulized saline or bronchodilators and then asking the patient to expectorate the sputum OR suctioning the back of the pharynx to collect sputum
▪ Since is difficult for an out-patient to provide 2 early morning specimens, spot-morning-spot samples are collected, i.e. a sample of sputum is collected on the spot when the patient attends the out-patient department and is then given a cup to collect the sputum of next day morning	b. Gastric aspiration – Classic method of culture collection in children – Usually, 3 gastric aspirates are collected first thing in the morning after an overnight fast c. Bronchoalveolar lavage (BAL) – Particularly helpful in patients in whom the cause of pulmonary disease or infection is not known

Advantages

- Simple, cheap, easy, reliable, confirmative and practical diagnostic test
- Helps to identify infectious cases[Q]
- Not only confirms the diagnosis but also helps in assessing the prognosis
- More objective and reliable than X-ray of chest and is 98% specific than X-ray
- Helps to categorize the patient by distinguishing between smear +ve and smear –ve patients (for patient to be +ve there should be at least 10,000 bacilli/mL of sputum[Q])
- Facilitates provision of appropriate treatment.

Significance

- Examination of sputum is first line of investigation and considered gold-standard test in adult tuberculosis[Q].

Ref:

1. Marais BJ, Pai M; Specimen collection methods in the diagnosis of childhood tuberculosis; Indian J Med Micrcbiol 2006:24;249-51.

6. Hepatitis B vaccine—schedule.

Refer Question No. 1 December 2014 (RS2) Paper II.

7. Oral rehydration therapy—indications.

- Oral rehydration therapy was introduced by WHO in 1971 with aim of preventing dehydration and reducing mortality.

Principle

- Glucose given orally enhances the intestinal absorption of salt and water[Q] and is capable of correcting the electrolytes and water deficit.

Composition of Oral Rehydration Fluids

a. Older WHO solutions

Composition	*Bicarbonate*	*Citrate*
Sodium chloride[Q]	3.5 g	3.5 g[Q]
Sodium bicarbonate	2.5 g	—
Trisodium citrate dehydrate[Q]	—	2.9 g[Q]
Potassium chloride[Q]	1.5 g	1.5 g[Q]
Glucose[Q]	20 g	20 g[Q]
Potable water[Q]	1 L	1 L[Q]

b. Newer WHO solution (reduced osmolarity ORS)

Low sodium ORS[Q]			
Composition[Q]		*Osmolar concentration*[Q]	
Sodium chloride	2.6 g	Sodium	75 mmol/ltr
Potassium chloride	1.5 g	Potassium	20 mmol/ltr
Sodium citrate	2.9 g	Chloride	65 mmol/ltr
Glucose	13.5 g	Citrate	10 mmol/ltr
Potable water	1 L	Glucose	75 mmol/ltr
Total	20.5 g	Total	245 mmol/ltr

c. Rehydration solution for malnourished (ReSoMal)

ReSoMal			
Composition		**Osmolar concentration**	
WHO ORS powder	1	Sodium	45 mmol/L
Potable water	2 L	Potassium	40 mmol/L
Glucose	50 g	Chloride	70 mmol/L
Electrolyte/mineral solution	40 g	Citrate	7 mmol/L
		Glucose	125 mmol/L
		Mg^{2+}, Zn^{2+}, CU^{2+}	4 mmol/L

d. Home made

Table salt	5 g	8 tablespoon	1 fistful
Sugar	20 g	1 tablespoon	3 pinch
Potable water	1 L	1 L	1 big glass

Oral Rehydration Therapy

Indications

a. Mild-to-moderate dehydration indicated by—sunken eyes/absence of tears/dry tongue/thirst/restlessness/loss of skin turgor
b. Diarrhoeal disorders—cholera, shigellosis, *E. coli* diarrhea, viral diarrhea, amoebiasis, infective diarrhea.
c. Hypovolemia
d. Vomiting
e. Excessive sweating
f. Inadequate fluid intake.

Procedure

- Any child with dehydration is assessed for degree of dehydration as follows:

	*Degree of dehydration**		
Signs	*A*	*B*	*C*
Look for			
▪ General condition#	Well, alert	Restless, irritable#	Lethargic, floppy#, unconscious
▪ Eyes	Normal	Sunken	Deeply sunken and dry
▪ Tears on cry$	Present	Absent	Absent
▪ Mouth and tongue	Moist	Dry	Very dry
▪ Thirst#	Not thirsty (drinks normally)	Thirsty# (drinks eagerly)	Very thirsty# (drinks poorly or unable to drink)
Feel for			
▪ Skin pinch@	Goes back quickly within a second	Goes back slowly#, taking 1–2 seconds	Goes back very slowly#, taking more than 2 seconds
▪ Anterior fontanel	Normal	Depressed	Very much depressed
Interpretation	No dehydration–Patient has no signs of dehydration	Some dehydration: Patient has 2 or more signs including at least 1 key sign#	Severe dehydration: Patient has 2 or more signs including at least 1 key sign#
Treatment	Plan A: With home available fluid to prevent dehydration	Plan B: With WHO recommended ORS solution to correct some dehydration	Plan C: With intravenous infusion urgently to correct severe dehydration and prevent death

#KEY signs
*Always move from column C to column A for assessment and management
@ Skin pinch is less useful in patients with malnutrition and obesity
$Tears on cry is a relevant only among infants and young children

Dosage

- Depending upon the degree of dehydration, age and weight of the child, the amount of ORS administered in 1st 4 hours is as follows:

Age	*<4 months*	*4–11 months*	*1–2 years*	*2–4 years*	*5–14 years*	*≥15 year*
Weight in kg	<5	5–8	8–11	11–16	16–30	>30
ORS in mL	200–400	400–600	600–800	800–1200	1200–2200	>2200
Local measure (glass)	1–2	2–3	3–4	4–6	6–11	12–20

Guidelines of ORS Therapy

a. Adults and older children
   – Gives as much ORS as they want preferably required amount within 4 hours and additional water.
b. Children below 2 years
   – Teaspoon every 1–2 minutes

– If child vomits, by again after 10 minutes slowly, i.e. spoonful every 2–3 minutes
– If child wants more ORS than estimated amount and does not vomit continue administering
– Disappearance of signs of dehydration denotes complete rehydration
– In case of breastfed children, continue nursing
– In one breastfed infants below 6 months, additional 100–200 mL of water should be given first 4 hours
– Use reconstituted ORS within 24 hours[Q.]

Advantages	*Disadvantages*
▪ It made domiciliary treatment possible ▪ The ingredients of ORS are in expensive, readily available ▪ It has reduced infant mortality significantly ▪ It is of modern scientific technology ▪ Preparation is easy and administration is also simple and safe ▪ It prevents hospitalization and thus reduces the treatment cost ▪ It involves mothers directly in the child care ▪ It has minimized antibiotic use ▪ It is free from side effects	▪ ORT cannot be given to those who have persistent vomiting or unconscious or in a state of shock due to severe dehydration ▪ It cannot be given to those who have paralytic ileus and marked abdominal distension ▪ It cannot also be given to those who have glucose malabsorption syndrome ▪ Its use among low birth weight babies has not been evaluated

Significance

- Oral rehydration therapy is a scientifically sound, practically adoptable, culturally acceptable and economically cheap thus is it is an appropriate technology which is one of the principles of primary health-care.
- Ors is the most important discovery of 20th century.

8. WHO classification of the severity of dengue infection.

Refer Question No. 12 June 2012 (RS2) Paper II.

9. Management of genital ulcers.

- Genital ulcer is a sexually transmitted disease characterized by formation of ulcerative lesion on genitals in both males and females

Common causes	*Common clinical signs*
▪ Syphillis (*Treponema pallidum*) ▪ Chanchroid (*Haemophilus ducreyi*) ▪ Genital herpes (herpes simplex virus) ▪ Lymphogranuloma venerum (*Chlamydia trachomatis*) ▪ Donovanosis (*Calymatobacterium granulomatosis*)	▪ Ulcer on penis or scrotum (in men) ▪ Ulcer on labia, vagina or cervix (in women)

Management of Genital Ulcers

- Sexually transmitted diseases such as genital ulcers are treated by syndromic approach
- This syndromic management is based on identification of consistent group of symptoms and easily recognizable signs.

Steps Involved in Syndromic Management of Genital Ulcers

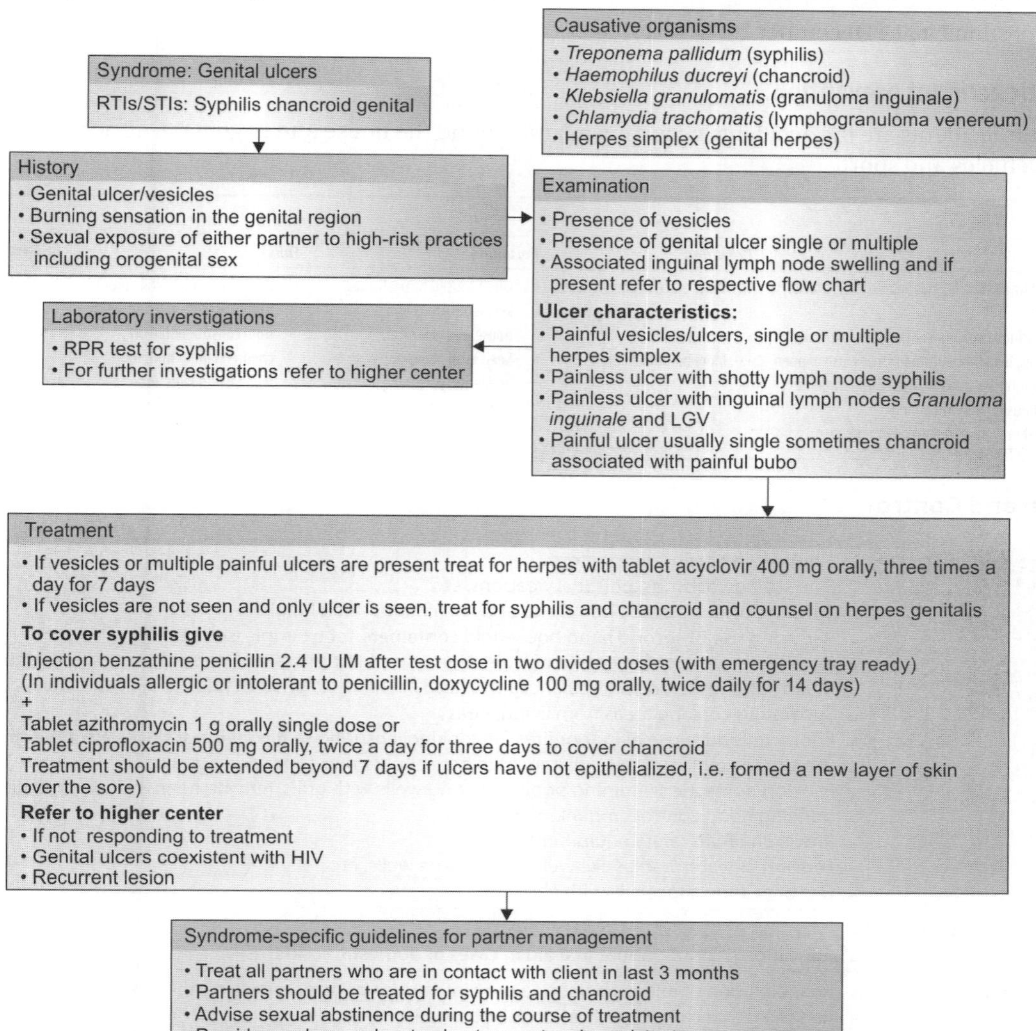

Management of pregnant women

- Quinolones (like ofloxacin, ciprofloxacin), doxycycline, sulfonamides are contraindicated in pregnant women
- Pregnant women who test positive for RPR should be considered infected unless adequate treatment is documented in the medical records and sequential serologic antibody titers have declined
- Injection benzathine penicillin 2.4 million IU IM after test dose (with emergency tray ready)
- A second dose of benzathine penicillin 2.4 million units IM should be administered 1 week after the initial dose for women who have primary, secondary, or early latent syphilis
- Pregnant women who are allergic to penicillin should be treated with erythromycin and the neonate should be treated for syphilis after delivery
- Tablet erythromycin 500 mg orally four times a day for 15 days
- (Note: Erythromycin estolate is contraindicated in pregnancy because of drug-related hepatotoxicity Only erythromycin base or erythromycin ethyl succinate should be used in pregnancy)
- All pregnant women should be asked history of genital herpes and examined carefully for herpetic lesions
- Women without symptoms or signs of genital herpes or its prodrome can deliver vaginally
- Women with genital herpetic lesions at the onset of labor should be delivered by cesarean section to prevent neonatal herpes
- Acyclovir may be administered orally to pregnant women with first episode genital herpes or severe recurrent herpes

Fig. 5: Steps involved in synodromic management of genital ulcers

10. Hypertension—"rule of Halves".

Refer Question No. 12 December 2008 (RS2) Paper II.

11. Domestic accident prevention.

- Domestic accidents are the accidents occurring in and around the house and in general, all accidents not related to traffic, vehicles and sport.

Classification

Burns	*Drowning*	*Poisoning*	*Falls*	*Injuries*
• May be by flames, hot liquids, electricity, crackers, chemical, etc. • Risk factors include cooking on open fires, explosion of pressure stoves, instability of small stoves, use of open fires during winter for warmth, use of inflammable materials in housing and furnishing • More amongst in women due to dowry menace	• Takes place in ponds, rivers and oceans or during flood and cyclones • More among children	• Often caused by pesticides, kerosene, drugs and household chemicals • Seen in all age groups but accidental poisoning is more common in children	• Occur from trees while picking fruits, coconut, tapping toddy, from construction work, children falling from roof while flying kites, etc. • Common in children and young adults	• Occur from falls, hitting with blunt or sharp objects and also from animal bites

Prevention and Control

a. Primary prevention	▪ Elimination of causative factors ▪ Safe storage of drugs, poisons, weapons, etc. ▪ Storing poisons outside home and above childrens head height ▪ Reducing use of second hand household containers, for example, soda bottles ▪ Introduction and enforcement of legislation to prohibit the sale of poisons in such containers ▪ Muscle strengthening and balance retraining in elderly to prevent falls ▪ Separating cooking areas from living areas ▪ Efforts to reduce use of indoor fires for cooking, ensuring that cooking surfaces are at heights, reducing the storage of flammable substances in households, and supervising young children more effectively ▪ Fencing domestic swimming pools, covering wells with grills, fencing nearby lakes or riverbanks, and building flood control embankments ▪ Provision of fire safety equipment ▪ Fencing of water bodies like well, ponds, bore wells, etc ▪ Use of caution especially with children
b. Secondary prevention	▪ Provision of accessible primary care ▪ Education of public about first aid in cases of domestic accidents
c. Tertiary prevention	▪ Rehabilitation of injured person to prevent, reduce or compensate disability and thus prevent handicap ▪ Rehabilitation can be medical, social, occupational, etc

Significance

- Domestic accidents are very common and best prevention for them is little caution.

12. Disaster management in India.

- 'Disaster management' is defined as a continuous and integrated process of planning, organizing, coordinating and implementing measures which are necessary or expedient to prevent danger or threat of any disaster, mitigation or reduce the risk or severity or consequences of any disaster, capacity-building and preparedness to deal with any disaster, prompt response to any threatening disaster situation or disaster, assessing the severity or magnitude of effects of any disaster, evacuation, rescue and relief, rehabilitation and reconstruction.

History of Disaster Management in India

- The late 1990s and the early part of this century marked a watershed in disaster management in India
- The 1990s were declared by the United Nations as the 'International Decade for Natural Disaster Reduction'
- Following the United Nations declaration, a permanent disaster management cell was established under the Ministry of Agriculture

- In 2002, the disaster management division of Ministry of Agriculture was shifted to the Ministry of Home Affairs (MHA)
- Based on the report submitted by the high powered committee was created in 1999 to review the existing mechanisms for disaster preparedness and mitigation and recommend measures to strengthen these mechanisms at the national, state and district levels, Disaster Management Act was enacted in 2005.

Disaster Management Act, 2005

- The Disaster Management Act specifies the responsibilities of the central, state and district governments in disaster management as follows.

Objectives

- Through the Disaster Management Act, the Government of India has decided to put in place, necessary institutional mechanisms for drawing up and monitoring the implementation of disaster management plans, ensuring measures by various wings of government for prevention of and mitigating the effects of disasters and for undertaking a holistic, coordinated and prompt response to any disaster situation
- More specifically, it aims to:
  - Promoting a culture of prevention, preparedness and mitigation
  - Establishing institutional and techno-legal frameworks
  - Mainstreaming disaster management into the developmental planning process
  - Developing contemporary forecasting and early warning systems
  - Ensuring efficient response and relief through dedicated decision support system
  - Undertaking reconstruction so that previous shortcomings are removed
- The act provides for establishing several institutions at the state and district levels with adequate financial and administrative powers keeping the NDMA at the top, creation of the National Disaster Response Force (NDRF) and of the National Institute of Disaster Management (NIDM) with the comprehensive mandate or planning and promoting training and research in the area of disaster management, documentation and development of national level information base relating to disaster management policies, prevention mechanisms and mitigation measures
- The act also provides guidelines for creation of National Disaster Response Fund, National Mitigation Fund, establishment of funds by State Government and allocation of funds by Ministries and Departments for Emergency Procurement.

Disaster Management Structure

See Figure 6

a. The National Disaster Management Authority (NDMA)
   - It will be the apex body with PM as the chairperson
   - It is to be responsible for drawing up and monitoring the implementation of disaster management plans and policies, ensuring measures for prevention and mitigation of disasters and for undertaking a holistic, coordinated and prompt response to any disaster situation.
   - It has the power to approve the national plans and the plans of the respective ministries and departments of Government of India.
   - The general superintendence, direction and control of National Disaster Response Force (NDRF) are vested in and will be exercised by the NDMA.

   Functions of NDMA
   - Laying down policy and guidelines for different ministries and departments of the Government of India for integration of the measures for prevention and mitigation of disasters in their development plans and projects
   - Lay down broad policies and guidelines for functioning of the National Institute of Disaster Management
   - Laying down guidelines for the minimum standards of relief to be provided to persons affected by disaster
   - Approve National Disaster Management (DM) Plan and DM Plans of Ministries and Departments
   - Ensure availability of funds and coordinate enforcement and implementation of disaster policy and plans

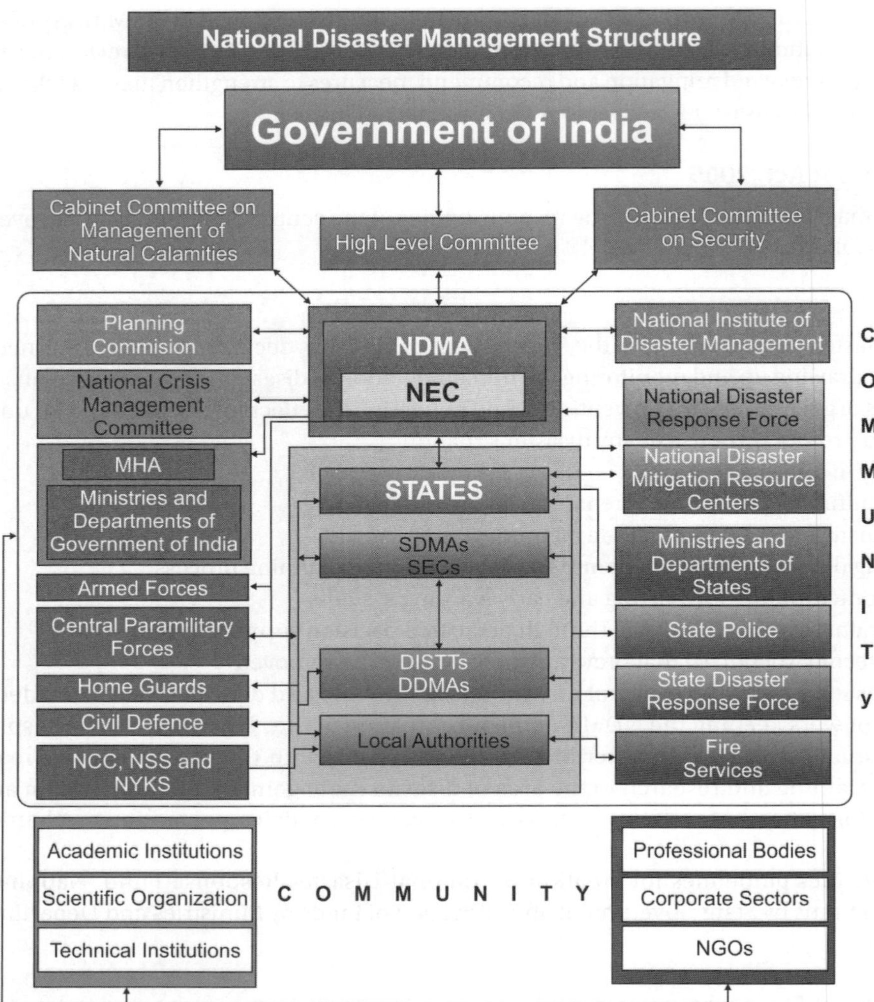

Fig. 6: Disaster management—structure in India

- Take measures for prevention, mitigation, preparedness and capacity building for dealing with potential disaster situations
- Exercise general superintendence, direction and control of National Disaster Response Force
- Give directions regarding relief in loan repayment or for grant of fresh loans on concessional terms as deemed appropriate by the authority
- Provide disaster management support to other countries affected by a major disaster, on direction from the Central Government.

b. National Executive Committee (NEC)
   - It is mandated to assist the NDMA in the discharge of its functions and further ensure compliance of the directions issued by the Central Government.
   - It consists of the Union Home Secretary as the chairperson, and the secretaries to the Government of India's various ministries/departments such as health, power, rural development, agriculture, atomic energy, defense, drinking water supply, environment and forests, finance (expenditure), science and technology, space, telecommunications, urban development, water resources and the chief of the integrated defense staff committee as members.
   - Special invitees include secretaries in the ministry of external affairs, earth sciences, human resource development, mines, shipping, road transport and highways and secretary, and NDMA.

Functions

- The National Executive Committee is responsible to prepare the national plan and coordinate and monitor the implementation of the national policy and the guidelines issued by NDMA
- It assists the NDMA to coordinate disaster management efforts, preparing a national plan for disaster management and monitoring the implementation of the disaster management guidelines formulated by the NDMA.

c. Central Level

i. Central Ministries

- Central ministries will continue with nodal responsibilities.
- The Ministry of Home Affairs (MHA) in the Central Government has the overall responsibility for disaster management in the country
- For some specific types of disasters the concerned ministries have the nodal responsibilities for management of the disasters:

Drought	*Ministry of Agriculture*
▪ Epidemics and biological disasters	▪ Ministry of Health and Family Welfare
▪ Chemical disasters	▪ Ministry of Environment and Forests
▪ Nuclear disasters	▪ Ministry of Atomic Energy
▪ Air accidents	▪ Ministry of Civil Aviation
▪ Railway accidents	▪ Ministry of Railways

ii. National Crisis Management Committee

- It includes cabinet secretary and secretaries of other departments that are in-charge of dealing with crises and giving directions to the Crisis Management Group.

iii. Crisis Management Group

- Reviews contingency plans formulated by the central ministries/departments.

d. State Level

i. State Disaster Management Authority (SDMA)

- It is headed by the chief minister
- It lays down policies and plans for disaster management in the state
- It performs the same duties as the NDMA at the national level
- It is mostly positioned in the revenue and relief department, which is the nodal authority for the state.

ii. State Executive Committee (SEC)

- It is headed by chief secretary
- It assists the SDMA in the implementation its policies and guidelines through coordinating and monitoring the implementation of the national policy, national plan and state plan.

iii. State Advisory Committee

- Consists of members with practical expertise on disaster management to make recommendations on the management of disasters.

e. District Level

i. District Disaster Management Authority (DDMA)

- It is headed by District Magistrate, with the elected representative of the local authority as the Co-Chairperson.
- DDMA is the planning, coordinating and implementing body for disaster management at district level.
- It will, inter alia prepare the district disaster management plan and monitor the implementation of the national and state policies and the national, state and the district plans.
- It is responsible for the on-site management of the disaster.

Composition

- District Magistrate—Chairperson
- Chairperson of Zila Parishad as Co-Chairperson—interface between government and public
- The local authorities include both the rural local self-governing institutions (Panchayati Raj Institutions) and urban local bodies (Municipalities, Cantonment Boards and Town Planning Authorities). These bodies will ensure capacity building of their officers and employees for managing disasters, carry out relief, rehabilitation and reconstruction activities in the affected areas and will prepare DM plans in consonance with guidelines of the NDMA, SDMAs and DDMAs.

f. Supporting Institutions
   i. National Disaster Response Force (NDRF)
      - It is the specialized force for disaster response which works under the overall supervision and control of the NDMA.
   ii. National Institute of Disaster Management (NIDM)
      - It has the mandate for human resource development and capacity building for disaster management within the broad policies and guidelines laid down by the NDMA
      - NIDM is required to design, develop and implement training programs, undertake research, formulate and implement a comprehensive human resource development plan, provide assistance in national policy formulation, assist other research and training institutes, state governments and other organizations for successfully discharging their responsibilities, develop educational materials for dissemination and promote awareness among stakeholders in addition to undertake any other function as assigned to it by the Central Government.

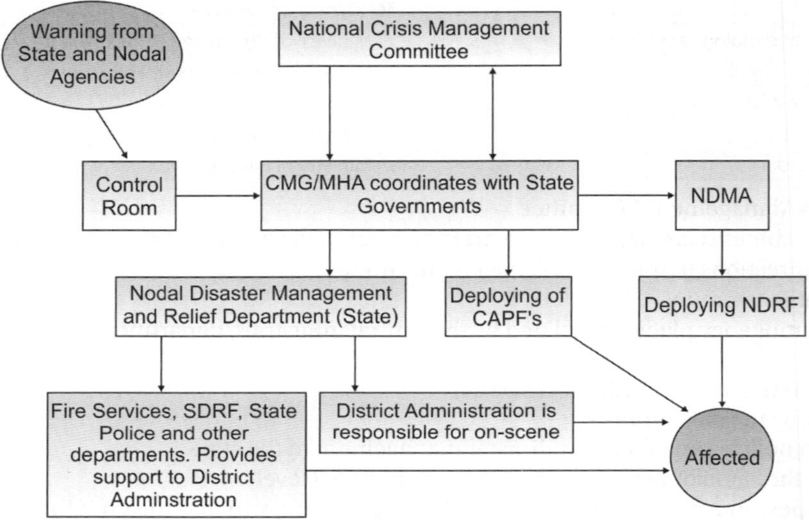

Fig. 7: Disaster response in India

Approach

- Paradigm shift from response centric to a holistic and integrated approach
- Backed by—institutional framework and legal authority
- Supported by financial mechanism, creation of new funds, i.e. response fund and mitigation fund at national, state and district levels.

Strategy

- A multi-dimensional strategy, focusing on:

Predisaster Phase	*Postdisaster Phase*
▪ Prevention ▪ Mitigation ▪ Preparedness ▪ Capacity Building and Awareness ▪ Community Based Disaster Management	▪ Prompt and efficient response—proactive ▪ Reconstruction to build back better

Funding

- The Ministry of Home Affairs is the nodal ministry for providing financial assistance in the aftermath of any disaster.

a. National Disaster Response Fund and State Disaster Response Fund
   – Based on the recommendations of the 13th Finance Commission, the schemes of the NDRF and SDRF were made operational for a period of five years from 2010 to 2015

- The funds from both are to be used only to provide immediate relief to people affected by cyclone, drought, earthquake, fire, flood, tsunami, hailstorm, landslide, avalanche, cloud burst and pest attack
- These funds are not for disaster preparedness, mitigation and restoration work, which must be met from the plan funds of the state
- The National Calamity Contingency Fund was merged with the NDRF and the Calamity Relief Fund was merged with the SDRF
- Central government was to contribute 75% of total yearly allocation to general category states and 90% of total yearly allocation to special category states in the form of non-plan grant to SDRF
- The balance was to be contributed by state governments
- Natural calamities that require expenditure in excess of the SDRF receive additional funding from the NDRF.

b. National Disaster Mitigation Fund and State Disaster Mitigation Fund
   - These two funds were to be created at the national and state levels respectively to fund mitigation efforts
   - The NDMF was to be placed at the disposal of NDMA
   - However, the NDMF is not operational as yet and only a few states have made their SDRFs operational
   - Therefore, at present, mitigation efforts are financed through state plans.

Significance

- Disaster management is essentially a dynamic process
- India is considered as the world's most disaster prone country
- Like many other countries in this region, India is plagued by various kinds of natural disasters every year, such as floods, drought, earthquakes, cyclones and landslides
- Millions of people are affected every year and the economic losses caused by natural disasters amount to a major share of the Gross National Product (GNP)
- Natural disasters are huge economic burdens on developing economies such as India. Every year, huge amount of resources are mobilized for rescue, relief and rehabilitation works following natural disaster occurrences
- Hence a clearly defined plan of action in events such as these is must to save human life as well avoid economic loss.

SHORT ANSWERS

13. Modes of transmission of typhoid fever.

Refer Question No. 10 June 2010 (RS2) Paper II.

14. Management of *Plasmodium vivax* malaria.

Refer Question No. 1 June 2013 (RS2) Paper II.

15. Urban rabies.

- Urban rabies is an epidemiological type of rabies.

Features

- Urban rabies is transmitted from bite of domestic animals like dogs
- In urban rabies cycle, domestic and stray dogs are the main reservoirs
- Transmission of virus amongst domestic animals is called urban cycle
- This cycle predominates in areas where the proportion of unvaccinated and semi-owned or stray dogs is high, such as some parts of Asia, Africa and Latin America.

Significance

- Urban rabies is the most common form of rabies seen in India
- Urban rabies can be easily controlled through measures like vaccination of stray and domestic dogs, registration of dogs, sterilization of stray dogs, etc.
- Other form of rabies is Sylvatic rabies which is transmitted by wild animals.

16. International certificate of vaccination.

- International vaccination certificate is a travel document issued by WHO
- Also called yellow card or *Carte Jaune*
- Since 2007, there has been revision in format and rules and since then it is now called "International Certification of Vaccination or Prophylaxis"
- It is not to be confused with yellow fever certificate.

Features	*Guidelines*	*Validity*	*Vaccines*
▪ Available in 2 versions, i.e. bilingual (English-French) and trilingual (English-French-Arabic) ▪ It contains personal details of traveler's like name, address, passport No., etc. ▪ There is also provision for providing medical history of traveler including history of previous vaccinations, contraindications to any vaccines, allergies, etc. ▪ Most important part of certificate is section on yellow fever	▪ Vaccination should be filled in with dates (in DD/MM/YYYY format), nature of vaccine and dose and should be signed by physician ▪ In order to make it international, it advised to mention complete details about vaccine under nature of vaccine	▪ It is recognized internationally and may be required for entry to certain countries where there are increased health risks for travellers ▪ It is valid as long as vaccine provides immunity	a. Mandatory – Yellow fever[Q] b. Recommended (depending upon country of travel) – Meningococcal meningitis – Japanese encephalitis – Hepatitis B – Typhoid – Cholera – Tick born encephalitis

Significance

- International vaccination certificate is an important travel document, as it important as passport that it is a medical passport of sorts.

Ref:

1. http://en.wikipedia.org/wiki/Carte_Jaune accessed on 4th June 2011.

17. Western blot test.

- Western blot test is a highly specific test for detecting HIV infection
- It is applied to weed out any false-positive cases detected on ELISA testing.

Principle

- Based on detection of specific antibody to viral core protein (p24) and envelop glycoprotein (gp41).

Procedure

- HIV proteins are separated according their electrophoretic mobility (and molecular weight) by polyacrylamide gel electrophoresis
- Then they are blotted onto strips of nitrocellulose paper retaining their relative position achieved on separation
- Antigen impregnated nitrocellulose is then cut into strips, each strip having full complement of vital proteins which were separated in the gel
- Each strip is then incubated with dilution of patient's serum
- Antibodies which attach to separated viral antigen on the strip are detected by enzyme linked tracer anti-human immunoglobulin antibodies
- Tracer antibodies are identified by adding substrate which changes color in presence of enzyme and permanently stains the strip
- Location or position on the strip at which a patient's antibodies attach to viral antigens indicates whether antibody is specific for viral antigens or directed against non-viral material from cells in which virus was grown.

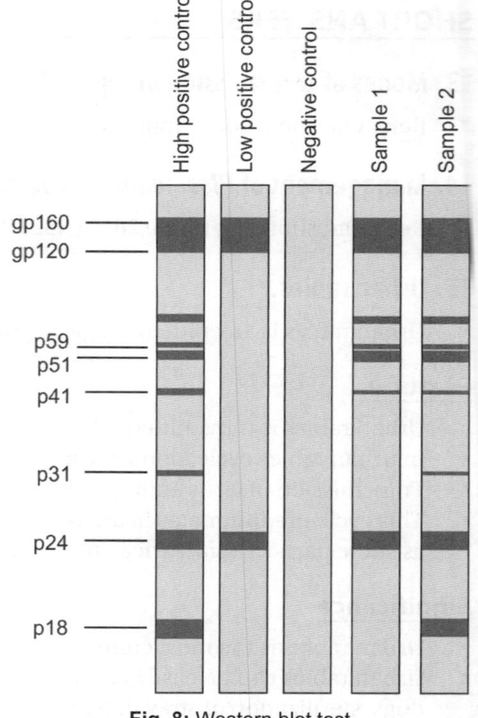

Fig. 8: Western blot test

Interpretation

Negative result	*Positive result*	*Indeterminate result*
▪ Weakly reactive p17 band may be considered negative (WHO)	▪ Bands seen with multiple proteins, typically p24 (gag gene, core protein), p31 (pol gene, reverse transcriptase) and gp41, gp120 or gp160 (env gene, surface antigen) ▪ Test is considered positive even with presence of 2 proteins representing three genes, gag, pol and env ▪ Bands representing all 3 genes is conclusive proof of HIV infection	▪ May arise from either insensitive detection of true reactivity (window period) or false reactivity with principally single band reactivity ▪ In such cases, western blot is repeated

Advantages	*Disadvantages*
▪ Highly specific test (specificity is >99.99% if combined with ELISA)	▪ More difficult to perform ▪ Require trained and experienced laboratory workers to interpret ▪ Indeterminate results with early HIV infection, HIV-2 infection, autoimmune disease, pregnancy and recent tetanus toxoid administration

Significance

- Western blot test is confirmatory test for HIV infection.

18. Screening of cancer cervix.

Refer Question No. 11 June 2013 (RS2) Paper II.

19. Measures for prevention of smoking.

- Smoking is an established modifiable risk factor for cardiovascular diseases like ischemic heart disease, hypertension, etc. and various cancers like lung cancer, oral cancer, etc.
- It is estimated that control of smoking alone would reduced the total burden of cancer by over a million cancers each year.

Measures for Prevention of Smoking

a. Health education and public information	▪ General population should be informed and educated about the hazards of smoking targeting the whole population in general but youth and school children in particular through mass media, internet and other sources of communication ▪ NGOs should be encouraged to start a nationwide anti-smoking campaign to change the life style associated with smoking ▪ National Health Policy should have curtailment of smoking as integral part
b. Taxation	▪ In recent years, Government has increased tax on tobacco and tobacco-related products in order to dissuade users from their use or at least curtain their use
c. Promotion of smoking cessation methods	▪ Establishment for smoking cessation clinics where individuals should be counseled to give up smoking ▪ These clinics should also relieve the smoker of abstinence symptoms ▪ They should be provided information about various smoking cessation methods or alternatives like electric cigarettes, nicotine gums or patches, etc.
d. Legislation	▪ India had started its anti-smoking campaign with "The Cigarettes (regulation of production, supply and distribution) Act, 1975 ▪ This act has further strengthened by a comprehensive tobacco control legislation titled "The cigarettes and other Tobacco products (Prohibition of Advertisement and Regulation of Trade and Commerce, Production, Supply and Distribution) Act, 2003 which become effective since 25th February 2004 ▪ Important provisions of both these act are: – Prohibition of smoking in public places like cinema, hospitals, education institutions, rest rooms, restaurants bus stand, railways, etc. and also at places of employment – Prohibition of direct or indirect advertisement of cigarettes and other products – Prohibition of scenes showing smoking in motion pictures – Prohibition of sale of cigarettes and other tobacco products to person under 18 years of age – Prohibition of sale of cigarettes and other tobacco products near education institutions – Mandatory depiction of statutory warning, i.e. "Cigarette smoking is injurious to health" including pictorial warning on cigarette packs – Mandatory depiction of tar and nicotine contents along with maximum permissible limits on cigarette packs – Prominent display of no smoking signs at all public places and places of work

Significance

- Some countries like Norway have developed ambitious programs to eradicate smoking completely by 2000
- However, in country like India, where tobacco-related products are a major source of revenue, complete stoppage of smoking requires political commitment besides public will.

20. Body mass index—uses.

Refer Question No. 4 June 2010 (RS2) Paper II.

21. Integrated Child Development Services (ICDS).

Refer Question No. 2 June 2010 (RS2) Paper II.

22. Nutrition Rehabilitation Center—concept.

- Application of concept of rehabilitation to nutritional disorders is called nutritional rehabilitation.

Principle	*Components*	*Practice (levels of action)*
▪ To encourage the child to eat as much as possible ▪ To re-initiate and/or encourage breastfeeding as necessary ▪ To stimulate emotional and physical development ▪ To prepare the mother or carer to continue to look after the child after discharge	▪ Guaranteed access to food ▪ Use of supplementary food mixtures, either traditional (kichidi, idli) or recommended (Hyderabad mix) ▪ Nutritional education in form of demonstration at institutional and domiciliary levels ▪ Provision of rehydration to those affected with diarrhea	▪ Hospital level ▪ Need in severe malnutritional cases ▪ Nutritional rehabilitation centers ▪ Provision of 3 times meal to malnourised children for about 1 week ▪ Ambulatory rehabilitation ▪ Out-patient treatment with home care

Significance

- Management of malnutrition is incomplete without rehabilitation services.

Ref:

1. http://whqlibdoc.who.int/monograph/WHO_MONO_62_(chp23).pdf accessed on 2nd Aug. 2011.
2. http://helid.digicollection.org/fr/d/Jwho77e/7.1.html accessed on 2nd Aug. 2011.
3. http://helid.digicollection.org/en/d/Jh0215e/4.6.2.1.html accessed on 2nd Aug. 2011.

MBBS PHASE III EXAMINATION

DECEMBER 2014

(Revised Scheme 2 & 3)

PAPER I

LONG ESSAYS

1. Enumerate the different types of randomized controlled trials (RCTs). Explain the steps involved in conducting a RCT.

Refer Question No. 2 June 2013 (RS2) Paper I.

2. Discuss natural history of disease with an example.

Refer Question No. 1 December 2007 (RS2) Paper I.

SHORT ESSAYS

3. Disability indicators.

Refer Question No. 1 June 2008 (RS2) Paper I.

4. Iodine deficiency disorders in India.

Refer Question No. 1 June 2013 (RS2) Paper I.

5. What are the effects of air pollution on health? How can it be prevented?

- Air pollution is the presence in the ambient atmosphere of substance generated by the activities of man in concentrations that interfere with human health safety or comfort or injurious to vegetations and animals and other environmental media resulting in chemicals entering the food chain or being present in drinking water and thereby constituting additional source of human source.

Sources

a. Automobiles	▪ Major source of air pollution ▪ Emit hydrocarbons, CO, lead, NO_2 and particulate matter ▪ In addition, diesel engines also emit black smoke and malodorous fumes
b. Industries	▪ Industries emit large amount of pollutants into the atmosphere ▪ Combustion of fuel to generate heat and power produces smoke, SO_2 No and fly ash ▪ Petrochemical industries generate hydrogen fluoride, HCl and organic halides ▪ Many industries discharge CO, CO_2, O_3, H_2S and SO_2 ▪ These wastes are discharged from the chimneys at high temperature and high speed
c. Domestic sources	▪ Combustion of coal, wood or oil in house is another major source of air pollution inform of smoke, SO_2 and NO
d. Human habits	▪ Most direct and important source of air pollution affecting the health is tobacco smoking ▪ It even affects those who do not smoke (passive smoking)
e. Miscellaneous	▪ Burning of refuse incinerators, pesticide spraying, natural sources and nuclear energy program

Air pollutant	*Source*	*Health effect*
NO, NO_2	Automobile exhaust, gas stoves and heaters, wood burning stoves, kerosene space heaters	Respiratory tract irritation, bronchial hypersensitivity, impai ed lung defences, bonchialitis obliterans
Hydrocarbons	Automobile exhaust, cigarette smoke	Lung cancer[Q]
Ozone	Automobile exhaust, high altitude cabins	Cough, sterna discomfort, bronchoconstriction, decreased exercise performance, respiratory tract irritation
SO_2	Power plants, smelters, oil refineries, kerosene space heaters	Exacerbations of asthma and COPD, respiratory tract irritations, hospitalization, death in severe exposure
Lead	Automobile exhaust	Impaired neuropsychological development in children

Effects

- Air pollution is the presence in the ambient atmosphere of substances generated by the activities of man in concentration that interferes with human health, safety and comfort or injurious to vegetation and animals and other environmental media resulting in chemicals entering the food chain or being present in drinking water thereby constituting additional source of human exposure.

Health effects of air pollution		*Social and economical effects*
Immediate and acute effects	*Delayed and chronic effects*	
▪ Irritation of conjunctiva, nose, throat and respiratory mucosa ▪ Conjunctivitis ▪ Allergic rhinitis ▪ Acute pharyngitis ▪ Acute bronchitis ▪ Episodes of acute attacks of bronchial asthma ▪ Death by suffocation	▪ Chronic bronchitis ▪ Bronchiectasis[Q] ▪ Emphysema ▪ Chronic obstructive pulmonary disease ▪ Bronchial asthma ▪ Lung cancer[Q] ▪ Impaired neuropsychological development in children	▪ Destruction of plants and animal life ▪ Corrosion of metals ▪ Damage to the buildings ▪ Cost of cleaning, maintenance and repairs ▪ Aesthetic nuisance ▪ Reduced visibility ▪ Soiling and damage to the clothing, etc.

Monitoring

- Air pollution monitoring comprises is daily monitoring of certain air pollutants.

Indicators of Air Monitoring

a. Sulfur dioxide index	▪ SO_2 gas is a major contaminant in many urban and industrial areas ▪ Its level is measured by lead peroxide device
b. Smoke or soiling index[Q]	▪ A known volume of air is filtered through a white filter paper under specified conditions and discoloration is measured by photoelectric meter ▪ Expressed as mg/m^3 of air as an average level over a period of time
c. Suspended particles (Grit and dust measurements)	▪ Grit, dust and other solids present in the volume of air is measured by an instrument Midget impinge on monthly basis ▪ Expressed as mg/m^3 of air
d. Coefficient of haze	▪ Amount of smoke or other aerosol per cubic meter of air
e. Air pollution index	▪ An arbitrary index taking into account one or more pollutants as a measure of the severity of pollution
f. Others	▪ Lead, CO, NO_2, oxidants are other parameters are also used

Prevention and Control

a. Containment	▪ It is the prevention of escape of toxic substances into the atmosphere by using variety of engineering methods such as enclosure, ventilation and air cleansing ▪ There has been development of arrestors for removal of contaminants
b. Replacement	▪ It is the replacement of the technological process that is causing air pollution with non hazardous or less hazardous process ▪ Increased use of electricity, natural gas, solar energy and central heating and biogas plants has substituted use of fossil fuel ▪ Development of unconventional sources of energy should be encouraged, e.g. hydroelectric power ▪ The lead content of the petrol is reduced in all the petrol dispensed in India

Contd...

Contd...

c. Dilution	▪ It is done by maintenance of green belt between and around the industries, in between industries and civilian habitats to filter the air pollutants and maintain air quality ▪ However, it is valid so long as it is within the self-cleansing capacity of the environment and its capacity is limited
d. Active community involvements	▪ Increasing the community awareness about air pollution, sources and effects of pollution and how avoid the same ▪ Regular maintenance of automobiles, use of arrestors to the exhaust from automobiles, complete combustion of fossil fuels, screening of windows, use of LPG, or natural gas or biogas, use of solar energy, proper effective ventilation in home and work place, maintenance of green belts, forbidding tobacco smoking, use of smokeless chullahs, maintenance of public spaces, cleanliness of streets and open spaces, etc. are many of the actions taken at individual or community level to prevent and control air pollution
e. Legislation	▪ The Government of India has enacted legislation "the Air (Prevention and control of pollution) Act in 1981 ▪ The act has laid down provisions such as height of chimneys power of local authorities to carry out investigations, research and education concerning air pollution, creation of smokeless zones and enforcement of standards for ambient air quality
f. International action	▪ To control air pollution who has established a network of laboratories for the monitoring and study of air pollution and one such laboratory is established in Nagpur[Q], India by WHO which issues warnings of air pollution where and when necessary

Status in India

- In India, air monitoring is done under agesis of National Air Quality Monitoring Program sponsored by Central Pollution Control Board
- It has generated data since last 14 years from 10 major Indian cities.

Significance

- Routine monitoring of air pollution is very important in control of air pollution
- Best indicator of air pollution are sulfur dioxide, smoke and suspended particles[Q].

6. Explain normal curve.

- normal curve or Gaussian curve is a curve obtained by graphical plotation of a frequency distribution
- It was developed independently by De Moirre and Gauss in 1733.

Characteristics

- It is a bell shaped[Q], smooth curve due to small and equal class intervals
- It is symmetrical in distribution[Q] variables on either side of mean are equal in number
- Its maximum height is at the mean
- The mean, median and mode are identical[Q]
- The curve has one peak and its skewness is zero[Q]
- Theoretically it does not touch the baseline
- Area under the curve is assumed to be 1.0
- Mean is presumed to be zero
- It has 2 curves convex central part and concave when it comes down on both sides
- Normal distribution curve depends on means and standard deviation[Q].

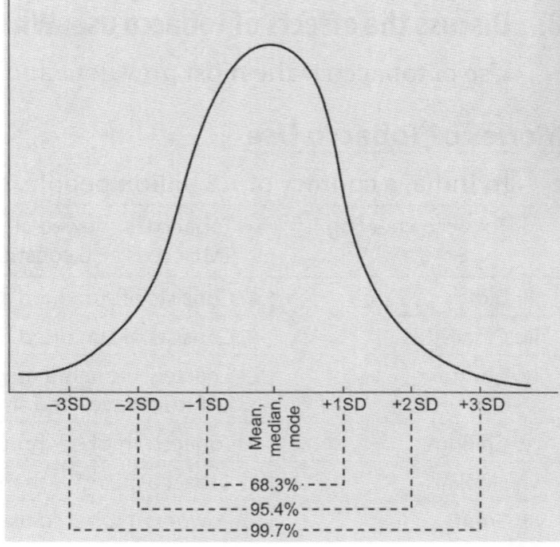

Fig. 1: Normal curve

Mathematic Formulae for Normal Curve[Q]

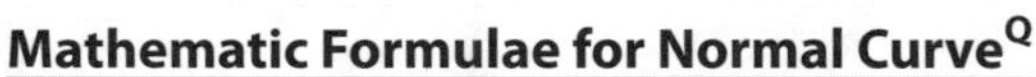

$$y = \frac{n}{\sigma 2\pi} e - x^2 / 2\sigma^2$$

Where

Y = An ordinate taken at any point on the baseline

n = Number of measures

π = 3.1416

e = 2.7193, the base of the system of natural logarithms

σ = Standard deviation of distribution
x = Deviation of any unit of measurement from the mean.

Applications

- Making probability statement about the number of individuals in any range of measurements
- Common/uncommon measurements.

Normal Distribution

- Normal distribution is continuous probability distribution defined by formula.

$$f(x) = \frac{1}{\sigma\sqrt{2\pi}} \ell^{-\frac{(x-\mu)}{2\sigma^2}}$$

Where
μ is mean
σ is standard deviation

- Also called Gaussian distribution.

Properties

- It is the only absolutely continuous distribution all of whose cumulants beyond first two (i.e. other than mean and variance) are zero
- It is also the continuous distribution with maximum entropy for a given mean and variance
- It is symmetric about its mean, and is non-zero over entire real line.

Significance

- Normal distributions are extremely important in statistics, and are often used for real-valued random variables whose distributions are not known.

7. Discuss briefly the approaches to health education.

Refer Question No. 5 December 2009 (RS2) Paper I.

8. Discuss the effects of tobacco use. What are the preventive measures?

- Use of tobacco is the most prevalent and preventable cause of disease and death.

Modes of Tobacco Use

- In India, a country of 1.2 billion people, a quarter (300 million) are tobacco users in one form or the other.

i. Tobacco chewing	▪ Tobacco is chewed alone or mixed with lime or in paan ▪ Tobacco is also constituent of pan masala, zarda and gutka
ii. Bidi	▪ Consists of sun dried and sun cured flakes hand rolled in dried leaves of "temburni"
iii. Cigarettes	▪ Consists of sun dried flakes rolled in a paper with filter at one end
iv. Chutta	▪ Coarsely prepared medium sized cigar made from cured tobacco leaves rolled and wrapped in dried tobacco/ jackfruit leaves and smoked with burning end inside mouth
v. Chillum	▪ Tobacco smoked through clay pipes
vi. Hookah	▪ Tobacco mixed with molasses is burnt and the smoke is passed through water before inhaled
vii. Snuff	▪ Powdered tobacco used for inhalation through nostrils

Constituents of Tobacco

- Tobacco contains several harmful constituents which include nicotine, many carcinogens, carbon monoxide and other toxins.

Carcinogenesis	*Tumor promoters*	*Irritation and toxicity to respiratory mucosa*	*Reduced oxygen transport*
▪ Tar ▪ Polycyclic aromatic hydrocarbons ▪ Nitrosamines	▪ Nicotine ▪ Phenol	▪ Formaldehyde ▪ Nitrogen oxide	▪ Carbon monoxide

- The harmful effects of smoking are related to a variety of factors, the most important of which is dose of exposure expressed in terms of pack years
- On cessation of smoking, the higher mortality slowly declines and the beneficial effect reaches the level of nonsmokers after 20 or more of smoke-free years.

Effects of Tobacco Use

A. Health aspects
 - Tobacco contains numerous toxic chemicals having adverse effects varying from minor throat irritation to carcinogenesis
 - Major diseases accounting for higher mortality in tobacco users include the following (in descending order of frequency)
   - Coronary heart disease
   - Cancer of the lung
   - Chronic obstructive pulmonary disease (COPD).

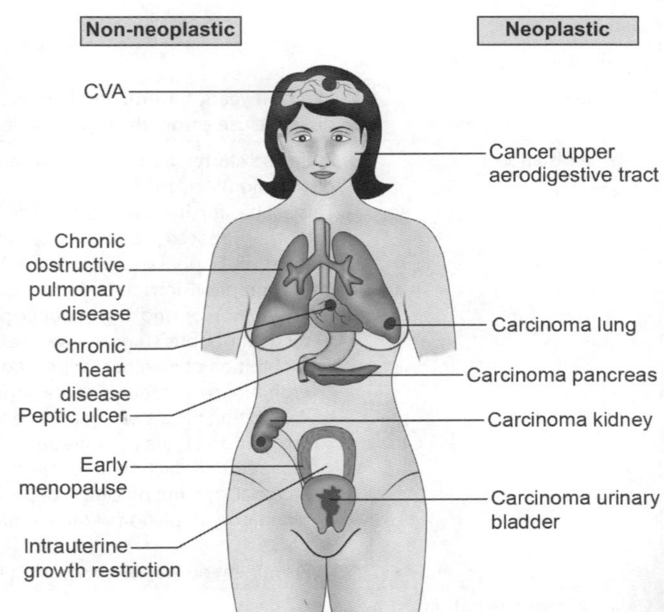

Fig. 2: Effects of tobacco use

Coronary heart disease	*Carcinoma*	*Non-neoplastic diseases*
▪ Cigarette smoking is one of the four major risk factors for myocardial infarction and acts synergistically with the other three—hypercholesterolemia, hypertension and diabetes mellitus ▪ There is more severe, extensive and accelerated atherosclerosis of coronary arteries and aorta in smokers, possibly due to increased platelet aggregation and impaired lung function that causes reduced myocardial oxygen supply ▪ Besides, the smokers have higher risk of development of atherosclerotic aortic aneurysm and Buerger's disease (thromboangiitis obliterans) affecting lower extremities	▪ Lung cancer ▪ Cigarette smoking is strongly implicated in evolution of lung cancer ▪ Oral cancers (lips, oral cavity) ▪ Oral cancers is common in people chewing tobacco, gutka ▪ Chutta smoking has strong association with squamous cell carcinoma of the oral cavity ▪ Cancer of larynx, esophagus, pancreas, urinary bladder and kidney ▪ Risk of cancers of larynx and esophagus increases with tobacco chewing ▪ Urinary bladder cancer is associated with combination of schistosomiasis and smoking (in Egypt)	▪ Chronic obstructive pulmonary disease (COPD) ▪ Includes chronic bronchitis and emphysema as the most common ▪ Peptic ulcer disease (70% higher risk in smokers) ▪ Early menopause ▪ Lower birth weight of fetus, higher perinatal mortality and intellectual deterioration of newborn (higher risk in smoking pregnant women)

B. Economic aspects
 - Economic loss due to tobacco use outweigh the economic benefits from it in form of employment and taxation revenue
 - It is very difficult to estimate the cost incurred to nation due tobacco-related diseases and also the manpower lost to its use
 - Tobacco use can also incur expenses to the family thus reducing their purchasing power, increases their health expenditure
 - Careless smoking leads to fires and accidents, loss due to which can be attributed to the smoking.

Prevention and Control

A. Primordial prevention	
a. Health education and public information	▪ General population should be informed and educated about the hazards of smoking targeting the whole population in general but youth and school children in particular through mass media, internet and other sources of communication ▪ NGOs should be encouraged to start a nationwide antismoking campaign to change the life style associated with smoking ▪ National Health Policy should have curtailment of smoking as integral part

Contd...

Contd...

B. Primary prevention	
a. Taxation	▪ In recent years, government has increased tax on tobacco and tobacco-related products in order to dissuade users from their use or at least curtain their use
b. Legislation	▪ India had started its antismoking campaign with "The Cigarettes (regulation of production, supply and distribution) Act, 1975 ▪ This act has further strengthened by a comprehensive tobacco control legislation titled "The cigarettes and other Tobacco products (Prohibition of Advertisement and Regulation of Trade and Commerce, Production, Supply and Distribution) Act, 2003 which become effective since 25th February 2004 ▪ Important provisions of both these act are: – Prohibition of smoking in public places like cinema, hospitals, education institutions, rest rooms, restaurants, bus stand, railways, etc. and also at places of employment – Prohibition of direct or indirect advertisement of cigarettes and other products – Prohibition of scenes showing smoking in motion pictures – Prohibition of sale of cigarettes and other tobacco products to person under 18 years of age – Prohibition of sale of cigarettes and other tobacco products near education institutions – Mandatory depiction of statutory warning, i.e. "cigarette smoking is injurious to health" including pictorial warning on cigarette packs – Mandatory depiction of tar and nicotine contents along with maximum permissible limits on cigarette packs – Prominent display of no smoking signs at all public places and places of work
C. Secondary prevention	
a. Promotion of smoking cessation methods	▪ Establishment for smoking cessation clinics where individuals should be counseled to give up smoking ▪ These clinics should also relieve the smoker of abstinence symptoms ▪ They should be provided information about various smoking cessation methods or alternatives like electric cigarettes, nicotine gums or patches, etc.

Significance

- Tobacco is one of the most commonly abused substance which places both financial and health burden on the individual besides the family, community and nation as a whole
- Every effort must be directed to curtail the use of tobacco for a progressive developed nation.

9. Medical measures to prevent occupational diseases.

Refer Question No. 2 June 2016 (RS2) Paper I.

10. What are the detrimental effects of iron deficiency anemia? Add a note on preventive measures.

Refer Question No. 10 June 2008 (RS2) Paper I.

11. Integrated vector control measures.

Refer Question No. 11 June 2010 (RS2) Paper I.

12. Ecological studies.

- Ecological studies are observational studies defined by the level at which data are analyzed, namely at the population or group level, rather than individual level
- Also called as correlational study
- They are often used to measure prevalence and incidence of disease, particularly when disease is rare
- These are studies of risk-modifying factors on health or other outcomes based on populations defined either geographically or temporally.
- Both risk-modifying factors and outcomes are averaged for the populations in each geographical or temporal unit and then compared using standard statistical methods.

Units of Study

- Population[Q]

Example

- Study by John Snow regarding a cholera outbreak in London is considered the first ecological study to solve a health issue.

Objectives

- To monitor population health so that public health strategies may be developed and directed
- To make large-scale comparisons, e.g. comparisons between countries
- To study the relationship between population-level exposure to risk factors and disease, or in order to look at the contextual effect of risk factors on the population
- Measurements at individual level are not available, e.g. confidentiality might require that individuals are anonymized by aggregation of data to small area level
- The disease under investigation is rare, requiring aggregation of data for any analysis to be carried out.

Types of Measurements

- In ecological studies health outcomes are aggregates of individual health data, e.g. prevalence, incidence, rate of disease, etc. to obtain one or more of the following:

Aggregate measures	*Environmental measures*	*Global measures*
▪ The data are summarize of individual level data ▪ Example: Mean DMFT, percentage of children with no caries, area-level deprivation indices	▪ Equivalent individual level data are conceivable ▪ Example: Mean annual exposure to fluoridation	▪ There are no equivalent individual level data ▪ Example: Number of dental practices, population density

Types of Ecological Studies

Geographical	*Longitudinal*	*Migration*
▪ This type of study compares one geography with another by assessing the health of the population of each ▪ Exposures for geographies may also be measured and included in analysis as well as other potential confounding variables such as demographic and socioeconomic information	▪ A population is monitored to assess changes in disease over time ▪ Again, confounding factors are often included in analysis	▪ Data of migrant populations are collected and analyzed ▪ The unit of interest is neither time nor place, but population type

Ecological Fallacy[Q]

- Ecological fallacy is a type of confounding specific to ecological studies
- Is an error of interpretation of statistical date in an ecological study, whereby characteristics are ascribed to a group of individuals which they may not posses as individuals
- It means that the findings for the groups may not apply to individuals in the group
- It occurs when relationships which exist for groups are assumed to also be true for individuals

Advantages	*Disadvantages*	*Precautions*
▪ Done in small time frame ▪ Inexpensive and easy to carry out, using routinely collected data ▪ Data can be used from population with different characteristics ▪ Can include the large number of people and large number of risk-modifying factors can be examined	▪ Prone to bias ▪ Socioeconomic confounding ▪ Ecological fallacy	▪ Because they are area-level studies, care must be taken when extrapolating either to individuals within the area level of measurement, or to a higher population level

Significance

- Although other study designs are generally considered more reliable, particularly in the inference of causation, the population context of individual characteristics determined by the ecological studies has been shown to be a stronger determinant of disease at population level than individual level risk factors.
- However, it is the least preferable observation/analytical study design[Q]

- Ecological studies have often found links between risk-modifying factors and health outcomes well in advance of other epidemiological or laboratory approaches.

Ref:

1. Levin KN. Study Design VI—Ecological Studies; Evidence-Based Dentistry. 2003;7: 60–1. http://www.bmj.com/about-bmj/resources-readers/publications/epidemiology-uninitiated/6-ecological-studies accessed on 1st Feb. 2015
2. Morgenstern H. Ecologic studies in epidemiology: concepts, principles, and methods. Annu Rev Public Health. 1995;16:61-81

SHORT ANSWERS

13. Epidemiological triad.

Refer Question No. 22 December 2010 (RS2) Paper I.

14. What are the functions of the family?

Refer Question No. 12 June 2013 (RS2) Paper I.

15. Sickness absenteeism.

Refer Question No. 5 June 2017 (RS2) Paper I.

16. Enumerate the dietary goals recommended by WHO.

Refer Question No. 4 June 2013 (RS2) Paper I.

17. Symposium.

Refer Question No. 2 June 2009 (RS2) Paper I.

18. Pellagra.

- Pellagra is a vitamin deficiency disorder:

Etiopathogenesis	*Clinical features (characterized by 3 D's)*	*Prevention*
Cause ▪ Due to deficiency of niacin (vitamin B_3) *Pathogenesis* ▪ Seen commonly in malnourished population subsisting mainly on maize or jowar diets which are rich in leucine ▪ Due to excess of leucine which interferes with conversion of tryptophan to niacin	a. Diarrhea – Often associated with anorexia, nausea, vomiting, dysphagia and dyspepsia b. Dermatitis – Bilaterally symmetrical – Seen on areas exposed to sunlight (back of hands, lower legs, face and neck) – Skin becomes pigmented, scaly and cracked – Often associated with itching and burning sensation c. Dementia (mental changes) – Includes depression, irritability and delirium	▪ Pellagra is preventable disease which can be prevented by consuming good mixed diet containing milk and/or meat ▪ Avoiding total dependence on maize or jowar as staple diet

19. Food adulteration.

Refer Question No. 21 June 2010 (RS2) Paper I.

20. What is matching in a case-control study?

Refer Question No. 1 June 2014 (RS2) Paper I.

21. Explain human development index.

Refer Question No. 3 December 2009 (RS2) Paper I.

22. Measures of central tendency.

Refer Question No. 3 December 2010 (RS2) Paper I.

MBBS PHASE III EXAMINATION

DECEMBER 2014

(Revised Scheme 2 & 3)

PAPER II

LONG ESSAYS

1. Describe the epidemiology, clinical picture and preventive measures of hepatitis B infection.

- Hepatitis B is an inflammatory disease of liver caused by a DNA virus, hepatitis B virus
- Also called as serum hepatitis[Q], Hippy hepatitis, Tattoo jaundice, Homologous serum jaundice.

Epidemiology

<table>
<tr><td>A. Agent factors</td><td></td></tr>
<tr><td>a. Causative agent</td><td>▪ Hepatitis B virus is a DNA virus, belonging to Hepadnaviridae family
▪ In serum, it appears in three forms
– Small spherical particles measuring 22 nm in diameter (used for making hepatitis B vaccine)
– Tubular particles of varying size and shapes
– Larger, double shelled, spherical particles of 42 nm diameter—Dane particle[Q] named after its discoverer (the only infective form)
▪ Antigenically complex virus, exhibiting three distinct antigens
<table>
<tr><th>Surface antigen or Australia antigen[Q] (HBsAg)—outer glycoprotein</th><th>Core antigen (HBcAg)—inner nucleoprotein</th><th>Envelope-antigen (HBeAg)</th></tr>
<tr><td>▪ First antigen to appear in serum—first evidence of infection[Q]
▪ Epidemiological marker of Hepatitis B infection[Q]</td><td>▪ Does not appear in serum alone[Q]</td><td>▪ Is a secretory form of HBcAg
▪ Indicates active viral replication[Q]
▪ Is a marker of infectivity for hepatitis B[Q]
▪ Persistence beyond 3 months indicates increased likelihood of chronic hepatitis B</td></tr>
</table></td></tr>
<tr><td>b. Reservoir of infection</td><td>▪ Humans are only known source of reservoir of infection
▪ Reservoir may be an active symptomatic case, inapparent subclinical case or even a carrier
▪ Persistent carriers (person with circulating surface antigen more than 6 months) are major reservoir of infection
▪ Risk of case becoming carrier is 50% in infants and 5–10% in adults and older children</td></tr>
<tr><td>c. Resistance</td><td>▪ Virus is quite stable and capable of surviving for days on environmental surfaces
▪ It can be easily destroyed by sodium hypochlorite or by autoclaving for 30–60 minutes</td></tr>
<tr><td>d. Infective material</td><td>▪ Contaminated blood is main source of infection
▪ However HBsAg is also present in body fluids of infected person such as saliva, semen, vaginal secretions, urine, CSF, ascitic fluid and synovial fluid
▪ Contaminated needles, syringes, surgical instruments or instruments are secondary sources</td></tr>
</table>

Contd...

Contd...

e. Incubation period	▪ 45–180 days[Q] (usually 60–90 days and Median <100 days[Q])—(6 weeks to 6 months) ▪ Lower the dose, longer the incubation period
f. Period of communicability	▪ Varies from several months to several years ▪ Person is communicable during last one month of incubation period, during acute phase of illness and until HBsAg disappears
g. Modes of transmission	▪ Hepatitis can be transmitted in all modes of transmission
	Parenteral route: ▪ Blood-borne infection is commonest route of transmission ▪ Disease can be transmitted by infected blood and blood products through transfusions, dialysis, handing of infected blood ▪ It can also be transmitted through contaminated needles, syringes, drip sets, etc.
	Percutaneous route: ▪ Accidental percutaneous inoculations can occur during surgical or dental procedures, mass immunization, traditional tattooing, ear piercing, nose piercing, ritual circumcision, acupuncture, etc. ▪ It may occur following use of contaminated razor, shaving brush, needles, etc.
	Vertical transmission: ▪ Direct vertical transmission of fetus by hepatitis B virus rarely happens ▪ Child usually gets infected during birth due to accidental leakage, ingestion or inoculation of maternal blood into baby (hence it is perinatal transmission[Q]) ▪ Risk of transmission of infection from mother to baby is dependent upon HBeAg status of mother ▪ Child may also be infected through breasts milk
	Direct contact: ▪ Other possible route of transmission is direct contact which includes kissing and sexual intercourse
	Horizontal transmission: ▪ Hepatitis B can be transmitted from child to child in presence of skin infections like scabies, impetigo or other injuries
B. Host factors	
a. Age	▪ Infection is acquired at early age in areas of high prevalence whereas it is acquired at later age (20–40 years) in areas of low prevalence
b. Sex	▪ Incidence is more amongst men
c. Occupation	▪ Surgeons, dentists, nurses, laboratory technicians and blood bank workers are at higher risk of contracting hepatitis B ▪ High incidence is also seen in homosexuals, sex workers, IV drug abusers and infants of HBV carrier mother
d. Concurrent infection	▪ Hepatitis B infection risk is more common in patients requiring repeated blood transfusion and on immunosuppressive therapy
e. Immunity	▪ Antibodies are produced 10 days after onset of jaundice ▪ Antibodies appear in order of anti HBcAg, anti HBeAg and lastly anti-HBsAg ▪ Anti HBsAg is protective and indicates recovery from illness and development of immunity
C. Environmental factors	▪ Hepatitis B is common in as elitist as doctors and also in drug abusers

Clinical Course

- Infection by hepatitis B virus may result in:

a. Asymptomatic infection (subclinical infection)
   - Manifestation free infection detected accidently by raised serum transaminases or presence of antibodies

b. Acute hepatitis (acute inflammatory involvement of entire liver)
   - Most common course of disease

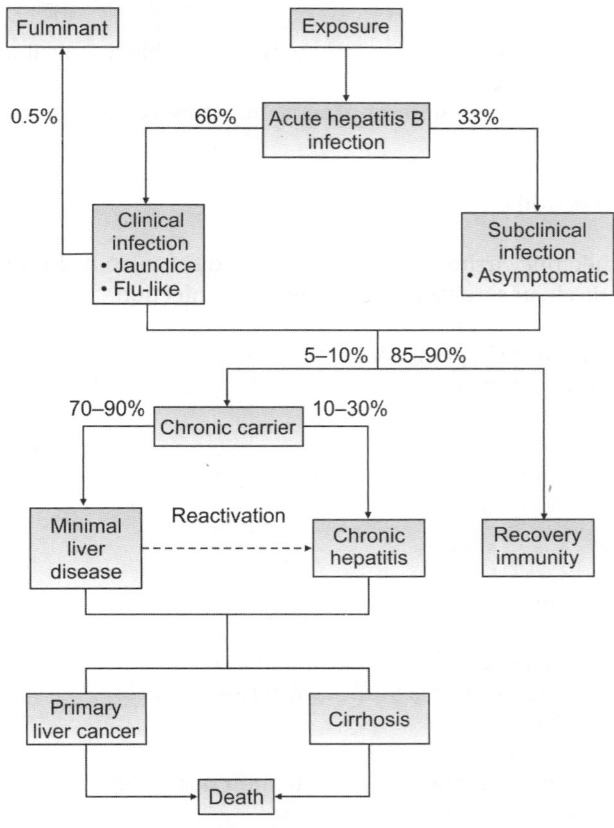

Fig. 1: Clinical course of hepatitis B

Clinical course

Incubation period	*Pre-icteric phase*	*Icteric phase*	*Post-icteric phase*
▪ 30–180 days (average 70 days) ▪ Asymptomatic but infective stage	▪ Prodromal symptoms like anorexia, nausea, vomiting, fatigue, malaise, arthralgia, headache ▪ Low grade fever preceding jaundice ▪ Transaminases elevated	▪ Lasts 1–4 weeks ▪ Onset of clinical jaundice ▪ Dark colored urine, clay colored stools, pruritus, weight loss, abdominal discomfort ▪ Deranged liver functions tests, positive serological markers	▪ Lasts 2–12 weeks resulting in clinical and biochemical recovery ▪ 1% cases may develop fulminant hepatitis and 5–10% progress to chronic hepatitis ▪ 10% of adults become carriers whereas 90% of infected neonates become carriers

c. Carrier state
   - Asymptomatic state without manifesting disease but harboring infection and capable of transmitting infection
   - Risk of case becoming carrier is 50% in infants and 5–10% in adults and older children.

Risk factors

▪ Age	Earlier the infection acquired, more likely the development of carrier state
▪ Sex	More common amongst males
▪ Diseases	Carrier state is more likely to occur in patients with Down's syndrome, lepromatous leprosy, chronic renal disease
▪ Immunosuprressive therapy	Patients on steroids are more likely to become carriers

d. Chronic hepatitis
   - Continuing or relapsing hepatic disease for >6 months with clinical, biochemical, serological and histopathological evidence of infection
   - Clinical spectrum from asymptotic to symptoms of acute hepatitis like fatigue, malaise, mild fever and sometimes jaundice.
e. Fulminant hepatitis
   - Most severe form of acute hepatitis.
f. Cirrhosis
   - Hepatitis B results in postnecrotic cirrhosis as progression of disease from chronic active hepatitis
   - 25% patients of postnecrotic cirrhosis give history of hepatitis infection.
g. Hepatocellular carcinoma
   - Hepatitis B infection predisposes to hepatocellular carcinoma by 200 times
   - Underlying mechanism may be integration of HBV-DNA into genome of tumor cells or inactivation of tumor suppressor oncogene p53.
h. Death
   - Mortality in hepatitis B infection may result due to untreated fulminant hepatitis or hepatocellular carcinoma

Prevention and Control

- Elimination of reservoir
- Not possible as there is no treatment
- Breaking chain of transmission
- Sterilization of syringes, needles, catgut, surgical instruments, etc.
- Avoiding sharing of toothbrush, razors, syringes among drug abusers, etc.
- Screening of blood donors for HBsAg
- Avoiding homosexuality and multiple sexual partners
- Instructions to carriers—not to donate blood, not to share their razors, bath brush, toothbrush, etc. with others and to use condoms during sex
- Sterilization of instruments before body modification procedures like tattooing, body piercing
- Protection of susceptible
   I. Active immunization (Hepatitis B vaccine)

Types

a. Plasma derived vaccine	
	▪ Sterile, liquid subunit vaccine[Q] ▪ Based on HBsAg
Preparation	▪ Surface antigen prepared from pooled plasma of HBV carriers (HIV negative) which are harvested, purified and residual virus inactivated by formalin
Advantages	▪ Safe, effective and widely effective
b. Recombinant DNA yeast derived vaccine	
	▪ Liquid, sterile, genetically engineered vaccine
Preparation	▪ Purified surface antigen prepared by recombinant DNA technology from yeast cloned with surface antigen HBsAg S-gene[Q]
Advantages	▪ Safe, effective and immunogenic ▪ Can be concomitantly given along with BCG, DPT, OPV and measles vaccine but on different site
Disadvantages	▪ Costlier ▪ No effect on carriers
Dose	▪ Adults—1 mL (contains 20 μg of HBsAg) ▪ Children <10 years—0.5 mL
Route of administration	▪ Intramuscularly in deltoid or anterolateral aspect of thigh in children[Q]
Schedule (regular)	▪ 3 doses at 0, 1 and 6 months followed by booster dose once in 5 years
Efficacy	▪ 95%

Immunity	▪ 3–5 years
Contraindications	▪ Preterm children with birth weight <2.0 kg (only vaccine contraindicated in low birth weight babies[Q])
Therapeutic uses	▪ Hepatitis B vaccine is used for pre- and postexposure prophylaxis of hepatitis B and D

Prophylaxis schedule

	Pre-exposure prophylaxis			*Post-exposure prophylaxis*
	Regular dosage schedule	*Rapid dosage schedule*	*Double dosage schedule*	
Indications	▪ General population	▪ High-risk individuals like surgeons, dentists, laboratory technicians in blood banks, etc.	▪ Chronic hemodialysis and immunocompromised patients	▪ Newborns born to HBV carriers mothers ▪ Individuals accidently exposed to needle stick injury or through transfusion, cuts and injuries ▪ Sexual contacts of acute hepatitis B patients
Schedule	▪ 3 doses at 0, 1 and 6 months and regular booster every 5 years	▪ 3 doses at 0, 1 and 2 months followed by booster dose at 12 months and regular booster once in 8 years	▪ 4 doses of 2 mL (40 µg) at 0, 1, 2 and 6 month followed by booster dose every 5 years	▪ Simultaneous active and passive immunization ▪ Started within 12 hours but not later than 48 hours

Significance

- Hepatitis B vaccine is the only vaccine available against any human cancer i.e. hepatocellular carcinoma.
- Vaccination with it also protects the vaccinee from hepatitis D.

II. Passive immunization (Hepatitis B immunoglobulin)
- Specific immunoglobulin prepared from immunized persons

Dosage	▪ 0.05–0.07 mL/kg body weight
Schedule	▪ 2 doses at interval of 30 days ▪ 1st dose ideally within 6 hours[Q] of exposure but not later than 48 hours
Immunity	▪ 3 months
Indications	▪ Required for immediate protection in: – Surgeons, nurse, laboratory workers – Newborn infants of carrier mothers – Sexual contact of acute hepatitis B patient
Therapeutic uses	▪ Post-exposure prophylaxis along with active immunization

Significance

- Prevention of hepatitis B is very important as there is no specific treatment and more risk of becoming carrier
- Vertical transmission of hepatitis B is an important factor for prevalence of disease in endemic areas thus prevention of neonatal infection by passive immunization in infants born to HBsAg positive mothers is very essential
- Ability of hepatitis B to make alliance with hepatitis D causing delta hepatitis is a new threat to world
- Longer incubation period and period of communicability, variable clinical course, carrier state and fatal outcome of disease makes hepatitis B a very grave danger to future of public health.

2. Describe the components of RCH (reproductive and child health) program and explain the various services provided to the mothers under this program.

Refer Question No. 1 Dec. 2008 (RS2) Paper II.

SHORT ESSAYS

3. Write briefly about measures to be taken to control a cholera outbreak.

- Cholera is an acute, infectious diarrheal disease of small intestine caused by *V. cholerae* 01 (classical or El-Tor) characterized by sudden onset of profuse, effortless, watery diarrhea following by vomiting, rapid dehydration, muscular cramps and suppression of urine
- Cholera is considered the father of public health[Q]
- It has been endemic in India since beginning of recorded history often resulting in sudden outbreaks periodically.

Control of Cholera Outbreak (WHO)

- Epidemics of cholera are characteristically abrupt and often create an acute public health problem
- They have a high potential to spread fast and cause death
- Epidemic reaches a peak and subsides gradually as force of infection declines
- Often times by the time control measures are instituted, epidemic has already reached its peak and is waning
- Thus cholera outbreak in a community is self-limiting.

A. Elimination of reservoirs
 – Consist of making infectious cases such as cases and carriers into noninfectious by giving treatment.
 a. Verification of diagnosis
  - Bacteriological diagnosis of cholera should be done quickly
  - All cases of diarrhea should be investigated at slightest suspicion
  - Identification of *V. cholerae* 01 in stool of patient is enough for confirmed diagnosis of cholera
  - Carriers are diagnosed only by stool culture report
  - In epidemic situation it is not necessary to make microbiological diagnosis of each and every case.
 b. Notification
  - Cholera is a notifiable disease locally, nationally and internationally[Q]
  - Any case of confirmed cholera should be notified to the local health authority
  - Cholera should be reported to WHO by national government within 24 hours of occurrence and daily and weekly reports of number of cases and fatalities need to be furnished to WHO till the area is declared cholera free (International Health Regulation)
  - An area is declared cholera free when 10 days (twice the incubation period) has elapsed since death, recovery or isolation of last case[Q].
 c. Early case finding
  - Aggressive case finding for cases with all severities should be carried at the earliest
  - It can be active case detection by house to house visit supplemented by passive case detection with static centers
  - It helps to detected infected household contacts and helps to decide specific intervention depending upon mode of spread.
 d. Treatment
  - Time is essence in treatment of cholera, hence no time should be lost to initiate treatment of confirmed cholera cases.
  i. Establishment of treatment centers
   - Treatment centers at the nearest subcenter, PHC or community health centers should be established to make treatment easily available to community
   - In areas with poor peripheral health services or epidemics is threatening, mobile teams should be employed to reach these areas
   - If no health infrastructure is available in convenient distance to transfer severe cases, nearest school or public building should be converted into treatment center because transportation of cases to far off areas may help spread the disease
   - Help of local volunteers like village health guide, multipurpose health workers, trained dai, anganwadi worker, local practitioners in organizing treatment.
  ii. Isolation
   - Patient should be isolated in hospital or at home till 2–3 consecutive stool culture report come negative.

iii. Rehydration therapy
   - Effective rehydration therapy is most important modality to treat cholera and has helped reduced mortality to <1%
   - 90–95% cases of cholera can be treated with ORS alone
   - Rehydration can be oral or intravenous
   - Mildly dehydrated patients can be treated with oral rehydration solution at home
   - Severely dehydrated patients require intravenous rehydration and should be shifted to nearest health infrastructure.

iv. Adjuvant therapy
   - Besides antibiotics, no other medication like antidiarrheals, antiemetics, antispasmodics or steroids should be prescribed for cholera cases
   - Antibiotics should be prescribed based on the sensitivity of the cholera or based on the response of patient to treatment
   - It should be started as soon as vomiting has stopped (usually within 3–4 hours of starting oral rehydration).

Dosage

Antibiotics[Q]	*Children*	*Adults*
Doxycycline (drug of choice for adults except pregnancy) Single dose	--	300mg
Trimethoprim + sulfamethoxazole (drug of choice for children) BD for 3 days	5 mg/kg + 25 mg/kg	160 mg + 800 mg
Furazolidone[Q] (drug of choice in pregnancy) QID for 3 days	1.25 mg/kg	100 mg
Tetracycline[Q] (chemoprophylaxis) QID for 3 days	12.5 mg/kg	500 mg
Erythrocycline or chloramphenicol (in case of non-availability of DOC or resistant bacteria)		

B. Breaking the chain of transmission
   – Chain of transmission of cholera can be broken by employing general sanitation measures
   – To define extent of outbreak and identify modes of transmission, epidemiological studies must be undertaken which helps to apply more effective and specific control measures
   – Epidemiological investigations
     - Initial cases give useful information about clustering of cases
     - Presence of widespread epidemic suggests massive contamination of common water source which should be collected and sent for examination
     - Epidemiological investigation is helpful in determining modalities to be applied for breaking chain of transmission
   – Sanitation measures
     - Since cholera is transmitted by feco-oral route, best way of breaking chain of transmission is by construction of sanitary barrier

i. Water control	▪ As water is most important and most common source of vehicle of transmission of cholera, it is paramount to ensure safe water to community for its domestic needs ▪ It is important to supply safe water quickly and with limited resources ▪ Various modalities are available for this but approach selected should be appropriate and acceptable to the community ▪ In urban areas, provision of property treated water containing free residual chlorine should be made available to all families ▪ In rural areas, water should be disinfected by boiling or chlorination ▪ Best and permanent solution is to supply piped chlorinated water supply on permanent basis and elimination of alternative unsafe water sources like pond, well, etc.

Contd...

Contd...

ii. Excreta disposal	▪ In case of cholera outbreak, sanitary latrines should be constructed with cooperation of community taking into consideration, the customs and practices of the locals, existing terrain and geology and available resources ▪ Besides, provision of sanitary latrine, community should be educated about proper use of such facilities, dangers involved in open air defecation on ground or near water source and importance of handwashing after defecation
iii. Food sanitation	▪ Food is another important vehicle of cholera transmission and thus measures should be taken to ensure proper food sanitation at home and in community ▪ Health education should be given regarding importance of eating cooked hot food, handling techniques for individual food, cleaning of cooking utensils ▪ Besides food sanitations, people should be also educated to prevent contact of food and flies which acts as mechanical vectors for cholera
iv. Disinfection	▪ Disinfection should be both concurrent and terminal ▪ Disinfectant should have Rideal-Walker coefficient of 5 or above (ideal and most effective is cresol) ▪ Alternatively good quality of bleaching powder can be used especially for chlorination ▪ Disinfection should be directed against, patients excreta and vomitus, clothes and personal items, latrine in patient's house and in neighborhood

C. Protection of susceptible
 - People living in close contact with the patient are most susceptible and should be prevented from getting infected
 - Chemoprophylaxis
   - Indicated only for household contacts or in a closed community[Q]
   - Mass chemoprophylaxis is not advised for total community
   - To prevent one case of cholera, 10,000 persons need to be given chemoprophylaxis.

Dosage

Drug	*Adults (>13 years)*	*4–13 years*	*0–3 years*
Tetracycline (drug of choice[Q]) BD for 3 days	500 mg	125 mg	50 mg
Doxycycline Single dose	300 mg	6 mg/kg	

 - Vaccination
   - Indicated for prophylaxis of community at large.

Types

	Parenteral vaccine	*Oral vaccines*	
		▪ Killed whole cell vaccine	▪ Live attenuated vaccine
Contents	▪ Saline suspension of 6,000 million each of classical Ogawa and Inaba serotypes of *V. cholerae* 01 per mL ▪ Killed and preserved by addition of 0.5% phenol	▪ Killed whole cell *V. cholerae* 01 in combination with a recombinant B subunit of cholera toxin (WC/rBS)	▪ Live attenuated, genetically manipulated classical *V. cholerae* strain CVD 103-HgR
Dose	▪ 0.5 mL (containing 6,000 million) ▪ 0.25 mL (for children <10 year)		
Schedule	▪ 2 doses 4–6 weeks apart	▪ 2 doses 10–14 days apart	▪ Single dose
Route of administration	▪ Intramuscularly	▪ Oral	▪ Oral
Immunity	▪ Develops within 15 days (hence no use in epidemics) ▪ Equally effective against El-Tor infections		
Efficacy	▪ 50% for 3–6 months	▪ 50–60% for 3 years	▪ 80%

Contd...

Contd...

	Parenteral vaccine	*Oral vaccines*	
Uses	▪ As chemoprophylactic measure before expected outbreak of epidemics such as fairs and pilgrimages ▪ Given in double the dose at least one month before		
Complications		▪ Hypersensitivity	▪ Hypersensitivity
Remarks	▪ Was only specific prophylactic available until recently ▪ Limitations ▪ Not effective in controlling epidemics (Waste of money, manpower and material) ▪ Do not prevent introduction of cholera into a country or interrupt the transmission ▪ Do not prevent development of carrier state or affect severity of disease ▪ Creates false sense of security of protection		▪ Avoid antibiotics and proguanil for one week before and after administration of live oral attenuated vaccine

– Health education
  - Health education is most effective prophylactic measure[Q]
  - It should be directed against poor and ignorant as cholera affects this group.

Components

– Routes of transmission of cholera and consequences of dehydration
– Effectiveness and simplicity of oral rehydration therapy with onset of diarrhea
– Benefits of early reporting for prompt treatment
– Food hygiene practices
– To avoid open air defection and to use sanitary latrine
– Handwashing with soap after defecation and before eating
– Benefits of cooked, hot food and safe water
– To control house flies, by keeping premises clean in and around the house
– To take cholera vaccine one month before going to places expected of cholera outbreak.

Significance

- Best way to control periodic cholera outbreaks is to develop and implement a sound practical national program for control of all diarrheal diseases because similarities shared by cholera and other diarrheal diseases in regards to epidemiology, pathophysiology, treatment and control.

4. Epidemiological determinants of diabetes mellitus.

Refer Question No. 1 June 2010 (RS2) Paper II.

5. Write a short note on strategies adopted for malaria control.

- With introduction of National Vector-Borne Disease Control Program, the existing Modified Modified National Malaria Control Program was merged into it along with other related health programs
- Currently under the new program, National Framework for Malaria Elimination is launched in February 2016.

Goals
- Eliminate malaria (zero indigenous cases) throughout the entire country by 2030
- Maintain malaria free status in areas where malaria transmission has been interrupted and prevent reintroduction of malaria

Objectives
- By 2022: Interrupt malaria transmission and attain zero indigenous cases (Categories 1 and 2 states/UTs)
- By 2024: Reduce malaria incidence to <1 case per 1000 population (all states/UTs)
- By 2027: Interrupt indigenous transmission of malaria (all states/UTs)
- By 2030: Eliminate malaria and prevent re-establishment (entire country)

Contd...

Contd...

Targets

2016	• Inclusion of malaria elimination in health policies and planning framework of all states/UTs
2020	• Completely interrupt malaria transmission and achieve Zero indigenous cases and deaths due to malaria—Category 1 states • Enter into elimination phase—Category 2 states • Reduce disease burden but continue to remain in Category 3—Category 3 states • Reduce estimated malaria burden at national level by 15–20%
2022	• Completely interrupt malaria transmission and achieve zero indigenous cases and deaths due to malaria – Category 1 and 2 states • Enter into Pre-elimination phase—Category 3 states • Reduce estimated malaria burden at national level by 30–35%
2024	• Reduce API <1 per 1000 population at risk, sustain zero malarial deaths and establish fully functional malaria surveillance to track, investigate and respond to each case • Interrupt malaria transmission, zero indigenous cases and deaths • Enter into elimination phase—Category 3 states
2027	• Interrupt indigenous malaria transmission and attain zero indigenous cases and deaths due to malaria
2030	• Sustain status of zero indigenous cases and deaths due to malaria for 3 consecutive years and initiate processes for certification of malaria elimination status

Activities

- Formulating policies and guidelines
- Technical guidance
- Planning
- Logistics
- Monitoring and evaluation
- Coordination of activities through states and UTs and in consultation with national organisation such as National Center for Disease Control, National Institute of Malaria Research
- Collaboration with international organization like WHO, World Bank, GFATM, etc.
- Training
- Facilitating research
- Coordinating control activities at state and international borders.

Organization

		Function
Central	Directorate Generate of Health Services, Ministry of Health and Family Welfare	Supply of DDT and larvicides
	↓	
	19 regional offices of NVBDCP at state levels	
State	Vector Borne Disease Control Division of Department of Health and Family Welfare	• Supervision, guidance and effective implementation • Coordination of activities with other states • Procurement of certain insecticides for indoor residual spray, spray equipment and certain antimalarials
	Health and Family Welfare Society	• Channelize funds from financing from central government to states and onwards to districts • District level planning and monitoring
District	District Health Office	• In-charge of activities in the district
	District Malaria Offices	• Key unit of planning and monitoring of program • Spray operations
	District Health Societies	• Assist management of funds and planning • Monitoring of program activities
PHC	Primary Health Center	• Supervision/ monitoring of activities • Surveillance and laboratory services • Supervise spraying
		• Work under MO of PHC
		• Case detection management and community outreach services

Infrastructure

	Location	***Manned by***	***Function***
Drug Distribution Centers and Fever treatment Depots	Subcenters	Voluntary worker from community	• Dispense anti-malaria tablets as per NMEP schedules • Collect blood slides from suspected fever cases
Laboratories (decentralized to minimize time lag between blood smear collection and their examination)	PHCs	Microscopists	• Reports blood slides collected at PHCs, subcenters or fever treatment depots

Strategies for Malaria Elimination

Principle

- Rapid reduction of transmission in areas with high malaria incidence
- Interruption of malaria transmission in low transmission areas
- Prevention of reestablish of malaria in areas with interrupted transmission.

Intervention

A. Reclassification of endemic areas
  - Under National Framework for Malaria Elimination, the endemic areas were reclassified into categories based on the annual parasite index (API) into:

Category	API (2014)	States/UTs	Intervention
0 (Prevention of re-establishment phase)	Zero indigenous cases	Non	▪ Detect any re-introduced case of malaria ▪ Immediately notify all detected cases of malaria ▪ Determine underlying causes of resumed local transmission ▪ Apply rapid curative and preventive measures ▪ Prevent re-introduction and possible re-establishment of malaria transmission ▪ Maintain malaria free status in these areas
1 (Elimination phase)	API <1 (in all districts)	HP, Punjab, JandK, Kerala, Manipur, Uttarakhan, Haryana, Sikkim, Rajasthan, Goa, Puducherry, Chandigarh, Delhi, Daman and Diu and Lakshadweep	▪ Interrupt local transmission in all active malarial foci ▪ Mandatory notification of each case of malaria (even from private sector) ▪ Establish adequate case-based surveillance and complete case management ▪ Investigation and classification of all foci of malaria ▪ Strict coverage of effective vector control in all active foci ▪ Prevent onward transmission by early detection and treatment ▪ Establish state and national level malaria elimination database ▪ Screening, management and prevention of malaria in mobile and migrant population ▪ Establish effective epidemic forecasting and response system ▪ Ensure rigorous quality assurance of all medicines and diagnostics ▪ Set up national level reference laboratory for confirmation of diagnosis and cross checking of all positive and fixed % of negative slides ▪ Notification of new cases in Category 0 states ▪ Training and certification of microscopists ▪ Screen all suspected cases of malaria during investigation of foci ▪ Surveillance of special groups, migrant populations and people living in vicinity of industrial area
2 (Pre-elimination phase)	API <1 but some districts API ≥1	Bihar, Tamil Nadu, Telangana, Uttar Pradesh, Karnataka, West Bengal, Andhra Pradesh, Assam, Maharashtra, Gujarat and Nagaland	▪ Setting up elimination surveillance system ▪ Initiating elimination phase activities in districts with API <1
3 (Intensified control phase)	API ≥1	Madhya Pradesh, Jharkhand, Arunachal Pradesh, Chattisgarh, Odisha, Megalaya, Tripura, Mizorum, Andaman and Nicobar, and Dadar and Nagar Haveli	▪ Massive scaling of existing disease management and preventive approaches and tools ▪ Screening of all fever cases suspected for malaria ▪ Tailored intervention based on geographical classification as per local malaria epidemiology and risk of transmission ▪ Strengthening of intersectoral collaboration ▪ One stop centers or mobile clinics on fixed days in tribal or conflict affected areas for malaria diagnosis and treatment and health education ▪ Reduce mortality by timely referral and treatment of severe cases ▪ Establishment of robust supply chain management system ▪ Maintain optimum surveillance using diagnostic measures ▪ Strengthening of health infrastructure and equipping them with diagnostic (microscopy and RDT) and treatment (injectable artemisinin derivatives) facilities

B. Surveillance
- Surveillance plays a key role in early detection of outbreaks
- It is aimed to target control interventions in high transmission areas and assessing their impact.

a. Active surveillance
- Active surveillance is a key component of malaria eradication program

Objectives
- Case detection through laboratory services and providing facilities for proper treatment.

Done by
- The case detection is carried out by the multipurpose health worker who has a population of 10,000 or approximately 2,000 houses under him
- There is a health assistant for 4 multipurpose health workers
- This population is 8,000 in difficult terrains.

Procedure
- The multipurpose health worker visits each house in area allotted to him once in a fortnight to enquire regarding:
  - Whether there is a fever case in the house including the members and guests
  - Whether there was a fever case in the house between his previous visit and the present visit
- If answers to any of this question is YES, then he should collect a blood film (thick and thin on same slide)
- He makes necessary entries in the stencil or the house card about his visit and dispatches the blood slides at least twice a week to the laboratory at PHC for microscopic examination
- He is also required to collect the slides from the subcenters and fever treatment depots and send them to laboratory
- If the report about blood film comes positive then he returns to the patient to administer a course of antimalaria treatment depending on the causative agent and chloroquine sensitivit.

b. Passive surveillance
- It is detection of malaria cases among the patients who seek medical care.

Done by
- The local health agencies such as ASHA, fever treatment depots, PHCs, subcenters, hospitals, dispensaries and local medical practitioners.

Procedure
- They collect blood smear from all fever cases and also from those with history of recent fever
- ASHA and other volunteer workers diagnose by RDTs where as at PHCs and other higher centers it is by examination of blood smears
- The result of blood examination is communicated to the local surveillance worker for institution of antimalaria treatment.

c. Sentinel surveillance
- Carried out in high endemic districts.

Done by
- 1–3 sentinel sites (large private hospitals).

Procedure
- Sentinel sites report all OP and IP cases of malaria and malaria-related deaths.

Parameters for epidemiological surveillance of malaria
- To evaluate the success of surveillance activity
  i. Annual parasite incidence[Q]
  ii. Annual blood examination rate[Q] (done for operational efficiency[Q])
  iii. Annual falciparum incidence[Q]
  iv. Slide positivity rate[Q]
  v. Slide falciparum rate[Q]

C. Urban Malaria Scheme
- Urban Malaria Scheme was launched to interrupt malaria transmission in towns and cities by intensive antilarval measure and drug treatment

- The criteria for inclusion of cities under the scheme are:
  - Population of more than 50,000
  - Slide positivity of more than 5.

  Interventions:
  - Implementation of civic bylaws to prevent mosquito breeding in domestic and peridomestic areas
  - Use larvivorous fish in water bodies and larvicides for water bodies unsuitable for fish use.

D. Tribal Malaria Action Plan
- Tribal Malaria Action Plan will cover Category 2 and 3 districts enabling concentration of available resources to high endemic areas.

Interventions
- Mobile-based surveillance
- Provision of hamlet-wise ASHA (instead of village-wise)
- Provide alternatives to ASHA like village headman, school teachers, forest department officials, etc.
- Mobile health services in areas with civic disturbances
- Involvement of NGOs
- Strengthening of health infrastructure with quality microscope facility
- On the spot species specific radical treatment of all positive cases
- Early referral of serious cases to PHCs with free transport
- Follow up and epidemiological tracking of all positive cases
- Integrated vector management
- Social marketing to increase use of mosquito nets
- Environmental engineering
- Intensive training of health cadres.

E. Antimalaria month campaign
- June to be observed as antimalaria month every year (prior to onset of monsoon and transmission season) to enhance awareness, encourage community participation and consolidate intersectoral collaborative efforts.

F. Intrasectoral collaboration
- Integrated disease surveillance project—provides early warning singles of malaria outbreaks
- Other vector-borne diseases—integrated of vector control activities
- Reproductive and child health—utilize antental visits to distribute mosquito nets.

G. Integrated vector management

Objective
- Achieve effective vector control by appropriate biological, chemical and environmental interventions of proven efficacy, separately or in combination as appropriate to the area through optimal use of resources.

Interventions

a. Antilarval measures
   i. Physical method (source reduction)
      - Consists of reduction in the sites of mosquito breeding like drainage of filing, deepening or flushing, management of water level, changing salt content of water and intermittent irrigation, etc. are some of the classical methods of malaria control
      - And if feasible, the major attention should be give to permanent reduction of sources by improvement of the environment.
   ii. Chemical method
      - Consists of application of larvicides over the breeding places
      - Before applying larvicides, the breeding places should be cleared of scum and vegetations so as to maximize the efficiency
      - Antilarval measures include oiling the collections of standing water or dusting them with paris green
      - Application of temephos confers long effect with low toxicity
      - However, larviciding must be repeated at frequent intervals making it a costly affair.
   iii. Biological method
      - Consists of using biocides such as using *Bacillus sphaericus* and *B. thuringensis*, which are effective against larvae of anopheline mosquitoes.

Significance
- Primary method of vector control in urban areas.

b. Antiadult measures
   i. Residual spraying
      - Spraying of indoor surfaces of houses with residual insecticides is still the most effective measure to kill the adult mosquito
      - It reduces the longevity of the vector to less than 10 days[Q]
      - DDT is most preferred insecticide and in areas resistant to DDT, most commonly used insecticides are organophosphates—malathion and fenitrothion

Insecticide	*Vector resistance*	*No. of round*	*Dosage (g/m^2 surface)*
DDT	Sensitive to DDT	2	1.0 g
Malathion	Resistant to DDT	3	2.0 g
Pyrethrin	Resistant to DDT and malathion	2 (6 weeks apart)	0.25 g

Disadvantages
- Spraying once applied may need to be continued for an indefinite period.

Significance
- Primary method of vector control in rural settings.

   ii. Space spraying
      - Ultraflow-volume method of pesticide dispersion in form of fog or mist using special equipment by air or on ground
      - It reduce vector population quickly.

Advantages
- Effective and economical.

c. Personal prophylaxis
   i. Insecticide treated bed nets
      - Use of insecticide treated bed nets resulted in significant decline in malaria incidence and API
      - Introduced newly in the program and scale up their use to replace indoor spraying as preferred antiadult measure
      - Population living in areas with API ≥ 5 will be covered by LLIN and those living in API ≥ 2 with conventional nets + Residual sprays.
   ii. Insect repellants
      - Chemicals that are rubbed on exposed parts of body to repel mosquitoes.

Revised Scheme 2 & 3

Significance

- National Framework for Malaria Elimination in India (2016–2030) is a bold step by the Government of India keeping in line with WHO Global Technical Strategy, however, its success is largely dependent upon the community participation.

6. Briefly discuss the principles of primary health care.

Refer Question No. 4 June 2012 (RS2) Paper II.

7. Explain demographic cycle with examples.

Refer Question No. 11 Dec. 2009 (RS2) Paper II.

8. Write briefly about AFP (acute flaccid paralysis) surveillance.

Refer Question No. 1 June 2014 (RS2) Paper II.

9. What are the responsibilities of WHO (World Health Organization)?

Refer Question No. 5 June 2009 (RS2) Paper II.

10. Enumerate the job descriptions of a female health worker.

Refer Question No. 10 Dec. 2007 (RS2) Paper II.

11. Discuss the various health problems of the aged in India.

Refer Question No. 2 June 2009 (RS2) Paper II.

12. What is cost-benefit analysis?

Refer Question No. 6 Dec. 2011 (RS2) Paper II.

SHORT ANSWERS

13. Mention the advantages of intrauterine contraceptive devices.

Refer Question No. 6 June 2009 (RS2) Paper II.

14. Objectives of school health services.

Refer Question No. 4 Dec. 2013 (RS2) Paper II.

15. Triage in disaster management.

Refer Question No. 16 June 2013 (RS2) Paper II.

16. Screening for cervical cancer.

Refer Question No. 11 June 2013 (RS2) Paper II.

17. Risk factors for coronary heart diseases.

Refer Question No. 11 June 2015 (RS2) Paper II.

18. Congenital rubella.

Refer Question No. 3 June 2011 (RS2) Paper II.

19. Measles vaccine.

Refer Question No. 1 Dec. 2010 (RS2) Paper II.

20. Enumerate the various levels of health-care services in India with examples.

Refer Question No. 11 June 2010 (RS2) Paper II.

21. Physical quality of life index (PQLI).

Refer Question No. 16 Dec. 2007 (RS2) Paper I.

22. Prevention of neonatal tetanus.

Refer Question No. 12 June 2013 (RS2) Paper II.

MBBS PHASE III EXAMINATION

JUNE 2015

(Revised Scheme 2 & 3)

PAPER I

LONG ESSAYS

1. Classify epidemiological studies. Describe time, place and person distribution with respect to descriptive studies.

- Epidemiological studies are studies carried out to find disease occurrence in a population and explore disease etiology.

Classification

Epidemiological studies			
Observational studies		Experimental or Interventional studies	
	Unit of study		Unit of study
a. Descriptive studies		a. Randomized control trials or Clinical trials	Patients
b. Analytical studies		b. Field trials	Healthy people
i. Ecological or Correlational	Population	c. Community trials	Communities
ii. Cross-sectional or Prevalence	Individuals		
iii. Case-control or Case reference	Individuals		
iv. Cohort or Follow-up	Individuals		

Descriptive Studies

- Descriptive studies are usually the first phase of an epidemiological investigation which are concerned with disease distribution or health-related characteristics in human populations and identifying the associated disease characteristics
- It basically tries to find the following characteristics of disease occurrence:
  - When—Time distribution
  - Where—Place distribution
  - Who—Person distribution.

Time Distribution

- Time distribution of disease is description of a disease in relation to the time of its occurrence, i.e. by week, month, year, the day of the week hour of onset, etc.
- It shows the relation of the disease with time, i.e. whether the disease is seasonal whether its shows periodic increase or decrease or does it follow consistent time trend.

Types

a. Short-term fluctuations (Epidemic)
   - Occurrence of number of cases clearly in excess of normal expectancy[Q]
   - Normal expectancy is derived from looking at average of number of cases of disease in previous 3–4 years in a geographic area
   - Statistically speaking Epidemic = Number of cases > Mean + 2SD.

   Types

Irregular fluctuations over short time	*Regular fluctuations over short time*
Diseases like common cold, diarrhea, acute respiratory infections show this trend in small communities	Disease here show rise and fall in frequency at a regular interval

b. Long-term fluctuations

Seasonal fluctuations	*Cyclic trend*[Q]
▪ It occurs due to climatic changes which change human life (herd immunity), life of animals involved in disease transmission, increase in the activity of vectors, climatic changes conductive for growth and development of organisms ▪ This phenomenon is common with many communicable diseases like measles[Q] and varicella[Q] peak in early springs, malaria in rainy seasons[Q] ▪ Upper respiratory tract infection show rise in winter months ▪ However some non infections diseases also exhibit seasonal fluctuations like sunstroke, hay fever, snake bite, etc.	▪ When the frequency of disease increases over a period of years usually less than 10 years[Q], it is called cyclic trends ▪ It occurs due to naturally occurring variations in herd immunity[Q] and for another attack to occur, there should be build up of susceptible[Q] in the herd and antigenic variation[Q] ▪ In prevaccination era, measles exhibited cyclic trend of 2–3 years[Q], rubella of 6–9 years[Q] and influenza pandemic of 10–15 years[Q]

c. Secular trends[Q] (Long-term fluctuations)
   - Secular trend is the change in the occurrence of disease over a long period of time generally several years or decades[Q]
   - The change may be either rising or falling in disease frequency
   - The noninfections, life style disease like diabetes, ischemic heart disease, etc. are showing rising secular bend where as due to vaccination disease like polio, measles are exhibiting decreasing secular trends.

   Significance of temporal variation
   - By surveillance and monitoring temporal variation, the emerging health problems can be identified and effectiveness of control measures for old diseases can be assessed
   - Etiological hypotheses can be formulated and assessed based on fluctuation is diseases frequency
   - Knowledge of the temporal variation of disease gives adequate time for community to take up preventive measures.

Significance

- Time distribution of disease gives important clues about the source or etiology of the disease, thereby suggesting potential preventive measures
- For example, cases of malaria increase during monsoon due to availability of breeding places for *Anopheles* mosquitoes and it can be prevented by getting rid of mosquito breeding places, antimosquito measures well before the monsoon.

Place (Geographic) Distribution

- Geographic distribution of disease means pattern of occurrence of a disease in different places.

Types

a. International variations
   - Many diseases have shown variations in disease pattern internationally depending upon the countries, they occur in

   Examples
   - Gastric cancer is common in Japan, rare in USA
   - Cervical cancer common in India but not so in USA, UK

- Breast cancer is low Japan and high in Western countries
- Yellow fever is limited to South American countries
- Sleeping sickness in found in African countries[Q].

Relevance in epidemiology
- These international variations stimulated research in cause and effect relationship between the environmental factors and disease thus identify factors which are crucial in cause and prevention of disease.

b. National variations
- Besides international variations, some diseases also show variations within the national boundary varying from region to region.

Examples
- Goiter is more in sub-Himalayan region
- Lathyrism is common Madhya Pradesh
- Leprosy cases are abundant in Tamil Nadu and Andhra Pradesh[Q].

Relevance in epidemiology
- National variations provides information needed to demarcate the affected areas for a particular disease and provide appropriate health care.

c. Rural-urban variations
- Extreme difference in the lifestyles, population density, education, sanitation, environment and healthcare facilities in rural and urban areas has manifested in rural-urban variations of diseases.

Examples
- Lifestyle diseases like diabetes, hypertension, mental illnesses, etc. are on rise in urban areas
- Zoonoses, soil borne diseases and other communicable diseases are prevalent in rural areas.

Relevance in epidemiology
- Rural-urban variations help to identify risk groups for a particular disease and provide healthcare to those needed for prevention and control.

d. Local distribution
- This studies the variations in disease frequency in a local area with aid of geographical spot maps.

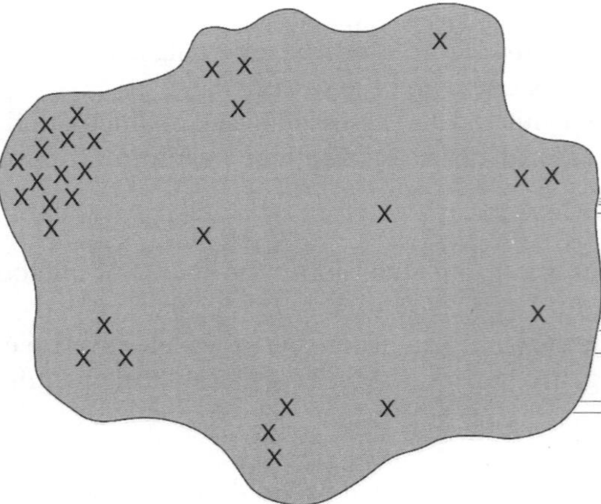

Fig. 1: Local distribution of disease on a spot map

Examples
- John Snow studied the 1854 cholera epidemic in London by spot maps to discover that the most cases were located around the common water pump in Broad Street, thus, he was able to identify the source of infection and therefore the local distribution of the disease in an area.

Relevance in epidemiology
- The study of local distribution of disease helps to identify the source of infection thus formulate etiological hypothesis.

Significance

- Study of geographic distribution of disease is an important dimension of descriptive epidemiology
- It helps to understand the variations in disease pattern between countries and also within a country from one state to another, from rural to urban areas and local area
- It provides evidence of source of disease and its mode of spread by relating these variations to agent, host and environmental factors
- It helps the medical professional to diagnose a certain condition depending upon geographical area of the patient.

Person Distribution

- Disease can be further described under host factors such as age, sex, occupation, marital status, habits, social class, etc. which helps to understand natural history of disease.

a. Age
   - Strongest host factor
   - Some diseases are more frequent in certain age groups like measles in childhood, cancer in middle age and atherosclerosis in old age
   - Prevalence of many chronic and degenerative diseases progressively increase with advancing age thus reflecting a persistent and cumulative exposure to a disease agent
   - Some diseases (Hodgkin's disease, leukemia and breast cancer) exhibit highest incidence in 2 separate age groups, which is called as Bimodality which suggests 2 distinct sets of causal factors responsible for disease
   - Uniform attack rate of a communicable disease in all age groups implies equal susceptibility of all age groups.

b. Sex
   - Diseases exhibit variation in disease frequency between sexes due to
   - Basic biological differences including sex-linked genetic inheritance
   - Cultural and behavioral differences
   - Diabetes, hyperthyroidism and obesity are more common in women
   - Lung cancer and coronary heart disease are more frequent in men.

c. Ethnicity
   - Disease occurrence differs in different population subgroups of different racial and ethnic origins
   - Sickle cell anemia is rare in African population.

d. Marital status
   - Marital status exhibited difference in mortality rates, i.e. married men and women exhibit lower mortality rates compared to unmarried counterparts
   - However, marital status can be a risk factor for some diseases and conditions
   - Incidence of cervical cancer is very low in nuns whereas it is very high in women with multiple sexual contacts and promiscuity.

e. Occupation
   - Occupation has an important bearing on health due to alteration in their behavior patterns and exposure to particular types of risks
   - Silicosis is more common in coal miners.

f. Social class
   - Health and diseases are not equally distributed in social classes
   - Upper social class people have a longer life expectancy and better health and nutritional status
   - Certain diseases (e.g. coronary heart disease, hypertension, diabetes) have a higher prevalence in upper classes.

g. Behavior
   - Human behavior is a major risk factor in modern day diseases such as coronary heart disease, cancer, obesity and accidents
   - These behavioral factors include cigarette smoking, sedentary life, over-eating and drug abuse.

h. Stress
   - Stress affects patient's response to disease agent, treatment, etc.

i. Migration
   - Due to urban migration of rural population, certain diseases like malaria, filariasis, leprosy have emerged as serious problem in urban areas also.

Significance

- Knowledge of the frequency of disease in certain subgroups of the population has lead to concept of "high-risk groups".

2. What is protein-energy malnutrition? Discuss the ecology and preventive and social measures to address the problem.

Refer Question No. 1 December 2012 (RS2) Paper I.

SHORT ESSAYS

3. What is social stratification? Discuss how social class affects health and utilization of health services.

- Social stratification is the process by which individuals and groups are ranked in a more or less enduring hierarchy of status.

Characteristics used for social stratification

a. Caste	• Indian society is based on caste therefore though this characteristic has lost its significance in modern India, it still is used for social stratification
b. Occupation	• Occupation is most widely used measure for social stratification as occupation to a great extent determines the lifestyle of as individual. **Occupational classes (The Registrar General of England)** i. Social class I—Professional ii. Social class II—Managerial iii. Social class III—Clerk and skilled iv. Social Class IV—Semiskilled v. Social class V—Unskilled **Disadvantages** • An individual may pursue two occupations simultaneously or may change their occupations
c. Education	• Education also determines one's lifestyle, and awareness regarding health therefore it is also used to stratify the population **Classification** i. Illiterate ii. Literate (Any person who is able to read and write with understanding in any language) iii. Primary education iv. Higher primary education v. Secondary education vi. Post graduate and professionals
d. Income	• If disclosed correctly income is a better method of social stratification however the income is always never disclosed correctly • Moreover the value of money changes always **Grading** i. Upper class ii. High middle class iii. Low middle class iv. High lower class v. Low lower class
e. Others	i. Religion ii. Purchasing power iii. Area of residence (urban/rural) iv. Type of house (kuccha/puckka) (owned/rented)

Significance

- We use social stratification for assessing the association between health and disease in society.
  a. Association with disease
    - Social factors have been long associated with disease causation
    - Diseases like protein-energy malnutrition, vitamin deficiency disorders, diarrheal diseases, respiratory infections are very common in low socioeconomic group
    - Similarly people from high socioeconomic class are more prone for ischemic heart disease, obesity, diabetes, peptic ulcer, etc.

Factors responsible for higher morbidity and mortality among the people of lower socioeconomic class are:
- Size of the family, which is usually bigger, resulting in overcrowding
- Early marriages, resulting in more frequent pregnancies depleting the maternal reserve
- Utilization of health services, which is less frequent
- Beliefs, such as diseases due to curse or punishment from God
- Physical environment, such as poor housing with poor lighting and ventilation, lack of protected water supply, etc
- Illiteracy and ignorance
- Genetic endowment, i.e. tendency for consanguineous marriages
- Attitude to disease which is usually indifferent, etc.

b. Identification of susceptible
- Because of close association between socioeconomic status and disease, it is easy to identify the at risk susceptible individuals for a particular disease.

c. Planning of health services
- Health services which are scare can be directed towards the susceptible to get maximum impact.

d. Utilization of healthcare services
- Utilization of healthcare services are very less in people from low socioeconomic groups; however they (BPL card holders) are provided the following benefits:
  i. Janani Suraksha Yojana (JSY) for pregnant mothers aged ≥19 years and up to two living children
  ii. National Maternity Benefit Scheme (NMBS) to provide better diet for pregnant women
  iii. Insurance of women workers by paying the premium of ₹ 200 per member; 50% of which is paid by social security fund. The insurance benefit is ₹ 20,000 for natural death, ₹ 50,000 for death/disability resulting from accident and ₹ 25,000 for partial disability
  iv. Bhagyalakshmi Scheme—Deposit of ₹ 10,000 for each of the first two female children, which will be returned with interest, after the child attains 18 years of age
  v. Social assistance such as old age pension scheme, family benefit scheme, widow pension scheme (widow should be 18 years old)
  vi. Prasooti Araike Scheme to promote antenatal care by giving ₹ 1,000 at 6th month of pregnancy and another ₹ 1000 at 9th month; a total of ₹ 2000.

4. Outline steps in outbreak investigation of food poisoning.

- Food poisoning is acute gastroenteritis caused by ingestion of food or drink contaminated with either living bacteria or their toxins or inorganic chemical substances and poisons derived from plants and animals
- It is characterized by:
  – History of ingestion of a common food
  – Affection of many people at the same time
  – Similarity in signs and symptoms of these people.

Investigation of An Outbreak

a. Secure complete list of people involved and their history
  – All the people who have consumed the suspected food should be interviewed by means of a questionnaire
  – The same rule applies to cooks, waiters and others working in a dining place
  – The questionnaires should include question to elicit information about
    - Total number of participants and total number of people affected
    - Personal data of affected people such as age, sex, residence, occupation and any other helpful information
    - Time of onset of symptoms
    - Symptoms of illness in order of appearance
    - Food eaten during previous 2 days
    - Place of consumption
    - Details of death if any.

b. Assessment of environmental factors
  – Inspection of eateries

- To assess sanitation of kitchen and dining hall
- To know the nature of the storage of food grains
- To know the nature of the storage of cooked foods
- To know the presence of rodents
– Interrogation and examination of food handlers and other employees regarding personal hygiene, habits and illness if any
– Questioning of food handlers regarding food preparation.

c. Laboratory investigation
– The samples of stool and vomit from the patients and also from the employees of the restaurant and food handlers as well as the suspected food is subjected to laboratory investigation to:
- Incriminate the causative agent
- Determine the total number of bacteria
- Determine relative number of each kind of bacteria involved
– The sample should be examined aerobically and anaerobically
– Serological test of blood of affected person for antibody titer (useful for retrospective diagnosis)
– Culture of stool and urine of food handlers and kitchen employees
– The laboratory investigation is not complete till phage typing of the organism.

d. Animal experiments
– Administering or feeding the remnants of food to the rhesus monkey
– Protection test, i.e. injection of saline filtrate of food stuff subcutaneously into mice protected with antitoxic sera.

e. Data analysis
– Data collected is analysed according to the descriptive methods of time, place and person distribution
– Food specific attack rate and case fatality rates are calculated
– Etiological hypothesis is formulated
– A case control study to be under taken to establish the epidemiologic association between illness and intake of a particular food.

Significance

- Investigation of food poisoning is a classical example of investigation of an epidemic.

5. Describe barriers to health communication.

Refer Question No. 5 June 2010 (RS2) Paper I.

6. Pneumoconiosis.

Refer Question No. 2 June 2012 (RS2) Paper I.

7. What are the detrimental effects of iron deficiency anemia? Add a note on its preventive measures.

Refer Question No. 10 June 2008 (RS2) Paper I.

8. Outline causes, clinical features and management of lead poisoning.

Refer Question No. 9 December 2011 (RS2) Paper I.

9. Benefits under ESI Act.

Refer Question No. 4 December 2012 (RS2) Paper I.

10. Describe the different methods for removal of hardness of water.

- Hardness is the soap destroying power of water or hard water is a one which does not readily form lather with soap
- Expressed in mEq/L
- 1 mEq/L of hardness producing ion is equal to 50 mg $CaCO_3$ (50 ppm) in 1 liter of water.

Types of hardness	*Causes (presence of any of following dissolved substance which form insoluble, sticky precipitates with soap)*	*Method of removal*
a. Carbonate (Temporary)	▪ Calcium bicarbonate ▪ Magnesium bicarbonate	▪ Boiling ▪ Addition of lime ▪ Addition of sodium carbonate ▪ Permutit process
b. Noncarbonate (Permanent)	▪ Calcium sulphate ▪ Magnesium sulphate ▪ Chlorides ▪ Nitrates	▪ Addition of sodium carbonate ▪ Base exchange process

Grading of hardness

Grading	*Level of hardness*
▪ Soft water (low buffering capacity and corrosive to plumbing)	▪ <1 mEq/L
▪ Moderately hard (used for domestic use)	▪ 1–3 mEq/L
▪ Hard water	▪ 3–6 mEq/L
▪ Very hard water	▪ <6 mEq/L

Removing of Hardness

Indication

- Hardness >3 mEq/L.

Method	*Principle*	*Remarks*
Boiling	▪ Removes temporary hardness by expelling CO_2 and precipitating insoluble calcium carbonate $Ca(HCO_3)_2 \rightarrow CaCO_3 + H_2O + CO_2$	Disadvantage ▪ Expensive on a large scale
Addition of lime (Clark's method)	▪ Absorbs CO_2 and precipitates insoluble calcium carbonate ▪ 1ounce of quick lime for 700 gallons of water for each degree (14.25 ppm) of hardness $Ca(OH)_2 + Ca(HCO_3)_2 \rightarrow 2CaCO_3 + 2H_2O$	Advantage ▪ Also reduces magnesium
Addition of Sodium Carbonate (Soda Ash)	$Na_2CO_3 + Ca(HCO_3)_2 \rightarrow 2NaHCO_3 + CaCO_3$ $Na_2CO_3 + CaSO_4 \rightarrow Na_2SO_4 + CaCO_3$	Advantage ▪ Removes both temporary and permanent hardness
Base (Ion) Exchange process (permutit process) (zeolite softening) **Fig. 2:** Ion exchange	▪ Sodium permutit (Sodium zeolite) is a complex compound of sodium, aluminium and silica ($Na_2\ Al_2\ Si_2O\ H_2O$) which has property of exchanging Na^+ for Ca^{2+} and Mg^{2+} in water ▪ Passing of hard water through the permutit, calcium and magnesium ions are entirely removed by base exchange and sodium permutit is converted into calcium and magnesium permutit ▪ Resultant water has zero hardness which as corrosive properties; hence a part of raw water is mixed with softened water to secure the desired hardness	▪ Permutit loses its effectiveness after repeated use but can be regenerated by treating it with concentrated solution of sodium chloride or brine and washing away the soluble calcium and magnesium chloride formed ▪ Advantages ▪ Removes both temporary and permanent hardness ▪ Used in automated treatment of large water supplies

Significance

- Drinking water should be moderately hard
- Hardness of water is dependent on regional geology (limestone regions have hard water and granite regions have soft water) and pollution with sewage and many other waste.

Advantages	*Disadvantages*
▪ Hardness of water is considered to be cardioprotective	▪ Consumes more soap and detergents ▪ Adversely affects cooking (soft water retains natural color and appearance of food and are more digestible) ▪ Reduces life of fabrics ▪ Causes irritation of skin and gastrointestinal system ▪ Causes precipitation of carbonates on boiling leading to furring or scaling of boilers resulting in great fuel consumption, loss of efficiency and may cause boiler explosions ▪ Unsuitable for numerous industrial processes (economic losses) ▪ Shortens life of plumbing pipes and fixtures by causing encrustation of water carrying system

11. Methods of assessment of nutritional status in a community.

Refer Question No. 2 June 2010 (RS2) Paper I.

12. Write a note on cold chain equipment present in a primary health center.

Refer Question No. 12 December 2007 (RS2) Paper I.

SHORT ANSWERS

13. Mental health services in India.

Refer Question No. 11 December 2016 (RS2) Paper I.

14. Guidelines for defining "at risk" groups.

- "At risk" approach is newer approach promoted by WHO wherein a target (at risk) group is identified by certain defined criteria and appropriate action is directed towards them
- It is a managerial device for increasing efficiency of healthcare services within the limits of existing resources.

Guidelines for Defining at Risk Groups

a. Biological situation	
i. Age groups	▪ Infants (LBW), toddlers, elderly
ii. Sex	▪ Females in reproductive age groups
iii. Physiological state	▪ Pregnancy, cholesterol levels, hypertension
iv. Genetic factors	▪ Family history of genetic disorders
v. Other health conditions	▪ Disease, physical functioning, unhealthy behavior
b. Physical situation	
i. Place of living	▪ Rural, urban slums
ii. Living conditions	▪ Overcrowding
iii. Environmental factors	▪ Water supply, proximity to industries
c. Sociocultural and cultural situation	▪ Social class ▪ Ethnic and cultural group ▪ Family disruption, education, housing ▪ Customs, habits and behavior (smoking, over eating, drug addiction, lack of exercise) ▪ Access to health services ▪ Lifestyles and attitudes

Significance

- Due to scarcity of resources, current approach in epidemiology is on identification of these risk groups as it helps to define priorities and direct the resources to those in most need
- At risk approach is "something for all but more for those in need—in proportion to the need".

15. Measures of central tendancy.

Refer Question No. 3 December 2010 (RS2) Paper I.

16. Differentiate between monitoring and surveillance with examples.

Refer Question No. 7 June 2009 (RS2) Paper I.

17. Effects and prevention of noise pollution.

Refer Question No. 4 December 2008 (RS2) Paper I.

18. Disaster cycle.

- Disaster is any occurrence that causes damage, ecological disruption, loss of human life or deterioration of health and health services on a scale sufficient to warrant an extraordinary response from outside of affected community or area (WHO).

Disaster Cycle

- Disaster cycle is cyclic management events following disaster.

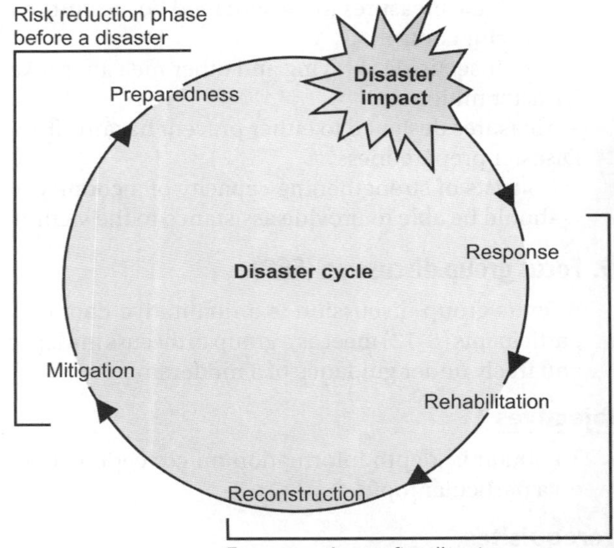

Fig. 3: Disaster cycle

Stages[Q]

a. Disaster impact and response
   i. Search, rescue and first aid
      - It is the uninjured survivors who come to immediate help. These survivors are organized, they come to rescue and provide first aid.
   ii. Field care
      - Food has to be provided at place of disaster. People are sheltered in tents, schools and community halls. Health resource persons and other volunteers, police, home guards are deployed to place. An enquiry center to be established to respond to patients, friends, relatives and family members. Dead victims need to be identified and adequate mortuary space to be provided.
   iii. Triage
      - Triage is a system of color coding causalities based on severity of injuries and chances of survival with medical supervision. It is carried out at the site and done as follows:

Priority I (Red color)	*Priority II (Yellow color)*	*Priority III (Green color)*	*Priority IV (Black color)*
Critically ill patients requiring immediate resuscitation within 6 hours	Moderately ill patients requiring medical attention within 24 hours	Ambulatory patients with minimum risk	Moribund patients or dead

   iv. Tagging
      - Identification of patients with tags providing information such as name, age, contact details, triage color, treatment given.
   v. Identification of dead
      - Dead bodies need to removed from the site of disaster, shifted to mortuary, identified and bereaved family members received.

b. Disaster containment (Stage of health and medical relief)
   - Most crucial phase

Primary phase (0–6 hours)	*Secondary follow up (6–24 hours)*	*Tertiary clean up (1–60 days)*
First aid, medical care	Transportation, sanitation and immunization	Food, clothing, shelter assistance, social service, employment, rehabilitation

c. Rehabilitation
   i. Water supply
      - Important and best way to provide water supply is by chlorination with residual chlorine concentration of 0.7 ppm. Survey the area to find source of water and protect it from contamination by animals and excreta
   ii. Sanitation and personal hygiene
      - Special emphasis is given for disposal of human excreta by construction of temporary trench latrines, separate for men and women. Provide facilities for bathing, washing and cleaning.
   iii. Food safety
      - Take measures to prevent food borne outbreaks like washing hands before eating food and after using toilets.
   iv. Vector control
      - Insecticide spraying and other measures taken immediately to control vectors.

d. Disaster mitigation[Q]
   - Measures designed to either prevent hazards from causing emergency or to lessen the effects of emergency.

e. Disaster preparedness
   - Consists of strengthening capacity of a country to manage efficiently all type of emergencies, so that resources, should be able to provide assistance to the victims and bring back life to normal.

19. Focus group discussion (FGD).

- A focus group discussion is a qualitative data collection method in which one or two researchers and several participants (6–12) meet as a group to discuss in-depth about a given research topic where members talk spontaneously and freely under guidance of a moderator.

Objectives

- To obtain in-depth information on concept, perceptions and ideas of group on a particular topic.

Prerequisites

- 6–12 participants who are willing to talk about the issue under discussion
- These participants should be as homogenous as possible with respect to their background characteristics
- There is a moderator conducting the discussion but not leading the discussion. He uses a predetermined pretested line of questioning to stimulate discussion among the participants in order to understand perceptions, interpretations and beliefs of a selected population to gain understanding of a particular issue from the perspective of the group's participants
- There is a recorder/note taker who notes down the proceedings and draws the sociogram (a pictorial representation of the way the interactions have occurred between various participants)
- There should be a predetermined FGD guide (written list of topics that need to be discussed in the group and consists of a series of open ended questions)
- It should not last more than an hour and half
- Recording equipment with a backup should be present as these sessions are usually tape recorded and sometimes videotaped.

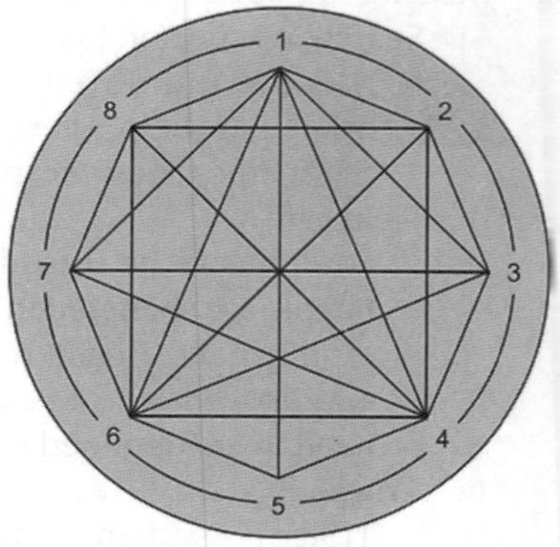

Fig. 4: Focus group discussion

Advantages	*Disadvantages*	*Application*
▪ They yield a large amount of information over a relatively short period of time ▪ They are also effective for accessing a broad range of views on a specific topic, as opposed to achieving group consensus	▪ Focus groups are not the best method for acquiring information on highly personal or socially sensitive topics	▪ Exploratory studies in health issues ▪ Testing ideas about acceptances of a new program ▪ Solving specific program problems ▪ Evaluating health programs

Significance

- Focus groups discussion is effective in helping researchers learn the social norms of a community or subgroup, as well as the range of perspectives that exist within that community or subgroup
- Focus groups seek to illuminate group opinion
- This method is especially well suited for socio-behavioral research that will be used to develop and measure health services that meet the needs of a community.

20. Differentiate between isolation and quarantine.

- Both isolation and quarantine are public health strategies that have proven effective in stopping the spread of infectious diseases.

Comparison between Quarantine and Isolation

	Quarantine	*Isolation*
Definition	▪ Quarantine is the separation and limitation of freedom of movements of such well persons or domestic animals exposed to communicable disease for a period of time not longer than the longest usual incubation period of the disease in such manner as to prevent effective contact with those not so exposed	▪ It is defined as separation for the period of communicability of infected persons or animals from others in such places and under such condition as to prevent or limit the direct or indirect transmission of the infectious agent from those infected to those who are susceptible or who may spread the agent to others
Separates whom	▪ It separates people who have been exposed to a specific illness (but aren't yet sick and don't have symptoms) from others. (Healthy contacts[Q])	▪ It separates those who are already ill or infected from those who are not. (cases)
Reason	▪ Some infections can be spread even before a person knows he or she is sick or has any symptoms	▪ Isolating sick people helps prevent the spread or transmission of disease
Benefits	▪ People around	▪ Cases themselves
Where	▪ A person is usually quarantined in his or her own home	▪ The location of isolation depends on how sick the person is. Isolation might take place at home, but if the illness is more serious or if the patient is already hospitalized, isolation might take place in the hospital
Level of prevention[Q]	▪ Primary (specific protection)	▪ Secondary (treatment)
Duration	▪ The individual and often the entire family will stay at home until the risk of developing the disease or its symptoms is over and health officials determine it is safe to end the quarantine. The length of time varies, depending on the disease and its incubation period ▪ Quarantine period = maximum incubation period of disease[Q]	▪ The duration of isolation will depend on the severity of the illness and how quickly the individual recovers (till recovery)
Public awareness	▪ If widespread quarantine is needed, people will be informed through public health news announcements made on TV, on radio, in newspapers or using other media	▪ A physician or public health official will write orders for an individual to be isolated, either at home or in a hospital, once he or she is diagnosed with or suspected to have the disease
Enforcement	▪ States generally have authority to declare and enforce quarantine within their borders	▪ In most cases, isolation is voluntary; however, federal, state and local governments have the authority to require isolation of sick people to protect the public
Examples	▪ Plague (quarantine was first applied for plague[Q]) in Europe where ships, crew and travelers where detained for 40 days	▪ Plague[Q], cholera[Q], chickenpox[Q], salmonellosis[Q] (in salmonellosis isolation is done till 3 stool cultures are negative[Q])

Ref:

1. http://www.marc.org/emergency/pdfs/IandQ-physicians.pdf
2. http://www.cdc.gov/ncidod/SARS/pdf/isolationquarantine.pdf

21. What is secondary attack rate?

- Secondary attack rate[Q] is the number of exposed persons developing the disease within the range of the maximum incubation period following exposure to a primary case[Q].

Calculation[Q]

$$\text{Secondary attack rate} = \frac{\text{Number of exposed persons developing the disease within the range of the incubation period}}{\text{Total number of exposed/susceptible contacts}} \times 100$$

- The primary case is excluded from both the numerator and denominator
- Denominator includes only those susceptible in close contact[Q].

Advantage	*Disadvantage*	*Application*
▪ Vaccinees and non-vaccinees from several families can be added to determine the overall attack rates in vaccinated and unvaccinated populations	▪ It is not useful in infectious diseases in which the primary case is infective for only a short period of time measured in days ▪ Identification of susceptible for denominator is difficult	▪ To measure the spread of an infection within a family, household or any closed aggregate of person having contact with case of disease ▪ To determine whether a disease unknown etiology s communicable or not (communicability of disease[Q]) ▪ In evaluating effectiveness of control measures such as isolation and immunization

Secondary Attack Rate of Few Diseases

Disease	*Secondary attack rate*
▪ Smallpox	30–45%
▪ Measles[Q]	>80%
▪ Chickenpox[Q]	~90%
▪ Mumps[Q]	~86%
▪ Pertussis	~90%

22. Integrated vector control measures.

Refer Question No. 11 June 2010 (RS2) Paper I.

MBBS PHASE III EXAMINATION

JUNE 2015

(Revised Scheme 2 & 3)

PAPER II

LONG ESSAYS

1. Write in detail about the epidemiology, clinical features and complications of measles. Add a note on measles vaccination.

Refer Question No. 1 December 2010 (RS2) Paper II.

2. National AIDS Control Program—explain in detail.

- Government of India launched National AIDS Control Program during 1987[Q] on recommendation of task force constituted to study problem of HIV in India
- Subsequently National AIDS Control Organization (NACO) was setup 1992 by Ministry of Health and Family Welfare to implement and monitor NACP activities
- In 2001, Government of India formulated National AIDS Prevention and Control Policy to further strengthen effort to control AIDS in India.

Objectives	*Targets*
▪ To reduce spread of HIV infection in India and to reduce morbidity and mortality associated with AIDS ▪ To strengthen India's capacity to responds to HIV/AIDS on long term basis	▪ 80% coverage of high-risk groups ▪ 90% coverage of schools and collages by education ▪ 80% awareness among rural population ▪ Reduction of transmission through blood to less than 1% ▪ Establishment of at least 1 voluntary testing counseling centre for every district ▪ Reduction of mother to child transmission ▪ Achieving zero level increase of HIV/AIDS new infection by year 2007

Phases

	Phase I (from 1987 to 1999)	*Phase II (from 1999 to 2006)*	*Phase II (from 2007 to 2012)*
	▪ Under NACO, surveillance activities were launched in 55 cities in 3 states	▪ Under Phase II, NACP became a 100% centrally sponsored scheme	▪ Started with primary goal of halting and reversing epidemic of AIDS in India over next 5 years by integrating programs for prevention, care, support and treatment
Salient features	▪ This phase created awareness, established state level structures for program implantation and blood safety	▪ Focus was shifted from raising awareness to changing behavior among high-risk groups ▪ There was decentralization of service delivery to states ▪ Voluntary counseling was encouraged, discouraging mandatory testing to protect human rights ▪ Operational research was supported ▪ Management research were encouraged	▪ Prevention of new infection in high-risk groups and general populations through ▪ Saturation of coverage of high-risk group with targeted interventions ▪ Scaled up interventions in general population ▪ Providing greater care, support and treatment to a large number of people living with AIDS ▪ Strengthening infrastructure, system and human resources in prevention, care, support and treatment programs at district, state and national level ▪ Strengthening a nationwide Strategic Information Management System

Strategies

- Strategies of National AIDS Control Program can be discussed as followed:

Prevention		*Care*	*Surveillance*
High-risk population	***Low-risk population***		
▪ Target intervention ▪ STI treatment ▪ Condom promotion ▪ Multisectoral collaboration ▪ Public private partnership	▪ Holistic IEC and social mobilization ▪ Safe blood ▪ Voluntary counseling and HIV testing ▪ AIDS vaccine initiative ▪ Sensitizing youth and adolescents ▪ Workplace interventions	▪ Low cost care and support ▪ Prevention of parent to child transmission ▪ Management of HIV-TB co-infection ▪ Treatment of opportunistic infections ▪ Piloting ART ▪ Postexposure prophylaxis	▪ Evidence-based planning ▪ Annual sentinel surveillance ▪ AIDS case detection ▪ Mapping of high-risk behavioral science

a. Target intervention
   - This consists of identifying high-risk groups and providing peer counseling, condom promotion, treatment of STIs and enabling environment
   - These measures are delivered through NGOs, community-based organizations and public sector.

Objectives	*Strategy*	*Components*	*Population covered*
▪ To reduce transmission of HIV amongst most vulnerable population	▪ Combine a comprehensive and integrated approach to vulnerable segment of population	▪ Behavior change ▪ Communication ▪ Treatment of STDs ▪ Create enabling environment to facilitate behavior change	▪ Sex worker ▪ Injecting drug users ▪ Truckers ▪ Homosexuals ▪ Migrant labourers ▪ Street children

b. STI treatment
   - STI treatment is one of major strategies to control HIV as STIs act as co-factor for HIV transmission and HIV is easily transmitted in presence of another STI
   - Objective is to reduce STIs and thereby control HIV transmission and to prevent morbidity and mortality due to STIs.

   Components
   - Development of adequate and effective program management
   - Promoting health education for control of STIs
   - Making arrangement for comprehensive care management through syndromic approach
   - Increasing access to healthcare by creating new structures.

c. Condom promotion
   - Condom promotion is very important in prevention of HIV as nearly 85% of HIV infection occur due to unprotected and multi partner sexual contacts
   - Correct and consistent use of condoms is most cost effective means of controlling STIs including AIDS
   - Besides protecting one from infection, it also prevents unwanted pregnancy and enhances pleasure associated with sex.

   Components
   - Sensitizing clients and commercial sex workers to use condoms
   - Making available low cost and good quality condoms to people at time and place, when they need it
   - Quality control of condoms (unlubricated condoms are phased out)
   - Social marketing of condoms (increasing acceptability and availability of condoms)
   - Involvement of NGOs in program.

d. Multisectoral collaboration
   - National AIDS Control Program is being funded by World Bank since several years
   - Bilateral cooperation has been extended by UK and USA
   - Other departments of India collaborating with NACP are
     - Department of youth and sports (under Ministry of Human Resource Development)
     - National Council of Education Research and Training (NCERT)
     - Nehru Yuvak Kendra
     - Directorate of audiovisual publicity, All India Radio and Doordarshan (under Ministry of Information and Broadcasting).

e. Public private partnership
   - NGOs are roped into program for providing care and support to people living with AIDS and their families.
f. Holistic IEC and social mobilization
   - Intensive health communication through IEC activities is imperative considering fact that health education is only time tested measure of prevention of HIV
   - It raises awareness about maintaining healthy practices and adoption of safe sex practices
   - Health education activities at national level are taken up by National AIDS Central Organization (NACO) but at state level, they have been decentralized.

   Components
   - Raising knowledge level of rural population regarding its transmission during pregnancy, delivery and breastfeeding, etc. through Family Health Awareness Campaign
   - Create awareness about services about availability for treatment of STIs, AIDS, etc.
   - Facilitate early diagnosis and prompt treatment.
g. Safe blood
   - Since 1st January 1998, professional blood donation has been prohibited and only voluntary blood donation is encouraged
   - Only licensed blood banks are permitted to operate in country
   - It has been made mandatory for detecting infection like HIV, hepatitis B and C, syphilis and malaria before blood donation.

   Components
   - Organising blood banking services
   - Education and motivation of population to donate blood voluntary
   - Enforcing quality control of blood before infusion.
h. Voluntary counseling and testing
   - Most important and innovative component of NACP
   - Voluntary counseling and testing center (VCTC) is a place where counseling and testing is done for HIV/AIDS.
   - It is an integral component of AIDS control program under NACO.

Objectives	*Location*	*Infrastructure*	*Staff pattern*
▪ To provide testing services to those who wish to know their HIV sero-status because of their exposure to risk or risk behavior ▪ To provide social and psychological support to those affected by HIV/AIDS ▪ To prevent HIV transmission to those at risk ▪ To establish linkage for care and treatment	▪ Blood banks, medical colleges, district hospitals, civil hospitals, CHC, PHC and village hospitals	▪ A well functioning laboratory ▪ Separate rooms for counseling ▪ Waiting space	▪ A microbiologist/ pathologist/ dermatologist as the officer in charge of VCTC ▪ One trained laboratory technician ▪ Two trained counselors (one male and one female)

Activities

i. Pretest counseling	▪ Pretest counseling prepares the clients for undergoing test and changing their behavior
ii. HIV testing	▪ A person tested for 3 different antigens before being declared positive ▪ The blood sample is tested with at least two ELISA and one rapid/simple test[Q] with different antigens ▪ A nominal fee of ₹ 10/- collected for testing
iii. Post-test counseling	▪ Post-test counseling prepares the client to understand the client to understand the meaning of positive and negative test and benefits of changing the risk behavior **Contents** *Negative result*: ▪ Providing information on staying negative ▪ Explaining the importance of undergoing test again after window period if there is history of recent exposure *Positive result*: ▪ Breaking the news gently to the patient ▪ Allowing the patient to react ▪ Discussing the treatment aspect and methods to reduce the risk of further transmission ▪ Encouraging the patient to tell spouse and getting them tested
iv. Follow-up counseling	▪ This is required for care and support of sero-positive cases ▪ Such people living with HIV/AIDS are referred to the physician for anti retroviral therapy and other supportive services
v. Postexposure prophylaxis	▪ Antiretroviral drugs are made available through voluntary counseling and testing center (VCTC) for postexposure prophylaxis

Significance
- HIV positive test has tremendous physical, psychological and social implications therefore HIV testing should be carried out on voluntary basis and with informed consent
- VCTC is a non-coercive, confidential and cost-effective approach that provides information, education and communication to motivate behavior change in HIV positive individuals.

i. AIDS vaccine initiative
- Vaccines against HIV are under various phases of clinical trial but none have proved effective
- More than 30 candidate vaccines have been tried since 1987.

Components
- Phase I and II provide date on safety of vaccine
- Phase III provides data on efficiency of vaccine.

j. Sensitizing youths and adolescents
- School AIDS education program is an important activity undertaken in NACP
- Training module called learning for life has been prepared and distributed in all states among higher secondary school children.

k. Low-cost care and support
- Home-based and community-based care programs are funded by central governments.

Components
- Protection of rights of people living with AIDS
- Proper care and support in hospitals and community
- Keeping confidentially of HIV status so as not to effect education and employment
- Encouragement and support for formation of self-help groups
- Encouragement for participation of NGOs
- Sensitization of medical and paramedical people not discriminate, stigmatize or deny of services
- Strict enforcement of biosafety and infection control measures in hospitals as per universal safety precautions guidelines

l. Prevention of parent to child transmission
- HIV positive pregnant women should be counseled properly enabling her to take an appropriate decision regarding continuation of pregnancy and childbirth
- There should be no forcible termination of pregnancy on grounds of HIV status

m. Piloting ART
- Antiretroviral treatment is a new initiative of program
- Under it, Government of India has decided to provide antiretorviral treatment at government hospitals, free of cost, for HIV cases in 6 high prevalence states[Q], i.e. Tamil Nadu, Maharashtra, Andhra Pradesh, Karnataka, Manipur, Nagaland and Delhi[Q]
- Cases have been prioritized according need of drug
- Pregnant women with HIV, children up to 15 years with HIV and full blown AIDS case are amongst high priority cases
- Under 3 by 5 target approach, it is devised to provide ART drugs to 3 million patients by 2005[Q].

n. 3 by 5 initiative[Q]
- Launched by WHO and UNAIDS on 1st December 2003.

Interim target	*Ultimate goal*	*Focus areas (5 pillars)*
▪ To provide ART to 3 million people living with HIV/AIDS in developing countries by end of 2005[Q]	▪ To provide universal access to treatment for HIV/AIDS to all those who need it	▪ Simplified, standardized tool to deliver ART ▪ New service to ensure an effective/reliable supply to medications and diagnostics ▪ Rapid identification, dissemination and application of new knowledge and successful strategy ▪ Urgent sustained support to countries ▪ Global leadership backed by strong partnership

o. Postexposure prophylaxis
- Postexposure prophylaxis is provided to people exposed to HIV as follows:
  - High-risk group—3 drugs (ZDV, lamivudine and saquinavir) for 4 weeks
  - Low-risk group—2 drugs (ZDV and lamivudine) for 4 weeks

p. HIV sentinel surveillance
   - Sentinel centers are identified and located at areas with high-risk population
   - Blood is collected from these sites at regular intervals through an unlinked anonymous procedure
   - Vulnerable groups are mapped out and taken care of.

q. Monitoring and evaluation
   - Activities conducted under NACP should be monitored regularly at centre level
   - NACO has been established for very same purpose but besides that there is need for performance and expenditure annual review to conducted.

Achievements

a. Prevention

– Targeted interventions	2100
– High-risk group reach	2.34 millions
– Adolescent education program	144,409 schools
– Condom promotion (sold)	3.5 billion/year
– Outlets selling condoms	3 million
– Safe blood units for transfusion	10 million/year

b. Care, support and treatment

– ICTCs setup	4995
– HIV tests	22 million/year (government) 12 million/year (private)
– Free ART supply to	300,000 (adults) 40,000 (children)

Recent Updates

National Strategic Plan for HIV/AIDS and STI, 2017–2024

Vision of the NACO

- Paving the way for an AIDS free India.

Goals—Three 'Zeros'

- Zero new infections
- Zero AIDS related deaths
- Zero discrimination

Targets by 2020

- 75% reduction in new HIV infections
- 90-90-90
  - 90% of those who are HIV positive in the country know their status
  - 90% of those who know their status are on treatment
  - 90% of those who are on treatment experience effective viral load suppression
- Elimination of mother-to-child transmission of HIV and syphilis
- Elimination of stigma and discrimination.

Targets by 2024

- 80% reduction in new HIV infections
- 95-95-95
  - Ensuring that 95% of those who are HIV positive in the country know their status
  - 95% of those who know their status are on treatment
  - 95% of those who are on treatment experience effective viral load suppression.

Expected Outcome—Ending of AIDS by 2030

- Enactment of the 'HIV/AIDS bill' as a law
- Implementation of the 'Test and Treat' policy.

Significance

- AIDS has become a pandemic and measures have been initiated by global health agencies like WHO, United Nations Program on HIV/AIDS (UNAIDS) and The Global Fund to Fight AIDS, Tuberculosis and Malaria (GFATM) which announced "3 by 5" initiative on 1st December 2003[Q], which plans to provide antiretroviral therapy to 3 millions in developing countries by end of year 2005[Q]
- Such massive global exercise requires grass root level support by countries which would benefit from it
- National AIDS Control Program is one step by Government of India towards this.

SHORT ESSAYS

3. Screening and diagnostic test.

- Screening test differ from diagnostic test in many ways.

Difference between Screening and Diagnostic Test

Point of comparison	*Screening test*	*Diagnostic test*
▪ Done on	Apparently healthy people[Q]	Sick people
▪ Number of people	Groups	Single individual
▪ Performed by	Epidemiologist	Physician
▪ Results	Arbitrary and final[Q]	Modifiable based on clinical correlation with history and examination
▪ Interpretation	Indicates possibility of disease or defect	Confirms presence of disease
▪ Based on	One criterion or cut off point	Evaluation of number of clinical features and laboratory findings
▪ Objective	To do community diagnosis, to launch a control program	To diagnose, to provide treatment
▪ Application in treatment	Not a basis of treatment[Q]	Used as basis of treatment
▪ Cost	Less expensive	More expensive
▪ Time consumed	Less	More
▪ Accuracy	Less accurate[Q]	More accurate
▪ Initiative	By epidemiologist or healthcare providing agency	By patient with complaints

Significance

- Screening tests and diagnostic tests are different but certain tests like blood picture for anemia, glucose tolerance (GTT) are certain tests which are common for both screening and diagnosis.

4. Primary immunization.

- Immunization is a mass means of protecting the greatest number of people through augmentation of the herd immunity by reducing the number of susceptible in the community making the infection more difficult to spread
- It also reduces the risk for those individuals who have escaped vaccination or those who have not developed satisfactory protection
- Immunization is achieved through 2 stages

Primary immunization	*Booster immunization*
▪ Eliciting primary immune response by exposing the body to live attenuated or killed pathogen or any immunogenic component of it ▪ May requires single dose or multiple doses to achieve seroconversion (production of antibodies)	▪ Done subsequently in high-risk age groups to maintain the protection by inducing antibody production

Primary Immunization

- Consists of injecting the vaccine to induce primary immune response.

Response

- After exposure to antigen, there is latent period of induction of 3–10 days before appearance of antibody

IgM type of response	*IgG type of response*
First antibody to appear is IgM which rises steadily during next 2–3 days or more and reaches peak level to decline almost as fast as it developed	If antigen stimulation is strong, then IgM type of response is followed by appearance of IgG in few days which reaches peak in 7–10 days and then gradually falls over a period of weeks or months

Outcome

- Education of reticuloendothelial cells
- Production of memory cells or primed cells by B and T lymphocytes which are responsible for immunological memory.

Factors Determining Primary Response

- Dose of antigen
  - Small dose of antigen only induces IgM type of response
  - Antigenic dose for production of IgG type of response is 50 times that of IgM type of response
- Route of administration
- Adjuvants
- Nutritional status.

Significance

- Primary immunization has to be planned according to the needs of the situation and local issues
- Ideal primary immunization schedule must be

Epidemiologically relevant	*Immunologically effective*	*Operationally feasible*	*Socially acceptable*
▪ Vaccinations should be included only against diseases which are public health problems and against which an effective vaccine exists	▪ Children must be vaccinated at an age when they can benefit from it, i.e. – When they are capable of forming defences – When they have lost the antibodies transmitted by the mother – Before they are exposed to possible infection	▪ Includes cost and ability to achieve a high percentage of coverage ▪ Schedule must minimize the number of visits, by simultaneous administration of vaccines	▪ Schedule must take into account the local customs, beliefs and practices, seasonal and climatic factors and daily work pattern of the community

5. Stop TB strategy.

- Stop TB strategy (2006–2015) is the global plan launched by WHO with objective of reducing incidence of tuberculosis
- It is to be implemented over the next 10 years as described in Global Plan to Stop TB 2006–2015
- It is adopted in India under Revised National Tuberculosis Control Program (RNTCP) since 2006.

Vision	Goal	Objectives	Targets
A TB free world	To dramatically reduce global burden of TB by 2015 in line with the Millennium Development Goals and the Stop TB Partnership targets	▪ Achieve universal access to high-quality care for all people with TB ▪ Reduce the human suffering and socioeconomic burden associated with TB ▪ Protect vulnerable populations from TB, TB/HIV and multidrug-resistant TB ▪ Support development of new tools and enable their timely and effective use ▪ Protect and promote human rights in TB prevention, care and control	▪ MDG 6, Target 8: Halt and begin to reverse incidence of TB by 2015 ▪ Targets linked to MDGs and endorsed by Stop TB Partnership ▪ By 2005: detect at least 70% of new sputum smear positive TB cases and cure at least 85% of these cases ▪ By 2015: reduce prevalence and deaths due to TB by 50% compared with a baseline of 1990 (Prevalence to <150 per million population and Deaths to <15 per million per year including TB-HIV cases) ▪ By 2050: eliminate TB as a public health problem (<1 case per million population)

Components

a. Pursue high-quality DOTS expansion and enhancement
   - Secure political commitment with adequate and sustained financing
   - Ensure early case detection and diagnosis through quality-assured bacteriology
   - Provide standardized treatment with supervision and patient support
   - Ensure effective drug supply and management
   - Monitor and evaluate performance and impact.

b. Addressing TB-HIV, MDR-TB, and needs of poor and vulnerable populations
   - Scale-up collaborative TB/HIV activities
   - Scale-up prevention and management of multidrug-resistant TB (MDR-TB)
   - Address needs of TB contacts and of poor and vulnerable populations

c. Contribute to health system strengthening based on primary healthcare.
   - Help improve health policies, human resource development, financing, supplies, service delivery and information
   - Strengthen infection control in health services, other congregate settings and households
   - Upgrade laboratory networks and implement the Practical Approach to Lung Health (PAL)
   - Adapt successful approaches from other fields and sectors and foster action on social determinants of health.

d. Engage all care providers
   - Involve all public, voluntary, corporate and private providers through Public-Private Mix (PPM) approaches
   - Promote use of International Standards for Tuberculosis Care (ISTC).

e. Empower patients and communities through partnership
   - Pursue advocacy, communication and social mobilization
   - Foster community participation in TB care, prevention and health promotion
   - Promote use of Patients' Charter for Tuberculosis Care.

f. Enable and promote research (diagnosis, treatment, vaccine)
   - Conduct program-based operational research
   - Advocate for and participate in research to develop new diagnostics, drugs and vaccines.

Significance

- Stop TB strategy focuses on 5 principal indicators used to measure the implementation and impact of TB control, i.e. case detection, treatment success, incidence, prevalence and deaths
- DOTS is the core element of Stop TB strategy
- It has created three specific research working groups devoted to new drugs, diagnosis and vaccine development respectively.

6. Modes of transmission of hepatitis B.

Refer Question No. 1 December 2014 (RS2) Paper II.

7. Prevention and control of food poisoning.

- Food poisoning is acute gastroenteritis caused by ingestion of food or drink contaminated with either living bacteria or their toxins or inorganic chemical substances and poisons derived from plants and animals.
- It is characterized by
  - History of ingestion of a common food
  - Affection of many people at the same time
  - Similarity in signs and symptoms of these people.

Prevention and Control

Food hygiene and handling	*Food handler*	*Environmental measures*
▪ Storing food in clean and dry place, free from rodents ▪ Leftover food should be immediately kept in cold storage, it should not be left in warm pantries ▪ Refrigeration of food below 4°C prevents bacterial multiplication and toxin production ▪ Protection of cooked food from rodents, insects and bare hands ▪ Avoiding handling of ready to eat foods with bare hands ▪ Reduction of time between preparation and consumption of food ▪ Stressing importance of rapid cooling and cold storage ▪ Pasteurization of milk and milk products and egg products ▪ Cooking food thoroughly ▪ Ensuring penetration of heat to center of food leaving no cool spots ▪ Examination of animal by veterinary staff before and after slaughter to ensure meat would be free from infection (meat inspection) ▪ Discouraging canned food consumption	▪ Maintaining high standards of personal hygiene among individuals engaged in handling, preparation and cooking of food ▪ Periodic medical inspection of food handlers to exclude workers suffering from infected wounds, boils, diarrhea, dysentery, throat infection, etc. ▪ Health educating food handlers in regards to importance of clean habits and personal hygiene such as frequent and thorough washing of hands, etc. ▪ Carriers should remain absent from duty till they are cured bacteriologically	▪ Maintaining clean and dry kitchen and dining hall ▪ Ensuring sanitization of all work surfaces, utensils and equipments ▪ Keeping food premises free from rats, mice, flies and dust

Significance

- With increasing rise in eateries, there is increasing trend of food poisoning and therefore proper health education of food handlers in regards to food handling is best way to prevent it
- However, golden rule to avoid food poisoning is still "Cook and eat same day".

8. Management of dengue hemorrhagic fever.

Refer Question No. 12 June 2012 (RS2) Paper II.

9. Multidrug therapy in leprosy.

Refer Question No. 5 December 2008 (RS2) Paper II.

10. Clinical manifestation of HIV infection.

- Acquired Immune Defeciency Syndrome (AIDS) is a fatal illness caused by a retrovirus known as the human immunodeficiency virus (HIV) which breaks down the body's immune system leaving the victim vulnerable to wide range of life-threatening opportunistic infections neurological disorders or unusual malignancies.
- Also called white disease[Q], slim disease.

Epidemiology	
A. Agent factors	
a. Agent	• Human immunodeficiency virus (HIV) is a lentivirus belonging to family retroviridae (as it contains an enzyme reverse transcriptase which synthesises DNA on an RNA template) • There are two types: HIV-1 and HIV-2, both of which are prevalent in India but HIV-1 is most common and most prevalent • It is easily killed by heat and chemicals like ether, ethanol • It is relatively resistant to ionising radiation and UV rays

Contd...

June 2015 (Paper-II)

Contd...

b. Reservoir of infection	• Cases and carriers are only reservoir of infection and once infected, person remains reservoir of infection throughout life • Carriers are highly infectious during "window period" i.e. period of 6–12 weeks between onset of infection and production of antibodies
c. Infective material	• Major infective materials are blood, semen, vaginal secretions and breast milk • However virus is also found in low concentration in CSF, saliva, tears, urine and joint fluids which may become infective if mixed with contaminated blood • Virus is also isolated from brain, bone marrow, lymph nodes and skin but they do not constitute infective materials
d. Period of infectivity	• Starts from 3rd month of infection and continues throughout life
e. Incubation period	• Varies from 5–10 years
B. Host factors	
a. Age	• Maximum incidence in sexually active and economically productive young age group of 15-40 years • Most common age group having AIDS cases is 30–44 years[Q]
b. Sex	• In India, male to female sex ratio is 3:1 with males accounting for 70% cases
c. Occupation	• Though HIV is not an occupational disease, but certain professions like healthcare workers, sex workers are at greater risk
d. Susceptibility	• Susceptibility to HIV is universal and nobody is immune
e. Presence of STDs	• Chances of HIV transmission in presence of STDs increase by 8–10 times[Q] • People suffering from genital ulcer, urethral discharge are at increased risk of acquiring and transmitting HIV
f. Frequency of exposure	• HIV to proportional to frequency of unprotected sex and number of sex partners
C. Environmental factors (social factors responsible for spread of HIV infection in India)	
a. Susceptible population	• Disease of sexuallyactive population which is in abundance in India
b. Presence of STDs	• Seen more commonly in presence of STDs which is quite prevalent practices
c. Sexual practices	• Visiting commercial sex worker is very common in India, evident from the fact that Sonagacchi, the sex district of Kolkatta is the largest in Asia
d. Urbanization	• Loss of income from agriculture and poor living standards are forcing people from rural India to migrate to cities in search of livelihood where they get entangled in high-risk behaviors like visiting commercial sex workers, drug abuse, etc.
e. Modernization	• Following the western culture indiscriminately without logic has seen rise in cases of homosexuality pre and extra marital relationships, drug abuse
f. High mobility	• Importance of India as a prime and cheap tourist destination for foreigners and for those seeking so called 'NIRVANA' has helped importing of more HIV cases thus widening its geographic span • Migration of the population by itself is not a risk factor, but their living conditions in urban slums predisposes to HIV infection. Longer working hours and relative isolation from the family may foster casual relationships making them vulnerable to STDs including HIV. The returning migrants do not their HIV status and thus may infect their sex partners in their community
g. Illiteracy	• Lack of knowledge in regards to modes of HIV transmission and above personal preventive measures has contributed extensively to spread of HIV.
h. Poverty	• Poverty can force women in prostitution making them susceptible to HIV infection. It can also force people to sell-infected blood for sake of money • It is also responsible for reuse of syringes poor people cannot afford disposable syringes
i. Addiction	• Alcohol increases they desire for sex but takes away the judgment capacity thus practice of safe sex is rare following alcohol consumption. • Addiction to other narcotics like heroin, etc. can lead to sharing of needles thus increasing the risk of transmission
j. Women's status in society	• Lower status of women in Indian society limits their ability to practice safer sex or ability to protect themselves • Increases number of HIV positivity among antenatal mothers is a worse indication • Poverty amongst women makes the situation worse • Further no women have the status to demand condom use from their husbands, even if she knows the HIV status of her husband
k. Separation from families	• Occupations like drivers, salesmen force people to remain away from the houses for long period making them prone for unsafe sexual practices
l. Cultural and ethnic practices	• Practices like circumcision or child delivery by unqualified persons increases the chances of infection
m. Social stigma	• The social stigma associated with AIDS forces people to conceal about their condition thus increasing the chances of spread
n. Lack of effective treatment	• The available drugs are costly and available at select centers • Moreover the treatment options are still in trial phase
o. Lack of vaccine	• Candidate vaccine is under trial but still no effective vaccine available
p. Quacks	• Quacks taking advantage of this situation and promising cure through so called herbal treatment providing false assurance • Quacks are unaware of safe injection practices thus aiding the transmission of HIV through parental route
q. Poor blood banks	• Unlicensed blood banks, trade in blood and blood products have compounded the problem
r. Lack of community involvement	• No health program is successful without involvement of the community • Poor management skills and poor involvement NGOs also add to the problem
s. Other risk practices	• Lack hygiene at hair cutting saloons, beauty parlours, tattoo shops, acupuncture clinics pose a problem
t. National health policies and expenditure	• There is a limited commitment on part of government to provide disposable syringes, free testing for HIV and free antiretroviral drugs to the needy

Contd...

Contd...

Modes of Transmission

- The HIV virus is transmitted from person to person through.

Route of transmission	*% of cases (in India)*	*Efficiency of route*
• By direct physical sexual contact (most common)	87[Q]	0.01-1%
• Blood contact (blood and blood products)	1Q	>90%
• Sharing needles/syringes	2	0.3%
• Mother to child transmission (Vertical transmission)	5	30%

a. Sexual transmission
   - It is one of the commonest and foremost modes of AIDS transmission
   - Any form of sex, i.e. vaginal, anal or oral can spread AIDS
   - Every single act of unprotected intercourse with an HIV infected person exposes the uninfected partner to the risk of infection

Factors determining risk

i. Type of sexual act	• The commonest mode of transmission is vaginal intercourse • Anal inter course carries higher risk of transmission as it is more likely to injure tissues of the uninfected partner • Even oral sex is a mode of transmission but less efficient • Risk of transmission increases by presence of abrasions on the skin and mucosa • Women are more vulnerable (twice) to risk of transmission because of a larger surface exposed and higher concentration of HIV in semen than in vaginal or cervical fluids[Q]
ii. Protection if any	• Use of condoms decreases the risk of transmission however, it is not full proof method
iii. Age and sex of the partner	• Exposed adolescent girls and women above 45 years of age are more prone to get HIV infection because in teenegers, the cervix is less efficient barrier to HIV than in mature genital tract of adult and after 45, this protective effect is lessened by thinning of mucosa postmenopause • Moreover, production of mucusin adolescent and post menopausal women is not as profilic as the women between this age group thus enhancing their susceptibility
iv. Presence of STDs	• Presence of a STD facilitates transmission of HIV in both HIV negative partners by easily passing into the ulceration due to STD of unifected partner. An STD also causes inflammation, T cells and monocytes/macrophages get concentrated in genital area • These are the cells which are carrier of the virus
v. Stage of illness of the infected partner	• An HIV infected person is more infections to others in early stage of disease before production of antibodiesm, i.e. in window period and when the infection is well advanced as these are two stages where level of virus in blood is higher than any other stages
vi. Virulence of the virus	• Higher the virulence of the virus, greater the chances of getting infected
vii. Period of menstruation	• For vaginal sex the risk is greater when woman is menstruating

b. Blood contact
   - HIV also transmitted by contaminated blood and blood products like whole blood cells, platelets and factor VII and IX
   - Contaminated blood is highly infections of introduced in large quantities directly into the circulation
   - Risk of contracting HIV is over 95% from transfusion of one unit of blood[Q]
   - Other modes of parentaral transmission are through contaminated needles, syringes or any other contaminated sharp instrument
   - However the risk is much lower compared to blood transfusion because likelihood of HIV transmission is dependent on the dose of virus injected
   - However repeated exposure to these modes like in IV drug abusers, the risk is significant
   - Any skin piercing instrument (needle, razor, etc.) if previously been used on an infected person and if not sterilized can transmit the virus
   - There is no evidence of transmission through other blood products like albumin, immunoglobulin or hepatitis vaccine

c. Maternal fetal transmission (Vertical transmission)
   - An infected mother may pass the virus to her child through placenta or during delivery or by breastfeeding
   - About 1/3rd of children of HIV positive mothers get infected through this route
   - Risk of transmission is higher if the mother is newly infected or has already developed AIDS
   - Once infected, children rapidly progress to AIDS.

Clinical Manifestations

A. Initial infection and antibodies production (Stage I : Acute retroviral syndrome—seroconversion)	▪ No clinical manifestations for first few years except a mild illness (fever, sore throat and rash) ▪ In this stage, patient appears healthy but is able to transmit the virus to others ▪ Once infected, patient remains infected for life ▪ After infection, between 2–12 weeks, anti-HIV antibodies appear in the blood-stream (up to 36 weeks) ▪ The period before production of antibodies is the "window period" during which, the patient tests negative with standard antibody blood tests although he infectious because of high viral load in blood

Contd...

Contd...

B. Asymptomatic carrier state (Stage II: CD4 count >500mm^3)	▪ Till development of full blown AIDS, patient shows no overt signs of disease, except persistent generalized lymphadenopathy ▪ Virus continues to replicate leading to progressive damage to the immune and nervous system ▪ Characterized by dermal manifestations (seborrheic dermatitis/pruritus/cellulitis/herpes zoster infection) and persistent generalized lymphadenopathy ▪ Blood shows leukopenia and thrombocytopenia ▪ Patient tests positive on standard antibody blood tests ▪ Asymptomatic carrier state lasts based on the immune status of the patient
C. AIDS-related complex (ARC) (Stage III: CD4 count 200–500 mm^3)	▪ Characterized presence of 2 or more of the following manifestations (including generalized lymphadenopathy) along with decreased T-helper lymphocyte count – Unexplained diarrhea lasting longer than a month – Fatigue and malaise – Loss of more than 10% body weight – Fever and night sweats – Milder opportunistic infections such as oral thrush, generalized lymphadenopathy or enlarged spleen
D. AIDS (End-stage of HIV infection) (Stage IV: CD4 count <200 mm^3)	▪ Characterized by number of opportunist infections and/or cancers due to unexplained defects in immunity ▪ Many people with AIDS have chronic diarrhea and severe weight loss along with a wasting syndrome, known as slim disease ▪ AIDS encephalopathy or AIDS dementia resembling senile dementia or Alzheimer's disease is seen in late stages when virus crosses the blood-brain barrier and directly acts on the brain ▪ Death is due to uncontrolled or untreatable infection
Opportunistic infections	
Early in the disease	
a. Persistent generalized lymphadenopathy	▪ Lymph nodes larger than 1 cm in diameter, in 2 or more sites other than the groin for a period of at least three months
b. Tuberculosis	▪ HIV positive individuals are more likely to develop active tuberculosis especially in endemic countries ▪ It is seen early in the disease where it the tuberculosis becomes active as the immune system breaks down ▪ Managed by individualized drug therapy following antibiotic sensitivity (because of multidrug resistance)
c. Kaposi sarcoma	▪ An opportunistic tumor appearing relatively early in the disease affecting both sexes across wide age range ▪ Characterized by generalized (in 2 or more places), invasive (rapidly progressive) reddish brown or purplish plaques or nodules on the skin and mucous membranes of mouth or gut
T helper cell count ≅ 100 (Late stage HIV disease)	
d. Oropharyngeal candidiasis (oral thrush)	▪ Caused by *Candida albicans*, a yeast fungus ▪ Presents with soreness and redness, with white plaques on the tongue and in the mouth and throat and sometimes a white fibrous layer covering the tonsils and back of the mouth
e. Pneumocystosis carinii pneumonia	▪ Symptoms include a dry, non-productive cough; inability to take a full breath and occasional pain on breathing; and weight loss and fever
f. Toxoplasma encephalitis	▪ Protozoal infection of CNS caused by *Toxoplasma gondii* ▪ Presents with focal neurological signs like mild hemiplegia or stroke, resulting from damage to part of the brain, seizures or altered mental status
g. Hairy leukoplakia	▪ White patches on the sides of the tongue, in vertical folds resembling corrugations
h. Cryptococcal meningitis	▪ A fungal infection of CNS presenting with fever, headache, vomiting and neck stiffness
i. Herpes-zoster (Shingles)	▪ Viral inflammation of CNS presenting with localized pain and burning sensations, followed by vesicle eruption and ulceration
j. Severe prurigo (Pruritic dermatitis)	▪ Chronic skin inflammation in form of a very itchy rash of small flat spots developing into blisters

Contd...

Contd...

k. Severe or recurrent skin infections	▪ Warts; dermatophytosis or ringworm and folliculitis
T helper cell count <50 (Advanced HIV disease)	
l. Cytomegalovirus retinitis	▪ Inflammation of the retina leading to blindness

Case Definition for AIDS Surveillance (WHO)

- An adult or adolescent (>12 years of age) is considered to have AIDS if at least 2 of the following major signs are present in combination with at least 1 of the minor sign listed below and if these signs are not known to due to a condition unrelated to HIV infection.

Major signs[Q]	*Minor signs*
i. Weight loss ≥10% of body weight[Q] ii. Chronic diarrhea for more than 1 month[Q] iii. Prolonged fever for more than 1 month[Q] (intermittent and constant)	i. Persistent cough for more than 1 month (major sign in tuberculosis patient) ii. Generalized pruritic dermatitis iii. History of herpes zoster iv. Oropharyngeal candidiasis v. Chronic progressive or disseminated herpes simplex infection vi. Generalized lymphadenopathy

- However, WHO expanded the definition to make it more simple and specific and also included a serological test.

Expanded WHO Case Definition for AIDS Surveillance

- An adult or adolescent aged above 12 years of age is considered to have AIDS if a test for HIV antibody gives a positive result and one or more of the following conditions are present.
  i. ≥10% body weight loss or cachexia with diarrhea or fever or both, intermittent for at least 1 month, not known to be due to a condition unrelated to HIV infection
  ii. Cryptococal meningitis
  iii. Pulmonary or extrapulmonary tuberculosis
  iv. Kaposi sarcoma
  v. Neurological impairment that is sufficient to present independent daily activities, not known to be due to a condition unrelated to HIV infection.
  vi. Candidiasis of the esophagus
  vii. Clinically diagnosed life threatening or recurrent episodes of pneumonia with or without etiological confirmation.
  viii. Invasive cervical cancer.

Epidemiological pattern of HIV epidemic in India (Type 4 pattern)

- Epidemic starts from highest risk group (commercial sex worker, homosexuals, drug users) to bridge population (clients of sex workers, STD patients, migrant population, partners of drug users) and then to general population

Prevention of HIV

- For prevention of AIDS, it is necessary to isolate the HIV not the person with HIV

A. Elimination of reservoir
   – Reservoir of infection in HIV infection are cases and carriers which can be treated but cannot be cured (eliminated)
   – These reservoir of infection are treated (controlled) by anti-retroviral therapy, personal measures and counseling
   a. Antiretroviral treatment
      - At present there is no vaccine to prevent and no drug to cure the HIV infection or AIDS
      - However there are antiviral drugs which are useful in prolonging the life of severely ill patients
      - They neither restore the immune system nor do they destroy the virus already installed in the cells

Commonly used drugs

Drugs	*Dosage*	*Indications*
Nucleoside reverse transcriptase inhibitors (NRTIs)		
Zidovudine (AZT)	500–600 mg orally daily in 2–3 divided doses	CD 4 £ 300 cells /mL or symptomatic disease or both
Didanosine (ddl)	125–300 mg orally BD	Intolerant to AZT or with progression of disease on AZT or combined with AZT

Contd...

Contd...

Drugs	***Dosage***	***Indications***
Zalcitabine	0.375–0.75 mg orally TID	Intolerant to AZT or with progression of disease on AZT or combined with AZT
Stavudine (d4T)	40–60 mg orally BD	CD 4 £ 300 cells /mL and intolerant to above drug
Lamivudine (3TC)	150 mg orally BD	
Abacavir (ABC)	300 mg orally BD or 600 mg orally OD	
Emtricitabine (FTC)	200 mg orally OD	
Non nucleoside reverse transcripatse inhibitors (NNRTIs)		
Nevirapine (NVP)	200 mg orally daily for 2 weeks followed by 200 mg BD	
Efavirenz (EFV)	600 mg orally OD	
Etravirine (ETV)	200 mg orally BD	
Delavirdine	400 mg orally TID	
Protease inhibitors (PIs)		
Saquinavir (SQV)	600 mg orally TID	
Ritonavir (/r)	400 mg orally BD	
Indinavir (IDV)	800 mg orally TID	
Atazanavir (ATV)	300 mg orally OD	
Darunavir (DRV)	600 mg orally BD	
Lopinavir (LPV)	400 mg orally BD	
Nelfinavir	750 mg orally TID	
Nucleotide reverse transcriptase inhibitors (NtRIs)		
Tenofovir	300 mg orally OD	
Integrase strand transfer inhibitors (INSTIs)		
Raltegravir (RAL)	400 mg orally BD	

- Nevirapine, zidovudine and lamivudine are supplied free through NACO to government hospitals[Q]

b. Personal measures
- Use of safe sexual practices like use of condom
- Refraining from multiple sexual partners
- Avoiding commercial sexual workers
- Avoiding blood donation, transfusion of safe blood or blood products
- Using disposable syringes and avoiding use of used syringes or sharing needles
- Avoiding breastfeeding if the mother has full blown AIDS
- Avoiding conception if the mother has AIDS
- Premarital AIDS testing of both the partners
- Use of gloves before handling any patient or biological material

c. Counseling
- Counseling is an integral part of management of HIV infection
- Counseling should be pre-test and post-test
- It includes information giving, assessing risk, providing psychological support and confidence building

B. Breaking chain of transmission
- Chain of HIV transmission is can be broken by any of the following:
  - By abstinence from sex
  - By having faithful and uninfected sexual partner
  - By adopting safe sexual practices like
    * Avoid sex with an unknown partner
    * Use condom while having sex with unknown partner
    * Use condom even with known partner if one of them has more than one sexual partner
    * Using condoms between HIV positive individuals (because each partner may be having different HIV and may retransmit HIV to each other which leads to rapid progression to AIDS)
  - By HIV screening for donors of blood, semen, organs and tissues
  - By adopting strict sterilization practices in all hospitals and clinics
  - By discouraging practice of tattooing
  - By prompt treatment of STDs
  - By giving heat treated coagulation factors VIII and IX for all hemophilics
  - By using presterilized, disposables syringes and needles for giving injections
  - By avoiding sharing of razors, tooth brushes, shaving brushes and bath brushes
  - By avoiding pregnancy among HIV positive woman

Contd...

Contd...

C. Protection of susceptible
   – Susceptibility is universal hence it should involve everyone with more emphasis on sexually active individuals and occupation with greater risk like healthcare workers, sex workers, etc.
   a. AIDS Vaccine
      - AIDS vaccine is still under development in clinical trials phase III
   b. Health education
      - Health education is one of the important strategies for prevention of HIV/AIDS[Q]
      - Health education is the only option till vaccine or cure for AIDS is discovered to enable people to make life saving choices such as:
         * Avoiding indiscriminate sex
         * Using condoms.
         * Avoiding use of shared razors or tooth brushes
         * Drug addicts should be informed that sharing of needles and syringes involve special risk
         * Women at risk of or suffering from AIDS should avoid pregnancy
      - Components
         * Modes of transmission of the virus
         * Risk behavior predisposing to HIV/AIDS
         * Social acceptance of the HIV/AIDS patients
         * About Parent to Child Transmission Program
         * Information regarding Voluntary Testing and Counseling Centers
      - It should cover following practices
         * By adopting safe sexual practices
         * By avoiding sharing of needles, syringes, razors, tooth brush, shaving brush, etc.
         * By avoiding direct contact with blood and body fluids of others
         * By adopting universal precautions and postexposure prophylaxis in high-risk groups
      - This can be done by
         * Making educational material guidelines for prevention widely available
         * Involving mass media like TV, radio, newspapers to educate people on nature, transmission and prevention of AIDS
   c. Universal precautions (standard precautions)
      - These are set of precautions designed to prevent transmission of blood borne infections
      - These are called universal because these should be employed, for every patient, every procedure considering as though he is HIV positive

Components

- Hand washing after any direct contact with patients
- Safe collection and disposal of needles (hypodermic and suture) and sharps (scalpel blades, lancets, razors, scissors), with required puncture- and liquid- proof safety boxes in each patient care area
- Wearing gloves for contact with body fluids, non-intact skin and mucous membranes
- Wearing a mask, eye protection and a gown (and sometimes a plastic apron) if blood or other body fluids might splash
- Covering all cuts and abrasions with a waterproof dressing
- Promptly and carefully cleaning up spills of blood and other body fluids
- Using a safe system for hospital waste management and disposal
- Do not recap the needle or recap with one hand only before disposal
- Resuscitator bags should be used preferably to mouth to mouth breathing
- Do not mouth-pipette; always use pipette with rubber bulb
- Process all laboratory specimens as potentially infectious

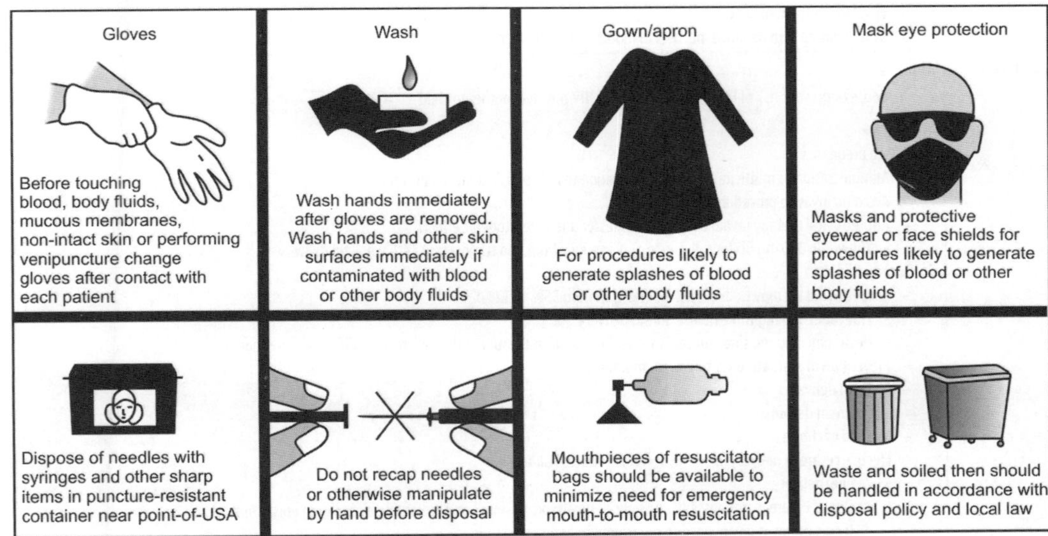

Fig. 1: Universal precautions

Contd...

Contd...

d. Postexposure prophylaxis
   - It refers to antiretroviral treatment started within hours following accidental exposure to the virus.
   - It aims at prevention of HIV infection of cells.

Recommended therapy
- AZT (200 mg 3 times daily) with Lamivudine (150 mg twice daily) for 4 weeks
- Indinavir (800 mg 3 times daily) OR Nelfinavir (750 mg 3 times daily) added if the contact has advanced AIDS

e. Prevention of mother to child transmission
   - Mothers with HIV can transmit HIV to their infants during pregnancy and childbirth (30–35% risk[Q]) or breastfeeding (10–15% risk)

Risk factors
- i. Maternal factors
  - Stage of maternal HIV disease
  - Maternal nutritional status
  - Disruption of placental barrier integrity
  - STDs during pregnancy
- ii. Obstetrical factors
  - Vaginal delivery has more risk than cesarean delivery
  - Preterm delivery
  - Breastfeeding
  - Early rupture of membranes
  - First born among twins has more risk
- iii. Child factors
  - Genetic factors of fetus increase the risk
- iv. Viral factors
  - HIV1 has more transmission rate

Prevention

Primary strategies	**Aim** • Preventing HIV infection among reproductive age group before they become pregnant Strategies i. Intensive health education to mothers about – Preventive measures for STDs – Informing about risk behaviors – Education to protect themselves from rape or sexual harassment – Education about reproductive health, safe sex and consequences of sexual behavior – Teacher training about teaching sex education at school ii. Increasing access to family planning method to avoid unwanted pregnancy – Extensive delivery of family planning services – Promotion of double contraceptive methods to prevent risk of pregnancy and protect from STDs iii. Expanding access to HIV conseling and testing – By identifying HIV infected mother in antenatal period – By referring them to VCTC – By motivating sero negative mothers to modify their behavior
Secondary strategies	**Aim** • To reduce or prevent risk of HIV transmission from HIV positive mother to child **Strategies** i. During pregnancy – Administration of multivitamin supplementation to reduce risk of low birth weight – Avoiding invasive procedures on uterus – Antiretroviral therapy (avoid during 1st trimester due to teratogenic effect) - Zidovudin 300 mg BD for full course of pregnancy from 2nd trimester or 34th week till delivery ii. During childbirth – Antiretroviral therapy (reduces risk of infection from 35% to 12%) - Zidovudin 300 mg three hourly during delivery - Nevirapine 200 mg single dose if mother brought during labor with no history of ART during pregnancy – Prevention of premature rupture of membranes – Mode of delivery - Cesarean delivery – Method of choice – Elective cesarean delivery in 36–38th week (reduces risk to 2%) - Vaginal delivery * Only if cesarean not possible and only by health professional and preferably by avoiding episiotomy * If episiotomy is given, need to be sutured as early as possible

Contd...

Contd...

	* Vaginal disinfection with 0.25% chlorhexidine * Do not milk umbilical cord – Care of newborn - Suction from throat first, followed by from nose to prevent swallowing of secretions - Wipe baby's body thoroughly with warm, clean towel to remove any blood stained secretions - Administer single dose nevirapine 2 mg/kg syrup orally to child within 72 hours[Q] after birth or zidovudine 4 mg/kg for 6 weeks - Follow-up baby to check for HIV infection after 18 months of age iii. During breastfeeding – Ensure adequate nutrition to mother during postnatal period – Advise mother on correct position and attachment to prevent sore nipple – Provide breast milk from uninfected lactating mother if possible – Practice exclusive breastfeeding only up to 3 months followed by animal milk or commercial infant formula – Inform mother to avoid breastfeeding if she has cracked nipples, mastitits or breast abscess

Control of HIV

- HIV cannot be cured but can be controlled by regular life long treatment with antiretroviral drugs and specific prophylaxis of secondary complication like opportunistic infections
- Control of HIV can only prolong life as long as CD4 count is maintained at desired level

a. Antiretroviral treatment (ART) for HIV positive individuals

WHO recommendations for ART

When to start	All adolescents and adults including pregnant women with HIV infection and CD4 counts of ≤350 cells/mm^{3}[Q], regardless of the presence or absence of clinical symptoms In presence of severe or advanced clinical disease (WHO clinical stage 3 or 4) irrespective of their CD4 cell count
Components	
First-line therapy	1 NNRTI + 2 NRTIs [one of which should be zidovudine (AZT) or tenofovir (TDF)]
Second-line therapy	1 ritonavir-boosted protease inhibitor (PI) + 2 NRTIs, [one of which should be AZT or TDF, based on what was used in first-line therapy]
Laboratory monitoring	Access to CD4 cell–count testing for all patients to optimize pre-ART care and ART management. HIVRNA (viral-load) testing is recommended to confirm suspected treatment failure Drug toxicity monitoring should be symptom-directed
HIV/TB coinfection	Started as soon as possible, irrespective of CD4 cell counts
HIV/HBV coinfection	Started irrespective of CD4 cell counts or WHO clinical stage First-line and second-line regimens for these individuals should contain TDF and either emtricitabine (FTC) or lamivudine (3TC)

Preferred First line ART

Target group	*Preferred option*	*Comments*
Adults and adolescents	AZT or TDF + 3 TC or FTC + EFV or NVP	Use fixed-dose combinations
Pregnant woman	AZT + 3 TC + EFV or NVP	Do not initiate EFV during first trimester TDF acceptable option
HIV/TB coinfection	AZT or TDF + 3 TC or FTC + EFV	Initiate ART as soon as possible
HIV/HBV coinfection	TDF + 3 TC or FTC + EFV or NVP	Consider HBsAg screening before starting ART Use of two ARVs with anti-HBV activity required
Children 3 years and over	NNRTI + 2 NRTI	
Infants not exposed to ARY	NVP + 2 NRTI	
Infants exposed to NVP	Boosted PI + 2 NRTI	
Infants with unknown ARV exposure	NVP + 2 NRTI	

Preferred Second line ART

Target Population	*Preferred option*	*Comments*
Adults and adolescents (including pregnant women)	TDF + 3 TC or FTC + ATV/r or LPVr	If d4T or AZT used in first-line therapy
	AZT + 3 TC + ATV/r or LPVr	If TDF used in first-line therapy
HIV/TB coinfection	Same as for adults and adolescents	If rifabutin available
	Same as for adults and adolescents plus LPVr or SQV/r with superboosted dosing of RTV	If rifabutin not available

Contd...

Contd...

Children 3 years and over	Boosted PI + 2 NRTI	
Infants not exposed to ARY	LPV/r + 2 NRTI	
Infants exposed to NVP	NNRTI + 2 NRTI	
Infants with unknown ARV exposure	LPV/r + 2 NRTI	

Caution
- Monotherapy or dual therapy should never be used (except for prevention of mother-to-child transmission and postexposure prophylaxis)
- Adhere to therapy for life
- Treat the side-effects promptly
- ART is costly and does not cure but only prolongs life

b. Specific prophylaxis
- The main aim of existing therapies of HIV infection is to treat or prevent secondary opportunistic infections

i. *P. carinii* pneumonia prophylaxis	Indicated in patients with CD4 count <200 cells/μL Trimethoprim—sulfamethoxazole/aerosolised pentamidine/dapsone Regimen can be changed or combined if the infection develops with one particular regime
ii. *M. avium* complex (1/3 of cases of AIDS)	Indicated in patients with <200 CD4 cells/μL Rifabutin decreases the incidence
iii. *M. tuberculosis* (most common opportunistic infection in India)	300 mg Isoniazid daily 9 months to one year Given to all HIV-infected patients with positive mantoux test
iv. Kaposi's Sarcoma	Interferon, chemotherapy or radiation
v. Cytomegalvirus retinitis	Ganciclovir
vi. Cryptococcal meningitis	Fluconazole
vii. Esophageal candidiasis or recurrent vaginal candidiasis	Fluconazole or ketoconazole
viii. Herpes simplex and herpes zoster	Acylovir or forcamet

c. Primary healthcare
- AIDS touches all aspects of primary healthcare including motor and child health, family planning and education
- Integration into countries primary healthcare system is essential

Significance

- AIDS has become a pandemic since its discovery in 1981 and has emerged as a global health problem of the 21st century and requires global effort to control it.

11. Risk factors of coronary heart disease.

- Coronary heart disease (CHD) is the impairment of heart function due to inadequate blood flow to the heart compared to its need, caused by obstructive changes in the coronary circulation to the heart.

Risk Factors

- Etiology of coronary heart disease is multifactorial
- There are numerous risk factors for development of coronary heart disease and the chances for development of coronary heart disease is proportional to the number of risk factors
- The important risk factors are:

Not modifiable[Q]	*Modifiable*[Q]
i. Age ii. Sex iii. Family history iv. Genetic factors v. Personality (Type A)	i. Cigarette smoking[Q] ii. High blood pressure[Q] iii. Elevated serum cholesterol[Q] iv. Diabetes mellitus[Q] v. Obesity vi. Sedentary habits vii. Stress and strains

Not modifiable[Q]	
a. Age	▪ Risk increases with age ▪ Peak incidence is seen in 51–60 years of age ▪ Occurs a decade earlier than with age incidence in developed nations
b. Sex	▪ Males are at more risk than females[Q]
c. Family history	▪ History of CHD in close family relatives increases the risk
d. Personality	▪ People with type A personality are more prone
Modifiable[Q]	
a. Cigarette smoking[Q]	▪ Cigarette smoking is a major modifiable coronary heart disease risk factor with several possible mechanisms – Carbon monoxide induced atherosclerogenesis – Nicotine stimulation of adrenergic drive raising both, blood pressure and myocardial oxygen demand. – Lipid metabolism with fall in protective high density lipoproteins, etc. ▪ Smoking is responsible for about 25% of CHD-related deaths in people under 65 years of age and particularly important in causing sudden death especially in men <50 years of age ▪ The degree of developing coronary heart disease is directly proportional to the number of cigarettes smoked per day[Q] ▪ Smoking exhibits synergistic effect when it combines with other risk factors like hypertension and hypercholesterolemia[Q] ▪ Risk of death from CHD decreases on cessation of smoking, so much so that after 10–20 years, it is the same as that of nonsmoker[Q]
b. Hypertension[Q]	▪ Hypertension is most commonly associated risk factor ▪ It accelerates atherosclerotic process, especially if hyperlipidemia is also present and contributes importantly to CHD ▪ Both diastolic and systolic blood pressure are predictor of coronary heart disease
c. Serum cholesterol[Q]	▪ There is a triangular relations between habitual diet, blood cholesterol and lipoprotein levels and CHD and these relationships causal ▪ Risk rises steadily with serum cholesterol concentration ▪ Of the various types of lipoproteins, levels of low density lipoprotein (LDL) cholesterol are most directly associated with CHD[Q]
	▪ Very low density lipoprotein (V and DL) is associated with premature atherosclerosis ▪ High density lipoprotein (HDL) cholesterol is protective against the development of CHD and therefore its level should be more than 30 mg/dL ▪ A total cholesterol/HDL ratio of less than 3.5 has been recommended as a clinical goal for coronary heart disease prevention[Q] ▪ Mean cholesterol level associated with high-risk of CHD is more than 200 mg/dL
Other risk factors	
a. Diabetes[Q]	▪ Risk is 2–3 times higher in diabetics than nondiabetics
b. Physical activity	▪ Sedentary lifestyle is associated with greater risk of development of premature CHD ▪ Regular physical exercise increases concentration of HDL cholesterol and are beneficial to cardiovascular health
c. Hormones	▪ Hyperestrogenemia is hypothesized as the common underlying factor that leads both to atherosclerosis and its complications such, CHD, stroke and peripheral vascular disease and may be the factor responsible for pronounced difference between male and female mortality from CHD
d. Alcohol	▪ Intake of alcohol more than 75 g/day is an independent risk factor for CHD, hypertension and all cardiovascular diseases
e. Oral contraceptives	▪ Oral contraceptive increases the systolic and diastolic blood pressure making women using them susceptible for development of CHD ▪ The risk is compounded by cigarette smoking
f. Miscellaneous	▪ Dyspnea on exertion of law vital capacity have been cited as possible risk factors

Prevention and Control (WHO Expert Committee)

a. Population strategy
   - Based on the principle that small changes in the risk factor levels in total population can achieve the biggest reduction in mortality and this strategy should be based on mass approach
   - Thus, the aim should be to shift the whole risk factor distribution on the direction of biological normality, which requires the mobilization and involvement of whole community to alter the life style practices that are associated with coronary heart disease in addition to medical means

   Specific Interventions

   i. Dietary changes (Prudent diet)
      - Reduction of fat intake to 20–30% of total energy intake[Q]
      - Reduction of saturated fat consumption to less than 10% of total energy intake[Q] (New guidelines <7%)
      - Reduction of cholesterol to below 100 mg/1000 Kcal/day
      - Increase in consumption of complex carbohydrates such as fruits, vegetables, whole grains and legumes
      - Avoidance of alcohol intake
      - Limiting salt intake to less than 5 g/day[Q]
      - Ultimate goal is to achieve cholesterol—HDL ratio <3.5

   ii. Smoking
      - A smoke free society should be achieved through following means
        * Effective information and education activity
        * Legislative restriction
        * Fiscal measures
        * Smoking cessation program

   iii. Blood pressure
      - Even a small reduction in the average blood pressure of whole community by a mere 2–3 mm Hg could produce large reduction in the incidence of cardiovascular complications
      - It can be achieved by multifactorial approach such as prudent diet, regular physical activity and weight control

   iv. Physical activity
      - Promotion of physical activity and making physical exercises as a part of normal daily life

   Primordial prevention
   - It involves prevention of emergence and spread of CHD risk factors and lifestyles that have not get appeared in the population
   - Thus the aim is to modify or control an many risk factors as possible

b. High-risk strategy
   i. Identifying the risk
      - Done by simple tests such as measurement of blood pressure, serum cholesterol blood sugar weight, etc.
   ii. Specific advice
      - Specific advice is given to bring the risk factors under preventive care and people are motivated to take positive action against all the identified risk factors

c. Secondary prevention
   - It aims at prevention of recurrence and progression of CHD
   - The principles governing secondary prevention are the same as that of primary, i.e. cessation of smoking, control of hypertension and diabetes, healthy nutrition, exercise promotion, etc.

Significance

- With improved living, the infectious diseases are on downside making way for the new lifestyle disease like CHD
- In prevention of such diseases, the population strategy has greatest potential.

12. Prevention of blindness.

Refer Question No. 12 December 2009 (RS2) Paper II.

SHORT ANSWERS

13. Salk polio vaccine.

- Salk polio vaccine is an inactivated polio vaccine developed by Dr Jonas Salk in 1955

a. Type	▪ Killed trivalent vaccine (inactivated by formaldehyde)
b. Formulation	▪ Liquid vaccine
c. Strains used	▪ WPV strains—Mahoney (Salk type-1), MEF-1 (Salk type-2) and Saukett (Salk type-3) grown in Vero cell culture or in human diploid cells
d. Composition (D-antigen, expressed only on intact poliovirus particles, is used to adjust concentration of individual viruses)	▪ 40 units of type-1 ▪ 8 units of type-2 ▪ 32 units of type-3
e. Seroconversion	▪ 90–95% after 2 doses and 99% after 3 doses

Contd...

Contd...

f. Immunity	▪ About 5 years (additional doses required at time of school entry and thereafter every 5 years till age of 18)
g. Efficacy	▪ About 50%
h. Route of administration	▪ Intramuscular (preferred) or subcutaneous
i. Dose	▪ 0.5 mL
j. Schedule	▪ First dose at 6 weeks followed by interval of 4–6 weeks ▪ Followed by 4th dose at 6–12 months after third dose
k. Reactions	▪ Local erythema, induration and tenderness
l. Advantages (in comparison to OPV)	▪ Stringent conditions are not required to maintain cold-chain (Thermostable) ▪ No risk of vaccine associated paralysis ▪ Safe to administer in – Immunodeficient patient – Corticosteroid and radiation therapy patient – Eldery (>50 years) receiving vaccine for first time – Pregnant women
m. Disadvantages (in comparison to OPV)	▪ Does not induce intestinal or local immunity (stimulates only humoral immunity) ▪ Do not prevent reinfection of the gut by wild viruses (protects only against the disease) ▪ Unsuitable in epidemics because ▪ Immunity is not rapidly achieved (more than one dose is required to induce immunity) ▪ Injections are to be avoided during epidemics (likely to precipitate paralysis) ▪ Does not help in the development of herd immunity ▪ Costly ▪ Requires the services of a trained person ▪ Short lasting immunity
n. Commercial preparations	▪ Stand alone vaccine ▪ Combination vaccine with diphtheria, tetanus, whole-cell or acellular pertussis, hepatitis B or HiB
o. Adulterants	▪ Formaldehyde, streptomycin, neomycin or polymyxin B ▪ Some versions contain phenoxy-ethanol (0.5%)—preservative

Significance

- With India achieving Polio Eliminated status, Government of India has introduced IPV in its National Immunization Program (Indradhanush) at 14 weeks along with the OPV.

14. Rotavirus.

- Rotavirus, a double stranded segmented RNA virus is the leading cause of severe, dehydrating diarrhea in under 5 children.

Epidemiology

a. Agent factors	
i. Agent (virus)	▪ Rotavirus is a double walled, Ds segmented RNA virus belonging to reoviridae family ▪ It has icosahedral capsid resembling little wheels with short spokes radiating from a wide hub to a clearly defined outer rim ▪ Group A virus incriminated in human diseases **Types** ▪ Complete or double shelled virus with smooth surface measuring 70 nm in diameter ▪ Incomplete or single shelled virus with rough surface measuring 60 nm in diameter
b. Host factors	
i. Age	▪ Children <5 years (largely limited to children aged 6–24 months) ▪ By the age 3 years almost all children suffer rotavirus infection at least once ▪ Median peak age is 6months to 1 year
ii. Socioeconomic status	▪ Low-income groups

Contd...

Contd...

iii. Immunity	▪ Neonates are immune due to transplacental transfer of maternal antibody and due to antibodies in the breast milk ▪ Most adults are immune though subclinical infection may occur
c. Environmental factors	
i. Seasons	▪ Peaks during winter (temperate climates)
d. Transmission	▪ Fecal-oral route, directly from person-to-person or indirectly via contaminated fomites
e. Incubation period	▪ 2–4 days

Clinical Features

- Vomiting is prominent early symptom followed by watery diarrhea (with flukes or mucus)
- Mild fever and respiratory symptoms in some cases
- Colicky abdominal pain, ill-defined tenderness and exaggerated bowel sounds are common
- Severe dehydration is not unusual
- Average duration of illness is 5–7 days.

Prevention

a. Health promotion
   i. Health education (about)
      - Improvement in the living condition
      - Sanitation in and around the house
      - To maintain personal hygiene
      - Correct weaning and feeding practices
      - To use protected water supply for drinking purposes
      - If not available, use boiled and cooled water for drinking
   ii. Sanitation measures to reduce transmission
      - Improved water supply
      - Improved excreta disposal
      - Improved domestic and food hygiene.

b. Specific protection
   i. Rotavirus vaccine

	Rotarix	*Rota Teq*
▪ Type	Live attenuated, lysophilized monovalent vaccine	Live attenuated pentavalent bovine-human reassortant vaccine
▪ Composition	Human rotavirus RIX 4414 strain, not less than 1060 CCID50	—
▪ Storage	2–8°C	—
▪ Protection	75–85% against rotavirus diarrhea 90–100% against rotavirus disease	75–85% against rotavirus diarrhea
▪ Indications	Infants of 2–4 months of age Not later than 24 weeks	Infants of 2–6 months of age Not later than 32 weeks
▪ Dose	2.0 mL	2.0ml
▪ Route of administration	Oral	Oral
▪ Schedule	3 doses at 6, 10 and 14 weeks	3 doses at 2, 4 and 6 months
▪ Usage	Reconstituted with liquid diluents and used within 24 hours	—
▪ Contraindications	Hypersensitivity to previous dose Congenital malformations like Meckel's diverticulum (predisposes to intussusceptions)	—

Significance

- Rotavirus is single most important cause of diarrhea in children and is associated with high fatality
- Thus as a measure to reduce IMR due to rota viral diarrhea, Government of India has introduced the rotavirus vaccine in National Immunization Program (Indradhanush).

15. Botulism.

- Botulism is a form of bacterial food poisoning.

Epidemiology

Agent	*Reservoir*	*Source*	*Incubation period*
Exotoxin of *Clostridium botulinum*, Type A, B or E	Dust and soil	Home preserved food such home-canned vegetables, smoked or pickled fish, homemade cheese and similar low acid foods containing spores of bacilli	18–36 hours

Clinical Features

- Under suitable anaerobic conditions, spores germinate into bacilli which preforms the toxin in food which acts on parasympathetic nervous system
- Prominent symptoms are dysphagia, diplopia, ptosis, dysarthria, blurring of vision, muscle weakness and quadriplegia
- Gastrointestinal symptoms are very slight
- Fever is generally absent and consciousness is retained
- Condition is fatal, death occurring 4–8 days later due to respiratory or cardiac failure
- Patients do not develop antitoxin in blood
- Infant botulism occurs in infants due to gut infection by *C. botulinum* with subsequent in vivo production of toxin.

Prevention and Control

Primary prevention	*Secondary prevention*
▪ Food sanitation—care of canned food, refrigeration ▪ Heating of food (100°C for a few minutes as toxin is thermolabile) before consumption ▪ Health education regarding proper cooking of canned food	▪ Polyvalent antitoxin ▪ 50,000–100,000 units IV to all individuals partaking suspected food ▪ Antitoxin is not useful if toxin is already fixed to nervous tissue ▪ Guanidine hydrochloride ▪ 15–40 mg/kg orally reverses neuromuscular block of botulism ▪ Active immunization with botulinum toxoid ▪ 3 doses of toxoid at 2 months interval

16. Hookworm—prevention.

Refer Question No. 9 Dec. 2017 (RS2) Paper I.

17. Malaria vaccine.

- An ideal malaria vaccine would be the one that prevents the infection at the first instance and if this is not possible, then should decrease the intensity of infection and should be successful in preventing malaria transmission
- Path of vaccine development has proved long and strewn with pitfalls, but there has been progress in forms of following vaccines.

Types

Type	*Features*	*Remarks*
a. Merozoite vaccine (Asexual blood stage vaccines)	Prepared from polypeptides of merozoites (blood stages) of *Pl. falciparum*	▪ Prevents infection of RBCs alone
b. Sporozoite vaccines	Prepared from antigens of sporozoites	▪ Prevents infection of both hepatocytes and RBCs
c. Gamete vaccines	Prepared from gametes	▪ Mosquito picks up antibodies produced in person, when it bites the vaccine which prevent fertilization of gametes inside the body of mosquito and thus arrests further development ▪ But the vaccinee is not prevented from getting infected
d. A synthetic cocktail vaccine (PfS 66)	Formulated as a peptide–alum combination	▪ Against *P. falciparum* (30% effective)
e. Transmission blocking vaccine (PfS 25)		▪ Under trial

Significance

- Despite considerable effort and expense, a generally available and highly effective malaria vaccine is not developed till date.

18. Prevention of neonatal tetanus.

Refer Question No. 12 June 2013 (RS2) Paper II.

19. Cancer registration.

Refer Question No. 16 June 2010 (RS2) Paper II.

20. Clinical classification of diabetes mellitus.

Refer Question No. 1 June 2010 (RS2) Paper II.

21. Accidentology.

- Accidentology is the research in accident prevention.

Components

- Gathering precise information about extent, type and other characteristics of accidents
- Correlating accident experience with personal attributes and environments in which accidents occur
- Investigating new and better methods of altering human behavior
- Seeking ways to make environments safer
- Precisely evaluating efficiency of control measures.

Significance

- Accidentology is future of accident prevention.

22. Reproductive and child health (RCH)—package.

Refer Question No. 1 December 2008 (RS2) Paper II.

MBBS PHASE III EXAMINATION

DECEMBER 2015

(Revised Scheme 2 & 3)

PAPER I

LONG ESSAYS

1. Write in detail about randomized controlled trials and add a note on "blinding".

Randomized Controlled Trial

- Randomized control trial is an assessment method which is really an epidemiological experiment
- It is so called because the patients who constitute the unit of the study are randomly allocated into study group[Q] or experimental group and control group depending upon whether they receive or do not receive the intervention[Q].

Objective

- To test the efficacy of a new drug or new drug regime or a new therapeutic or surgical procedure.

Basic Steps

a. Drawing up a protocol
   - This means specifying the following basic information before commencement of clinical trial like
     - Aims and objectives of study
     - Criteria for selection of study group and control group
     - Size of sample
     - Procedures for allocation into study group and control group
     - Intervention to be done or methodology of procedure
     - Cooperation of participants till end of study.

b. Selecting reference and experimental population
   - Reference population is target population to which results if found successful are expected to be applicable
   - Reference population, depending upon study could be all suffering from particular disease under experiment.

c. Randomization (selection of study and control group)
   - This is central component of randomized controlled trial and is known as Heart of a trial[Q]
   - It provides every individual from reference population, an equal opportunity to be selected into either study group or control group.

Selection of study group (experimental group)	*Selection of control group*
▪ It is actual population derived randomly from reference population, participating in experiment voluntarily, still retaining same characteristics as reference population ▪ Study group receives interventions or undergo experimental procedure ▪ Criteria for selection of study group ▪ It should be true representative of reference population ▪ They must give informed consent after being fully informed about procedure and possible dangers of trial ▪ They must be susceptible to disease under study	▪ Another group of individuals of same size as experimental group, selected randomly from reference population, maintaining similar characteristics as study group ▪ Control group does not receive intervention

Significance

- Randomization eliminates bias and allows comparability.

d. Manipulation or intervention
   - Study group is deliberately application or withdrawal or reduction of causal factor like new drug where as control group is put on inert (placebo) or old drug.

e. Follow-up
   - Follow-up is periodic and regular examination of both groups at define intervals of time framed
   - Results of this examination are submitted to statistician
   - Loss of follow-up due to death or migration of any individual is called attrition, which if substantial affects outcome of study.

f. Assessment of outcome
   - It is final step of clinical trial
   - It may be positive, i.e. new drug may be better and safe or may be negative, i.e. new drug is not effective or hazardous.

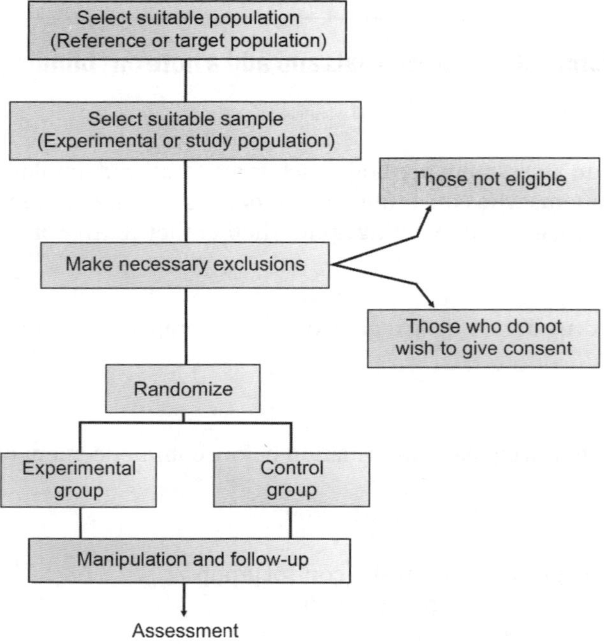

Fig. 1: Randomized trial—steps

Advantages

- Random allocation eliminates selection bias[Q]
- Double blinding eliminates investigator's bias[Q]
- Baseline characteristics of intervention and control group are similar[Q].

Application

- It is used to evaluate methods of treatment and prevention[Q].

Types of randomized controlled trials

Types	*Concerned with*
a. Clinical trials	▪ Evaluation of a therapeutic agent or procedure
b. Preventive trials	▪ Trials of primary preventive measures such as vaccines or chemoprophylactic drugs
c. Risk factor trials	▪ Trials of risk factors involving risk factor modification
d. Cessation experiments	▪ Termination (cessation) of a habit which is considered causally related to a disease
e. Trial of etiological agents	▪ Trials to confirm or refute etiological hypothesis
f. Evaluation of health services	▪ Assessment of effectiveness and efficiency of health services

Significance

- Randomized control trial is the most used method of evaluation of new programs and new therapies.

Blinding in Randomized Controlled Trials

- Randomized control trial is an assessment method which is really an epidemiological experiment
- Even in randomized controlled trials, bias can creep in, affecting final outcome of study, hence blinding technique is adopted.

Methods

Single blind trial	*Double blind trial*	*Triple blind trial*
▪ Participant is not aware whether he belongs to study group or control group but investigator knows who belongs to which group ▪ Helps overcome subject variation	▪ Neither investigator nor participant is aware about group allocation and treatment administered however statistician knows the group allocation ▪ Avoids both observer and subject bias[Q] ▪ Participants and drugs are coded ▪ Most commonly used method and is scientifically sound	▪ Participant, investigator and statistician are blind ▪ Most ideal method

Significance

- Application of blinding in randomized controlled trial ensures objective assessment of final outcome.

2. Explain the steps in "investigation of an epidemic" with suitable examples.

- Epidemic is defined as the occurrence in a community or region of cases of an illness or other health-related events clearly in excess of normal expectancy
- It is a short-term fluctuation of disease.

Investigation of an Epidemic

- Occurrence of an epidemic signals some significant shift in existing balance between the agent, host and environment and calls for prompt and thorough investigation to uncover the responsible factor and to guide in advocating control measures to prevent further spread.

Objectives

- To define magnitude of the epidemic outbreak or involvement in terms of time, place and person
- To determine the particular conditions and factors responsible for occurrence
- To identify the cases source of infection and modes of transmission to determine measure necessary to control the epidemic
- To make recommendations to prevent recurrences.

Steps or procedure of epidemic investigation

a. Verification of diagnosis[Q]	▪ It is the first step[Q] ▪ It is necessary to have the verification of diagnosis on spot as quickly as possible ▪ It is necessary to examine all cases but clinical examination of a sample of cases suffice ▪ Wherever applicable laboratory investigations are most useful to confirm the diagnosis
b. Confirmation of the existence of an epidemic	▪ An epidemic is confirmed by comparing the disease frequencies during the same period of previous year ▪ If the number of cases observed is in excess of the expected frequency for that population based on previous experiences, then it is labeled as epidemic ▪ An arbitrary limit of two standard errors from the endemic occurrence is used to define the epidemic threshold for common diseases ▪ Common source epidemics such as cholera need no comparison ▪ However modern epidemics such as cardiovascular diseases need comparison with previous experience

Contd...

Contd…

c. Defining the population of risk	
i. Obtaining a map of the area	▪ A current map of the area showing details such as natural landmarks, roads and location of all dwellings is necessary ▪ It the map is not available, it should be prepared ▪ The area should be divided into segments using natural landmark as boundaries and again subdivided into smaller sections ▪ In each section dwelling into smaller sections
ii. Counting the population	▪ Population helps in computing the attack rates in various groups and subgroups ▪ This entire population or subgroup forms the denominator ▪ The denominator can be related to total events ▪ Without an appropriated denominator of population at risk attack rates cannot be calculated
d. Rapid search for all cases and their characteristics	
i. Medical surveys	▪ A medical survey should be carried out in the defined area to identify all cases including those who have not sought medical help or those probably exposed to the risk ▪ The lay health worker can collect relevant data through "epidemiological case sheet or questionnaire ▪ A complete health survey will pick up all affected individuals with signs and symptoms of the disease
ii. Epidemiological case sheet	▪ It is a case sheet or interview form used for collection data from cases and from people apparently exposed but unaffected ▪ It should include following questions to collect relevant information: – Name, age, sex – Occupation – Social class – Travel – History of previous exposure – Onset of disease – Signs and symptoms – Personal contacts at home, work school – Social gatherings attended and food eaten – Exposure to common vehicle like water, milk, food – Visits out of community – History of receiving injections or blood products ▪ However, information collected should be relevant to the disease under question ▪ In cases of large outbreaks, random samples should be examined and data collected
iii. Searching for more cases	▪ More cases can be searched by asking the patient if he knew of other cases in home, family, neighborhood, school work place, etc. having an onset within the incubation of the index case ▪ Cases admitted in the local hospital should be considered which may reveal additional cases and also information about person-to-person spread ▪ This activity should be carried out everyday till the area is declared epidemic free, i.e. no new case should be detected in period twice the incubation period of disease since occurrence of last case
e. Evaluation of ecological factors	▪ To prevent further transmission of the disease an investigation into the circumstances involved is must ▪ They can be: – Sanitary status of eating establishments, milk and water supply – Breakdown in the water supply system – Movement of the human population – Atmospheric changes such as temperature humidity and air pollution – Population dynamics of insects and animal reservoirs ▪ This study helps to determine the source of infection, reservoirs and modes of transmission
f. Further investigations of population at risk	▪ Additional information can be obtained by study of population at risk by medical examination screening tests, examination of suspected food, feces or blood sample, biochemical studies assessment of immunity status, etc. ▪ The approach may be prospective or retrospective.
g. Data analysis	▪ Using the classical epidemiological parameters like time, place and person (Agent–Host–Environment if causative agent is known) the collected data is analyzed on ongoing basis ▪ It is done to identify common events or experience and to delineate the group involved in common experience.
i. Time	▪ An epidemic curve is constructed by plotting dates of onset in chronological order to suggest: – A time relationship with exposure to a suspected source – Whether it is a common source or propagated epidemic – Whether it is a seasonal or cyclic pattern suggestive of a particular infection

Contd…

Contd...

ii. Place	▪ A spot map of detected cases is prepared showing their relationship with possible source of infection if possible ▪ Clustering of cases, suggest common source epidemic
iii. Person	▪ Data collected is analyzed by age, sex, occupation and other risk factors ▪ Case fatality rate or attack rate is determined for those exposed and those not exposed and according to host factors
h. Formulation of hypotheses	▪ On basis of data collected a hypotheses are formulated in order of relative likelihood to explain the epidemic in terms of: – Possible source – Causative agent – Modes of spread – Environmental factors
i. Testing of hypotheses	▪ All reasonable hypotheses need to be considered and weighed by comparing the attack rate in various groups for those exposed and those not exposed to each suspected factor ▪ This helps to ascertain which hypothesis is consistent with all the known facts
j. Writing the report	▪ The report should be complete and convincing

Short Essays

3. Tools of measurement in epidemiology.

- Magnitude of a disease in a community is expressed in terms of rates, ratio and proportions which are called the Basic tools in epidemiology.

a. Rate
   - Measures occurrence of some particular event in a population during a given time period
   - Expressed per 1000 mid year population.

   Examples:
   - Death rate = No. of deaths in a given area in an year × 1,000/mid year population of the area

   Types

– Crude or unstandardized rate	Actual observed rates like birth rate, death rate, etc.
– Specific rate	Actual observed rates due to specific cause or occurring in specific groups or during specific time periods
– Standardized rate	Obtained by direct or indirect methods of standardization or adjustments

b. Ratio
   - An expression of a relation in size between two random quantities, i.e. numerator is not a component of denominator or simply it is a result of dividing one quantity by another
   - Numerator and denominator may involve a time interval or may be instantaneous in time
   - Expressed in form of X : Y or X/Y.

   Example:
   - Doctor patient ratio, sex ratio, etc.

c. Proportion
   - Ratio which indicates relation in magnitude of a part of whole, i.e. numerator is always included in denominator
   - Always expressed in percentage.

   Example
   - Proportions of juvenile delinquents = No. of delinquents × 100/total no. of juveniles.

4. Cold chain.

Refer Question No. 12 December 2007 (RS2) Paper I.

5. Dietary antioxidants.

- Antioxidants are substances which counter or negate the oxidative stress produced by free radicals or reactive oxygen species.

Dietary Antioxidants

- Vitamins E, C, β-carotene and minerals such as selenium, iron, copper and zinc.

Sources	*Daily requirement*	*Functions*
▪ Vegetables, fruits, legumes, spices, beverages (green tea and wine) and cereals	▪ Amount of antioxidants to be consumed daily to protect against risk factors cannot be quantitatively fixed at present ▪ However, in healthy subjects, dietary antioxidants from a balanced diet with adequate fruits and vegetables ranging from 500–600 g/d will probably be enough to take care of oxidant damage and repair cellular and tissue defects	▪ Antioxidants reduce oxidative adverse effects of reactive oxygen species (ROS) and nitrogen species generated during physiological or pathological conditions

Significance

- Antioxidants play an important preventive role in diseases such as cardiovascular, cancer, cataract, diabetes, neurodegenerative disorders and age-related masculopathy
- Though numerous food articles are rich in antioxidants, but scientific evidence of protective role of dietary antioxidants is available only for vegetables and fruits.

6. Egg—a reference protein.

- Egg contains all the nutrients except carbohydrate and vitamin C.

Nutritive Value

- A single egg of hen weighing 60 g contains 6 g of protein (ovalbumin)
- Egg protein is biologically a complete protein (it contains all the essential amino acids in right proportions) and net protein utilization (NPU) is 100 (i.e. high biological value and high digestibility coefficient)
- Therefore, egg-protein is called a 'reference protein.'

Application

Egg protein is used for assessment of protein quality as follows

a. Amino acid (chemical) score
   - Measure of concentration of each essential amino acid in test protein expressed as a percentage of that amino acid in the reference protein

$$\text{Amino acid score} = \frac{\text{mg of amino acid/g of test protein}}{\text{mg of same amino acid/g of reference protein}} \times 100$$

   - Amino acid score is somewhere between 50–60 for starches and 70–80 for animal foods

b. Net protein utilization (NPU)
   - Product of digestibility coefficient and biological value divided by 100
   - Gives a more complete expression of protein quality than the amino acid score
   - It is a biological method requiring special laboratory facilities

$$\text{Net protein utilisation (NPU)} = \frac{\text{Nitrogen retained by the body}}{\text{Nitrogen intake}} \times 100$$

   - 1 g of protein is assumed to be equivalent to 6.25 g of N
   - NPU of egg protein is 100
   - NPU of protein of Indian diets is about 50–80.

7. Balanced diet.

Refer Question No. 4 June 2013 (RS2) Paper I.

8. Iodine deficiency disorders and their prevention.

Refer Question No. 1 June 2013 (RS2) Paper I.

9. Comfort zones.

Refer Question No. 11 December 2011 (RS2) Paper I.

10. Effects of noise pollution.

refer Question No. 4 December 2008 (RS2) Paper I.

11. Adverse health effects of smoking.

- Smoking is a form of tobacco consumption in forms of inhaling the smoke of burning tobacco through cigarettes, beedis, cigars or hookah.

Adverse Health Effects of Smoking

Immediate effects		
▪ Feeling of relaxation, sharpness, calmness and alertness ▪ Unpleasant experience will be nausea, cough, dizziness, rapid heartbeat which vanish once dependency over nicotine develops		
Delayed effects		
Lungs ▪ Bronchogenic carcinoma ▪ Chronic obstructive pulmonary disease (COPD) ▪ Asthma exacerbation ▪ Predisposition to respiratory tract infection like tuberculosis **Heart** ▪ Coronary heart disease ▪ Ischemic heart disease ▪ Atherosclerosis ▪ Myocardial infarction ▪ Arrhythmias ▪ Cardiomyopathy **Carcinomas of** ▪ Respiratory—larynx, lungs ▪ GIT—oral cavity, esophagus, stomach, pancreas, colorectal ▪ Genitourinary—kidney, bladder ▪ Reproductive—vulva, cervical ▪ Blood—AML	**Reproduction** ▪ Infertility (azoospermia) ▪ Impotency (erectile dysfunction) ▪ Miscarriages ▪ Premature menopause **Foetus (maternal smoking)** ▪ Growth retardation ▪ Prematurity ▪ Still birth ▪ Birth defects ▪ Mental retardation ▪ Sudden infant death syndrome (SIDS) **Blood vessels** ▪ Arteriosclerosis ▪ Peripheral vascular disease ▪ Buerger's disease **Skin** ▪ Premature wrinkling ▪ Psoriasis	**Bones** ▪ Degeneration of disk ▪ Osteoarthritis ▪ Osteoporosis ▪ Delayed healing of fractures ▪ Musculoskeletal injury **Brain** ▪ Transient ischemic attack (TIA) ▪ Stroke ▪ Multiple sclerosis **Miscellaneous** ▪ Cataract ▪ Macular degeneration ▪ Snoring ▪ Peptic ulcers ▪ Crohn's disease ▪ Periodontal disease ▪ Leukoplakia ▪ Immunity impairment

Significance

- Smoking besides being a health problem, is also a social and economic problem
- Besides affecting the smoker, it also adversely affects the bystanders due to second hand smoke (passive smoking).

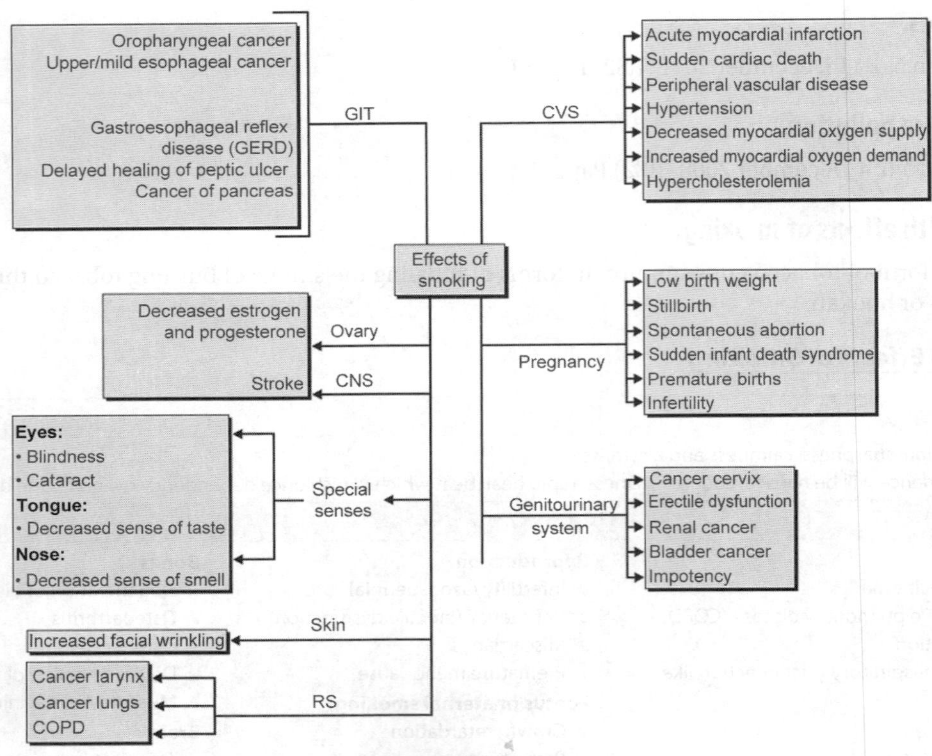

Fig. 2: Effects of smoking

Abbreviations: GIT, gastrointestinal tract; CVS, cardiovascular system; CNS, central nervous system; COPD, chronic obstructive pulmonary disease

12. Standard deviation.

Refer Question No. 9 June 2016 (RS2) Paper I.

SHORT ANSWERS

13. Relative risk.

Refer Question No. 1 December 2016 (RS2) Paper I.

14. Toxoids.

- Toxoid is a type of subunit vaccine produced by detoxification of the toxin produced by the pathogen
- Thus toxoid is a modified (detoxified) toxin which only posses only antigenicity but not the pathogenicity (toxicity).

Examples.

- Tetanus toxoid
- Diphtheria toxoid.

Mechanism

- On administration of toxoids, antibodies are produced against the toxin
- On subsequent infection, antibodies produced neutralize the toxic moiety produced during infection.

Advantages	*Disadvantages*
▪ Highly efficacious and safe	▪ Offers no protection from infection ▪ Acts only on toxin; not on pathogen ▪ Require multiple doses in primary course followed by booster doses

15. Nalgonda technique.

- Nalgonda technique[Q] is a method of chemical deflourination of the water at domestic level
- It is developed by National Environmental Engineering Research Institute, Nagpur, Maharashtra, India.

Procedure

- This is carried out in a bucket with a tap 3–5 cm above the bottom of the container
- 40 liters of raw water is taken the bucket, mixed slowly with alum[Q] (500 mg/L), followed by lime[Q] or sodium carbonate (30 mg/L) and bleaching powder[Q] (120 mg/40 L)
- Water is stirred slowly for 10–20 minutes and allowed to settle for nearly one hour (Flocculation)
- The settled sludge will be below the tap level and the supernatant water becomes less in fluorine content and is withdrawn through tap for consumption (Sedimentation)
- The settled sludge is discarded (Filtration).

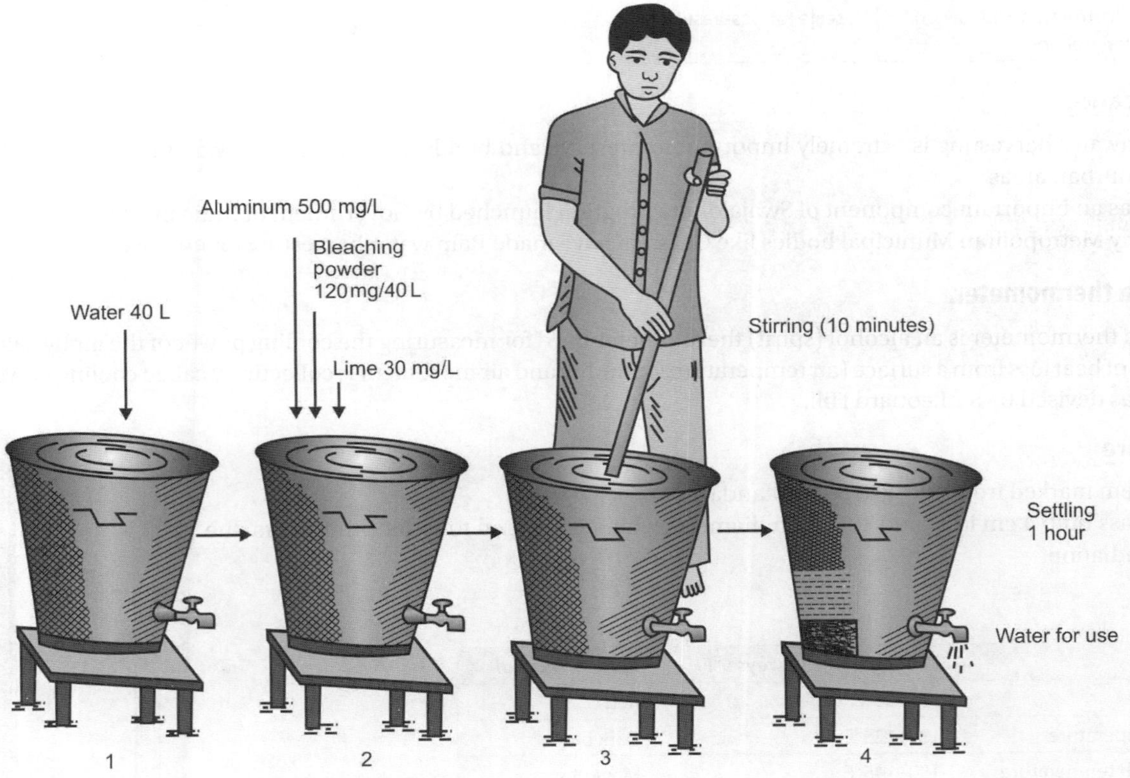

Fig. 3: Nalgonda technique of deflourination

Significance

- Nalgonda technique is a example of appropriate technology of primary health care.

16. Rain water harvesting.

- Rain water harvesting simply means catching and holding rain where it falls and using it
- It is a method of water conservation consisting of diverting rainwater from rooftops and courtyards into soaking pits or trenches, instead of drains
- Rainwater can also be cleaned and filtered before diverting it into existing tube wells or wells.

Design

- Open spaces, roof tops and ground are used as catchment areas
- Water collected from here is brought into large underground pits by PVC pies
- Underground pits are large pits or tanks filled in layers with big stones, followed by gravel and sand
- Rainwater is filtered through these layers and sent through PVC pipe connecting bottom of the pit into nearby well or tube well.

Advantages	*Disadvantages*
▪ Recharges ground water ▪ Economical (minimal construction and low on maintenance)	▪ Liable for contamination ▪ Needs to be done on large scale for best results

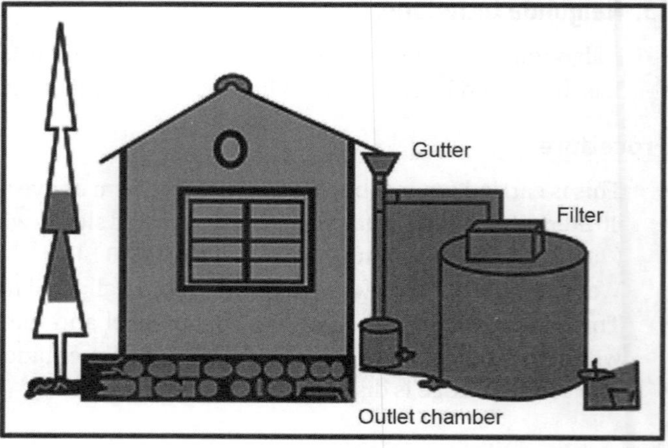

Fig. 4: Rain water harvesting

Significance

- Rainwater harvesting is extremely important to preserve and builds up underground water reserves in urban and semiurban areas
- It was an important component of Swajaldhara program launched by Government of India in 2002
- Many Metropolitan Municipal bodies like Chennai have made Rain water harvesting mandatory.

17. Kata thermometer.

- Kata thermometer is an alcohol (spirit) thermometer used for measuring the cooling power of the air by calculating rate of heat loss from a surface (air temperature, humidity and air movement is collectively called cooling power of air)
- It was devised by Sir Leonard Hill.

Structure

- A stem marked from 100°F to 95°F (Standard)
- A glass bulb 4 cm long and 1.8 cm in diameter which is silvered to reduce the errors due to radiation.

Types

	Cooling range (always 5°F)	*Color of alcohol*
Standard	100–90°F	Red
High temperature	130–125°F	Dark blue
Extra high temperature	150–145°F	Magenta

Method to Use

- 2 Kata thermometer are used—dry Kata and wet Kata (bulb covered with a wet muslin cloth)
- Before taking readings, bulbs are warmed slightly above 130°F by immersing them in hot water thus raising alcohol into a small reservoir at the top of the instrument
- Bulb of dry Kata is wiped dry and of wet Kata is covered with wet muslin cloth
- Both the instruments are suspended in air at point of observation and time (in sec) taken for level to fall from 100°F to 95°F is noted
- Repeat this at least 4 times and take average of last 3 readings
- Length of time depends upon cooling power of the air
- Each instrument has a Kata factor (predetermined by manufacturer) marked on their stem.

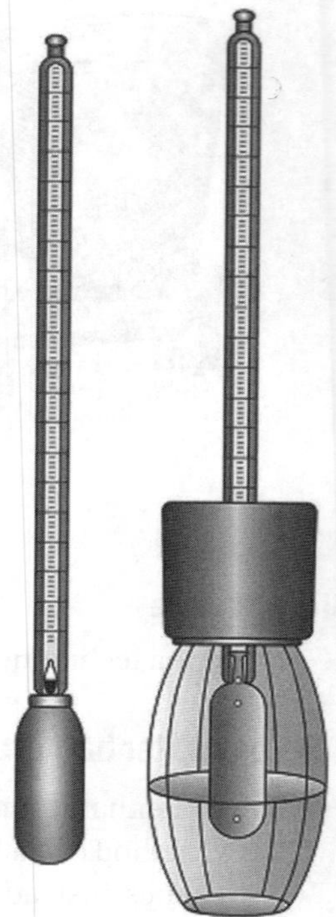

Fig. 5: Kata thermometer

Calculations

- Rate of cooling (millicalories/cm^2/sec) = Kata factor/Average cooling time.

Inference (indices of thermal comfort)

	Indices of thermal comfort	*Determines rate of cooling by*
▪ Dry kata	≥6	Radiation and convention
▪ Wet kata	≥20	Radiation, convention and evoparation

Significance

- Kata thermometer through originally devised for measuring cooling power of air, is now largely used for recording low air velocities (instead of an anemometer).

18. Disinfection of air.

- Disinfection of air is modality to reduce microbial air pollution.

Methods

Natural	
Mechanical ventilation	▪ This reduces vitiated air and bacterial density
Artificial	
Ultraviolet radiation	▪ Effective in special situations such as operation theaters and infectious disease wards ▪ Ultraviolet lamps are shaded and located in the upper portion of the rooms near the inlet of air (direct exposure to ultravoilet rays is dangerous to the eyes and skin) ▪ Ultraviolet rays have proved effective for general use in public assembly and school rooms
Aerosols (Chemical mists)	▪ They act by collision with and absorption by organisms or condensation of vapor on bacteria—carrying particles quickly destroying their bacterial content ▪ Ideal aerosol should be non-irritating to the mucosa, non-toxic even after prolonged exposure, invisible, inodorous, noncorrosive, noninflammable, highly bactericidal in low concentrations and capable of penetrating organisms in dried secretions such as saliva ▪ 3 groups viz. hypochlorites, resorcinols and glycols *Advantage* ▪ Disinfection of air in enclosed places due to their penetration to the remote corners of rooms
Dust control	▪ Application of oil to floors of hospital wards reduces the bacterial content of the air

Significance

- Air disinfection is still in the experimental stage.

19. Antimosquito measures.

Refer Question No. 11 June 2010 (RS2) Paper I.

20. Bar charts.

Refer Question No. 17 December 2008 (RS2) Paper I.

21. Chi-Square test.

Refer Question No. 4 June 2008 (RS2) Paper I.

22. Barriers of communication.

Refer Question No. 5 June 2010 (RS2) Paper I.

MBBS PHASE III EXAMINATION

DECEMBER 2015

(Revised Scheme 2 & 3)

PAPER II

LONG ESSAYS

1. Describe in detail about directly observed treatment short course (DOTS) chemotherapy in tuberculosis.

Refer Question No. 2 December 2012 (RS2) Paper II.

2. Explain in detail the National Program for Control of Blindness.

- National Program for Prevention (control) of Blindness was launched in the year 1976 as 100% centrally sponsored program and incorporates the earlier trachoma control program of 1968
- The ultimate goal of the program is to reduce prevalence of blindness from 1.4% to 0.3% by providing comprehensive eyecare through primary healthcare[Q]
- Current prevalence is 1.05% (2007)
- India was the first country in the world to launch a National Program for Control of Blindness[Q]
- India is the single largest contributor to global blind pool.

Objectives	*Targets (under 10th five-year plan)*
▪ To reduce backlog of blindness through identification of cases and their treatment ▪ To strengthen the quality of service delivery ▪ To develop human resource for providing eyecare facilities ▪ To promote out reach activities and public awareness ▪ To develop institutional capacity ▪ To establish eyecare facilities for every 5 lakhs persons ▪ To secure the participation of voluntary organization in the provision of eyecare services	▪ Reduce prevalence of blindness to 0.5% by 2010[Q] (National Health Policy) ▪ Increase the rate of cataract surgery rate to 450 operations per lakh population[Q] ▪ Increase the rate of IOL implantation to more than 80% among the cataract surgery by 2007[Q] ▪ Develop 50 pediatric ophthalmology units[Q] ▪ Improve facilities for early diagnosis and treatment of glaucoma and diabetic retinopathy ▪ Setting up 20,000 vision centers in rural areas ▪ Developing 25 fully operational eye bank network ▪ Develop human resources and institutional capacity for eyecare by providing training to eye surgeons and other personnel at various levels and supplying ophthalmic equipments and grants to NGOs

Administrative Setup

Level	*Members*	*Function*
Central	Ophthalmology section, Directorate General of Health Services, Ministry of Health and Family Welfare, New Delhi, India National institute of Ophthalmology, New Delhi, India	Formulation of policies and guidelines for all activities related to eyecare
Regional	Regional Institute of Ophthalmology (Apex institute for Ophthalmology in the region)	Man power development, research and referral care
State	State Ophthalmic cell, Directorate of Health and Family Welfare Services, medical colleges designated as training centers	Mobile units attached to medical colleges provided eyecare in rural areas
District	District Blindness Control Societies comprising of representative from government, non-government and private sectors under chairmanship of District Collector or Deputy Commissioner	Organizing eye camps, providing mobile eyecare through district mobile units attached to the Government General Hospitals
Sub-District	Medical officer of a PHC and Paramedical Ophthalmic Assistants	Organizing mobile eye camps

Components

a. Cataract surgery	▪ It is restore the vision of the affected persons so that they can return to normal life. ▪ The major thrust of the program is on cataract surgery
b. Eye screening	▪ Under school eye screening program, the children are first screened by the trained teachers[Q] and in suspected children by ophthalmic assistance to prescribe corrective spectacles – Focus is on middle school (V-VII class) covering age of 10–14 years[Q] – 150,000 children are screened per block – Teachers are trained at nearest PHC[Q] and one trained teacher can handle 150 students[Q] – Teacher is provided with visual kit containing vision screening cards, referral cards, tape/rope to measure 20 feet ▪ Screening of diabetic for ophthalmic complications of diabetes
c. Eye donation	▪ Under hospital retrieval program, eye donations are motivated through the relatives of terminally, ill patients, accident victims and other grave diseases ▪ Eye donation fortnight is organized every year from 25th August to 8th September to promote eye donation.
d. Voluntary organization	▪ Voluntary organizations such as Rotary International, Lions International and such others are promoted to provide eyecare through conducting eye camps, eye health education, preventive, promotive, curative and rehabilitative services for control of blindness
e. Vitamin A prophylaxis	▪ 5 mega doses of vitamin A is administered for all pre-school children for prevention of blindness
f. Training	▪ All ophthalmic surgeons are provided training in IOL implantation since 1996 through the faculty members of medical colleges ▪ District eye surgeons, nurses and ophthalmic assistance are also provided training in their respective fields in regards to eyecare
g. IEC activities	▪ Prototype information, education and communication material is provided to all the states in their regional languages ▪ Adequate funds are provided to district societies to carry out IEC activities ▪ World Sight Day is celebrated every year on 2nd Thursday of October.

Strategy

- Undertaking blindness surveys
- Performing cataract operations
- Providing postoperative care
- Establishing eye banks
- Establishing training and IEC facilities
- Providing supportive facilities.

Revised Strategy[Q]

- To make National Program for Central Blindness (NPCB) more comprehensive by strengthening the services for other causes of blindness like corneal blindness, glaucoma and refractive errors among school going children, improving follow up services of cataract operated persons and treating other causes of blindness like glaucoma
- To shift from the eye camp approach to a fixed facility surgical approach[Q] and from conventional surgery to IOL implantation for better quality of post operative vision in operated patients
- To expand the World Bank project[Q] activities like construction of dedicated eye operation theaters, eye wards at district level, training of eye surgeons in modern cataract surgery[Q] and other eye surgeries and supply of ophthalmic equipments, etc. to the whole country
- To strengthen participation of voluntary organization in the program to earmark geographical areas to NGOs and government hospitals to avoid duplication of effort and improve the performance of government units like medical colleges, district hospitals, subdivisional hospitals, community health centers, PHCs, etc.
- To enhance the coverage of eyecare services in tribal and other under served areas through identification of bilateral blind patients, preparation of village wise blind register and giving preference to bilateral blind patients for cataract surgery.

Achievements

- Rate of cataract surgery is increasing steadily
- IOL implantation has raised from 20% to 83%
- Rate of detection of refractive errors in school going children is increased
- Involvement of PHC medial officers in implementation of the program is increased
- About 84% of cataract operated cases receive free spectacles.

SHORT ESSAYS

3. Uses of screening.

Refer Question No. 1 December 2010 (RS2) Paper I.

4. Congenital rubella.

Refer Question No. 3 June 2011 (RS2) Paper II.

5. Tuberculin test.

Refer Question No. 1 December 2009 (RS2) Paper II.

6. Pentavalent vaccine.

- Pentavalent vaccine is a combined vaccine
- Also called as Easy Five Vaccine
- It is so called as it active against 5 vaccine preventable diseases.

Contents	▪ Diphtheria toxoid, tetanus toxoid, whole cell pertussis vaccine, conjugated *Haemophilus influenzae* type B vaccine and hepatitis B surface antigen
Preparation	▪ All contents are adsorbed on aluminum phosphate, suspended in isotonic saline solution, using thiomersal as preservative
Formulation	▪ Liquid vaccine
Storage	▪ 4–8°C
Dose	▪ 0.5 mL IM on lateral aspect of thigh
Schedule	▪ Primary course—6th, 10th and 14th week after birth
Indications	▪ Simultaneous active immunization against diphtheria, tetanus, pertussis, *Haemophilus influenzae* type B (Hib) and Hepatitis B among infants
Contraindications	▪ Acute febrile illness (Immunization is postponed) ▪ History of hypersensitivity reaction to previous dose of DPT or Easy Four or Easy Five ▪ History of any CNS disorder (contraindication for pertussis component)
Application	▪ As part of UIP in 2 states i.e. Kerala and Tamil Nadu instead of DPT since December 2011 ▪ Then expanded to 6 states, i.e. Haryana, Jammu and Kashmir, Gujarat, Karnataka, Goa and Puducherry in 2012–2013 ▪ Will involved 11 more states in October 2014 and entire country from April 2015
Precautions	▪ Shake the vial before use to get an uniform suspension
Advantages	▪ DPT and hepatitis B vaccination require 6 injections to deliver primary doses ▪ With introduction of pentavalent vaccine, a new antigen, i.e. Hib has been added which protects against haemophilus *influenzae* type B (associated with pneumonia and meningitis) and the number of injections are reduced to 3
Disadvantages	▪ Cannot be used for booster doses (booster with tetravalent vaccine only – DPT + Hib)

Significance

- Introduction of pentavalent vaccine has reduced the number of pricks for the infant from 6 to 3 with added advantage of protection against *Haemophilus influenzae*.

7. Tribal malaria.

- Tribal malaria is an epidemiological types (pattern) of malaria.

Epidemiology

- Tribal areas contribute about 50% of *P. falciparum* cases
- There is an Intermediate level of stability in prevalence of tribal malaria in Tribal settlements of in following states—Andhra Pradesh, Telangana, Gujarat, Jharkhand, Madhya Pradesh, Chhattisgarh, Maharashtra, Odisha, Rajasthan, Meghalaya, Mizoram
- In these states, high incidence is seen in tribals living in foothills, forested or conflict affected areas

Risk groups	*Factors responsible for sustaining tribal malaria*	*Factors favoring transmission of tribal malaria*
▪ Infants, young children and pregnant women ▪ Mobile tribal population engaged in forest-related activities	▪ Limited health infrastructure ▪ Lack of drugs at village level ▪ Orthodox health beliefs ▪ High degree of mobility ▪ Outdoor sleeping habits ▪ Inadequate clothing ▪ Forest-based economy	▪ Climatic diversity favoring growth and proliferation of the parasite and vector ▪ Efficient vectors ▪ Triple insecticide resistance ▪ Innumerous breeding sites ▪ Highly susceptible human population ▪ Poor utilization of health services

Control (Under Tribal Malaria Action Plan)

- Tribal Malaria Action Plan will cover Category 2 and 3 districts enabling concentration of available resources to high endemic areas.

Interventions

- Mobile-based surveillance
- Provision of hamlet wise ASHA (instead of village wise)
- Provide alternatives to ASHA like village headman, school teachers, forest dept officials, etc.
- Mobile health services in areas with civic disturbances
- Involvement of NGOs
- Strengthening of health infrastructure with quality microscope facility
- On site treatment of laborers of development projects by the contractors
- On the spot species specific radical treatment of all positive cases
- Early referral of serious cases to PHCs with free transport
- Follow up and epidemiological tracking of all positive cases
- Integrated vector management
- Social marketing to increase use of mosquito nets
- Environmental engineering like de-silting of drainage, filling pits and ditches
- Intensive training of health cadres
- Community mobilization through Information-Education-Communication.

Significance

- India has set goal of malaria elimination by 2030 under National Framework for Malaria Elimination adopted in 2016
- However tribal malaria is a major problem in achieving this goal; hence these tribal dominated States/UTs and districts need special attention
- Improving socioeconomic status of the community in the long run will have a great impact on the incidence of malaria.

8. Control of trachoma.

- Trachoma (Greek—Rough eye) is a chronic communicable infectious disease of the eye and the leading cause of the world's infectious blindness
- It is a chronic communicable keratoconjunctivitis of insidious or abrupt onset, characterized by conjunctival inflammation with lymphoid follicles and papillary hyperplasia associated with vascular invasion of the cornea (pannus) and in its later stages by conjunctival cicatrization which may lead to gross deformity of the eyelids, progressive visual disability and blindness.

Epidemiology

Agent factor	
a. Causative agents	• *Chlamydia trachomatis* – Types A, B or C—Classical endemic trachoma – Types D, E, F, G, H, I, J or K—Inclusion Conjuctivitis • Morax-Axenfeld diplobacillus—Most innocuous • Koch-Weeks bacillus— Most widespread • *Gonococcus* —Most dangerous
b. Reservoir	• Children with active disease, chronically infected older children and adults
c. Source of infection	• Ocular discharges of infected persons and fomites
d. Communicability	• Low infectivity • Infective as long as active lesions are present in the conjunctiva, but not after complete cicatrization
Host factors	
a. Age	• Children aged 2–5 years most infected
b. Sex	• Equal in younger age groups, in adults, more preponderance in females
c. Predisposing factors	• Direct sunlight, dust, smoke and irritants such as *kajal* or *surma*
Environmental factors	
a. Seasons	• Incidence of active trachoma is high during April-May and again July-September • Higher temperature and rainfall favors increase in population of eye-seeking flies
b. Quality of life	• Trachoma thrives in conditions of poverty, crowding, ignorance, poor personal hygiene, squalor, illiteracy and poor housing • As living conditions improve, the disease tends to regress
c. Customs	• Custom of applying *kajal* or *surma* to the eyes is a positive risk factor
Mode of transmission	• Eye to eye transmission in endemic areas by direct or indirect contact with ocular discharges or fomites • Mechanical transmission via eye-seeking flies (e.g., *Musca* species, *Hippefatus* species) • Venereal transmission by genital localisation of *C. trachomatis* in cases of sporadic cases
Incubation period	• 5–12 days

Diagnostic criteria (at least 2 of the following)

- Follicles on the upper tarsal conjunctiva
- Limbal follicles or their sequelae, Herbert's pits
- Typical conjunctival scarring (trichiasis, entropion)
- Vascular pannus, most marked at the superior limbus

Environmental risk factors

- Six Ds [Dry, Dusty, Dirty, Dung, Discharge and Density (overcrowding)]
- Five Fs [Flies, Feces, Face (eyes), Fingers and Fomites]

WHO Grading

Stage	*Clinical features*
a. Trachomatous inflammation; Follicular (TF)	Five or more follicles of >0.5 mm on the upper tarsal conjunctiva
b. Trachomatous inflammation; Intense (TI)	Papillary hypertrophy and inflammatory thickening of the upper tarsal conjunctiva obscuring more than half the deep tarsal vessels
c. Trachomatous trichiasis (TT)	At least one ingrown eyelash touching the globe, or evidence of epilation (eyelash removal)
d. Corneal opacity (CO)	Corneal opacity blurring part of the pupil margin

Control of Trachoma

Objective

- Prevention of blindness.

Target population (communities with blindness rate >0.5%)

- Communities with substantial prevalence of blinding trachoma indicated by:
  - Corneal blindness
  - Trachomatous trichiasis and entropion
  - Moderate and severe trachomatous inflammation.

SAFE Strategy

- World Health Organization (WHO) has set a goal of eliminating blinding trachoma as a public health concern by 2020, using the SAFE strategy.

Components[Q]

S – Lid surgery for those at immediate risk of blindness[Q]
A – Antibiotics to treat individual cases and to reduce infection in a community[Q]
F – Facial cleanliness and hygiene promotion to reduce transmission[Q]
E – Environmental improvements such as provision of water and household sanitation[Q]

S—Surgery	▪ Active search for individuals with lid deformities (trichiasis, entropion) and performing necessary surgical procedures and follow up has immediate impact on preventing blindness ▪ Surgery reverses the in-turned eyelashes of people with severe trachoma ▪ Lid surgery is a fairly simple procedure that can be offered in the community or at health centers ▪ Offering community-based surgery is the best way to encourage people suffering with trichiasis to seek help ▪ Lid surgery takes away the pain of lashes scraping against the eyes and prevents further damage, but does not restore sight that was already lost
A—Antibiotic therapy	*Objective* ▪ To reduce severity, lower the incidence and in the long run decrease the prevalence of trachoma *Antibiotics* ▪ Tetracycline (drug of choice) 1% oint or oily suspension ▪ Erythromycin ▪ Rifampicin *Types* i. Mass treatment (blanket treatment)—given to entire community – Indicated in community with prevalence of >5% severe and moderate trachoma in children under 10 years – Application of 1% tetracycline ointment for all children ❖ Daily twice for 5 days each month or Once daily for 10 days for 6 consecutive months ❖ 60 consecutive days Disadvantage – Need for repeated applications over long periods of time ii. Selective treatment—given to person with active trachoma (after population screening) – Indicated in communities with a low to medium prevalence
F—Facial cleanliness	▪ Dirty faces are associated with active trachoma ▪ Children with dirty faces are more likely to transmit trachoma if they have an active infection or to get trachoma if they are not infected ▪ Discharge from the eyes and nose attracts flies that can bring the infection or carry it to other people ▪ Wiping or rubbing dirty eyes with cloths, bed sheets, or a mother's shawl can contribute to the transmission of trachoma ▪ With support from the Carter Center Trachoma Control Program, communities are educated on the importance of clean faces
E—Environmental improvement	▪ Trachoma persists where people live in poverty with crowded living conditions and without water, sanitation, and proper waste disposal ▪ Transmission of trachoma occurs where these conditions exist and should be expected to return after antibiotic treatment if the conditions are not changed ▪ Improvements like construction of household pit latrines and hand-dug wells will bring about sustainable elimination of trachoma

Significance

- India is now free from infective trachoma

	Elimination criteria (WHO)	*National Trachoma Survey Report (2014–2017) findings*
Prevalence of active trachoma infection among children (<10 years)	<5%	<0.7%

- Trachoma is no longer a public health problem in India
- India has met the goal of trachoma elimination (WHO GET 2020)
- SAFE strategy has major role in achieving this
- Now the government has directed its efforts to eliminate trachomatous trichiasis from the country.

9. Syndromic management of vaginal discharge.

- Syndromic approach diagnosis is innovative management approach for sexually transmitted diseases
- It is based on the identification of syndromes, which are combinations of the symptoms the patient reports and the signs the physician observes
- Using set of flowcharts, the treatments are recommended which are effective for all the diseases that could cause the identified syndrome
- Provides single dose treatment as far as possible

Components	*Advantages*	*Disadvantages*	*Patient education*
• History taking including sexual history • Clinical examination • Syndromic diagnosis • Syndromic treatment • Counseling and education • Promotion and provision of condoms • Partner management • Referral for ICTC and VDRL test • Follow-up	• Fast—the patient is diagnosed and treated in one visit • Highly effective for most of the syndromes • Relatively inexpensive since it avoids use of laboratory tests • No need for patient to return for lab results • All possible STIs are treated at once • Scientifically tested in globally • Easy for health workers to learn and practice • Integrated into primary healthcare services more easily • Can be used by providers at all levels • Simple to treat with good drug compliance • Effective against mixed infections • Goes beyond pharmaceutical treatment to include client education and counseling	• Not useful in asymptomatic individuals • Over-treatment in patient with one STI that causes a syndrome • Financial cost of over-treatment, side-effects • Increases potential for antibiotic resistance especially if full course not completed • Not effective in some cases such as vaginal discharge	• Taking the full course of treatment will cure most STIs • Avoid sex during treatment period to prevent spread of STIs • Help sexual partners to get treatment • Condom use to stay uninfected • Reduce risk of acquiring new infection by having one sex partner • Protect against HIV/AIDS • In case of pregnancy, report to antenatal clinic to protect both mother and baby

Significance

- Syndromic management of STDs has come into vogue because traditional approach of etiological diagnosis by microscopic examination and culture of materials is not only expensive but also time consuming in obtaining results. Added to this, is the lack of facilities in rural areas.

Ref: http://www.indmedica.com/journals.php?journalid=3andissueid=75andarticleid=975andaction=article

Syndromic Management of Vaginal Discharge

Syndrome: Vaginal discharge

Vaginitis trichomoniasis cervical herpes cervicitis

Causative organisms

Vaginitis
- *Trichomonas vaginalis (Tv)*
- *Candida albicans*
- *Gardnerella vaginalis, Mycoplasma* causing bacterial vaginosis (Bv)

Causative organisms cervicitis
- *Neisseria gonorrhoeae*
- *Trichomonas vaginalis*
- *Chlamydia trachomatis*
- Herpess simplex virus

History
- Menstrual history to rule out pregnancy
- Nature and type of discharge (amount, smell, color, consistency)
- Genital itching
- Burning while passing urine, increased frequency
- Presence of any ulcer, swelling on the vulval or inguinal region
- Genital complaints in sexual partners
- Low backache

Examination

Per speculum examination to differentiate between vaginitis and cervicitis

a). Vaginitis:
- Trichomoniasis greenish frothy discharge
- Candidiasis curdy
- White discharge
- Bacterial vaginosis–adherent discharge
- Mixed infections may present with atypical discharge

b). Cervicitis:
- Cervical erosion/cervical ulcer/mucopurulent cervical discharge
- Bimanual pelvic examination to rule out pelvic inflammatory disease
- If speculum examination is not possible or client is hesitant treat both for vaginitis and cervicitis

Laboratory investigations (if available)
- Wet mount microscopy of the discharge for *Trichomonas vaginalis* and clue cells
- 10% KOH preparation for *Candida albicans*
- Gram stain of vaginal smear for clue cells seen in bacterial vaginosis
- Gram stain of endocervical smear to detect gonococci

Treatment

Vaginitis (Tv+Bv+Candida)
- Tablet secnidazole 2 g orally, single dose or tablet tinidazole 500 mg orally twice daily for 5 days
- Tablet metoclopramide taken 30 minutes before tablet secnidazole, to prevent gastric intolerance
- Treat for candidiasis with tablet fluconazole 150 mg orally single dose or local clotrimazole 500 mg vaginal pessaries once

Treatment for cervical infection (Chlamydia and gonorrhea)
- Tablet cefixim 400 mg orally, single dose
- Plus azithromycin 1 g, 1 hour before lunch. If vomiting within 1 hour, give antiemetic and repeat
- If vaginitis and cervicitis are present treat for both
- Instruct client to avoid douching
- Pregnancy, diabetes, HIV may also be influencing factors and should be considered in recurrent infections
- Follow up after one week

Specific guidelines for partner management
- Treat current partner only if no improvement after initial treatment
- Advise sexual abstinence during the course of treatment
- Schedule return visit after 7 days
- If partner is symptomatic, treat client and partner using above protocols
- Provide condoms, educate about correct and consistent use

Management in pregnant women

Per speculum examination should be done to rule out pregnancy complications like abortion, premature rupture of membranes

Treatment for vaginitis (Tv+Bv+Candida

In first trimester of pregnancy
- Local treatment with clotrimazole vaginal pessary/cream only for candidiasis. Oral fluconazole is contraindicated in pregnancy
- Metronidazole pessaries or cream intravaginally if trichomoniasis or Bv is suspected in second and third trimester oral metronidazole can be given
- Tablet secnidazole 2 g orally, single dose or tablet tinidazole 500 mg orally, twice daily for 5 days
- Tablet metoclopramide taken 30 minutes before tablet metronidazole, to prevent gastric intolerance

10. Prevention of coronary heart disease.

Refer Question No. 11 June 2015 (RS2) Paper II.

11. Vision 2020.

Refer Question No. 5 June 2013 (RS2) Paper II.

12. Integrated counseling and testing centers.

Refer Question No. 2 June 2015 (RS2) Paper II.

SHORT ANSWERS

13. Assessment of dehydration.

Refer Question No. 7 June 2014 (RS2) Paper II.

14. Screening for cervical cancer.

Refer question No. 11 June 2013 (RS2) Paper II.

15. Treatment of amoebiasis.

- Amoebiasis is a clinical condition of harboring the protozoan parasite *Entamoeba histolytica* with/without clinical manifestations (WHO)

Epidemiology	
Agent factors	
a. Agent	• *E. histolytica*, a protozoal parasite **Forms** • Trophozoite (Pathogenic form)—Colonize large intestine, cause bowel ulceration • Cyst (Infective form)
b. Reservoir of infection	• Man is the only reservoir of infection • Healthy and convalescent carrier state occurs • Immediate source of infection is the feces containing the cysts
c. Source of infection	• Food and drink contaminated with human feces
d. Period of communicability	• As long as cysts are excreted (may be several years if left untreated)
Host factors	
a. Age	• Occurs at any age
b. Sex	• Equal distribution
c. High-risk groups	• Travelers, migrants, immigrant workers, immunocompromized individuals, prisoners and children in daycare centers • Severe infections occur in very young children, pregnant women, malnourished and people taking corticosteroids
d. Immunity	• Cell mediated immunity prevents recurrence of invasive amoebiasis
Environmental factors	
a. Socioeconomic status	• Seen more in poor communities • Overcrowding favors spread of disease
b. Seasons	• Higher incidence during rains (cysts may survive longer)
c. Sanitation	• Closely related to poor sanitation (indiscriminate defecation) • Sewage seepage into the water supply results in epidemics • Use of nightsoil for agricultural purposes favors the spread of the disease
Mode of Transmission	
a. Feco-oral route	• Through contaminated food (vegetables irrigated with sewage polluted water) or water (contamination of drinking water supply) • Through contaminated hands (Viable cysts present on the hands and under finger nails)
b. Sexual route	• By oral-rectal contact especially among male homosexuals
c. Vectors	• Cyst carrying flies, cockroaches and rodents can contaminate food and drink

Incubation period	• About 2–4 weeks or longer
Clinical features	
a. Intestinal disease	• Spectrum varies from mild abdominal discomfort and diarrhoea to acute fulminating dysentery • Lower abdominal pain and tenesmus is common and tenderness over caecum and colon • 10–12 stools per day containing little fecal material and consists blood and mucous • Fever is usually absent
b. Extraintestinal amoebiasis	• Includes amoebic liver abscess (commonest), involvement lungs, brain, spleen, skin, etc. • Amoebic liver abscess commonly affects the posterior lobe of the liver and presents as right upper quadrant pain associated with hepatomegaly • Fever is common, jaundice rare • Complications include pleuropulmonary involvement, hepatobronchial fistula and rupture in peritoneum or pericardium

Prevention and Control

a. Primary prevention (Breaking chain of transmission, i.e. preventing contamination of water and food with human feces)

Sanitation	Water supply	Food hygiene	Health education (Beneficial for long term)
Safe disposal of human excreta coupled with the elementary sanitary practice of washing hands after defecation and before eating	Protection of water supplies against fecal contamination Water filtration (sand filters) and boiling are more effective than chemical treatment of water (cysts are not killed by routine chlorination)	Disinfection of uncooked vegetables and fruits with aqueous solution of 5–10% acetic acid or full strength vinegar Thorough washing with detergents in running water Periodic examination, treatment and education of food handlers regarding food hygiene practices such as hand washing	Must emphasize on Always wash hands thoroughly with soap and water before eating or preparing food, after using the toilet, and after changing diapers After changing diapers, wash the child's hands as well as your own Avoid open air defection and dispose of feces in a sanitary manner Avoid sexual practices that may permit fecal – oral transmission Do not eat fruit that already has been peeled or cut Drink only pasteurized milk or dairy products

b. Secondary prevention (Elimination of reservoir)

Early diagnosis	Treatment		
	Symptomatic cases	Asymptomatic infections	
		In endemic areas	In non-endemic areas
Demonstration of trophozoites containing RBCs is diagnostic Microscopy of freshly passed mucus per rectum also shows trophozoites Serological tests such as Indirect hemagglutination test (IHA) (most sensitive), counter immunoelectrophoresis (CIE) and ELISA technique are positive in extraintestinal amoebiasis (negative in intestinal amoebiasis)	Metronidazole (Drug of choice) 30 mg/kg/day, divided into 3 doses orally after meals or IV, for 8–10 days Tinidazole (alternative) 2 g OD for 3 days	No treatment (due to very high probability of reinfection) Treatment only if he is food handler	Diiodohyroxyquin, 650 mg TDS (adults) or 30–40 mg/kg/day (children) for 20 days orally Diloxanide furoate, 500 mg TDS for 10 days orally (adults) Paromomycin, 500 mg TDS for 10 days orally Iodoquinol, 650 mg TDS for 20 days orally

Significance

- Amoebiasis is often called a social disease and requires invention at community levels rather than mere treatment of cases alone.

16. Dengue shock syndrome.

Refer Question No. 12 June 2012 (RS2) Paper II.

17. Demographic gap.

Refer Question No. 15 June 2008 (RS2) Paper II.

18. International Red Cross Society.

- Red Cross is an independent, nongovenmental, nonpolitical, international organization concerned with offering humanitarian assistance in war time and peace time disastrous situations
- It was founded by John Henry Dunant[Q], a Swiss businessman 1864 in form of International Committee of Red Cross with headquarters at Geneva[Q].

Objectives	*Activities*
▪ Providing relief and rehabilitative services to the wounded and disabled individuals afflicted by war, famine, earthquake, floods and other natural or manmade disasters	▪ Providing service to the armed forces ▪ Providing service to war veterans ▪ Disaster services ▪ First aid and nursing ▪ Health education ▪ Maternity and child welfare services

Significance

- Red Cross is the biggest relief organization in the world with about 200 million members and tens of thousands employees.

19. Record linkage.

Refer Question No. 12 June 2014 (RS2) Paper I.

20. Danger signals of cancer.

Refer Question No. 12 December 2007 (RS2) Paper II.

21. Adolescent Reproductive and Sexual Health (ARSH) or SNEHA Clinics.

- Adolescent Reproductive and Sexual Health (ARSH) strategy is a component of Reproductive and Child Health (RCH) Phase II.

SNEHA Clinics

- These are the adolescent friendly clinics conducted on fixed days and timings at subcenters, PHCs, Community Health Centers and District Hospitals of Karnataka
- Similar clinics are called with separate names in other states such as MAITRI in Maharasthra, UDAN in Uttarakhand, etc.

Objectives

- Providing information and services on promoting safe sexual behavior including abstinence, delayed age at onset of sexual course, preventing unwanted and early pregnancies and preventing STIs including HIV/AIDS.

Location (Target Districts)

- In districts where >60% girls marry before the age of eighteen (based on incidence of teenage pregnancy).

Services

Distribution of	*Information about*	*Treatment of*
▪ Weekly iron and folic acid supplementation and Albendazole ▪ Sanitary napkins ▪ Contraceptives ▪ Medicines	▪ Counseling on nutrition, menstrual disorders, personal hygiene, menstrual hygiene, use of sanitary napkins, use of contraceptives, sexual concerns, depression, sexual abuse, gender violence, substance misuse and promoting healthy behavior to prevent non communicable diseases	▪ Severe malnutrition ▪ Common RTI/STI problems ▪ Menstrual disorders ▪ Sexual concerns of males and females ▪ Depression (Mental health services) ▪ Noncommunicable diseases and other common ailments ▪ Injuries related to accidents and violence ▪ Substance misuse ▪ Noncommunicable diseases like hypertension, stroke, cardio-vascular diseases and diabetes

Levels of Healthcare Delivery

Levels	*Subcenter*	*PHCs/ CHCs*
Service provider	Healthcare worker—female	Health assistant—female Medical officer
Target group	Married males and females Unmarried males and females	Unmarried males and females
Mode of delivery	During routine subcenter clinics	Once a week 2 hour adolescent clinic
▪ Services	▪ Enroll newly married couples ▪ Provision of spacing methods ▪ Routine ANC and institutional delivery ▪ Referral for easy and safe abortion ▪ STI/HIV/AIDS prevention, education ▪ Nutrition counseling including anemia prevention ▪ Distribution of sanitary napkins	▪ Contraceptives ▪ Management of menstrual disorders ▪ RTI/STI prevention, education, management ▪ Counseling and services for pregnancy termination ▪ Nutritional counseling and management of anemia ▪ Counseling for sexual problems ▪ Distribution of sanitary napkins

Significance

- SNEHA clinics are a befitting example of community clinics where a package of services including preventive, promotive, curative and counseling services are provided under one roof.

22. Enumerate the illnesses managed under Integrated Management of Neonatal and Childhood Illnesses (IMNCI).

Refer Question No. 10 June 2008 (RS2) Paper II.

MBBS PHASE III EXAMINATION

JUNE 2016

(Revised Scheme 2 & 3)

PAPER I

LONG ESSAYS

1. What is sampling? Explain different sampling techniques with suitable examples.

- Sampling is the procedure of obtaining a group of people or items for a study involving a large proportion of individuals or items or units, however, the people selected must be representative of the whole population is study.

Sampling Techniques

Probability sampling	*Non-probability sampling*
i. Simple random sampling ii. Stratified random sampling iii. Systematic random sampling iv. Multistage random sampling v. Multiphase sampling vi. Cluster sampling vii. Point or line sampling	i. Accidental or incidental sampling ii. Judgment sampling or purposive sampling or deliberate sampling iii. Quota sampling iv. Convenience sampling v. Sequential sampling

Methods

a. Simple random sampling (unrestricted random sampling)
   - A random sample is a sample selected in such a way that every item in the population has an equal chance of being included[Q]
   - This method is applicable when population is small, homogenous and readily available[Q] such as a village, a household or an individual in a community
   - Here, the sample is selected from the known population randomly and to ensure randomness of selection, any of the following method is adopted.
     i. Lottery method
        - This is the simplest and most popular method of obtaining a random sample
        - Under this method, various units of population are numbered on small and identical slips or papers, which are folded and mixed together in a drum thoroughly
        - A blindfold selection is made of the number of slips required to constitute the desired size of the sample
        - Another way of doing it is to draw a slip, note the number and replace the slip back in drum. Reshuffle and draw a second slip and go on doing it till the desired sample size is obtained. However reject the cards that are drawn for the second time
        - Even numbers on the currency notes can be used in place of paper slips
        - Control sample can also be drawn in similar way.

     ii. Random number tables
        - The other common method of drawing sample is by making use of published tables of random numbers.

        Commonly used random tables
        - Tippets random number table

- Fisher and Yates table
- Rand Corporation random number table

Example

- To select a random sample of 25 students from a class of 75 students.

Procedure

- All the 75 students are arranged in an order say in the alphabetical order of their names and they are numbered from 1 to 75. This is known as "Sampling frame"
- Twenty units from the serial numbers are obtained as detailed below by referring the Tippets random number table which has 50 columns of single digit numbers, in each table. Out of these a row and a column are selected at random, say 8th row and 6th column core is selected. The corresponding number of the crossing of row and column is 6
- The total population size is two digits i.e. 75 and hence two adjacent columns are to be clubbed together i.e. 6th and 7th columns are clubbed and read as two digit numbers, which becomes the starting number. In this table, it corresponds to 61
- Starting from 61, the numbers in the list are read downwards and all the numbers less than or equal to population size are noted down
- When the last row of these columns is reached, then the corresponding number of next two columns is selected i.e. 8th and 9th column and the procedure is repeated till 25 unduplicated numbers are obtained.
- Thus numbers selected are:
  61, 62, 02, 31, 51, 11, 56, 64, 21, 01, 16, 39, 06, 38, 26, 34, 08, 65, 22, 52, 07, 29, 30, 14 and 18
  The students with these numbers constitute the sample.

Advantages	*Disadvantages*
▪ Scientific method ▪ More representative (as the sample size increases, it becomes more representative) ▪ More economical	▪ It needs complete list of study population, which is often difficult to obtain[Q] ▪ If the sample size is small, this sample will not be a true representative of the universe ▪ Cases selected by random sampling tend to be widely dispersed geographically and the time and cost of collecting data becomes too large

b. Systematic random sampling
   – This method is preferred when the population is large, scattered and not homogenous such as number of houses in a village or town
   – Here, no prenumbering is necessary as in simple random sampling
   – The sample size is selected by picking the unit of sample at a regular interval[Q]

   Example
   – Filariasis survey in a town requires 10% sample
   – The houses are numbered
   – The sampling interval is calculated as follows:
     - R = Total population/desired sample size which becomes 10 in this case
     - Then a number is selected between 1 to 10, randomly say 2
     - Then every 10th number is selected from that point onwards i.e., 2, 12, 22, 32, etc.

Advantages	*Disadvantages*
▪ Simple and convenient to adopt ▪ Time and labor involved in the collection of sample is relatively small	▪ Suitable when there is no unique variation in the universe

c. Stratified random sampling[Q]
   – This method of sampling used when the population is not homogenous and is composed of diverse segments[Q]
   – Here the entire population is divided into certain homogenous subgroups or strata depending upon the characteristics to be studied and simple random sampling is drawn independently from each sub group or strata[Q]
   – This technique gives more representative sampling than a simple random sampling in a given large population
   – In practice, geographical, sociological and economical characters are often used for stratification, for example, workers like skilled workers and unskilled workers, religion wise, age group wise, etc.

– Then the size of the sample from each strata can either be proportional or disproportional to the size of each stratum.
 i. Proportional size: Here, a given percentage of units are selected from each stratum
 ii. Disproportional size: It is recommended if the different strata reveal different levels of within strata variability

Example[Q]

– In case of study of religion, we may select only 10% from a large group like Hindu whereas select more like 50% from a small group like Christians and select few less like 25–30% from medium group like Muslims so that the sample in each stratum should not be less than 30 in size[Q].

Advantages	*Disadvantages*
▪ It is more representative ▪ It gives estimates with increased precision ▪ As the population is more concentrated geographically, the time and money will be saved ▪ Stratification is more advantageous when the distribution of the universe is skewed	▪ It is very difficult task to divide the population into homogenous strata. This may require considerable time and money and statistical expertise ▪ The supplementary information to set up strata is not available sometimes ▪ Sometimes the different strata may overlap and the sampling would not be representative

d. Multistage sampling
– As the name implies, this method consists of sampling procedure carried out in several stages, using random sampling technique
– Under this method, the random selection is made of primary, intermediate, final units from a given population
– Thus, the area of investigation is scientifically restricted to a small number of ultimate units, which are representative of whole
– This is convenient when the population of entire district or state or country is to be studied, within limited resources
– To bring down the cost involvement the size of sample is reduced progressively in stages till a conveniently representative sample is obtained.

Example

– For hookworm survey in a district, 10% of talukas are selected, followed by 10% of villages in these talukas
– Finally all people in 10th house of these villages are subjected to stool examination.

Advantages	*Disadvantages*
▪ This method is very helpful in many large scale surveys where population list preparation is difficult ▪ It is less expensive and less time-consuming ▪ This method introduces flexibility in sampling ▪ It enables the use of existing divisions and subdivisions and thus saves the extra labor involved in independent enumeration or census ▪ It permits available resources to be concentrated on a limited number of units of the frame, which results in a lower cost per unit of the enquiry and in preparing a complete sampling frame	▪ Sampling error is usually increased ▪ Sampling units will be of unequal size at various stages resulting in analytical difficulties

e. Multiphase sampling
– In this method, the study is carried out in several phases
– A part of information is collected from the whole sample and part of information from sub-sample.

Example

– For a cross-sectional study of nutrition, all the families in the original sample are covered for KAP (Knowledge, Attitude and Practice) study in the first phase
– A sub-sample of the families is then surveyed for dietary intake in the second phase
– Then a sub-sample of family members covered in the second phase is subjected to anthropometric examination in third phase
– A further sub-sample of members covered in third phase is subjected to biochemical examination in the fourth phase
– Thus in multiphase sampling, the number of subject or units gets reduced in every succeeding phase, thereby reducing the magnitude of the complicated and costly procedure reserved for the last phase.

Advantages

– Less expensive

- Less time consuming
- Less laborious
- More purposeful

f. Cluster sampling
- Cluster is the smallest unit into which the population can be described
- We can simplify it as the randomly selected group of individual[Q], e. g. villages, wards, etc.
- Cluster sampling allows small number of target population to be sampled which the data provides is statistically valid at 95% confidence limits
- This type of sample is used for national surveys commonly for determining vaccination coverage under Universal Immunization Program[Q].

Example
- Immunization status of children in a PHC jurisdiction is done as follows:
  i. Identification of total population and geographical area
     - It is the total population of the area to which PHC caters.
  ii. Identification of age group to be included
     - The age group selected in this case (immunization) is children age 1 year[Q].
  iii. Listing of all villages
     - It is done alphabetically
  iv. Tabulation
     - The population of each village is tabulated.
  v. Sampling interval (SI)
     - Sampling interval is determined by following interval.

$$SI = \frac{\text{Total cumulative population}}{\text{Total of clusters}}$$

  vi. Selection of starting point
     - This is a random number which is equal to or less than sampling interval which is selected by using a random number or by using the number of currency drawn.
     - The first village in which this figure equals or less than the cumulative population is taken as first cluster.
  vii. Selecting subsequent clusters
     - Subsequent clusters are selected using following formula:
       * C_2 = Random number + sampling interval
       * $C_3 = C_2$ + sampling interval
       * And so on
  viii. Selecting first household in a cluster
     - This done by random method.
  ix. Information collection
     - In each household following enquiry is made.
       * Number of persons living in the household
       * Any infant below age of 1 year living in the household.
       * If yes whether the infant has received vaccine according to his age.

Advantages
- It is useful when the list of sampling units is not available

g. Point or line sampling
- On the map or aerial photograph of the area to be studied random horizontal and vertical lines are drawn
- The points where these lines intersect are included in the sample
- People residing at these points are included into the sample.

Nonprobability Sampling

a. Accidental or incidental sampling
- The people who are assembled in one place with a common interest or accidentally are surveyed.

Example
- Studying prevalence of blood pressure in a population who are assembled to watch a movie

b. Judgmental sampling
- This is also called deliberate sampling or purposive sampling
- Here the sample selection is based on the judgment of the person entrusted with the job
- The work of this method will depend on the sampling design and purpose of representativeness
- Here an expert in the field needs to exercise proper judgment
- Therefore, the knowledge and attitude of the investigator will decide the effectiveness of the sampling.

c. Quota sampling[Q]
- This is stratified random sampling minus randomization, i.e. here we select the strata
- Here the surveyor tries to complete the quota assigned to them by supplementing new respondents in place of those not available or uncooperative but among the selected ones only

d. Convenience sampling[Q]
- It is said to have been used when the selection is made from an available source like that of telephone directory, stock exchange directory, etc.
- It is so called because getting sample is convenient
- However, the correctness of the procedure depends upon the purpose of the enquiry
- They represent certain characteristics group of people like the literate group, intelligent group, etc.

e. Sequential sampling
- Here number of sample lots are drawn one after another from a population depending upon the results of earlier samples
- So this sampling is used as quality control
- If the first sample is clearly acceptable, no new sample is needed
- If it is completely unacceptable, the lot is rejected straightaway
- If the initial sample is doubtful or marginal in character, second, if needed third sample of large size may be drawn.

f. Snowball sampling
- It is technique for developing a research sample where existing study subjects recruit future subjects from among their acquaintances, thus the sample groups to grow like rolling snowball
- Is often used in hidden population[Q] which are difficult for researchers to access (e. g. drug abusers, commercial sex workers).

Significance

- Sampling offers a representative sample of the study population thus minimizing the effort and making the study economical and faster.

2. Classify the various occupational diseases. Describe the measures for prevention of occupational diseases.

- Occupational diseases are diseases arising out of or in the course of employment.

Classification

Agent	*Disease*
a. Diseases due to physical agents	
i. Heat	▪ Heat hyperpyrexia (body temperature <102°F) ▪ Heat exhaustion (body temperature >106°F) ▪ Heat syncope (body temperature up to 110°F) ▪ Heat cramps ▪ Burns ▪ Local effect such as prickly heat
ii. Cold	▪ Trench foot ▪ Frost bite ▪ Chilblains

Contd...

Contd...

Agent	***Disease***
iii. Light	▪ Occupational cataract ▪ Miner's nystagmus
iv. Pressure	▪ Caisson's disease ▪ Air embolism ▪ Explosion
v. Noise	▪ Occupational deafness
vi. Radiation	▪ Cancer ▪ Leukemia ▪ Aplastic anemia ▪ Pancytopenia
vii. Mechanical factors	▪ Injuries ▪ Accidents
viii. Electricity	▪ Burns
ix. Vibration	▪ Vibration sickness ▪ Neurogenic damage
b. Diseases due to chemical agents	
i. Gases	▪ Poisoning by CO_2, CO, HCN, CS_2, NH_3, H_2S, HCl, SO_2, etc.
ii. Dusts (pneumoconiosis) Inorganic dusts	
❖ Coal dust	▪ Anthracosis
❖ Silica	▪ Silicosis
❖ Asbestos	▪ Asbestosis, cancer lungs
❖ Iron	▪ Siderosis
Organic dust	
❖ Cane fiber	▪ Bagassosis
❖ Cotton dust	▪ Byssinosis
❖ Tobacco	▪ Tobacossis
❖ Hay or grain dust	▪ Farmer's lung
iii. Metals and their compounds	▪ Poisoning by lead, mercury, cadmium, manganese, beryllium, arsenic, chromium, etc.
iv. Chemicals (acids, alkalis, pesticides)	▪ Poisoning, burns
v. Solvents (carbon bisulfide, benzene)	▪ Dermatitis, cancers
c. Diseases due to biological agents	▪ Brucellosis ▪ Leptospirosis ▪ Anthrax ▪ Actinomycosis ▪ Hydatid disease ▪ Psittacosis ▪ Tetanus ▪ Encephalitis ▪ Fungal infection
d. Occupational cancers	▪ Cancer of skin, lungs, bladder
e. Occupational dermatosis	▪ Dermatitis, eczema
f. Diseases of psychological origin	▪ Industrial neurosis ▪ Hypertension ▪ Peptic ulcer

Prevention of Occupational Diseases

A. Primary prevention
  a. Health promotion
    i. Preplacement examination
      - Preplacement or pre-employment examination is the medical examination done at the time of employment
      - Based on the results the person may be totally rejected or given a job suited to his physical and mental abilities.

Components	*Objectives*	*Examples*
▪ Worker's medical, family, occupational and social history ▪ Thorough physical examination and ▪ Battery of biological and radiological examinations	▪ Objective of preplacement examination is to place the right man in the right job[Q] so that the worker can perform his duties efficiently without detriment to life of him or others	▪ A person with color blindness cannot be employed as driver for public transport, railways, etc. ▪ Similarly there are some conditions wherein person suffering from which are not employed in certain industries, for example, people with active or healed tuberculosis of lung or chronic lung disease are not employed in silica industry

Significance

- Preplacement examination is the foundation of an efficient occupational health services
- It helps to place a right man in the right job
- It improves the efficiency of the worker
- It improves the satisfaction and confidence of the worker
- It also serves a useful benchmark for future comparison thus helps in early detection of any departure from health
- It separates high-risk individuals from potentially dangerous environments.

ii. Provision of healthy physical environment (Engineering Measures)

▪ Building	▪ Should be structurally safe to withstand the stress and strain of the machineries ▪ Protected from solar radiation and conducted heat and noise ▪ Should be away from the residential areas ▪ There should not be overcrowding inside the building nor the area be congested with machine (area per worker: 400 cu. Ft)
▪ Lighting	▪ Sufficient light in the factory (natural, artificial or both), to enable clear vision ▪ No glare ▪ Excessive brightness avoided ▪ Obtain uniform light from the sun because defective illumination predisposes for accidents and nystagmus ▪ Periodic white washing of walls to keep the room bright and help proper diffusion of light ▪ Indirect illumination reflecting from the ceiling is best ▪ Use fluorescent lights for artificial lighting
▪ Ventilation	▪ Proper ventilation of the working place must ▪ Arrange adequate artificial ventilation if natural ventilation is not adequate ▪ Ventilatory openings should be in the proportion of 5 sq. feet for each worker ▪ Prefer exhaust system of ventilation especially in rooms where dust is generated ▪ Good ventilation minimizes the occurrence of pneumoconiosis ▪ The Indian Factories Act has prescribed a minimum of 500 cu-ft of air space for each worker
▪ Thermal comfort	▪ Comfort-zone is a one wherein the worker feels comfortable for doing this work Criteria of comfort zone ▪ Corrected effective temperature 25–27°C ▪ Relative humidity 30–65% ▪ Dry Kata reading ≥6 ▪ Wet Kata reading ≥20 ▪ Predicted 4 hour sweat rate (P4SR) 1–3L
▪ Control of dust	▪ Prevent or to reduce the formation of dust by wet method, oiling, etc. ▪ Prevent the escape of dust by hoods, enclosures, to trap the dust ▪ Remove the dust by exhaust ventilation, suction fans, etc. ▪ Control the dust by wet-mopping of the floors

▪ Good house-keeping	▪ Regularly clean the floor with wet-mopping or vacuum cleaning ▪ Regular white washing and painting of the industry ▪ Keep the premises clean and tidy
▪ Water supply	▪ Provide protected water supply to the workers in the industry ▪ Install drinking water fountains, at convenient points ▪ Provide about 5 liters of water per head per day
▪ Latrines and urinals	▪ One sanitary latrine for 25 workers and one urinal for 50 workers is must ▪ These should be separate for men and women and located in a convenient place
▪ Disposal of sewage	▪ Own sewage treatment plant in large industries ▪ Release sewage into the river water only after treatment ▪ Re-circulation can be done if necessary

iv. Machine safety and process control
- Accidents are common among those, who are working with unguarded improperly installed, carelessly operated or defective machineries
- Take following precautionary measures
- Use standard machinery and equipment
- Leave sufficient space all around the machinery
- Have built in safety device in machinery
- Fence or guard the dangerous parts of the machine
- Proper installation of the machines
- Periodical cleaning of the machine
- Properly earth all electrical connections
- Control the manufacturing process so as to expose the worker to the least amount of noxious substances
- Mechanization of the plant to protect the workers from dangers
- Substitution of harmful substances by less harmful

v. Health education
- This is also an important health promotive measure and envisages at both—the worker and the management
- Worker is educated about the risks involved and the measures to be taken for self-protection
- They are also educated of personal hygiene and also the importance of maintaining a healthy social relationship with the co-workers and the management

vi. Safety education and training
- All workers are given safety education by the Welfare officer (Safety officer) and the Factory Physician (Industrial Medical Officer) about the dangers of the machine and the materials they are handling and their self-protection
- Workers are also given education on first-aid
- They must also be given "Job training", which in turn promotes their health.

vii. Working hours
- 8 hours a day with a break for 1 hour during lunch hours, for 6 days in a week and 1 day preferably Sunday to be holiday

viii. Other health promotional activities
- Recreational, play and cultured activities
- Provision of quarters, lunch rooms and retiring rooms
- Incentives and reward for initiative, craftsmanship and the like
- Family welfare advice and services
- Creches for the children of employed mothers
- Insurance facilities against loss of job, illness and disablement.

ix. Environmental monitoring
- Environmental monitoring specially with reference to thermal conditions, lighting, ventilation, dust concentration, etc. by periodical survey goes a long way in reducing occupational hazards.

x. Notification
- Notifiable diseases as The Factories Act should be notified to the Chief-Inspector of Factories, who makes an epidemiological enquiry and gets compensation

- The main purpose of notification in industry is to initiate measures for protection of the workers by investigating the working conditions and to prevent such recurrences.

b. Specific protection
   - When it is not possible or practical to control the environment in which a person works, personal protective measure become necessary which are as follows:
     i. Personal protective equipments
        - Head protection: By wearing helmet of correct size which should not be heavy and made up of noncombustible material and non-conductor of heat and electricity
        - Eyes protection: By suitable protective goggles, heat treated lenses, eye-shields, visors etc.
        - Ear protection: By using ear-plugs, ear-muffs, etc.
        - Skin protection: By using protective clothes against chemicals, asbestos suit against heat, lead apron of 0.5 mm against radiation[Q], etc. protective ointments such as barrier creams against carcinogens, personal cleanliness by daily bath and frequent washing of hands with soap
        - Leg protection: By using safety shoes, gum boots
        - Respiratory protection: By using gas masks and respirators.
     ii. Personal health habits
        - Smoking and alcoholism must always be avoid
        - Nutrition must be adequate
        - Food should never be taken in the work-room, but only in the place meant for it
        - Moderate exercise like early morning walk keeps the worker healthy, active and energetic.
     iii. Immunization
        - The workers should protect themselves against communicable diseases such as cholera, tetanus, typhoid, hepatitis B, and also against rabies among workers in the veterinary hospitals.

B. Secondary prevention
   a. Periodic examination
      - Periodic medical examination is the medical examination of the industrial worker at fixed intervals depending upon the nature of the job and risk involved in it.

Components	*Frequency*
▪ Examination of the worker should include thorough physical examination and biochemical and serological and radiological investigations of necessary ▪ The health data from the preplacement examination serves as a useful guide for comparison and early detection of deviation from health in an individual worker	▪ The frequency of examination hence is variable (depends upon the type of occupational exposure) ▪ In radioactive contaminated areas, it should be done daily, in glass manufacture and lead industries monthly, quarterly in pesticide exposure, half yearly in exposure to carbon disulfide fumes otherwise at least every year in other industries ▪ Particular attention should be given to workers going on or returning from the medical leave in regards to nature and degree of any disability and suitability for returning to the same job

Significance
   - Most of the occupational diseases are insidious in onset, requiring long periods to manifest. Hence, it is vital that the worker is subjected to periodical medical check-ups with necessary investigations
   - The knowledge of the hazards likely to occur, exact nature of job, mode of exposure, earliest, etc. should be known for recommendation of solutions to the problem.

   b. Prompt treatment
      - As soon as the diagnosis is made, the worker is shifted from further exposure of the risk to a safer job and treated promptly to prevent the development of disability.
   c. Personal monitoring
      - This is specially important among those who are exposed to radiation hazards, by wearing Dosimeter on shirt collar, which gives an information about the cumulative dose of the radiation the worker has received.

C. Tertiary prevention
   a. Disability limitation
      - This consists of limiting the development of further disability which occurs usually among the chronic patients and middle aged persons by giving intensive treatment and aid to enable the worker to continue working effectively till retirement.

b. Rehabilitation
- Careful attention must be given to those workers who become physically handicapped during the course of their employment, either by accident or injury
- Such persons are rehabilitated and given a suitable job, so that his/her psychological trauma is countered and becomes a useful person to himself, to the family and country.

SHORT ESSAYS

3. Differences between a screening test and diagnostic test.

Refer Question No. 3 June 2015 (RS2) Paper II.

4. Indicators of human development index.

Refer Question No. 3 December 2009 (RS2) Paper I.

5. Surveillance of drinking water quality.

- Surveillance of drinking water quality is an essential measure of health promotion or disease prevention.

Objective

- To protect public from water-borne diseases.

Elements

A. Sanitary survey
– On-the-spot inspection and evaluation of entire water supply system by a qualified person.

Objective
– Detection and correction of faults and deficiencies.

Significance
– Essential for adequate interpretation of laboratory results.

B. Sampling
– Carried out by competent and trained personnel in strict accordance with methods and frequency of sampling prescribed by WHO or ICMR.

Methods

i. Tap water	▪ Taps in regular use—open the tap fully and let water run for atleast 2 minutes and then fill sample bottle from gentle stream of water (avoiding splashing) holding bottle near the base with one hand ▪ Taps not in regular use—Sterilize the tap (by heating) and then collect as in regular use taps ▪ Avoid collection from leaky taps
ii. Rivers, lakes, reservoirs and wells	▪ Best source is point of draw off (not too near the bank or too far away) ▪ Sterilized bottle with string attached to neck is lowered into water and allowed to fill up OR hold the bottle by bottom and plunge its neck downwards below water surface and slowly brought upwards
iii. Transport and storage	▪ If bacteriological examination of water cannot begin immediately then sample is stored/transported in ice for up to 48 hours

Significance
– Results of analysis depends upon the method of sampling hence, it should be done with aseptic precautions.

C. Bacteriological surveillance
– Bacteriological examination of water is a very delicate and sensitive test for detecting contamination of drinking water by feces or sewage.

Methods

a. Presumptive coliform count
- Presence of coliform organisms[Q] is taken as indicator of feacal pollution of water.
- It is the primary and most reliable indicator for water quality[Q]

- *E. coli*[Q] are chosen because
  - Human intestine secret *E. coli* in abundance about 1 lakhs to 1 million per mL of feces
  - They cannot survive outside human intestine for long period but survive longer than the pathogens of fecal origin
  - They are easy to detect and culture in laboratory[Q]
  - They are always foreign to natural waters
  - They offer greater resistance to forces of natural purification.

Methods

i. Multiple tube method
   - It is done on lactose bile salt medium (MacConkey's broth)[Q]
   - It is based on estimating the most probable number of coliform organisms in 100 mL of water[Q].
   - Bromocresol purple[Q] is used as indicator
   - 16 test tubes containing single or double strength MacConkey's fluid medium are sterilized.
   - Add different quantities of water to be tested as follows.
     * 50 mL of water to 50 mL double strength medium one tube
     * 10 mL of water to 10 mL double strength medium in each of 5 tubes
     * 1 mL of water to 5 mL single strength medium in each of 5 tubes
     * 0.1 mL of water to 5 mL single strength medium in each of 5 tubes
   - Incubate all 16 test tubes for 48 hours
   - From the number of tubes showing acid and gas, an estimate of most probable number of coliform organisms in 100 mL of sample water is obtained from McCrandy's table[Q].
   - It is called presumptive count because the actual number of organism in the sample of water is not counted and the presumption being each tube showing fermentation contains coliform organisms.

   Confirmatory test (Eijkman test[Q]*)*
   - Confirmation of the presence of coliform organisms in each tube showing a presumptive positive reaction is required in chlorinated water
   - It is done by Eijkman's test where each presumptive positive tube is subcultured in 2 tubes of brilliant green bile broth
   - One of this tube is incubated at 37°C for 48 hours and other at 44°C and inspected after 6 hours and 24 hours.
   - *E. coli* is the only coliform organism capable of producing gas from lactose at 44°C
   - Further confirmation can be done by indol production at 44°C.

   WHO recommendations
   - No sample should have *E. coli* in 100 mL[Q]
   - No sample should have more that 3 coliforms per 100 mL[Q]
   - Not more than 5% samples throughout the year should have coliforms in 100 mL. [For large urban areas]
   - Not two consecutive samples should have coliform organism in 100 mL.

ii. Membrane filtration technique
   - In some countries, measured volume of water sample is filtered through a membrane especially made of cellulose ester
   - All the bacteria present in water are retained on the membrane, which is inoculated with face upward on suitable media and at appropriate temperature
   - The colonies produced after 20 hour incubations are counted

b. Detestation of fecal streptococci and *Cl. perfringens*[Q]
   - Presence of fecal streptococci and *Cl. perfringens* provide useful confirmatory evidence of fecal pollution[Q] of water in doubtful cases[Q]

Detection of fecal streptococci	*Detection of Cl. perfringens*
▪ Using glucose azide broth – Multiple portions of water are inoculated into tubes of glucose azide broth and incubated at 37°C for 3 days – Production of acid confirms presence of fecal streptococci	▪ Using DRC medium – Water heated at 75°C for 10 minutes (to destroy nonsporing organisms) is inoculated into differential reinforced clostridium medium in a screw capped bottle at 37°C for 2 days

Contd...

Contd...

Detection of fecal streptococci	*Detection of Cl. perfringens*
▪ Using BAGG medium – Multiple portions of water are inoculated into tubes of buffered azide glucose glycerol broth and incubated at 45°C for 2 days – Production of acid confirms presence of fecal streptococci ▪ Membrane filtration technique – After filtration, membrane placed on well dried plate of glucose azide agar and incubated at 37°C for 4hrs and then at 44°C for 44 hours – All red and maroon colored colonies considered fecal streptococcal colonies **Significance** ▪ Presence of fecal streptococci indicates recent contamination of water[Q]	– Blackening of medium due to reduction of ferrous sulfite and precipitation of ferrous sulfide indicates positive reaction ▪ Sulfite reduction method – Volume of water mixed with melted medium incubated at 37°C for 2 days – Development of black colonies indicate contamination with *Cl. perfringes* **Significance** ▪ Presence of *Cl. perfringens* indicates remote contamination of water[Q]

c. Colony count (plate count)
   - Colony count on nutrient agar at 37°C and 22°C are frequently used in bacteriological examination of water.

Procedure
- Two sterile petri dishes with 1cc of water to be tested are taken, over which 10 cc of nutrient agar is poured
- One petri dish is incubated at 37°C for 2 days and other at 22°C for 3 days.

Observation
- At end of 3 days, count colonies appearing in plates with hand less and expressed as numbers of bacteria per mL of water.

Inference (Recommended plate)

Water at point of consumption	*Plate count*	
	After 2 days at 37°C	*After 3 days at 22°C*
Disinfected	0	20
Not disinfected	10	100

Significance
- It provides an estimate of the general bacterial purity of water
- A single count is of little value but counts from the same source at frequent interval is of considerable value
- A sudden increase in the colony count gives earliest indication of contamination.

Significance
- Bacteriological examination of water both routine or random is very important preventive measure for breaking chain of transmission of feco-oral infections
- Periodicity of routine bacteriological examination is as follows:

Population served	*Minimum interval between successive samples*
<20,000	1 month
20,000–50,000	2 weeks
50,000–100,000	4 days
>100,000	1 day

D. Biological examination
   - Water plankton (microscopic organisms such as algae fungi, yeast, protozoa, rotifers, crustaceans, minute worms) which produce objectionable taste and odor in water
   - They are an index of pollution and degree of pollution is assessed qualitatively and quantitatively by noting type and number of organisms prevailing in water.

E. Chemical surveillance
   - Include basic test such as tests for pH, color, turbidity, chlorides, ammonia, chlorine demand and residual chlorine

– Complete chemical analysis would also include analysis for toxic metals, pesticides, persistent organic chemicals and radioactivity.

Significance

- Surveillance of drinking water is essentially a health measure intended to protect the public from water-borne diseases.

6. Prevalence vs incidence.

Refer Question No. 3 June 2014 (RS2) Paper I.

7. Merits of case control study.

Refer Question No. 1 June 2014 (RS2) Paper I.

8. Natural history of disease.

Refer Question No. 1 December 2007 (RS2) Paper I.

9. Measures of dispersion.

- Measures of dispersion or measures of variations are the calculated variation in a given data of a large group of individuals or even within a single individual
- The widely known measures of dispersion[Q] are:
  a. Range[Q]
  b. Mean[Q] or average deviation
  c. Standard deviation[Q].

Measures of Dispersion

a. Range
   - Range is the difference between the highest and lowest figures in a given sample
   - It is by far the simplest measure of dispersion
   - It is not of much practical importance because it indicates only the extreme values between the two values and nothing about the dispersion of values between the two extreme values.

   Example:
   - In a simple data, it is calculated by subtracting the lowest value from the highest value of the given sample. In case of grouped data, the range is taken as the difference between the midpoints of the extreme categories.

b. Mean deviation
   - It is the average of the deviation from the arithmetic mean
   - It is calculate by the following formula.

$$\text{Mean deviation} = \frac{\sum(x - X)}{\eta}$$

Where
x = single in a given sample
X = arithmetic mean
η = total number of values

Example:
- The mean deviation in the following data of weight of 10 individuals in the age group 40 is calculated as follows:

Weight (x)	Arithmetic mean $= \frac{\Sigma x}{\eta}$ (x)	Deviation from the mean (x – X)
62	64	62 – 64 = - 2
60	64	60 – 64 = - 4
58	64	68 – 64 = - 6

54	64	54 – 64 = - 10
61	64	61 – 64 = - 3
67	64	67 – 64 = 3
80	64	80 – 64 = 16
62	64	62 – 64 = - 2
66	64	66 – 64 = 2
70	64	70 – 64 = 6
		Σ(x – X) = 54

$$\text{Arithmetic mean} = \frac{\sum x}{\eta} = \frac{62+60+58+54+61+67+80+62+66+70}{10} = \frac{640}{10} = 64$$

$$\text{Therefore mean deviation} = \frac{\sum(x-X)}{\eta} = \frac{54}{10} = 5.3$$

c. Standard deviation
- Standard deviation is "Root – Means – Square – Deviation of values from their means
- It is denoted by the Greek letter sigma
- It is the most frequently used measure of deviation[Q] and is also most appropriate
- It is calculated by the following formula
  a. For sample size more than 30[Q]

$$\sigma = \sqrt{\frac{\Sigma(x-X)^2}{\eta}}$$

  b. Sample size less than 30 (Requires substitution of denominator n with η - 1)

$$\sigma = \sqrt{\frac{\Sigma(x-X)^2}{\eta - 1}}$$

- If is an abstract number that gives an idea of the spread of the dispersion, i.e. larger the standard deviation greater the dispersion of values about the mean.

Example:

- For the given weights of individuals in the example the standard deviation is calculated as follows:

x	X	(x – X)	(x – X)²
62	64	- 2	4
60	64	- 4	16
58	64	- 6	36
54	64	- 10	100
61	64	- 3	9
67	64	3	9
80	64	16	256
62	64	- 2	4
66	64	2	4
70	64	6	36

10. Primordial prevention.

Refer Question No. 1 December 2007 (RS2) Paper I.

11. Chlorination.

- Chlorination of water is not mere addition of chlorine to water.

Principles of Chlorination (Prerequisites for Chlorination of Water)

a. Quality of water	▪ Water to be chlorinated should be clear and free from turbidity (turbidity impedes efficient chlorination)
b. Chlorine demand	▪ Chlorine demand of water is difference between amount of chlorine added to water and amount of residual chlorine remaining at end of specific period of contact (usually 1 hour) at given temperature and pH of water ▪ Chlorine demand of water should be calculated before chlorination and addition of chlorine beyond chlorine demand (break point) results in appearance of free chlorine in water
c. Contact period	▪ Contact period is time interval from chlorination till it is free of all bacteria and viruses and is suitable for drinking ▪ It requires atleast 60 minutes to kill all bacteria and viruses (however chlorine has no effect on spores, protozoal cysts and helminthic ova except at higher concentration)
d. Free chlorine	▪ Free chlorine is chlorine beyond chlorine demand of water and is essential to provide margin of safety against subsequent microbial contamination that may occur during storage and distribution ▪ 0.5 mg/L for 1 hour is minimum recommended concentration of free chlorine

Significance

- Chlorination of water is one of the greatest achievements in sanitation and provision of safe potable water
- However, it is futile without following principles of chlorination (prerequisites for chlorination of water).

12. Determinants of health.

- Health is multifactorial and factors which influence health lie both within the individual and externally in the society in which he or she lives.

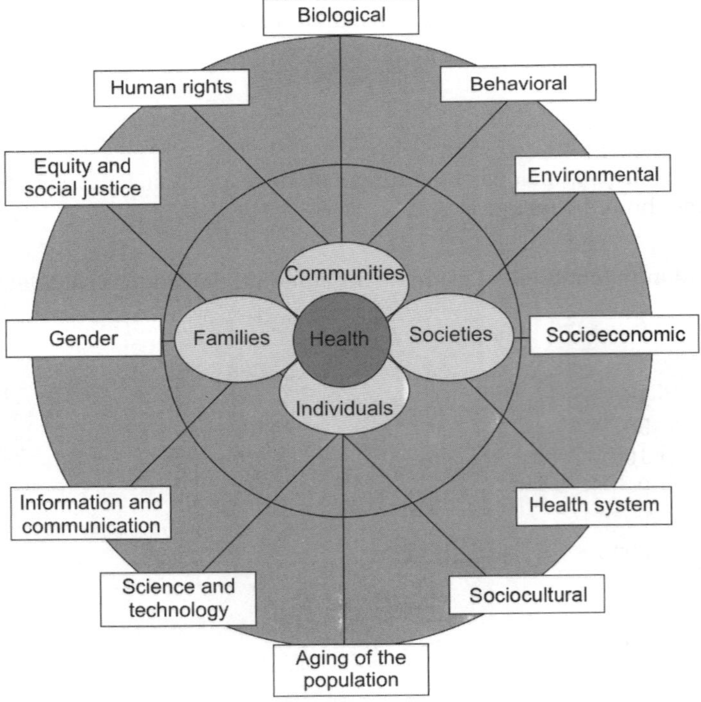

Fig. 1: Determinants of health

Determinants of Health

a. Biological determinants
   – The state of health of an individual depends partly on his genetic constitution

- From the genetic stand-point, health may be defined as that "state of the individual which is based upon the absence from the genetic constitution of such genes as correspond to characters that take the form of serious defect and derangement and to the absence of any aberration in respect of the total amount of chromosome material in the karyotype or stated in positive terms, from the presence in the genetic constitution of the genes that correspond to the normal characterization and to the presence of a normal karyotype"
- Medical genetics offers hope for prevention and treatment of a wide spectrum of diseases, thus the prospect of better medicine and longer, healthier life
- It plays a particularly important role in genetic screening and gene therapy.

b. Behavioral and sociocultural conditions
   - The term lifestyle, reflecting a whole range of social values, attitudes and activities is composed of cultural and behavioral patterns and lifelong personal habits that have developed through processes of socialization
   - Lifestyles are learnt through social interaction with parents, peer groups, friends and siblings and through school and mass media
   - Health requires the promotion of healthy lifestyle
   - There is considerable evidence indicating an association between health and lifestyle of individuals
   - Many health problems especially in the developed countries like coronary heart disease, obesity, lung cancer, drug addiction are associated with lifestyle changes
   - In developing countries such as India where traditional lifestyles still persist, risks of illness and death are connected with lack of sanitation, poor nutrition, personal hygiene, elementary human habits, customs and cultural patterns
   - However, it may be noted that not all lifestyle factors are harmful and there are many that can actually promote health like adequate nutrition, enough sleep, sufficient physical activity, etc.
   - Thus achievement of optimum health demands adoption of healthy lifestyles.

c. Environment
   - Environment is classified as "internal" and "external".

Internal environment	*External environment*
▪ The internal environment of man pertains to "each and every component part, every tissue, organ and organ-system and their harmonious functioning within the system" ▪ It is the domain of internal medicine	▪ The external or macro-environment is defined as all that which is external to the individual human host and consists of those things to which man is exposed after conception ▪ It can be divided into physical, biological and psychosocial components, any or all of which can affect the health of man and his susceptibility to illness

   - Environment has a direct impact on the physical, mental and social well-being of those living in it
   - The environmental factors range from housing, water supply, psychosocial stress and family structure through social and economic support systems, to the organization of health and social welfare services in the community.
   - If the environment is favorable to the individual, he can make full use of his physical and mental capabilities.

d. Socioeconomic conditions
   - People's health status is also determined by their level of socioeconomic development, e.g. per capita GNP, education, nutrition, employment, housing, the political system of the country, etc.

Components

Economic status	*Education*	*Occupation*	*Political system*
The per capita GNP is the most widely accepted measure of general economic performance	A second major factor influencing health status is education (especially female education)	The very state of being employed in productive work promotes health, because the unemployed usually show a higher incidence of ill health and death because for many, loss of work may mean loss of income and status causing psychological and social damage	Health is also related to the country's political system because often the main obstacles to the implementation of health technologies are not technical, but rather political. Decisions concerning resource allocation, manpower policy, choice of technology and the degree to which health services are made available and accessible to different segments of the society are examples of the manner in which the political system can shape community health services

e. Health services
   - The term health and family welfare services cover a wide spectrum of personal and community services for treatment of disease, prevention of illness and promotion of health

  - The purpose of health services is to improve the health status of population
  - To be effective, the health services must reach the social periphery, equitably distributed, accessible at a cost the country and community can afford and socially acceptable.
f. Aging of the population
  - A major concern of rapid population aging is the increased prevalence of chronic diseases and disabilities both being conditions that tend to accompany the aging process and deserve special attention.
g. Gender
  - Action for promoting women's health should cover nutrition, reproductive health, the health consequences of violence, aging, lifestyle related conditions and the occupational environment.
h. Other factors
  - The development of information and communication offers tremendous opportunities in providing an easy and instant access to medical information once difficult to retrieve
  - It contributes to dissemination of information worldwide, serving the needs of many physicians, health professionals, biomedical scientists and researchers, the mass media and the public
  - Other contributions to the health of population derive from systems outside the formal health care system, i.e. health-related systems (e.g. food and agriculture, education, industry, social welfare, rural development) as well as adoption of policies in the economic and social fields that would assist in raising the standards of living
  - This would include employment opportunities, increased wages, prepaid medical programs and family support systems.

Significance

- In short, medicine is not the sole contributor to the health and well-being of population
- The potential of intersectoral contributions to the health of communities is increasingly recognized.

SHORT ANSWERS

13. Define epidemic.

Refer Question No. 4 December 2016 (RS2) Paper I.

14. National Immunization schedule for Under-5.

Refer Question No. 20 December 2007 (RS2) Paper II.

15. Odds ratio.

Refer Question No. 1 June 2014 (RS2) Paper I.

16. Prevention of drug dependence.

Refer Question No. 10 December 2007 (RS2) Paper I.

17. Characteristics of reference adult Indian woman.

- Concept of reference man/woman was first devised by FAO committee for calorie requirement in 1950 and has been in use ever since.

Characteristics of Indian Reference Woman (as defined by ICMR)

Characteristic	*Reference adult woman*	*Reference adult man*
Age	18 to 29 years[Q]	18 to 29 years[Q]
Weight	55 kg	60 kg[Q]
Height	1.61 m	1.73 m
Body mass index	21.2	20.3

Contd...

Contd...

Characteristic	Reference adult woman	Reference adult man
Body surface area	1.4 m^2	1.62 m^2
Basal metabolic rate (BMR)	31.6 K cal/hour/m^2	35.5 K cal/hour/m^2
Associated conditions	Non pregnant and non-lactating Free from disease and physically fit and mentally alert	Free from disease and physically fit and mentally alert
Type of work	Moderate activity	Moderate activity[Q]
Daily activities	8 hours of work 8 hours sleeping in bed 4-6 hours of sitting and moving around 2 hours of walking and active recreation/household duties	8 hours of work[Q] 8 hours sleeping in bed[Q] 4–6 hours of sitting and moving around 2 hours of walking[Q] and active recreation/household duties
Energy requirement	1900 Kcal of energy per day[Q] and 60 gms of protein per day[Q]	2400 Kcal of energy per day[Q] and 60gms of protein per day[Q]

Significance

- Concept of reference man/woman is adopted universally for estimating the energy needs of a person based on weight, body surface area, BMR and activities.

18. Types of communication.

- Communication is countless ways that humans have of keeping in touch with one another.

Types of Communication

Type	Features	Remarks
a. One-way communication (Didactic Method)	One way flow of communication from communicator to audience	Disadvantage ▪ Formal method ▪ Knowledge is imposed ▪ Learning is authoritative ▪ Little audience participation ▪ No feedback ▪ Does not influence human behavior
b. Two-way communication (Socratic method)	Both communicator and audience take part Audience may raise questions and add their own information, ideas and opinions to the subject	Advantages ▪ More informal ▪ Active learning ▪ Democratic ▪ Instant feedback ▪ Influences behavior
c. Verbal communication	Word of mouth	▪ Traditional ▪ Persuasive ▪ May be loaded with hidden meanings
d. Non-verbal communication	Includes a whole range of bodily movements, postures, gestures, facial expressions (smile, raised eye brows, frown, staring, gazing, etc.)	▪ Effective as silence speaks louder than words
e. Formal and informal communication	Formal (follows lines of authority)—circulars Informal (grape-vine)—gossips	
f. Visual communication	Comprises charts and graphs, pictograms, tables, maps, posters, etc.	
g. Telecommunication and internet	Process of communicating over distance using electromagnetic instruments designed for purpose	Mass media—Radio, TV and internet ▪ Advantage: Large number reached in short time ▪ Disadvantage: Not very effective in bringing about changes Point-to-point system: Telephone and telegraph ▪ Advantage: Very effective

19. Record linkage.

Refer Question No. 12 June 2014 (RS2) Paper I.

20. Employees State Insurance Act.

Refer Question No. 4 December 2012 (RS2) Paper I.

21. Warning signals of poor mental health.

Refer Question No. 6 June 2009 (RS2) Paper I.

22. Panel discussion.

Refer Question No. 2 June 2009 (RS2) Paper I.

MBBS PHASE III EXAMINATION

JUNE 2016

(Revised Scheme 2 & 3)

PAPER II

LONG ESSAYS

1. Discuss the various modes of transmission of communicable diseases.

Refer Question No. 1 June 2009 (RS2) Paper I.

2. Describe the epidemiology of road traffic injury. Describe the prevention and control of accidents in India.

- Accident is an unpremeditated event resulting in recognizable damage (WHO).

Road Traffic Accidents

- Road traffic accidents is highest contributor of accidental deaths and for every road traffic death, 10–15 are seriously injured.

Epidemiological Factors

a. Agent factors	
i. Type of vehicle	▪ More common with 2 wheelers because they are unstable and provide less protection to their riders
ii. Speed of vehicle	▪ Over speeding increases risk of accident manifold
iii. Maintenance of vehicle	▪ Poorly maintained vehicles usually get involved in accidents
b. Host factors (Human factors)	
i. Age	▪ Incidence high in age group of 15–34 years
ii. Sex	▪ Usually common in males
iii. Pedestrians	▪ Pedestrians are more affected than riders
iv. Medical conditions	▪ Existing medical conditions like epilepsy, vertigo, refractory errors, etc. contribute to accidents
v. Habits	▪ Habits like smoking, alcoholism, talking on phone etc play significant role in road accidents
vi. Other factors	▪ Fatigue, boredom, anxiety, hurry predispose individual to road accidents ▪ Lack of protective equipment is related to chances of morbidity and mortality in an accident
vii. Psychological factors	▪ Delayed judgment, faulty perception, mental condition at time of accident
c. Environmental factors	
i. Relating to road	▪ More common in urban areas ▪ Defective, narrow roads, curvy or slippery roads contribute to accidents ▪ Presence of cross roads, poor signaling and poor lighting also play important role
ii. Relating to vehicles	▪ Overloading may cause accidents ▪ Low driving standards also contribute to accidents
iii. Season	▪ More common in rainy season and winter (due to fog and poor weather)
iv. Mixed traffic	▪ Common where pedestrians and animals easily get onto roads
v. Legislation	▪ Ignorance about rules ▪ Lax implementation of traffic rules ▪ Fraudulent issue of driving licenses

Prevention and Control

a. Seat belts	▪ Use of seat belts approximately by 50% number of fatalities and non-fatal injuries ▪ Their use has been made mandatory in major cities across India
b. Safety helmets	▪ Use of helmets reduces the risk of head injury by 30% and fatalities by 40% ▪ Their use by a two wheeler rider is compulsory as per Motor Vehicle Act and Government of Karnataka has made it mandatory in corporation limits of Bengaluru, Mysore, Mangaluru, Belgavi and Karnataka ▪ A good helmet is one which – Covers the maximum area of head and face – Provides thermocol padding of atleast 22 mm – Is visible clearly, i.e. of yellow or orange color or has reflective stripes on back and side
c. Leather clothing and boots	▪ Leather clothing and boots reduces the risk of extensive superficial soft tissue injury and therefore their use should be encouraged
d. Children	▪ Children should remain seated in a vehicle and they should not be seated in front seats
e. Use of headlights	▪ Headlights be used in day to enhance visibility of the vehicle and thus reduces the chance of accident ▪ Even in night, the headlights should be on low beam to avoid dazzling the oncoming vehicle
f. Drinking and driving	▪ Education of people and strict law enforcement can reduce alcohol related accidents
g. Mobile phones	▪ Use of mobile phones while driving should be prohibited as it diverts the attention
h. Use of proper glass in wind screen	▪ Indian vehicles should use laminated wind shield rather than toughened glass to avoid excess damage
i. Pneumatic bus doors	
j. Curb parking	

Significance

- Accident is one of the major causes of death in most countries and these deaths can be prevented by following safety measures.

SHORT ESSAYS

3. Epidemiological indices in tuberculosis.

Refer Question No. 1 December 2009 (RS2) Paper II.

4. Typhoid vaccines.

Refer Question No. 10 June 2010 (RS2) Paper II.

5. Socioeconomic effects of smoking.

- Smoking has been incriminated in numerous diseases and is a major health care concern
- However, besides being a health care issue, it also affects social and economic dimension of a person's life
- Smoking besides affecting the smoker, also affects the people in vicinity due to passive smoking which is a major social problem associated with smoking
- With increasing health awareness about passive smoking, smokers have become social outcasts
- Smoking also takes toll on the finances of the smoker as, to discourage smoking, Government has levied numerous taxes on the cigarettes
- Smoker also incurs additional expenses on the health care for the diseases resulting from smoking
- Smoking and also passive smoking decrease the productivity of workers
- Illness due to smoking leads to sickness absenteeism which is an economical loss the nation besides the employee (smoker)
- Fires related to cigarette smoking are the leading cause of civilian fire deaths and health care cost for burn patients is also substantial
- So, it is obvious that non-smoking would save health care-related money.

Ref: Kim YW; The socioeconomic effects of tobacco smoking, J Korean Med Assoc. 2004 March;47(3):209–13.

6. Ebola fever.

- Ebola fever (Ebola hemorrhagic fever) is a new emerging fatal viral hemorrhagic fever
- Viruses target small capillaries, causing leak of blood eventually leading to multiorgan failure.

Agent factors	*Incubation period*	*Case fatality rate*	*Reservoirs*
Ebola virus, a ssRNA virus of family Filoviridiae group	2–21 days (non-infective)	70–90%	Monkeys, fruit bats, chimpanzees, gorillas

Transmission

- Animal to human transmission through direct contact with blood, organs, body secretions or other body fluids of infected animals
- Human to human transmission through blood or body fluids of infected symptomatic person or exposure to contaminated objects
- Not transmitted through air, water or food.

Clinical Features

- Sudden onset of fever, intense weakness, muscle pain, headache, sore throat, vomiting, bloody diarrhoea, impaired renal and hepatic functions
- A rash appears within a week and hemorrhagic spots appear over trunk and mucous membranes
- Bleeding—both internally and externally
- Gastrointestinal bleeding is common and often profuse leading to shock and death
- Profound leukopenia and thrombocytopenia are observed.

Prevention and Control

Primary prevention		*Secondary prevention*
Health education	*Specific protection*	*Early diagnosis and treatment*
▪ Health education during epidemics about modes of spread of diseases	▪ No vaccine ▪ Use of universal precautions by health care workers	▪ No specific treatment ▪ Intensive supportive care (reduces mortality and disease transmission)

Significance

- Ebola virus being a highly contagious virus with no specific treatment or vaccine has been forefront of research in medical treatment and also in biological weapon.

7. Srivastava committee.

Refer Question No. 6 June 2010 (RS2) Paper II.

8. UNICEF.

Refer Question No. 8 June 2010 (RS2) Paper II.

9. Community needs assessment approach.

- Community needs assessment approach is a newer, innovative method of family planning promotion
- Implemented since April 1996
- Here, the health workers consult target couples to assess their needs and preference at start of the year to work out a yearly program and workload for themselves
- Contraceptive requirement of PHC is sum of all the requirements of the ANMs in their jurisdiction.

Special features	Advantages	Disadvantages
▪ Program is target free ▪ Evaluation is based on population goals	▪ Reflects user preference ▪ Feedback mechanism regarding preference of contraceptive in a particular age group or region ▪ Improved quality of service and care ▪ Higher compliance ▪ Genuine performance stastitics	▪ Success based on highly motivated voluntary health worker ▪ Requirements calculated by health workers themselves ▪ Difficult to evaluate ▪ Possibility of falsification of data

Significance

- Community needs assessment approach is a novel idea based on the concept of Cafeteria Approach where community is provided based on their preference and requirements.

10. "Lifestyle" as etiology of diseases.

- Lifestyle denotes the way people live reflecting a whole range of social values, attitudes and activities
- It is composed of cultural and behavioral patterns and life-long personal habits that have developed through processes of socialization, i.e. learnt through social interactions with parents peer, group, friends and siblings and through school and mass media
- Health requires promotion of healthy lifestyle
- Many current day health problems especially in the developed countries are associated with lifestyle changes, e.g. coronary heart disease, obesity, lung cancer, drug addiction, etc.
- In developing countries, lifestyle pattern such as lack of sanitation, poor nutrition, personal hygiene, elementary human habits, customs and cultural patterns are the risk factors for illness and death
- But it must be noted that not all the lifestyle factors are harmful. There are some which actually promote heath, e.g. adequate nutrition, enough sleep, sufficient physical activity, etc.
- In short adoption of healthy lifestyle helps to achieve optimum health.

Lifestyle factors promoting health	Lifestyle factors causing disease
▪ Adequate nutrition, yoga exercises, meditation, enough sleep, etc.	▪ Use of alcohol, drugs, tobacco ▪ Sedentary lifestyle

Significance

- Lifestyle changes that promote health can be influenced by health education
- Health education is a basic element of all health activity
- It is of paramount importance in changing views, behavior and habits of people (critical awareness and lifestyle changes[Q])
- The health education is the responsibility of the individual, community, physician and health worker in particular.

11. Integrated approach for vector control.

Refer Question No. 11 June 2010 (RS2) Paper I.

12. Integrated disease surveillance project.

- Integrated disease surveillance system is a decentralized, state based, surveillance program in the country started in 1998.
- It is called integrated because there is incorporation of:

Health sectors	Diseases	Health systems	Health Agencies
▪ Public sector ▪ Private sector ▪ Community participation	▪ Communicable ▪ Noncommunicable	▪ Rural health system ▪ Urban health system	▪ Medical colleges ▪ International health agencies like WHO, CDC, NIH, USAID, DFIS and others

Objectives

- To establish a decentralized surveillance system in the country
- To detect early warning signals of impeding outbreak
- To initiate control measures early, by allocating the health resources more efficiently
- To study the disease pattern and to identify new emerging diseases
- To involve all stakeholders (public and private sector and community) in surveillance
- To involve paramedical personnel in surveillance system.

Surveillance Methods

Surveillance classification	*Diagnosis by*	*Based on*	*Case classification*
a. Syndromic	Paramedical worker/community member	Clinical pattern	Suspect case
b. Presumptive	Medical officer or private doctor	History and clinical examination	Probable case
c. Laboratory	Laboratory test	—	Confirmed case

Diseases and Conditions Covered Under Integrated Disease Surveillance System

Category	*Disease and condition*
▪ Regular surveillance	
i. Vector-borne disease	▪ Malaria
ii. Water-borne disease	▪ Acute diarrheal disease (Cholera[Q]) ▪ Typhoid
iii. Respiratory disease	▪ Tuberculosis[Q]
iv. Vaccine preventable diseases	▪ Measles ▪ Polio
v. Other conditions	▪ Accidents
vi. Other international commitments	▪ Plague
vii. Unusual clinical syndromes	▪ Meningoencephalitis[Q] ▪ Respiratory distress[Q] ▪ Hemorrhagic fevers ▪ Other undiagnosed conditions
▪ Sentinel surveillance	
i. STIs/Blood borne diseases	▪ HIV ▪ Hepatitis B ▪ Hepatitis C
ii. Other conditions	▪ Water quality ▪ Outdoor air quality
• Regular periodic survey[Q]	
i. Noncommunicable risk factors	▪ Anthropometry ▪ Physical activity ▪ Blood pressure ▪ Tobacco ▪ Nutrition ▪ Blindness
▪ Public health emergency	▪ Other unusual health emergencies

Significance

- Integrated disease surveillance system is an effective tool for early identification and effective control of epidemics.

SHORT ANSWERS

13. Triage.

Refer Question No. 16 June 2013 (RS2) Paper II.

14. Syndromic management of urethral discharge.

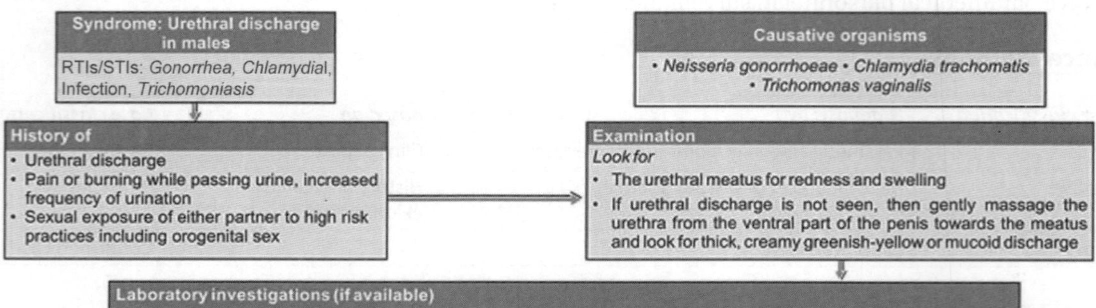

Laboratory investigations (if available)

- Gram stain examination of the urethral smear will show Gram-negative intracellular diplococci in case of gonorrhea
- In nongonococcal urethritis more than 5 neutrophils per oil immersion field (1000X) in the urethral smear or more than 10 neutrophils per high field in the sediment of the first void urine are observed

Treatment

As dual infection is common, the treatment for urethral discharge should adequately cover therapy for both, gonorrhea and chlamydial infections.

Recommended regimen for uncomplicated gonorrhea + chlamydia

Uncomplicated infections indicate that the disease is limited to the anogenital region (anterior urethritis and proctitis).

- Tablet Cefixime 400 mg orally, single dose Plus Tab Azithromycin 1 g orally single dose under supervision
- Advise the client to return after 7 days of start of therapy

When symptoms persist or recur after adequate treatment for gonorrhea and chlamydia in the index client and partner(s), they should be treated for *Trichomonas vaginalis.*

If discharge or only dysuria persists after 7 days

- Tablet Secnidazole 2 g orally, single dose (to treat for *T. vaginalis*)

If the symptoms still persists

- Refer to higher center as early as possible

If individuals are allergic to Azithromycin, give Erythromycin 500 mg four times a day for 7 days

Syndrome specific guidelines for partner management

- Treat all recent partners
- Treat female partners (for gonorrhea and chlamydia) on same lines after ruling out pregnancy and history of allergies
- Advise sexual abstinence during the course of treatment
- Provide condoms, educate about correct and consistent use
- Refer for voluntary counseling and testing for HIV, Syphilis and Hepatitis B
- Schedule return visit after 7 days

Follow-up
After seven days

- To see reports of tests done for HIV, syphilis and Hepatitis B
- If symptoms persist, to assess whether it is due to treatment failure or reinfection
- For prompt referral if required

Management of pregnant partner

Pregnant partners of male clients with urethral discharge should be examined by doing a per speculum as well as per vaginal examination and should be treated for gonococcal as well as chlamydial infections

- Cephalosporins to cover gonococcal infection are safe and effective in pregnancy
- Tablet Cefixime 400 mg orally, single dose or
- Ceftriaxone 125 mg by intramuscular injection +
- Tablet Erythromycin 500 mg orally four times a day for seven days or
- Cap Amoxicillin 500 mg orally, three times a day for seven days to cover chlamydial infection
- Quinolones (like ofloxacin, ciprofloxacin), doxycycline are contraindicated in pregnant women

15. Causes for blindness in India.

Refer Question No. 12 December 2009 (RS2) Paper II.

16. Vaccines for cancer.

- Vaccines for primary prevention of cancer at the forefront of Medical Research
- Currently only vaccines available are for prevention of hepatic cancer and cervical cancer.

Vaccines for Cancer

a. Hepatic carcinoma
   – Hepatic carcinoma is linked to infection with Hepatitis B virus hence it could be prevented by hepatitis B vaccine

For hepatitis B vaccine

Refer Question No. 1 December 2014 (RS2) Paper II.

b. Cervical cancer
   – Human papilloma virus (HPV) has been incriminated as the important cause of cervical cancer
   – Currently 2 vaccines are available for immunisation against cervical cancer, one of which is approved by Food and Drug Administration (FDA).

HPV vaccine

	Gardasil	*Cervarix*
Status	Approved by FDA (2006)	--
Type	Killed vaccine	Killed vaccine
Contents	HPV types 6, 11, 16 and 18 (Quadrivalent)	HPV types 16 and 18 (Bivalent)
Formulation	Liquid vaccine	Liquid vaccine
Storage	2–8°C but not frozen	2–8°C but not frozen
Protection	100%	100%
Dose	0.5 mL	0.5 mL
Route	Intramuscular (Deltoid)	Intramuscular (Deltoid)
Schedule	3 doses at 0, 1 and 6 months	3 doses at 0, 1 and 6 months
Indications	Immunisation of girls and women aged 6 to 26 years	Immunization of girls and women aged 6 to 26 years
Timing	Before acquiring any HPV infection (i.e. before sexual debut)	Before acquiring any HPV infection (i.e. before sexual debut)
Effective against	Cervical cancer, vulvar and vaginal precancers (caused by HPV types 16 and 18) Genital warts (caused by HPV types 6 and 11)	Cervical cancer, vulvar and vaginal precancers (caused by HPV types 16 and 18)

Disadvantages

– Costly
– Specific to certain cancers, i.e. does not cover the 30% of cancers attributed to other HPV types.

Status in India

– Trials are under study to observe its efficacy and safety
– Challenges for introduction of HPV vaccine in India include:
  - Relatively high cost
  - Reaching the target population
  - Poor health care infrastructure, inadequate maintenance of cold chain and injection safety
  - Competition faced from other newer vaccines like Hib, pneumococcal, rotavirus, meningococcal, JE vaccines, etc.
  - Poor success of secondary prevention methods like HPV screening, Pap testing, etc.
  - Religious barriers, cultural taboos and misconceptions influencing acceptance by the public at large
  - Lack of political will.

Significance

- Cancer is a major cause of mortality besides the morbidity and vaccines against cancer would a major accomplishment in reduction of death rate of a country and improving quality of life

17. Infant Mortality Rate.

Refer Question No. 2 June 2011 (RS2) Paper II.

18. HAART (Human Aids Antiretro Viral Therapy).

- Treatment protocol consisting of atleast three antiretroviral drugs used in treatment of AIDS is called Highly Active Antiretroviral Therapy (HAART)
- HAART therapy is known to suppress HIV replication and it has demonstrated superiority in reducing the virus to less than detectable level in the blood.

Principle

- Three drugs are used in order to reduce the likelihood of the virus developing resistance.

HAART Regimen (WHO 2015)

	First line regimen	*Second line regimen*
Principle	▪ TDF + 3TC (or FTC) + EFV at standard doses (600 mg/day) is the preferred first-line regimen for treatment initiation in antiretroviral therapy (ART)-naïve adults and adolescents because this approach has clinical, operational and programmatic benefits when compared with other NNRTI- and PI-based options ▪ Dolutegravir (DTG) and EFV at lower dose (400 mg/day) are included as new alternative options in first-line regimens ▪ AZT and NVP are maintained as alternative drug options	▪ Simple second-line regimens includes the combination of 2 NRTIs + a heat stable boosted protease inhibitor ▪ LPV/r and ATV/r heat stable co-formulations are the preferred PI options for second line therapy, and DRV/r is recommended as an alternative option
Preferred option	TDF+XTC3+EFV_{600}	2 NRTI+ATV/r or LPV/r
Alternative options	AZT+3TC+EFV_{600} AZT+3TC+NVP TDF+XTC+NVP TDF+XTC+DTG TDF+XTC+EFV	2 NRTI+DRV/r LPV/r+RAL
Note	▪ FDCs are the preferred approach ▪ XTC = 3TC or FTC	▪ Recommended sequence of 2nd line NRTI backbone options – If failure with TDF+XTC in 1st line, use AZT+3TC – If failure with AZT+3TC in 1st line, use TDF+XTC – Use of NRTI backbones as FDCs is recommended as the preferred approach ▪ 2 Heat stable FDCs of boosted PIs are the preferred approach

Key

	Drug	*Class*
TDF	Tenofovir Disoproxil Fumarate	NRTI
3TC	Lamivudine	NRTI
AZT	Zidovudine	NRTI
FTC	Emtricitabine	NRTI
EFV	Efavirenz	NNRTI
NVP	Nevirapine	NNRTI
ATV/r	Atazanavir + Ritonavir	Protease inhibitor
LPV/r	Lopinavir + Ritonavir	Protease inhibitor
DRV/r	Darunavir + Ritonavir	Protease inhibitor
DTG	Dolutegravir	Integrase inhibitor
RAL	Raltegravir	Integrase inhibitor

Advantages	*Disadvantages*
▪ Reduced mortality and morbidity rates among HIV-infected people ▪ Lower risk of opportunistic infections ▪ Improved quality of life	▪ Long-term commitment to high levels of adherence ▪ Short- and longer-term side-effects ▪ Drug–drug interactions ▪ Potential for development of resistant viral strains

Significance

- Ever since the advent of HAART in 1996 there has been a drastic reduction in opportunistic infections.

19. Severe acute respiratory syndrome.

- SARS or severe acute respiratory syndrome is an acute, highly infectious respiratory disease caused by a new strain of corona virus usually transmitted by droplet infection, common among adults, clinically characterized by short incubation period, mild prodromal symptoms followed by respiratory symptoms rich as cough, breathlessness and progressive hypoxemia.
- Earliest case was reported from China[Q].

Epidemiology

Agent factors	▪ SARS virus is a deadly new strain, belonging to coronavirus family, closely related to common cold virus ▪ It is a single stranded, RNA virus, non-segmented and enveloped, 80–140 nm in size ▪ It has projections on the surface known as peplomers giving it an appearance of halo ▪ Human pathogens belong to 229E and OC-43 serogroups ▪ The envelop has S (spike) protein, M (matrix) protein and HF (hemagglutinin)
Reservoir	▪ Humans are the only reservoirs and there is no known animal reservoir
Age incidence	▪ Common in age group above 25 years
Sex incidence	▪ More common amongst males than females
Mode of transmission	▪ Transmitted by droplet nuclei ▪ Other suspected mode of transmission is through fomites
Infectious material	▪ Nasal and throat secretions are highly infectious ▪ Virus has also been found in urine and stool samples
Period of infectivity	▪ SARS patients are infectious during the period of illnessQ but there is no data about their infective status during incubation period and during convalescent period.
Incubation period	▪ 2–7 days (maximum 10 days)

Clinical features	*Investigations*	*Treatment*
a. Prodromal phase – Characterized by mild to moderate high fever associated with chills, rigors, headache, malaise and myalgia lasting for two to four days b. Respiratory phase – Characterized by dry cough, breathlessness, features of atypical pneumonia, progressing to hypoxemia – Few respiratory crackles are heard – Anorexia, confusion, muscular stiffness are also present – Death due to progressive respiratory failure	a. X-ray chest – Febrile phase – Normal – Respiratory phase – Generalized patchy infiltrations b. CT scan – Ground glass opacification in peripheral subpleural areas c. Hematological findings – Lekopenia, lymphopenia, thrombocytopenia d. Biochemical findings – Hyponatremia, hypokalemia, elevated levels of serum ALT, LDH and CPK e. Specific tests – Electron microscopy, culture on Vero cell lines, indirect immunofluorescent test, PCR test	▪ No specific treatment ▪ Antiviral agent Ribavirin with steroids promises good results

Prevention and Control

a. Surveillance (WHO case definition for surveillance purpose)	i. Suspect case – A person presenting after 1st November 2002 with history of: ❖ High fever (>38°C) ❖ Cough or breathing difficulty ❖ One or more of these features - Close contact with a suspect or probable case of SARS history of travel to SARS affected area - Residing in an affected area ii. Probable case – A suspect case with radiographic evidence of infiltrates consistent with pneumonia or respiratory distress on chest X-ray
b. Early detection of infection	▪ IEC activities to be carried out vigorously ▪ Heightened index of suspicion among the patient giving H/O contact with SARS patients or H/O travel to SARS endemic areas ▪ Segregation of symptomatic ▪ Notification ▪ Visual alert
c. Containment of infection	▪ Segregation of suspect cases until confirmation of diagnosis ▪ Isolation of SARS patients in designated wards, having a negative pressure room ▪ Doors always kept closed ▪ No visitors ▪ Maximizing natural ventilation by opening the windows and also by using exhaust fans ▪ Minimizing people traffic in hospital ▪ Dedicated staff to take care of the patient ▪ Barrier nursing to all the SARS patients ▪ Concurrent disinfection of respiratory secretions, line, utensils, etc. ▪ Treatment protocol
d. Personal protective attire	▪ Respiratory protection by N-95 masks ▪ Eyes protection by goggles ▪ Contact protection by gloves and gowns
e. Care of environment	▪ Disinfection of soiled linen ▪ Safe disposal of biohazard waste
f. Other measures	▪ Avoid use of nebulizer ▪ Limit the patient movements ▪ Place mask or gown on the patient during transportation

Significance

- SARS is a new emerging infectious disease posing a problem to entire medical fraternity around the world today.

20. DOTS agents.

- DOTS agents are health workers who administer antitubercular treatment under direct supervision
- Ideal DOTS agents are accessible and acceptable to patients and accountable to health system
- Family members are not effective DOTS agents.

Examples	*Incentives (per patient completed treatment)*	*Job responsibility*
▪ Health worker (male), ASHA, teachers, anganwadi workers, social workers, ex-patients, members of nongovernmental organizations (NGOs)	₹ 1,000 for Category I ₹ 1,500 for Category II ₹ 5,000 for drug resistant TB	▪ Direct observation of the TB patient swallowing every dose of anti-TB drugs – Intensive phase: All at a time, preferably empty stomach – Continuation phase: First dose of the week and checking the returned multiblister combipack for compliance ▪ Motivating and supporting the TB patient to continue and complete the course

Revised Scheme 2 & 3

Significance

- DOTS agents are the backbone of the Revised National Tuberculosis Program (RNTCP) and are instrumental in its success.

21. Principles of primary health care.

Refer Question No. 4 June 2012 (RS2) Paper II.

22. Assessment of obesity.

Refer Question No. 4 June 2010 (RS2) Paper II.

MBBS PHASE III EXAMINATION

DECEMBER 2016

(Revised Scheme 2 & 3)

PAPER I

LONG ESSAYS

1. Describe a cohort study with a suitable example.

- Epidemiology is the study of the distribution and determinants of health related states or events in specified populations, and the applications of this study in control of health problems.

Types of Epidemiological Studies[Q]

Observational studies		*Experimental studies intervention studies*
Descriptive studies[Q] (done for diseases who etiology is unknown[Q])	Analytical studies • Ecological[Q] • Cross sectional • Case control • Cohort	• Randomized controlled trials • Field trials • Community trials

Cohort Study

- Cohort study is a type of analytical study usually undertaken to obtain additional evidence to refute or support the existence of an association between suspected cause and disease.

Also known as (**Synonyms[Q]**)	*Characteristics*	*Indications*
▪ Prospective study ▪ Forward looking study ▪ Cause to effect study ▪ Exposure to outcome study ▪ Risk factor to disease study ▪ Incidence study ▪ Follow up study	▪ The cohorts are identified prior to the appearance of the disease under investigation ▪ The study groups so define are observed over a period of time to determine the frequency of disease among them ▪ The study proceeds forward from cause to effect	▪ When there is good evidence of an association between exposure and disease, as derived from clinical observations and supported by descriptive and case control studies ▪ When exposure is rare but the incidence is high among exposed ▪ When attrition of study population can be minimized ▪ When ample funds are available

Cohort Selection

- Cohort is a group of people who share a common characteristic or experience within a define time period
- For selecting a cohort, following facts should be considered:
  - Cohorts must be free from the disease under study
  - Both the study and control cohorts should be equally susceptible to the disease under study or efficiently reflect any difference in disease occurrence
  - Both the cohort must be comparable in respect to all possible variables which may influence the frequency of disease
  - Diagnostic and eligibility criteria of the disease must be defined before hand.

Framework of a Cohort Study

- Basic design of simple cohort study is as follows:

Cohort	*Disease*		*Total*
	Yes	*No*	
Exposed to putative etiological agent	a	b	a + b
Not exposed to putative etiological agent	c	d	c + d

- It consists of two cohorts:
  – Study cohort consisting of people exposed to a particular agent thought to be related to disease occurrence
  – Control cohort consisting of people not exposed to that particular agent.

Types of Cohort Studies[Q]

a. Prospective cohort studies[Q]	▪ A prospective or current cohort study is one in which the outcome has not yet occurred at the time the investigation begins ▪ Also known as current cohort study or concurrent cohort study ▪ Most prospective studies begin in the present and continue into future ▪ Investigator look for development of same disease in both exposed and non-exposed groups *Examples* ▪ Framingham heart study ▪ Doll and Hills prospective study on smoking and lung cancer
b. Retrospective cohort studies[Q]	▪ A retrospective or historical cohort study is one in which the outcomes have all occurred before the start of the investigation ▪ Also known as historical cohort study or non-concurrent cohort study ▪ The investigator goes back in time, sometimes 10–30 years, to select his study groups from existing records of past employment, medical or other records and traces them forward through time, from a past date fixed on the records, usually up to the present ▪ Sample size required is same as that of prospective cohort study ▪ Retrospective cohort studies are generally more economical and produce results more quickly than prospective cohort studies ▪ It combines advantages of both cohort study and case control study *Examples* ▪ Effect of fetal monitoring on neonatal deaths ▪ PVC exposure and angiosarcoma of liver
c. A combination of retrospective and prospective cohort studies[Q] (mixed cohort study)	▪ In this type of study, both the retrospective and prospective elements are combined, i.e. the cohort is identified from past records, and is assessed of date for the outcome and is followed up prospectively into future for further assessment of outcome ▪ Also known as mixed cohort study ▪ Combines designs of both prospective cohort study and retrospective cohort study *Examples* ▪ Court Brown and Doll study on effects of radiation therapy

Steps of Cohort Study

- Selection of study subjects
- Obtaining data on exposure
- Selection of comparison groups
- Follow-up
- Analysis.

A. Selection of study subjects
- The subjects of a cohort study are usually assembled from:

General population	Special groups	
	Select groups	Exposure groups
▪ When the exposure or cause of death is fairly frequent in the population, cohorts may be assembled from the general population, residing in well defined geographical, political and administrative areas ▪ If the population is very large, an appropriate sample is taken, so that the results can be generalized to the population sampled	▪ These may be professional groups, insured persons, obstetric population, college alumni, government employees, volunteers, etc. ▪ These groups are usually a homogeneous population and also offer advantages of accessibility and easy follow-up for a protracted period	▪ If the exposure is rare, a cohort of persons known to have experienced the exposure to physical, chemical and other disease agents is selected ▪ A readily accessible source of these groups is workers in industries and those employed in high-risk situations ▪ Such selection, it facilitates classification of cohort members according to the degree or duration of exposure to the suspected factor for subsequent analytical study

B. Obtaining data on exposure
- Information about exposure is obtained directly from the any one or all the following sources

Cohort members	Review of records	Medical examination or special tests	Environmental surveys
▪ Through personal interviews or mailed questionnaires ▪ Since cohort studies involve large numbers of population, mailed questionnaires offer a simple and economic way of obtaining information	▪ Certain kinds of information like dose of radiation, kinds of surgery, or details of medical treatment can be obtained only from medical records	▪ Some types of information like blood pressure, serum cholesterol, etc. can be obtained only by medical examination or special tests	▪ This is the best source for obtaining information on exposure levels of the suspected factor in the environment where the cohort lived or worked

- Information about exposure should be collected in a manner that will allow classification of cohort members.
  - According to whether or not they have been exposed to the suspected factor
  - According to the level or degree of exposure, at least in broad classes.
- In addition to the above, basic information about demographic variables which might affect the frequency of disease under investigation, should also be collected
- Such information will be required for subsequent analysis.

C. Selection of comparison groups
- There are many ways of assembling comparison groups

Internal comparisons	External comparisons	Comparison with general population rates
▪ In some cohort studies, the comparison groups are in-built. ▪ That is, single cohort enters the study, and its members may, on the basis of information obtained, be classified into several comparison groups according to the degrees or levels of exposure to risk before the development of the disease in question. ▪ The groups, so defined, are compared in terms of their subsequent morbidity and mortality rates	▪ When information on degree of exposure is not available, it is necessary to put up an external control, to evaluate the experience of the exposed group, e.g. smokers and nonsmokers ▪ The study and control cohorts should be similar in demographic and possibly important variables other than those under study	▪ If none is available, the mortality experience of the exposed group is compared with the mortality experience of the general population in the same geographic area as the exposed people ▪ Rates for disease occurrence in subgroups of the control cohort by age, sex, and other variables considered important may be applied to the corresponding subgroups of the study cohort (exposed cohort) to determine the expected values in the absence of exposure ▪ The ratio of observed and expected values provides a measure of the effect of the factor under study

Limitations

- Non-availability of population rates for the outcome required
- Difficulties of selecting the study and comparison groups which are representative of the exposed and non-exposed segments of the general population.

D. Follow-up
- Regular follow-up is one of the problems in cohort studies and therefore, at the start of the study, methods should be devised depending upon the outcome to be determined (morbidity or death), to obtain data for assessing the outcome.

Components

- Periodic medical examination of each member of the cohort (yields the greatest amount of information)
- Reviewing physician and hospital records
- Routine surveillance of death records
- Mailed questionnaires, telephone calls, periodic home visits—preferably all three on an annual basis.

Limitations

- However, inspite of best efforts, a certain percentage of losses to follow-up are inevitable due to death, change of residence, migration or withdrawal of occupation
- These losses may bias the results
- It is therefore necessary to build on outcome for those who cannot be followed up in detail for the full duration of the study
- The safest course recommended is to achieve as close to a 95 per cent follow-up as possible.

E. Analysis
- The data are analyzed in terms of:
  - Incidence rates of outcome among exposed and non-exposed
  - Estimation of risk—relative risk, attributable risk, absolute risk, population attributable risk.

a. Incidence rates[Q]
- In a cohort study, we can determine incidence rates directly in those exposed and those not exposed as follows:

Smoking	*Developed lung cancer*	*No lung cancer*	*Total*
Yes	60	5940	6000
No	2	1998	2000
Total	62	7938	8000

Incidence rates

- Among smokers = 60/6000 = 10 per 1000
- Among non-smokers = 2/2000 = 1 per 1000

b. Estimation of risk (risk measurement)
- Estimation of the risk of outcome (e.g. disease or death) in the exposed and non-exposed cohorts is done in terms of relative risk and attributable risk.

i. Relative risk[Q]
- Relative risk is the ratio of the incidence of the disease (or death) among exposed and the incidence among nonexposed
- It is a direct measure (or index) of the strength of the association between suspected cause and effect[Q].

Calculation

$$\text{Relative risk} = \frac{\text{Incidence of disease (or death) among exposed}}{\text{Incidence of disease (or death) among nonexposed}}$$

- In the above example, the relative risk of lung cancer = 10/1 = 10

Interpretation

Relative risk	*Interpretation*[Q]		*Example*	
			Risk factor	*Disease*
1	$I_{exp} = I_{nonexp}$	No association (Chances/incidence of disease development is same among exposed as compared to non-exposed)	Smoking	HIV/AIDS
>1	$I_{exp} > I_{nonexp}$	Positive association (so many times chances/incidence of disease development is more among exposed as compared to non-exposed)	Smoking	Lung cancer
<1	$I_{exp} < I_{nonexp}$	Negative association (chances/incidence of disease development is less among exposed to compared to nonexposed)	Vitamin A intake	Epithelial cancer

- The larger the relative risk, the greater the strength of the association between the suspected factor and disease[Q], however, risk does not necessarily imply causal association.
- Significance
- Estimation of relative risk is important in etiological enquiries.

ii. Attributable Risk
- Attributable risk is the difference in incidence rates of disease (or death) between an exposed group and nonexposed group[Q].
- Attributable risk is often expressed as a per cent.
- Attributable risk indicates to what extent the disease under study can be attributed to the exposure.

Calculations

$$\text{Attributable risk} = \frac{\text{Incidence of disease rate among exposed - incidence of disease rate among non-exposed}}{\text{Incidence rate among exposed}} \times 100$$

- In above example, attributable risk of lung cancer[Q] = 10- 1/10 × 100 = 90%

Significance
- Attributable risk suggests the amount of disease that might be eliminated if the factor under study could be controlled or eliminated.
- Attributable risk signifies potential for prevention[Q]

iii. Absolute risk
- It the risk of developing the disease, irrespective of exposure to the risk factor and is expressed in percentage[Q].

Calculations

$$\text{Absolute risk} = \frac{\text{Incidence of disease rate among exposed + incidence of disease rate among non-exposed}}{\text{Total study population}} \times 100$$

- In the above example, absolute risk of Ca lung in nonsmoker[Q] = (62/8000) × 100 = 0.77%

iv. Population attributable risk
- It is the difference between the incidence of the disease occurring in the total population of both the groups irrespective of risk factor and incidence among the control group.

Interpreation[Q]
- If risk factor is modified or eliminated, there will be so much annual reduction in incidence of disease in given population

Revised Scheme 2 & 3

Advantages of cohort study	Disadvantages of cohort study (Problems)
▪ Incidence can be calculated[Q] ▪ Several possible outcomes related to exposure can be studied simultaneously ▪ Provide a direct estimate of relative risk[Q] ▪ Dose-response ratios can also be calculated ▪ Certain forms of bias can be minimised like misclassification of individuals into exposed and unexposed groups, since comparison groups are formed before disease develops[Q]	▪ Involve a large number of people ▪ Generally unsuitable for investigating uncommon diseases or diseases with low incidence in the population ▪ Long time to complete the study and obtain results and thus posing a difficulty of keeping a large number of individuals under medical surveillance indefinitely ▪ Administrative problems such as loss of experienced staff, loss of funding and extensive record keeping ▪ Loss of a substantial proportion of the original cohort due to migration, loss of interest in the study or simple refusal to provide any required information ▪ Selection of comparison groups which are representative of the exposed and unexposed segments of the population ▪ Changes in the standard methods or diagnostic criteria of the disease over prolonged follow-up. ▪ Difficult to introduce new knowledge or new tests later, after establishment of study protocol. ▪ Expensive[Q] ▪ Alternation in people's behavior during the study period ▪ Ethical problems of varying importance ▪ Practical considerations dictate concentration on a limited number or factors possibly related to disease outcome

Significance

- A well-designed cohort study is considered the most reliable means of showing an association between a suspected risk factor and subsequent disease because it eliminates many of the problems of the case control study and approximates the experimental model of the physical sciences.

2. Write in detail about "adverse events following immunization—AEFI" and the precautions to be taken.

- No immunization process is free from the risk of adverse reactions or remote sequels.
- An adverse event following immunization (AEFI) is any untoward medical occurrence which follows immunization and which does not necessarily have a causal relationship with the usage of the vaccine.
- It could be any unfavorable or unintended sign, abnormal laboratory finding, symptom or disease.

Types (WHO/CIOMS)

Cause-specific type	Definition
a. Vaccine product-related reaction	An AEFI caused or precipitated by a vaccine due to one or more of the inherent properties of the vaccine product
b. Vaccine quality defect-related reaction	An AEFI caused or precipitated by a vaccine that is due to one or more quality defects of the vaccine product, including its administration device as provided by the manufacturer
c. Immunization error-related reaction (formerly "program error")	An AEFI that is caused by inappropriate vaccine handling, prescribing or administration and thus by its nature is preventable
d. Immunization anxiety-related reaction	An AEFI arising from anxiety about the immunization
e. Coincidental event	An AEFI caused by something other than the vaccine product, immunization error or immunization anxiety

Adverse Events following Immunization

a. Reactions inherent to inoculation	▪ May be local or general reactions – Local Pain, swelling, nodules, sterile abscess, redness, tenderness at the site inoculation – General Fever, malaise, headache, etc. ▪ Most killed bacterial vaccines produce local or general reactions
b. Reactions due to faulty techniques	▪ Faulty production of vaccine (inadequate inactivation or detoxification) ▪ Too much vaccine given in one dose ▪ Improper route of vaccination ▪ Faulty reconstitution of vaccine (with incorrect diluents, wrong amount of diluents) ▪ Improper preparation of vaccine for immunization (adsorbed vaccine not shaken before use) ▪ Contaminated vaccine or diluents ▪ Improper handling of vaccine (not stored as recommended) ▪ Ignoring contraindications ▪ Reusing the same vaccine in multiple sessions ▪ Use of improperly sterilized needles or syringes
c. Reactions due to hypersensitivity	▪ These can be immediate or delayed ▪ Immediate reaction is called anaphylactic shock is very dangerous and is characterized by hypotension, rapid thready feeble pulse, perspiration, cyanosis, cold extremities and collapse ▪ Delayed reaction is called serum sickness which is characterized by pyrexia, arthralgia, myalgia, urticaria and edema
d. Neurological involvement	▪ Administration of certain vaccines may produce neurological complications which are often fatal: – BPL anti-rabies vaccine Post vaccination encephalitis, post vaccination neuroparalysis – Swine influenza vaccine Güillian-Barre syndrome – Measles vaccine Sub-acute sclerosing pan encephalitis (SSPE)
e. Provocative reaction	▪ These are reactions, i.e. occurrence of disease which is totally unconnected with the immunizing agent. ▪ Provocative polio is a well known example of provocative reaction following vaccination with APT or PTAP against diphtheria ▪ Administration of the vaccine shortens the incubation of period of infectious period of the infectious agent in an individual which already harbours the infectious agent or otherwise it may convert a latent infection into clinical attack
Others	▪ Damage to the fetus following rubella vaccination of pregnant woman ▪ Toxic shock syndrome due to contamination of measles vaccine with *Staphylococcus aureus* ▪ Displacement in age distribution of a disease
Miscellaneous	▪ Sudden infant death syndrome ▪ Autism (MMR vaccine) ▪ Multiple sclerosis (hepatitis B vaccine) ▪ Inflammatory bowel disease (MMR vaccine) ▪ Diabetes (Hib vaccine) ▪ Asthma

Management of Immediate AEFI

- Observe the patient for 30 minutes after any serum injection
- In event of anaphylaxis inject 0.5 mL IM immediately, followed by 0.5 mL every 20 minutes if the systolic BP is <100 mmHg
- Administer 10–20 mg of CPM (chlorpheniramine maleate) IM to minimize the after-effects such as urticaria or edema
- Oxygen if available
- External cardiac massage if central pulse is not palpable
- Antipyretics for pain and fever.

Reporting AEFI

- In case of serious AEFI refer the patient to appropriate health facility, inform the supervisor immediately—document the type of vaccine(s), batch number, expiry date, and full address of the child
- Report all serious AEFIs to the MO I/C

Precautions to be Taken

a. Test for sensitivity reaction before administration of antiserum or antitoxin

Methods

- Instilling a drop of the preparation into the conjunctival sac. A sensitized person will develop pricking of the conjunctiva
- Intradermal injection of 0.2 mL of antiserum diluted 1 : 10 with saline. A sensitized patient will develop a wheal and flare within 10 minutes at the site of injection (more reliable).

For anaphylaxis/Hypersensitivity

- Keep adrenaline (1:1000 solution) ready when giving foreign serum.

b. Proper immunization practices

- Proper sterilization of syringes and needles
- Proper selection of the subject and the product
- Exercise due care in carrying out the procedure
- Reconstitute the vaccines (especially measles and BCG) only with the diluent supplied by the manufacturer
- Discard the reconstituted vaccine at the end of each immunization session and never retain it for use in subsequent sessions
- Don't store any other drug or substance besides the vaccines in the refrigerator of the immunization center
- Ensure proper training of immunization worker and their close supervision
- Carry out careful epidemiological investigation in case of adverse event following immunization to find out the cause of the incident and to correct immunization practices.

SHORT ESSAYS

3. Survival rate.

Refer Question No. 4 December 2007 (RS2) Paper I.

4. Types of epidemics and epidemic curve.

Epidemic

- Epidemic is the occurrence in a community or region of cases of an illness or other health-related events clearly in excess of normal expectancy[Q]
- Normal expectancy is derived by looking at average of no. of cases of the disease in previous 3–5 years in that geographical area
- If NE = 0 then even one case is epidemic
- Statistically speaking epidemic is when no. of cases > Mean + 2 SD[Q]
- Epidemic is also occurrence of a new disease or recurrence of an eliminated or eradicated disease in population (as NE = 0).

Epidemic Curve

- Epidemic curve is graphical representation of time distribution of epidemic cases
- It gives, probable date of onset of epidemic, its duration, how cases started increasing, when did they reach peak, how long peak was maintained, when and how did epidemic start declining, when did it reach endemic level.

Types of Epidemics

Common source epidemics		*Propagated epidemics*			Slow or modern epidemics
↓	↓	↓	↓	↓	
Single exposure or point source epidemics	Continuous or multiple exposure epidemics	Person to person	Arthropod vector	Animal reservoir	
Examples: Food poisoning	Examples: Cholera	Examples: Polio, measles	Examples: Plaque	Examples: Ebola	Examples: Diabetes, Hypertension

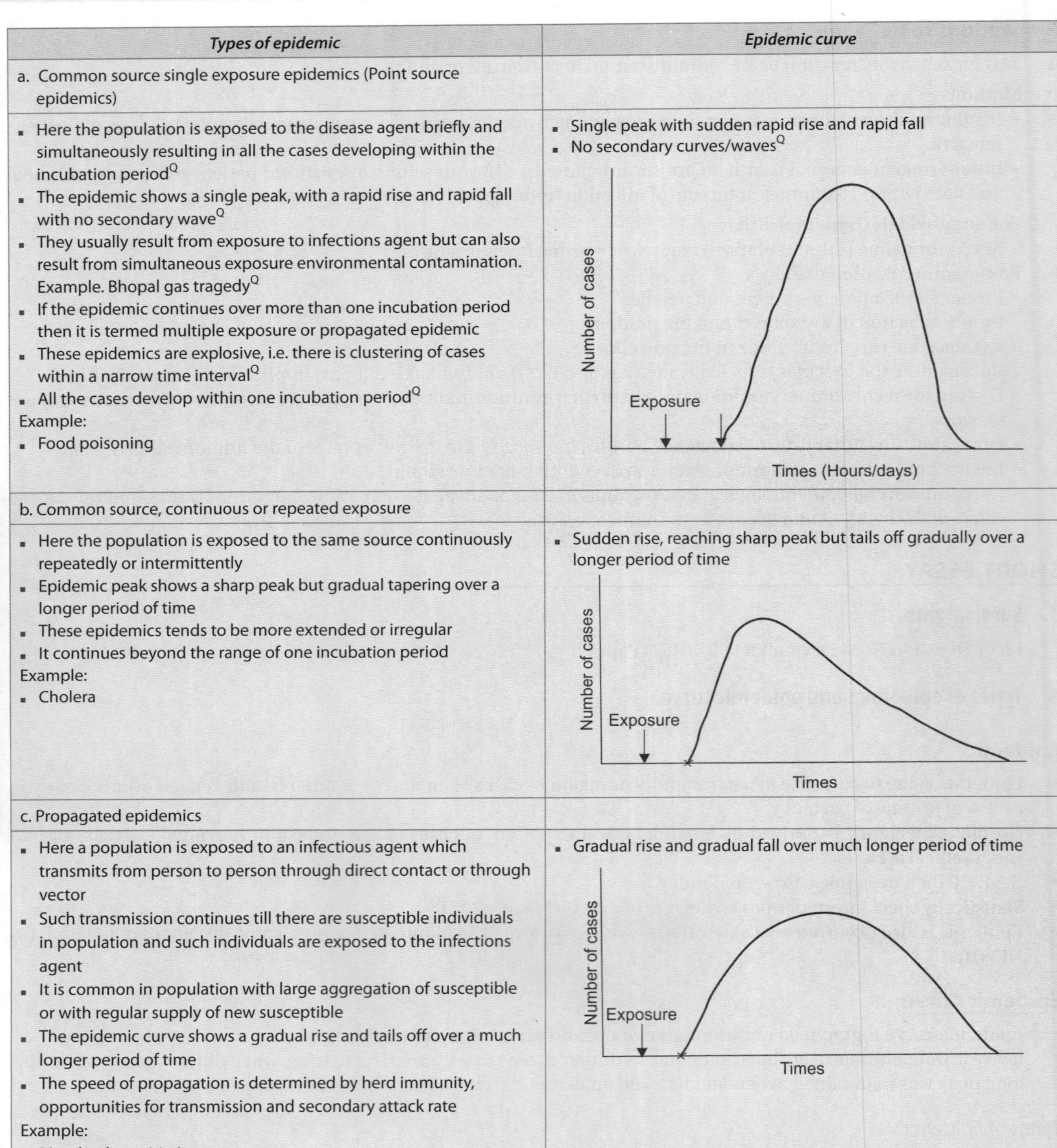

Types of epidemic	*Epidemic curve*
a. Common source single exposure epidemics (Point source epidemics)	
▪ Here the population is exposed to the disease agent briefly and simultaneously resulting in all the cases developing within the incubation period[Q] ▪ The epidemic shows a single peak, with a rapid rise and rapid fall with no secondary wave[Q] ▪ They usually result from exposure to infections agent but can also result from simultaneous exposure environmental contamination. Example. Bhopal gas tragedy[Q] ▪ If the epidemic continues over more than one incubation period then it is termed multiple exposure or propagated epidemic ▪ These epidemics are explosive, i.e. there is clustering of cases within a narrow time interval[Q] ▪ All the cases develop within one incubation period[Q] Example: ▪ Food poisoning	▪ Single peak with sudden rapid rise and rapid fall ▪ No secondary curves/waves[Q]
b. Common source, continuous or repeated exposure	
▪ Here the population is exposed to the same source continuously repeatedly or intermittently ▪ Epidemic peak shows a sharp peak but gradual tapering over a longer period of time ▪ These epidemics tends to be more extended or irregular ▪ It continues beyond the range of one incubation period Example: ▪ Cholera	▪ Sudden rise, reaching sharp peak but tails off gradually over a longer period of time
c. Propagated epidemics	
▪ Here a population is exposed to an infectious agent which transmits from person to person through direct contact or through vector ▪ Such transmission continues till there are susceptible individuals in population and such individuals are exposed to the infections agent ▪ It is common in population with large aggregation of susceptible or with regular supply of new susceptible ▪ The epidemic curve shows a gradual rise and tails off over a much longer period of time ▪ The speed of propagation is determined by herd immunity, opportunities for transmission and secondary attack rate Example: ▪ Measles, hepatitis A	▪ Gradual rise and gradual fall over much longer period of time

Applications

- To study time relationship with exposure to a suspected source
- To know whether it is common source or propagated epidemic
- To find out type of epidemic based on cyclic or seasonal pattern of a particular infection.

Significance

- Epidemic curve is very easy method of analyzing and understanding a epidemic.

5. Quarantine.

- Quarantine (meaning 40 days) is the limitation of freedom of movements of such well person or domestic animals exposed to communicable diseases for period of time not longer than the longest usual incubation period of the disease[Q], in such manner as to prevent effective contact with those not so exposed
- It applies to those who have exposed to a contagious disease but how may or may not become ill, i.e. it applies to healthy contacts of an infectious disease (in contrast to Isolation)
- Quarantine was first applied to plague[Q] in 14th Century Europe.

Types

Absolute quarantine	*Modified (partial) quarantine*	*Segregation*
▪ Limitation of freedom of movements to prevent effective contact with those not so exposed ▪ It was practiced against smallpox, plague, cholera and yellow fever ▪ Outdated now	▪ Selective partial limitation of the movement, such as exclusion of children from school during period of treatment ▪ Practiced against scabies, diphtheria, chickenpox, etc.	▪ Separation for special consideration, control of observation of some part of a group of person or domestic animals from the others to facilitate control of a communicable disease, such as removal of susceptible children to homes of immune persons

Significance

- In earlier days, quarantine was the only means to prevent import of exotic diseases in the country and any traveler suspected of suffering from disease or those travelling without international certificate of vaccination would be quarantined at the international seaports or airports
- It also applicable to animals (e.g. dogs for rabies)
- However, quarantine failed in its objective because of the lack of scientific knowledge regarding the causation and mode of spread of disease
- Moreover 40-day detention obstructed and caused serious inconveniences to international trade and travel
- Thus quarantine has been currently replaced by active surveillance.

6. Pentavalent vaccine.

Refer Question No. 6 December 2015 (RS2) Paper II.

7. Iron deficiency anemia and its prevention.

Refer Question No. 10 June 2008 (RS2) Paper I.

8. Dietary goals.

Refer Question No. 4 June 2013 (RS2) Paper I.

9. Break point chlorination.

- Break point chlorination is the point at which the chlorine demand is met and the residual chlorine starts appearing and when all combined chlorines has been completely destroyed and the corresponding dosage is the break point dosage.

Mechanism

- As chlorine is added it combines with ammonia to form chloramines which is combined residual chlorine
- Addition of further chlorine then oxidizes ammoniacal compounds
- Addition of next increment of chlorine results in destruction of chloramines, resulting in release of free residual chlorine
- This point is called break-point chlorination.

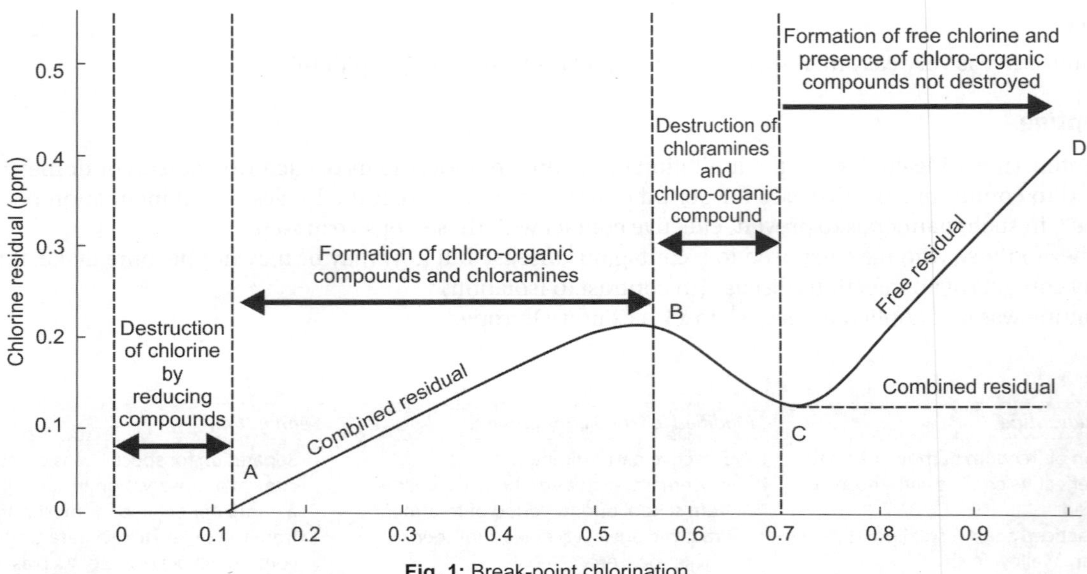

Fig. 1: Break-point chlorination

Features

- Free chlorine is released in water after break point chlorination[Q]
- Contact period of 1hr is necessary[Q].

Significance

- Break point chlorination achieves the same results as super chlorination in a rational manner and can therefore be constructed as controlled super chlorination.

10. Lightning standards.

- Good lighting is essential for efficient vision
- If lighting conditions are not ideal, eyes are put to strain leading to general fatigue and loss of efficiency.

Lightning Standards

- Illumination to which eye responds ranges from bright sunlight (100,000 lux) to full moonlight (0.1 lux)
- Due to adaptive ability of the eye, there is considerable confusion about standards.

Currently Accepted Lightning Standards (Illuminating Engineer Society)

Visual task	*Illumination (lux)*
▪ Casual reading	100
▪ General office work	400
▪ Fine assembly	900
▪ Very severe tasks	1,300–2,000
▪ Watch making	2,000–3,000

Significance

- Visual efficiency increases with increase of illumination but at higher level, the curve flattens out (law of diminishing return)
- Standard illumination level is 30 times higher than the level at which task can just be done (rule of thumb)

- As there are no universally accepted lightening standards, it usually better to err on side of much light, provided glare can be avoided.

11. Mental health services in India.

- Mental health services in a community are concerned not only with early diagnosis and treatment, but also with preservation and promotion of good mental health and prevention of mental illness
- Provision of basic mental health services is basic objective of national mental health program.

Components

- Early diagnosis and treatment
- Rehabilitation
- Group and individual psychotherapy
- Mental health education
- Use of modern psychoactive drugs
- After-care services.

Delivery of Mental Health Services

Tier	*Health care provider*	*Functions*
a. 1st tier	Paramedical worker at village and sub center level	▪ Recognizing and providing first aid to psychiatric emergencies ▪ Following up diagnosed cases in their home environment for ensuring continuity of treatment ▪ Providing basic advise to patient and family ▪ Health education of community members on basic preventive procedures
b. 2nd tier	Medical officers at PHC level	▪ Diagnose and treat common psychiatric illnesses ▪ Refer complicated cases to higher centers
c. 3rd tier	Psychiatrist at district hospital or private practitioners	▪ Deals with referred cases ▪ Provide guidance and training to lower level health personnel ▪ Provide necessary inputs to district health administration for planning mental health care services in the district
d. 4th tier	Psychiatrist at super-specialized centers such as medical colleges, mental health institutes	▪ Take care of complicated/referred cases ▪ Organize epidemiological research and surveys for planning and evaluating the services

Significance

- With increasing stress, mental health is has become major public health problem which has been rightly identified by WHO through their World Health Day theme of 2017 – "Depression – Let's talk"
- India also has taken step in right direction to provide better mental health care by passing the Mental Health Care Act in 2017.

12. Notification of diseases.

- Notification is compulsory reporting of a disease under legal provisions under certain times or at all times to the health authorities
- Notification of diseases is the first health information sub-system to be established
- The list of notifiable disease varies from country to country.

Status in India

- In India, there is no legal provision except Epidemic Disease Act, 1897.
- The main agent responsible for notifying a disease in India is village health guide and multipurpose health worker.

Notifiable Diseases

As per WHO	*As per Ministry of Health, Govt of India*[1]	*As per The Factories Act, 1948*[2]
▪ Notifiable diseases[Q] ▪ Cholera[Q] ▪ Plague[Q] ▪ Yellow fever[Q] (*Child Playing with Yellow ball*) Diseases under suveillance[Q] ▪ Louse borne typhus ▪ Relapsing fever[Q] ▪ Polio ▪ Influenza ▪ Malaria[Q] ▪ Rabies[Q] ▪ Salmonellosis	▪ AIDS ▪ Anemia ▪ Cerebrospinal fever ▪ Chickepox ▪ Cholera ▪ Dengue fever ▪ Diphteria ▪ Dysentery ▪ Fever syndrome more than 6 days ▪ Hepatitis A ▪ Hepatitis B ▪ Herpes zoster ▪ Influenza ▪ Iodine deficiency ▪ Leprosy ▪ Malaria ▪ Malnutrition ▪ Measles ▪ Plague ▪ Polio ▪ Rabies ▪ Scarlet fever ▪ Small pox ▪ Tetanus ▪ Tuberculosis ▪ Typhoid fever ▪ Viral encephalitis ▪ Vitamin A deficiency ▪ Whooping cough	▪ Poisoning or its sequele – Lead, lead tetra-ethyl, phosphorus, mercury, manganese arsenic, nitrous fumes, carbon bisulphate, benzene and its derivatives, poisoning or its sequelae, halogens or its derivatives of hydrocarbons, beryllium, carbon monoxide, phasgene, isocyanates ▪ Chrome ulceration or its sequelae ▪ Anthax ▪ Pneumoconiosis – Silicosis, Byssinosis, Asbestosis, Coal miner's pneumoconiosis ▪ Pathological manifestation due to radium, radioactive substances, or X-rays ▪ Primary epitheliomatous cancer of the skin ▪ Toxic anemia ▪ Toxic jaundice due to poisonous substances ▪ Oil acne or dermatitis due to mineral oil or its derivatives in any form ▪ Occupational or contact dermatitis caused by direct contact with chemical or paints. It could be primary irritants or allergic sensitisers. ▪ Noise induced hearing loss ▪ Occupational cancers ▪ Toxic nephritis

Advantages	*Disadvantages*
▪ Notification of disease helps in prevention and/or control of the diseases ▪ It is a valuable source of morbidity data, i.e. it presents incidence and distribution of a particular disease ▪ It provides valuable information about fluctuations in the disease frequency ▪ It also provides for early warnings about new occurrences or outbreaks of disease	▪ Notification of disease reflects only a small part of the total sickness in the community ▪ It suffers from a good deal of under reporting ▪ Many cases especially atypical and subclinical cases escape notification due to non-recognition like rubella, non-paralytic polio, etc. ▪ Correct diagnosis and notification depends upon the facilities for bacteriological, viriological and serological examination which are lacking in rural areas

Ref:

1. http://health.puducherry.gov.in/details_of_notifiable_diseases.htm accessed on 2nd Feb. 2015.
2. http://nihfw.nic.in/ndc-nihfw/html/Legislations/TheFactoriesAct1948.htm accessed on 2nd Feb. 2015.

SHORT ANSWERS

13. Anthropozoonoses—give an example.

- Anthropozoonoses is a type of zoonoses
- Here infections are transmitted from vertebrate animals to human being (Vertebrate → Man)

Example

Disease	Source animal
Rabies	Dogs
Plague	Rats
Kyasanur forest disease	Monkeys
Brucellosis	Cattle
Japanese encephalitis	Pigs
Hydatid disease	Pigs

14. Killed vaccines.

- Killed vaccines a type of vaccine produced by killing the virus or bacteria grown in culture media using heat or chemicals (formalin, phenol, β-propiolactone) to stimulate active immunity.

Route of administration	Contraindication	Examples	
		Bacterial	Viral
▪ Subcutaneous or intramuscular route	▪ Severe hypersensitivity (local or general) to a previous dose	▪ Typhoid vaccine ▪ Pertussis vaccine ▪ Cholera vaccine ▪ Plaque vaccine	▪ Salk polio vaccine ▪ Rabies vaccine ▪ Influenza vaccine ▪ JE vaccine ▪ KFD vaccine ▪ Hepatitis A vaccine

Advantages	Disadvantages
▪ Usually safe ▪ Can be used in immunodeficient individual ▪ More stable (than live vaccine) ▪ Not affected by circulating antibodies ▪ Minimal adverse reactions	▪ Less effective and less potent (than live vaccines) ▪ Requires 2–3 primary doses for adequate antibody response (production) ▪ Only stimulates IgG production ▪ Induction of mucosal and cell mediated immunity is poor ▪ Requires boosters later in life (in most cases) ▪ Shorter duration of immunity (months to years)

15. Xerophthalmia.

Refer Question No. 12 December 2012 (RS2) Paper I.

16. Epidemic dropsy.

- Epidemic dropsy is a food toxicity produced due to a toxic alkaloid, sanguinarine from argemone seeds[Q]
- It is commonly seen when there is contamination of mustard oil with argemone oil either accidently or deliberately as the seeds of *Argemone mexicana* closely resemble mustard seeds and they too become mature is march when the mustard crop is harvested.

Toxin	Pathogenesis	Clinical manifestations	Diagnosis
▪ A toxic alkaloid, sanguinarine from argemone seeds	▪ Sanguinarine interferes with oxidation of pyruvic acid and lactic acid which accumulates in blood ▪ This leads to dilatation, engorgement and ↑ permeability of capillaries, ↓ blood viscosity, ↑ in hydrostatic pressure, hyperdynamic circulatory state, all features of toxic vasculites, leading to transudation of fluid into skin and subcutaneous tissue resulting in edema	▪ Incubation period—1–2 weeks ▪ Manifests as sudden, non-inflammatory bilateral swelling of legs often associated with diarrhoea[Q] ▪ Edema is due to protinuria (specifically loss of albumin) ▪ Dyspnea, cardiac failure[Q] and death may follow and mortality varies 5–50%. ▪ Some patients develop glaucoma[Q] ▪ Affects all ages except breast fed infants ▪ It may sometimes manifest as sarcoids (dilatation of skin capillaries)	▪ Confirmation of epidemic ▪ Large number of cases of pedal edema in the same family/community ▪ History of consumption of mustard oil ▪ Demonstration of argemone oil in the mustard oil ▪ Detection of sanguinarine in the serum or urine Lab test ▪ Spectrofluorophotometric method (using silica gel G)—detects sanguinarine in the serum and urine of the affected persons

Prevention and Control

- Argemone oil is orange in color with an acrid odor and can be detected by following tests:

Nitric acid test[Q]	*Paper chromatography test*[Q]	*Ferric chloride test*
Development of brown to orange-red color in a test tube of oil added with HNO_3 indicates argemone oil	Most sensitive and specific test[Q] detecting 0.0001 % of aregemone oil	Highly specific test where addition of ferric-chloride gives orange-red precipitate

- Removing the argemone weeds growing among the oil seed crops
- Strict enforcement of prevention and Food Adulteration Act to deal with culprits
- Detoxification of sanguinarine from edible oil
  - Edible oil is shaken with phosphoric acid and activated Fuller's earth followed by filtration and neutralization of phosphoric acid with precipitated chalk
  - Shaking the oil with Fuller's earth at 140°C
- Avoiding mustard oil altogether in presence of epidemic in locality
- Extensive public awareness including health education.

17. Balwadi nutrition program.

- The Balwadi Nutrition Program is community Nutrition Program, initiated in 1970 by the Ministry of Social Welfare, Government of India

Objective	*Target population*	*Components*
▪ To improve the nutritional status of children enrolled in Balwadi centers with daily food supplement	▪ Children in age group of 3–6 years in rural areas	▪ Food supplement providing 300 kcal and 10–12 grams of protein per child per day ▪ Grand of funds to 4 national level organizations such as Indian Council of Child Welfare to implement the program ▪ Funding of voluntary organizations actively involved in day-to-day management

Significance

- With universalization of ICDS, Balwadis are being phased out and merged into ICDS since 1975.

18. Backwashing.

- Backwashing is the process of cleaning the filter bed of rapid sand filter.

Indications

- Loss of head approaches 7–8 feet in rapid sand filters.

Mechanism

- Water or compressed air is passed in reverse direction or below upwards so that the filter bed of sand is elevated to loosen the sand bed and dislodge the impurities to be washed away
- Backwash rates of 42–54 $m^3/m^2/h$ is used to clean the filters
- Washing is stopped when clear sand is visible or wash water is clear which usually takes 15 minutes
- After backwashing, filter bed is put to use immediately (unlike slow sand filter which requires waiting period of 24 hours for formation of biological film).

Significance

- To maintain the efficiency of the rapid sand filter, backwashing needs to be done frequently like several times per day.

19. Control of ebola virus disease (EVD).

Refer Question No. 6 June 2016 (RS2) Paper II.

20. Birth and death registration.

Refer Question No. 13 December 2008 (RS2) Paper II.

21. Focus group discussion (FGD).

Refer Question No. 19 June 2015 (RS2) Paper I.

22. Sampling methods.

Refer Question No. 1 June 2016 (RS2) Paper I.

MBBS PHASE III EXAMINATION

DECEMBER 2016

(Revised Scheme 2 & 3)

PAPER II

LONG ESSAYS

1. What are the common problems of the elderly? Write about the social security measure for the elderly in India.

For Common Problems of Elderly

Refer Question No. 2 June 2009 (RS2) Paper II.

For Social Security

Refer Question No. 2 December 2009 (RS2) Paper I.

2. Discuss the epidemiology of tuberculosis. Add a note on the Revised National Tuberculosis Control Program.

For Epidemiology of Tuberculosis

Refer Question No. 1 December 2009 (RS2) Paper II.

For Revised National Tuberculosis Control Program

Refer Question No. 2 December 2012 (RS2) Paper II.

SHORT ESSAYS

3. Mass Drug Administration.

Refer Question No. 11 June 2011 (RS2) Paper II.

4. Chandler's index.

- Chandler's index is an endemic index of hookworm infection based on the average number of hookworm eggs per gram of stools[Q].

Interpretation

Average no. of hookworm eggs per gram of stool	*Public health importance*
<200	Not of much significance
200–250	Potential danger
250–300	Minor public health problem
>300	Major public health problem

Application

- Comparison of worm load in different population groups
- Comparing degree of reduction of egg out after mass treatment.

Significance

- Chandler's index is an indicator used to assess the severity of public health problem of ancylostomiasis
- It also helps to evaluate the control measures of ancylostomiasis following mass treatment.

5. Natural history of measles.

Refer Question No. 1 December 2010 (RS2) Paper II.

6. Epidemiology of STDs.

- Sexually transmitted diseases are a group of communicable diseases that are predominately by sexual contact.

Epidemiology of STDs

Agent	*Sexually transmitted diseases*
A. Agent factors (Classification of STDs)	
a. Bacteria	
i. *Treponema pallidum*	▪ Syphilis ▪ Yaws ▪ Pinta
ii. *Haemophilus ducreyi*	▪ Chancroid
iii. *Neisseria gonorrhoeae*	▪ Gonorrhea ▪ Urethritis ▪ Cervicitis ▪ Epididymitis ▪ Saphingitis ▪ Pelvic inflammatory disease (PID)
iv. *Calymmatobacterium granulomatis*	▪ Granuloma inguinale
v. *Chlamydia trachomatis*[Q] (L_1, L_2, L_3)	▪ Lymphogranuloma venereum
vi. *Chlamydia trachomatis* (D to K)	▪ Nongonococcal urethritis ▪ Cervicitis
vii. *Mycoplasma hominis*	▪ Nongonococcal urethritis
viii. *Ureaplasma urealyticum*	▪ Nongonococcal urethritis
ix. *Shigella* species	▪ Proctocolitis
x. *Campylobacter* species	▪ Proctocolitis
xi. Bacterial vaginosis associated organism	▪ Bacterial vaginosis
xii. Group B streptococci[Q]	▪ Vaginitis ▪ Urethritis ▪ Cervicitis ▪ Balanitis ▪ Cystitis
b. Viral	
i. Human α herpes virus 1 and 2	▪ Herpes genitalis
ii. Human β herpes virus 5	▪ Cervicitis ▪ Nongonococcal urethritis
iii. Hepatitis B virus[Q]	▪ Serum hepatitis
iv. Human papillomavirus	▪ Genital warts
v. Molluscum contagiosum virus	▪ Genital molluscum contagiosum
vi. Human immunodeficiency virus (HIV)	▪ Acquired immunodeficiency syndrome (AIDS)

c. Protozoa	
i. *Entamoeba histolytica*	▪ Amoebiasis
ii. *Giardia lamblia*	▪ Giardiasis
iii. *Trichomonas vaginalis*	▪ Trichomoniasis
d. Fungi	
i. *Candida albicans*[Q]	▪ Vaginal candidiasis
e. Ectoparasites	
i. Pthirus pubis	▪ Pubic pediculosis
ii. *Sarcoptes scabiei*	▪ Genital scabies
B. Host factors	
a. Age	▪ Highest incidence is observed in 20–24 years old, followed by 25–29 and 15–19 years age groups ▪ Most serious morbidity is observed during fetal development and in the neonates
b. Sex	▪ Morbidity rate is higher in men but morbidity caused by infection is much more severe in women
c. Marital status	▪ Higher frequency amongst single, divorced and separated persons than among married couples
d. Socioeconomic status	▪ Highest morbidity rate in individuals from the lowest socioeconomic groups
e. Occupation	▪ High incidence in commercial sex workers, truck drivers
C. Social factors	
a. Prostitution	▪ Prostitutes or commercial sex workers are the reservoirs of infection
b. Broken homes	▪ Broken homes are the sources of promiscuous women
c. Sexual disharmony	▪ Married people with strained relations, divorced and separated persons are often victims of STDs
d. Poverty	▪ Extreme poverty forces women to go astray and become prostitution as it is an occupation with easy money
e. Illiteracy	▪ Illiteracy associated with emotional immaturity predisposes girls to become easy victims of STDs
f. Urbanization and industrialization	▪ Long working hours, relative isolation from the family and geographical and social mobility due to urbanization and industrialization foster casual relationships
g. Social disruption	▪ Social disruption due to disasters, wars and civil unrest have increased the spread of STDs
h. International travel	▪ Travelers can import and export infection
i. Changing behavioral patterns	▪ Relaxation of moral and cultural values, idea of intendance, freedom from supervision and equal rights for both sexes have produced a tendency to break away from traditional ways of life especially among the youths
j. Social stigma	▪ Social stigma attached to the STDs account for non-detection of cases, not disclosing the sources of contacts, dropping out before treatment is complete, going to quacks for treatment, self medication
k. Alcoholism	▪ Alcohol has indirect effect by encouraging risk taking behavior like unprotected sex and promoting prostitution
l. Type of marriage	▪ Polygamy and polyandry predisposes to prevalence of STDs
m. Co-education and co-work	▪ Foster casual sexual relationships thus aiding STDs
D. Demographic factors (contributing to increase in STDs)	▪ Population explosion and marked increase in the young age population ▪ Rural to urban migration ▪ Increasing educational opportunities for women delaying their marriage and increasing STD risks

Significance

- STDs are becoming a major public health problem in India and they have a profound impact on sexual and reproductive health
- Social stigma attached to it and ignorance about their causation and prevention are major factors responsible for people not seeking medical attention thus further spreading the disease in the community.

7. Define acute flaccid paralysis.

Refer Question No. 1 June 2014 (RS2) Paper II.

8. Food and Agricultural Organisation.

- Food and Agricultural Organisation (FAO) is a specialized agency of United Nations set up in 1945 with a mission of achieving food security for all.

Structure	*Objectives*	*Departments*	*Activities*
▪ Headquarters at Rome[Q] ▪ FAO is governed by Conference of Member Nations, which meets every two years to review the work carried out ▪ Conference elects a Director-General and Council of 49 Member Nations (on 3 years rotation basis) to act as an interim governing body	▪ To help nations raise living standards ▪ Improve nutritional status of world population by adequate food distribution ▪ To increase efficacy of farming, forestry and fisheries to increase food production to keep pace with ever growing world population ▪ To better the conditions of rural people and through all there means to widen opportunity of all people for productive work	▪ Agriculture and consumer protection ▪ Economic and social department ▪ Fisheries and aquaculture ▪ Forestry ▪ Human, financial and physical resources ▪ Knowledge and communication ▪ Natural resource management ▪ Environment and technical cooperation	▪ Ensuring consumption of food by the needy, in sufficient quantities and in right proportion to develop and maintain a better state of nutrition throughout the world ▪ Collaborating with other international agencies in applied nutrition programs ▪ Conduct nutritional surveys, training courses, seminars ▪ Coordinate research programs on brucellosis and other zoonoses

FAO in India

- Regional of FAO for India is at Bangkok which provides regular support in field of Food Security and Nutrition.

Activities

- Plant production activities, forestry, fisheries, nutrition and food quality and safety (current focus)
- Vulnerability mapping through establishment of a Food Insecurity and Vulnerability Information and Mapping System (FIVIMS) and preparation of a Nutrition Country Profile for India
- Supports design of a large scale maize production scheme (Special Program for Food Security)
- Undertaking following projects in India (Under its technical cooperation program)
  - Transfer of technology for vegetative propagation of walnuts in Jammu and Kashmir
  - Development of integrated plant nutrition systems methodology
  - Training in sea safety development programs
  - Greenhouse technology for floriculture
  - Food quality control.

9. Healthcare delivery indicators.

- Healthcare delivery indicators are positive indicators reflecting availability of health manpower and other health resources in a community and thus provision of healthcare to a population.

Healthcare Delivery Indicators

Indicators	*Suggested in India*
▪ Doctor-population ratio	1:2500
▪ Nurse-population ratio	1:5000
▪ Health worker-population ratio	1:3000
▪ Pharmacist-population ratio	1:10000
▪ Lab technician-population ratio	1:10000
▪ Doctor-nurse ratio	1:2
▪ Population-bed ratio	50 per 10000
▪ Population per health center	1 per 30000
▪ Population per subcenter	1 per 3000
▪ Population per trained birth attendant	

Significance

- Healthcare delivery indicators reflect equity of distribution of health resources in different parts of country and of provision of healthcare
- They reflect pattern of distribution of resources in urban and rural areas
- They point towards national health policy and political commitment for healthcare delivery
- It helps compare healthcare delivery personnel and infrastructure among different countries and also among different parts of a country
- They not only reflect availability and distribution of resources but help to understand utilization pattern of resources by community
- WHO has listed it as one of the categories of indicator to monitor progress of Goals of Health for All by 2000.

10. Demographic cycle.

Refer Question No. 11 December 2009 (RS2) Paper II.

11. Prevention of rheumatic fever.

- Rheumatic fever is a febrile disease affecting connective tissues particularly in heart and joints initiated by infection of throat by group A β-hemolytic streptococci
- Rheumatic heart disease is the ultimate, squeal and crippling stage of Rheumatic fever
- Though it is not a communicable disease, it results from communicable pharyngitis thus prevention is targeted towards prevention of streptococcal pharyngitis.

Prevention of Rheumatic Fever

A. Primordial prevention
   Defined as measures directed towards prevention of communication of streptococcal infection in high risk population
   a. Health promotion
      - Improvement in living conditions
      - Prevention of over crowding
      - Improvement in sanitation in and around the house
      - Prevention of malnutrition among children
      - Improvement in socioeconomic condition
      - Health education of the people regarding dangers of sore throat
      - Health fair should be conducted in the schools to make children health conscious
   b. High risk strategy
      - Periodic surveys of random samples (of 20,000–30,000 children) in school-going children in age group of 6–14 years at 5-year intervals

B. Primary prevention
- Defined as adequate antibiotic therapy of group A streptococcal pharyngitis to prevent an initial attack of acute rheumatic fever.

Objective
- To prevent first attack of rheumatic fever, by identifying all patients with streptococcal throat infection and treating them with penicillin (Practically not feasible).

Early diagnosis and treatment

Antibiotic	*Administration*	*Dose*
Benzathine benzyl penicillin[Q]	Single IM injection	Adults—1.2 million units Children—600,000 units
Penicillin V	Orally 2–4 times/day for 10 days	Adults—500 mg BD Children—250 mg BD

Significance
- Primary prevention of rheumatic fever is impractical due to impossible logistics coupled with enormous financial constraints forcing to concentrate on secondary prevention.

C. Secondary prevention
- Continuous administration of specific antibiotics to patients with a previous attack of rheumatic fever or a well-documented rheumatic heart disease.

Objective
- To prevent colonization or infection of upper respiratory tract (URT) with group A β-hemolytic streptococci and development of recurrent attacks of rheumatic fever
- Mandatory for all patients, who have had an attack of rheumatic fever, whether or not they have residual rheumatic valvular heart disease.

Specific protection

Antibiotic	*Administration*	*Dose*
Benzathine benzyl penicillin	Single IM injection every 3–4 weeks	Adults—1.2 million units Children—600,000 units
Penicillin V	Oral	250 mg BD

Duration

Cases with rheumatic fever	Atleast 5 years or until child reaches 18 years of age (whichever is later)
Cases with carditis	Atleast 10 years after last attack or until age of 25 years (whichever is later)
Cases with sever valvular disease or post valve surgery	Lifelong treatment

Advantage
- Practically feasible, inexpensive and cost effective than primary prevention.

Disadvantages
- Patient compliance for a long-term prophylaxis.

D. Tertiary prevention

Disability limitation
- Limiting disability development by intensive treatment with
  - Aspirin for joint pains
  - Prednisolone for carditis
  - Benzathine Penicillin, 1.2 million units, once in 3 weeks life long
  - Balloon valvotomy or valve replacement

Rehabilitation
- By social, vocational and psychological measures.

Significance

- Though a noncommunicable disease, rheumatic fever can be prevented by breaking chain of transmission of streptococcal infection by treating the patients already suffering from it
- Thus secondary prevention is a better cost effective and practically feasible method of preventing rheumatic fever.

12. Diseases transmitted by soft ticks.

- Ticks are blood sucking ectoparasites belonging to class Arachnida family Argasidae.

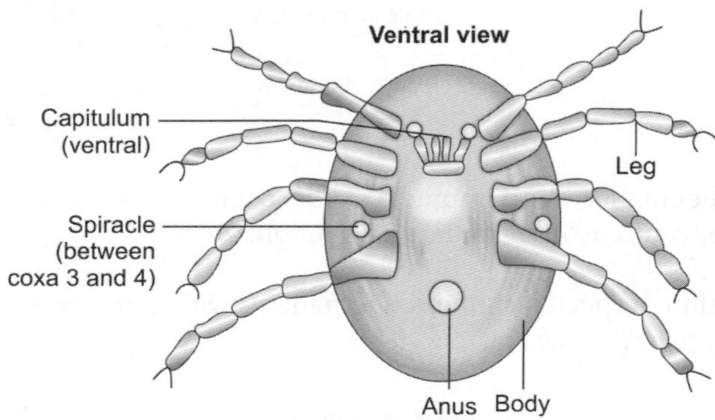

Fig. 1: Soft tick (argasidae)

Important Species

- *Ornithodorus moubata*—transmits relapsing fever
- *Ornithodorus lahorensis*
- *Ornithodorus crossi.*

Features

- Males are smaller than females
- Oval shaped body, measuring 1 cm, not distinctly separated into head, thorax and abdomen
- Head (Capitulum) is present ventrally (on underside), entirely invisible from above
- Possess 4 pairs of pointed legs terminating in claws but no antennae
- Dorsal surface doesn't exhibit scutum (a chitinous shield) contributing to their softness.

Feeding Habits

- Hide in cracks and crevices during day and emerge at night to feed
- Require intermittent blood meal
- Can withstand starvation for several months.

Life History

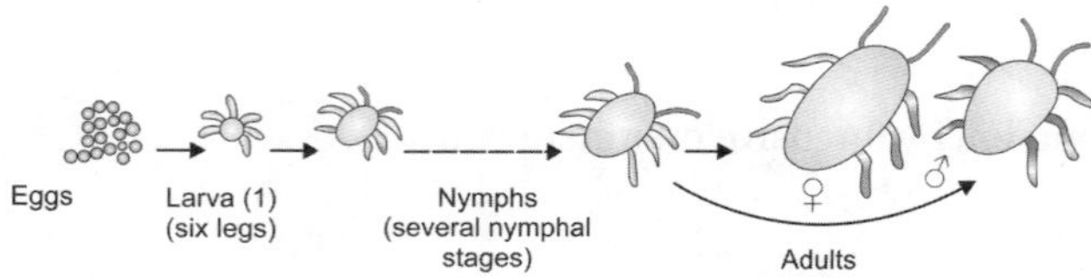

Fig. 2: Life cycle of soft tick

Egg *Hatch in 1–3 weeks*	*Larva (seed tick)* *Lasts 2–13 days*	*Nymph* *Lasts 6 weeks*	*Adult* *Egg become adults in 9-10 months*
▪ Lays eggs on ground in batches of 20-100 over a long period	▪ Possesses 3 pairs of legs ▪ Lies in wait among grass and herbiage till a suitable host appears to which it attaches itself ▪ After a blood meal, it drops off and in course of time moults to become a nymph	▪ Resembles adult in having 4 pairs of legs but has no genital pore ▪ Are all blood suckers and attach themselves to suitable hosts for a blood meal ▪ Undergoes 5 nymphal stages	▪ Live for a year or more (longer compared to hard tick) ▪ Attaches to host by means of its mouth parts ▪ Rostrum is burrowed into skin to enable it to suck blood and secreting neurotoxin containing saliva at the same time ▪ Mature ticks, especially gravid female ticks remain attached for a comparatively long time but male usually drops off after a few days ▪ As it feeds, it gradually becomes engorged with blood

Disease Transmitted

Infective forms	*Mode*	*Diseases*
Adults, larva and nymph (exhibit trans-stadial and transovarian transmission)	By biting	Q fever, relapsing fever and KFD

Control Measures

Insecticidal control	*Personal protective measures*	*Habitat management*
Disinfestation of animals by application of insecticides (tickcides) such as lindane or malathion in form of dusting powder or solution Application of insecticides on vegetations and floors and walls	Use of fully covering cloths and protective clothing impregnated with an insect repellent such as indalone and diethyl toluamide Health education	Environmental control measures includes removal of shrubs and vegetation near dwellings

SHORT ANSWERS

13. Advantage and limitation of insecticides as method of vector control.

Refer Question No. 2 June 2014 (RS2) Paper I.

14. Define acute flaccid paralysis.

Refer Question No. 1 June 2014 (RS2) Paper II.

15. Objectives of multidrug therapy in leprosy.

Refer Question No. 5 December 2008 (RS2) Paper II.

16. Screening methods for cancer of breast.

Refer Question No. 11 June 2013 (RS2) Paper II.

17. Net reproduction rate.

Refer Question No. 18 June 2013 (RS2) Paper II.

18. Triage.

Refer Question No. 16 June 2013 (RS2) Paper II.

19. Xenodiagnosis.

- Xenodiagnosis is a method of filiarial survey
- This consists of collection of mosquitoes and their larvae and dissecting them to detect filarial larvae

Method of Collection

Mosquitoes	*Larvae*
▪ A person is made to sleep inside a bigger, outer curtain with a flap opened on one side to allow mosquitoes to get inside ▪ At certain intervals (1-2 hours), flap of outer curtain is closed and all mosquitoes resting inside are collected using a special pipette ▪ This is expressed as number of mosquitoes per ten man hour catch (i.e. 10 persons exposed for 1 hour or 5 persons exposed for 2 hours or 1 person exposed for 10 hours) ▪ Mosquitoes are carefully maintained alive for 10–14 days in a clean paper cup covered with a gauze and fed on a sugar soaked cotton wool placed over the gauze ▪ After 14 days (of extrinsic incubation period), mosquitoes are identified, killed by chloroform vapor and dissected for filarial larvae ▪ The data is anlayzed and expressed as filarial indices	▪ Mosquito larvae are collected either by dipping a bowl or by using a nylon net attached to an iron ring or by pipetting ▪ In case of Mansonia larvae, acquatic plant is uprooted and shaken in a bucket of water so that the larvae are detached ▪ Addition of sodium hydroxide to water helps in detachment of larvae and their easy collection

Significance

- Xenodiagnosis may help detect low density microfilaremia (when other methods fail).

20. Program evaluation review technique.

Refer Question No. 6 December 2011 (RS2) Paper II.

21. Absolute contraindications of oral contraceptive pill.

Refer Question No. 5 June 2012 (RS2) Paper II.

22. Define primary healthcare.

Refer Question No. 4 June 2012 (RS2) Paper II.

MBBS PHASE III EXAMINATION

JUNE 2017

(Revised Scheme 2 & 3)

PAPER I

LONG ESSAYS

1. Define health education. Enumerate the principles of health education. Write briefly about communication process.

For health education

Refer Question No. 2 December 2011 (RS2) Paper I.

Communication Process

Communication is a complex process in which a source of information gives the information through various channels to the audience and in turn gets the feedback to know the effect of the process.

Components[Q]

Sender (source)	▪ Communicator or originator of message ▪ He should know the audience, the message to be given and methods or channels to communicate
Message (content)	▪ Technical know how of information being communicated to the audience Properties of good message ▪ Should be clear, understandable, interesting, meaningful, related to the objective, specific and accurate, timely and adequate, culturally and socially acceptable by the audience
Media (channel)	▪ Channel which bridges between the sender and the receiver Types i. Interpersonal (face to face) communication – Most common and personal and direct – More persuasive and effective in influencing decisions of undecided persons ii. Mass media – Through TV, radio, press, etc – Can reach wider audience in shortest time – But is one way communication with poor feedback mechanism iii. Traditional or folk media – Include traditional events such as Yakshagana (Karnataka), Burrakatha (AP), Kathakali (Kerala), Nautanki (UP), etc. – Important channels of communication being close to the cultural values of the rural population as they are principal instruments of preserving the cultural heritage
Audience (receiver)	▪ May be a single person or a group of persons with common interest (controlled) or gathered out of curiosity (uncontrolled or free) ▪ It is the element of audience and their frame of mind (opinions, attitudes, prejudices) which lends meaning to all the different types of communication
Feedback (effect)	▪ Reverse flow of information or remarks made by audience about the message to the sender so that sender can make modification and improve communication to make it more effective and acceptable to the audience

Significance

- Communication is a two way process
- It is the main weapon to change the behavior of the people and its final goal is to change the people's knowledge, attitude, behavior and practices.

2. Define epidemiology. Classify epidemiological study designs. Write about the advantages and disadvantages of cohort study.

Refer Question No. 1 December 2016 (RS2) Paper I.

SHORT ESSAYS

3. Child guidance clinic.

- Child guidance clinic is meat for those children/adolescents who for one reason as other are not fully adjusted to their environment[Q]
- Was first started in Chicago[Q].

Objective

- To prevent children from the possibility of becoming neurotics and psychotics in later life.

Features

- Health team comprises of a psychiatrist, a clinical psychologist, psychiatric social worker, public health nurses, pediatrician, speech therapist, occupational therapist and a neurologist.
- Head of the team is the psychiatrist who is helped by others to arrive at correct diagnosis and formulate the line of treatment
- Pediatrician takes care of child's physical health
- Psychotherapy is the core of therapy; to take care by restoring positive feeling in child by various measures such as play therapy, counseling, easing parental tension, reconstruction of parental attitudes, etc.

Significance

- Child guidance clinic is based on philosophy that if sound foundations of mental health are laid in childhood, the same would continue into adulthood.

4. Sampling methods.

Refer Question No. 1 June 2016 (RS2) Paper I.

5. Sickness absenteeism.

- Sickness absenteeism is absence from work on account of sickness which may be real or certified by the physician.

Causes

Causes			*Prevention*
Economical	*Social*	*Medical*	
▪ Availing paid sick leaves if available to them	▪ Social and family obligations like wedding, festivals, etc. ▪ Visits to native places especially during festivals or sowing harvest season ▪ Addictions to drug and alcohol ▪ Poor interpersonal relations	▪ Occupational accidents ▪ Respiratory alimentary illnesses ▪ Pyrexia of unknown origin ▪ Nutritional disorders	▪ Application of principles of ergonomics ▪ Adequate preplacement and periodic examination ▪ First Aid provision ▪ Selective employment and rehabilitation ▪ Health education ▪ Good employer and employee relation ▪ Provision of welfare and safety procedures ▪ Elimination of stressful conditions ▪ Psychological counseling

Significance

- Sickness absenteeism is considered as a sensitive index of work satisfaction
- Higher absenteeism is due to job dissatisfaction, poor environment, poor ergonomics, poor interpersonal management and vice versa
- Serves as a useful index to assess the health status of industrial workers[Q] and their physical, mental and social well-being[Q]
- Frequency of absenteeism is inversely proportional to worker's age and size of urban area, i.e. lower the age and larger the population, higher the rate of sickness absenteeism
- More common in women than men
- In poor environment worker tries to find as excuse to be away from job by declaring himself sick or producing false certificates
- This results in poor quality and quantity of finished product more labor turnover, more industrial sickness, strikes and lockouts and the poverty and poor development of community at large
- Rate of sickness absenteeism in India is 8–10 days per head per year[Q]
- It is an important problem in occupational health and results in loss of number of working days and thus leads to decreased production.

6. Disability indicators.

Refer Question No. 1 June 2008 (RS2) Paper I.

7. Uses of screening.

Refer Question No. 1 December 2010 (RS2) Paper I.

8. Bar charts.

Bar diagram is a method of diagrammatic representation of data.

Concept

- It is simple diagram with rectangular bars drawn along the graph sheet
- Height of each bar or rectangle corresponds to the frequencies in the data and the width corresponds either to the class interval of variable in quantitative data or to various groups in qualitative data
- The bars can be arranged either vertically or horizontally, in ascending or descending order, etc.
- However, bars should stand on the same line and possess same width and a suitable scale should be chosen to present the length of the bars
- The spacing between the two consecutive bars should be equal to the half of the width of the bar.

Types

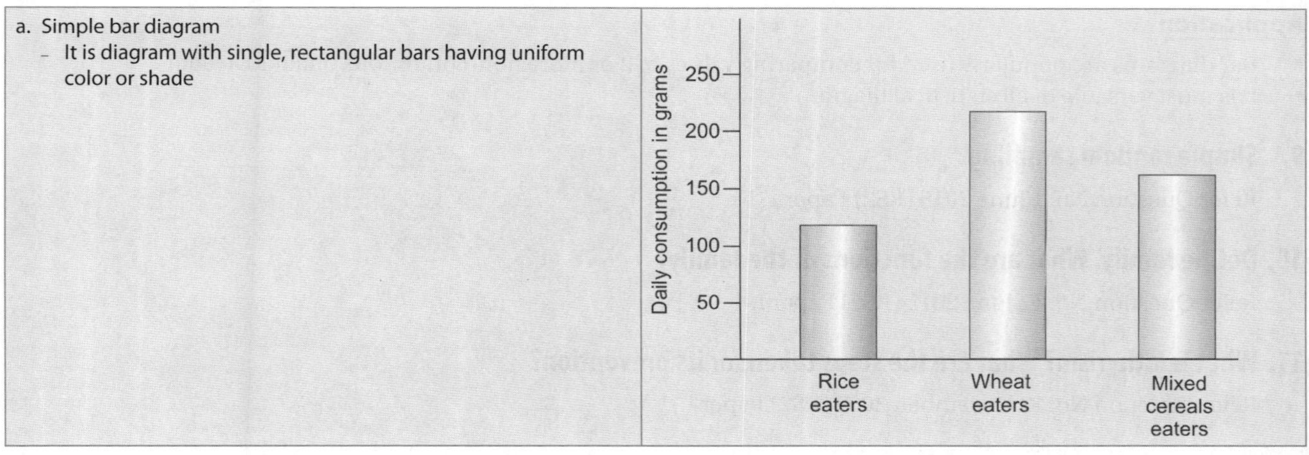

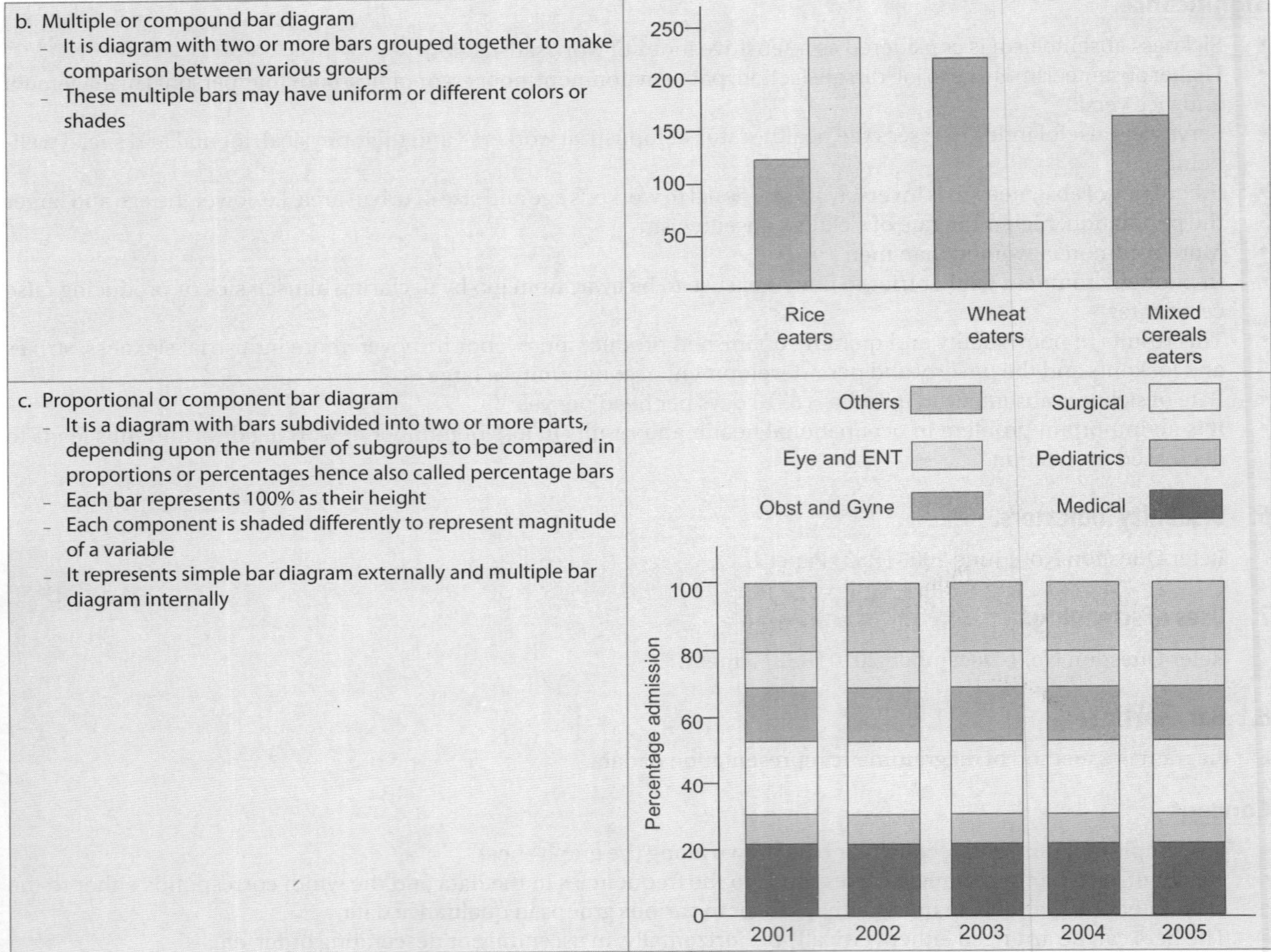

b. Multiple or compound bar diagram – It is diagram with two or more bars grouped together to make comparison between various groups – These multiple bars may have uniform or different colors or shades	
c. Proportional or component bar diagram – It is a diagram with bars subdivided into two or more parts, depending upon the number of subgroups to be compared in proportions or percentages hence also called percentage bars – Each bar represents 100% as their height – Each component is shaded differently to represent magnitude of a variable – It represents simple bar diagram externally and multiple bar diagram internally	

Advantages	*Disadvantage*
▪ Easy to prepare and understand ▪ Enables visual comparison of the variables	▪ Cannot be used for data with various variables

Application

- Bar diagrams are popularly used for comparing values of 2 or more non-continuous qualitative data
- It is most versatile of all statistical diagram[Q].

9. Simple random sampling.

Refer Question No. 1 June 2016 (RS2) Paper I.

10. Define family. What are the functions of the family?

Refer Question No. 12 June 2013 (RS2) Paper I.

11. What is lathyrism? What are the steps taken for its prevention?

Refer Question No. 12 December 2009 (RS2) Paper I.

12. Prevention of iodine deficiency disorders.

Refer Question No. 1 June 2013 (RS2) Paper I.

SHORT ANSWERS

13. Human development Index.

Refer Question No. 3 December 2009 (RS2) Paper I.

14. Criteria for selection of anganwadi worker.

Refer Question No. 2 June 2010 (RS2) Paper II.

15. Enumerate job responsibilities of ASHA.

Refer Question No. 2 June 2014 (RS2) Paper II.

16. Properties of normal curve.

Refer Question No. 6 December 2014 (RS2) Paper I.

17. Discuss the effects of tobacco use. What are the preventive measures?

Refer Question No. 8 December 2014 (RS2) Paper I.

18. What is triage?

Refer Question No. 16 June 2013 (RS2) Paper II.

19. Write briefly about beri-beri.

- Beri beri (Sinhalese = I cannot) is a vitamin deficiency disorder.

Cause

- Deficiency of thiamine (Vitamin B1).

Clinical Features (common to all)

- Anorexia, nausea, vomiting
- Weight loss, lassitude
- Rise in blood pyruvate level

Dry or neurotic beri beri (predominant CNS manifestations)	Wet or edematous beri-beri (predominant CVS manifestations)	Infantile beri-beri
▪ Hyperesthesia, paralysis and blindness (due to inflammation of peripheral nerves) ▪ Lesion in ventral horn of spinal cord, inflammation of dorsal root ganglia ▪ Loss of deep reflexes ▪ Mental confusion and anxiety	▪ Edema of legs, face, trunk and serous cavities ▪ Palpitation and breathlessness (due to enlarged heart) ▪ Tender calf muscles are tender ▪ Pulsatile and distended neck ▪ Low diastolic BP and increased systolic BP ▪ Fast and pounding pulse ▪ Weak heart resulting in heart failure	▪ Seen in infants born to mothers suffering from thiamine deficiency ▪ Characterized by sleeplessness, restlessness, vomiting ▪ Convulsions and bouts of screaming resembling abdominal colic ▪ Death due to cardiac failure

Prevention

- Dietary supplementation in high-risk groups like lactating mothers
- Health education about well-balanced diet, consumption of thiamine rich food, stoppage of alcohol.

20. List out 6 contraindications for oral contraceptive pills.

Refer Question No. 5 June 2012 (RS2) Paper II.

21. Measles vaccine.

Refer Question No. 1 December 2010 (RS2) Paper II.

22. Chi-square test.

Refer Question No. 4 June 2008 (RS2) Paper I.

MBBS PHASE III EXAMINATION

JUNE 2017

(Revised Scheme 2 & 3)

PAPER II

LONG ESSAYS

1. Describe the epidemiology, clinical features, prevention and control of measles in a community.

Refer Question No. 1 December 2010 (RS2) Paper II.

2. Describe the causes of maternal mortality in india. Suggest preventive and control measures for reduction of MMR.

Refer Question No. 2 June 2012 (RS2) Paper II.

SHORT ESSAYS

3. Describe the epidemiology and prevention of accidents.

Refer Question No. 2 June 2016 (RS2) Paper II.

4. What are the principles and elements of primary health care?

Refer Question No. 4 June 2012 (RS2) Paper II.

5. What are the different types of hormonal contraceptives? Write a note on mode of action, contraindications and complications of oral contraceptive pills.

Refer Question No. 5 June 2012 (RS2) Paper II.

6. Briefly explain the modes of transmission of hepatitis B infection.

Refer Question No. 1 December 2014 (RS2) Paper II.

7. Mention the steps involved in eradication of poliomyelitis.

Refer Question No. 1 June 2014 (RS2) Paper II.

8. What are the measures for control of sexually transmitted diseases?

Refer Question No. 8 June 2012 (RS2) Paper II.

9. Cancer registries.

Refer Question No. 9 June 2012 (RS2) Paper II.

10. Write a note on cold chain equipment present in primary health center.

Refer Question No. 12 December 2007 (RS2) Paper I.

11. Describe the case finding tool for diagnosis of tuberculosis under Revised National Tuberculosis Control Program (RNTCP). Add a note on reasons for 'false positivity' and 'false negativity'.

Refer Question No. 1 December 2009 (RS2) Paper II.

12. Describe the salient epidemiological features of dengue syndrome.

Refer Question No. 12 June 2012 (RS2) Paper II.

SHORT ANSWERS

13. What is exclusive breastfeeding? Enumerate the advantages.

Refer Question No. 13 June 2012 (RS2) Paper II.

14. What is a blocked flea?

Refer Question No. 14 June 2012 (RS2) Paper II.

15. Mass drug administration for filariasis.

Refer Question No. 11 June 2011 (RS2) Paper II.

16. What is network analysis?

Refer Question No. 6 December 2011 (RS2) Paper II.

17. Treatment for leprosy.

Refer Question No. 5 December 2008 (RS2) Paper II.

18. Case definition used for diagnosis of AIDS.

Refer Question No. 10 June 2015 (RS2) Paper I.

19. What is Chandler's index?

Refer Question No. 4 December 2016 (RS2) Paper II.

20. What is rule of halves in hypertension?

Refer Question No. 12 December 2008 (RS2) Paper II.

21. Preventive measures in Ebola virus disease (EVD)—disease transmission.

Refer Question No. 6 June 2016 (RS2) Paper II.

22. Juvenile delinquency.

Refer Question No. 10 December 2012 (RS2) Paper I.

MBBS PHASE III EXAMINATION

DECEMBER 2017

(Revised Scheme 2 and 3)

PAPER I

LONG ESSAYS

1. Describe in detail, the various health problems due to industrialization.

- Industrialization implies the transformation of a peasant society into a community dependent upon the industries
- Industrialization causes a social and economic revolution in the culture of a nation and any such revolution is bound to cause some health problems.

Health Problems Due to Industrialization

a. Communicable diseases
   - Industrial areas show high prevalence of tuberculosis, venereal diseases and food and water-borne infections
   - Areas with industries without proper sewage disposal are also prone for mosquito-borne diseases like filariasis owing to breeding of mosquitoes in contaminated water
   - All these are in addition to certain specific diseases associated with specific industries like pneumoconiosis, occupational cancer, etc.

b. Foodborne diseases
   - Food sanitation standards are lowered due to industrialization leading to rise in incidence of typhoid fever and viral hepatitis
   - With industrialization, increasing demand of ready to eat food and use of modern techniques has leads to various diseases like mechanical refining of flour has resulted in decreased fiber intake, causing numerous diseases associated with this condition and refined sugar intake is well known risk factor for diabetes
   - To increase self-life food processing industry is relying heavily on chemical additives which are foreign to human body leading to allergic conditions.

c. Mental health
   - Industrialization has leads to migration of people villages to alien urban life which requires certain adjustments
   - Failure to adjust to altered living conditions leads to mental illness, psychoneurosis, behavior disorders, and delinquency, etc.

d. Noncommunicable diseases
   - With industrialization and rapid urbanization, there is increasing level of affluence (modernization) which has lead changes in the lifestyle leading to high prevalence of chronic noncommunicable diseases or lifestyle disorders
   - Machines have decreased the need for physical energy expenditure by man, leading to obesity which is risk factors for ischemic heart diseases, diabetes.

e. Accidents
   - Accidents are on rise in industrial towns due to congestion, vehicular traffic and increased momentum of life
   - Then there are accidents that occur in the factories due to worker's fatigue, mechanical problems, etc.

f. Diseases due to poor environmental sanitation
   i. Housing
      - Most of the migrant labors in industrial towns live in slums with poor standards of living, overcrowding, poor lightening and ventilation and insanitary conditions leading to high prevalence of communicable diseases in these slums often leading to epidemics.

ii. Water pollution
   - Discharge of toxic industrial waste without treatment into water bodies which are main source of drinking water for the industrial towns has leads to numerous water-borne diseases besides skin infections in people using these water bodies for other purposes like bathing, etc.

iii. Air pollution
   - Industries are notorious for polluting air with toxic fumes, gases, smoke and dust into atmosphere
   - Moreover burning of more fuel for transport, cooking and electricity needed by more people means higher air pollution
   - Thus, there is a rapid increase in incidence of respiratory disorders like chronic obstructive pulmonary disease (COPD), asthma in population especially children and elderly living in industrial towns.

iv. Noise pollution
   - Noise pollution like other pollutants is also a by-product of industrialization leading to hearing loss, tinnitus, mental stress, etc.

v. Sewage disposal
   - Rapid urbanization and uncontrolled growth of slums has caused enormous pressure on existing sewage disposal infrastructure
   - Improper sewage disposal is major risk factor for spread of diseases due to water pollution, soil pollution, vector breeding, etc.

vi. Vector problem
   - Collections of water, in and around industries and residential areas, become the potential breeding places for the mosquito vectors.

g. Diseases due to social problems
   - Social problems like alcoholism, drug addiction, prostitution, etc. have lead to increased incidences of certain diseases.

h. Morbidity and mortality
   - Industrial areas are characterized by high morbidity and mortality from certain diseases like chronic bronchitis and lung cancer
   - Crude death rate and infant mortality rate has increased in industrial areas.

Prevention

a. Town planning/zoning
   - Numerous health problems of industrialization can be prevented or resolved with proper town planning or zoning.

b. Sewage and effluent treatment
   - Proper sewage disposal methods or strengthening of existing sewage treatment plants helps in reduction in vector breeding
   - Dilution or treatment of industrial effluents can contain water pollution.

c. Improving public health infrastructure
   - Establishment of urban health centers in slums help in rapid detection of communicable diseases and prevent their spread to before they become epidemics.

d. Food hygiene
   - Improvement of food hygiene, consumption of fresh food and less reliance of processed food or ready to eat food will prevent many of the food-borne diseases or allergies.

e. Ergonomics
   - Healthy working environment will improve mental health of the workers.

Significance

- In race to become developed nation, India has promoted industrialization; however, policy makers have blind sided with the concurrent development of public health
- Thus due to low level of public health, the average expectation of life in India is less than that in industrially advanced countries.

2. Classify and describe the various methods of health communication. Enlist the advantages and disadvantages of the different methods.

Refer Question No. 2 June 2009 (RS2) Paper I.

SHORT ESSAYS

3. Characteristics of a normal distribution curve.

Refer Question No. 6 December 2014 (RS2) Paper I.

4. Attributable risk and population attributable risk.

Refer Question No. 1 December 2016 (RS2) Paper I.

5. Prevention of indoor air pollution in India.

- Indoor air pollution is the degradation of indoor air quality by harmful chemicals and other materials.

Principal Sources

- Combustion, building material, and bioaerosols.

Prevention and Control

a. Health education and public awareness
   - Most important steps in prevention of indoor air pollution is health education, i.e. spreading awareness among people about the issue and the serious threat it poses to their health and wellbeing
   - It should help people in finding different ways of reducing exposures with better kitchen management and protection of children at home
   - People should be educated about the use of alternative cleaner sources of energy to replace direct combustion of biomass fuel
   - Besides public, other stakeholders like politicians and administrators also should be educated to ensure their commitment and increase their awareness about health effects of indoor air pollution.

b. Change in pattern of fuel use
   - Factors determining preferred fuel include individual habit, availability and affordability of the fuel
   - Majority of low income families rely solely on direct combustion of biomass fuels for their cooking needs as this is the cheapest and easiest option available to them
   - This scenario can be improved by promoting use of cleaner energy sources such as Gobar Gas which utilizes cow dung to produce gas for cooking.

c. Modification of design of cooking stove
   - Traditional smoky and leaky cooking stoves should be modified to fuel efficient, smokeless stoves with an exit (e.g. chimney)
   - National Biomass Cookstoves Initiative, of the Ministry of New and Renewable Energy designed a new stove under a Special Project on Cookstove during 2009–2010, with the primary aim of enhancing the availability of clean and efficient energy for the energy deficient and poorer sections of the country.

d. Improvement in ventilation
   - Provision for adequate ventilation should be made during the construction of a house
   - For poorly ventilated houses, measures such as a window above the cooking stove and cross ventilation though doors should be instituted

e. Intersectoral coordination and global initiative
   - Indoor air pollution can only be controlled with coordinated and committed efforts between different sectors concerned with health, energy, environment, housing, and rural development.

Significance

- It is essential to prevent and control indoor pollution as due to contained areas, pollutants can build up more thus can be up to 10 times worse than outdoor air pollution
- Tackling indoor air pollution and providing universal access to clean household energy is a great opportunity to improve health, reduce poverty, and protect our environment; thus, contributing significantly to achieving the Millennium Development Goals.

Ref: Kankaria A, Nongkynrih B, Gupta SK. Indoor Air Pollution in India: Implications on Health and its Control. Indian Journal of Community Medicine 2014;39(4):203-20.

6. Sampling techniques.

Refer Question No. 1 June 2016 (RS2) Paper I.

7. Role of legislation in reducing alcoholism in the society.

- Legal control on the distribution of alcohol, when effectively applied has been and remains an important approach in the prevention of alcoholism.

Legislation Methods for Reducing Alcoholism

a. Partial restriction
  - Minimum age at which minors may legally have access to alcoholic beverages is raised in some countries, like in India, it is 21 years
  - Limited drinking hours at bars or drinking in public places discourages alcoholics.

b. Complete non-availability
  - Countries like Saudi Arabia have absolute ban on alcohol where it is completely not available.

c. Controlling manufacture
  - Almost all countries control alcohol manufacturers through licensing.

d. Promotion
  - Banning advertisements of alcohols on electronic media.

e. Distribution
  - There is also legislation controlling the distribution of alcohol in some countries
  - Retail distribution of alcohol also requires licence which is strictly controlled by the government
  - In India, it is illegal to sell alcohol within 500 meters of National Highways to prevent drunken driving.

f. Increase price
  - Many countries levy numerous taxes on the price of alcohol to increase its price thus deter the alcoholics.

g. Prohibit alcohol
  - Many Islamic countries have prohibited consumption of alcohols to its citizens
  - In India, state of Gujarat, Bihar, Nagaland, Manipur, Lakshwadeep and district of Wardha have alcohol prohibition.

h. Legislation
  - Almost all countries have drunken driving as a serious offence inviting jail term
  - Maximum legal BACs also show a wide variation ranging from 30–70 mg% in different countries
  - In India legal limit of alcohol is 30 mg/dL.

8. Methods of pasteurization of milk.

Refer Question No. 6 December 2009 (RS2) Paper I.

9. Modes of transmission of diseases.

Refer Question No. 1 June 2009 (RS2) Paper I.

10. Define rate, ratio and proportion using appropriate examples.

- Rate, ratio and proportion are basic tools in measurement of disease magnitude in a community
- They help to compare disease frequency with that of other countries or other groups of population in the same country

	Rate	*Ratio*	*Proportion*
Definition	▪ Rate is a measure of occurrence of a event (disease incidence or death) in a population during a given time period ▪ It is a statement of the risk of developing a condition and indicates the change in some event that takes place in a population over a period of time ▪ It is basically a proportion, but with an added relationship with time	▪ Ratio is a relation in size between two random quantities obtained by dividing one quantity by another	▪ Proportion is a ratio which indicates the relation in magnitude of a part of the whole
Expressed as	▪ Expressed per 1000 or some other round figure (10,000; 100,000) selected according to the convenience or convention to avoid fractions	▪ Expressed as x: y or x/y	Expressed as percentage
Components	▪ Numerator (usually a component of denominator) ▪ Denominator ▪ Time specification (usually a calendar year) ▪ Multiplier	▪ Numerator (not a component of denominator) ▪ Denominator Both may involve an interval of time or may be instantaneous in time	▪ Numerator (always a component of denominator) ▪ Denominator
Example (in a hypothyroidism study)	Rate of hypothyroidism in females = Total No. of female patients in a year/Total female study population × 1000	Ratio of female patients to male patients = No. of females/No. of males	Proportion of female patients = No. of female patients/Total no. of patients
Other examples	▪ Death rate, birth rate, Infant mortality rate	▪ Maternal mortality rate, ▪ Sex-ratio, doctor-population ratio, child-woman ratio, etc.	▪ Under 5 proportional mortality rate, proportional mortality rate
Significance	▪ Rate helps the epidemiologist compare frequency or rate of a particular event in a community with that of another community	▪ Ratio gives idea of another very important measure, i.e. the odds	▪ Proportion gives idea of a important measure in research methodology, i.e. the probability

11. Implications of false-positive and false-negative results in clinical practice.

- In relation to a screening test, epidemiologist thinks in terms of sensitivity and specificity whereas the clinician thinks in terms of false-negatives and false-positives

	False-negatives	*False-positives*
Definition	▪ Percentage of diseased people wrongly identified as not having the disease, because the test result is negative	▪ Percentage of healthy people wrongly identified as having the disease, because the test result is positive
Features	▪ False-negative result means that patients who actually have the disease are told that they do not have the disease, i.e. they are falsely given negative reports ▪ Amounts to giving them a false reassurance	▪ False-positive result means that patients who do not have the disease are told that they have the disease, i.e. they are falsely given positive reports ▪ Amounts to giving them a false anxiety

Implications in clinical practice	▪ Patient with a "false-negative" test result might ignore the development of signs and symptoms and may postpone the treatment ▪ This could be detrimental if the disease in question is a serious one and the screening test is unlikely to be repeated within a short period of time	▪ Normal healthy people may be subjected to further diagnostic tests, at some inconvenience, discomfort, anxiety and expenses ▪ False-positives not only burden the patients and diagnostic laboratories, but they also bring discredit to practicing physician
Related to	▪ Sensitivity (Lower the sensitivity, larger the number of false-negatives)	▪ Specificity (Higher the specificity, lower the number of false positives)

Significance

- False-positives and false-negatives help calculate predictive value of a screening test
- False-positives and false-negatives have to confirmed by the gold-standard test (test with high validity).

12. Different types of association.

- Association is the concurrence of two variables more often than would be expected by chance
- It does not necessarily imply a causal relationship.

Types

a. Spurious association
b. Indirect association
c. Direct (causal) association
   i. One-to-one causal association
   ii. Multifactorial causation.

Spurious Association

- Spurious association is an observed association between a disease and the suspected factor which is not fact
- Such association may result from
  - Chance
  - Ecological correlation
  - Selection bias, i.e. disparity between the study group and the control group.

Example

- In a study in UK, it was observed that the perinatal mortality was more in hospital deliveries than home deliveries thus wrongly interpreting that the domiciliary deliveries are safer
- This kind of spurious association resulted because home deliveries were compared with hospital deliveries which are usually high risk thus associated with high perinatal mortality.

Prevention

- In a epidemiological study, the study group and control group should be comparable, i.e. there should be no selection bias to avoid such spurious associations.

Indirect Association

- Indirect association is a statistical association between a characteristic (or variable) of interest and a disease due to presence of third factor (known or unknown) which is common to both the characteristic and the disease
- This third common factor is called as "confounding factor"
- Common confounding variables include age, sex, social class and they are potentially and probably present in all data
- They represent a formidable obstacle to overcome in trying to assess the causal nature of relationship.

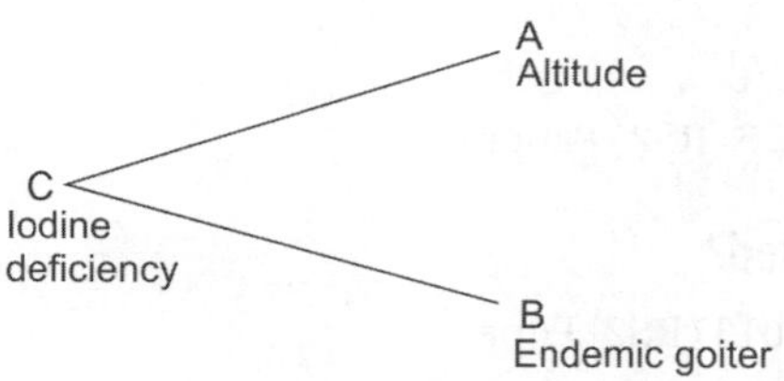

Example

- Endemic goiter is associated with high altitude, however, there is no direct association between these two variables unless the common (compounding) factor of iodine deficiency is taken into consideration.

Significance

Indirect association is only a statistical association which does not necessarily mean causation.

Direct (Causal) Association

a. One-to-one causal relationship
   - This means if causative factor (A) is present, disease (B) must result and conversely when disease (B) is present, causative factor (A) must be present
   - It is significant in communicable diseases.
   - Usually single causative agent results in single disease
     - Example: Tubercle bacilli is the causative agent of tuberculosis
       Tubercle bacilli ↔Tuberculosis
   - However, in some instances single causative factor (A) can result in more than one disease (B, C, D)
     - Example: Hemolytic streptococci results in tonsillitis, scarlet fever and erysipelas.

   Significance
   - This concept of one-to-one causal relationship is the essence of Koch's postulates of germ theory
   - However, though ideal in disease etiology, it does not explain every situation.

b. Multifactorial causation
   - In noncommunicable diseases more than often, multiple factors are involved, which may act independently or synergistically
   - A complex interaction of various causal factors are involved in disease causation
   - In certain diseases like independent risk factors can produce disease independently
     - Example: In lung cancer independent risk factors like smoking, air pollution, etc., can produce the disease independently

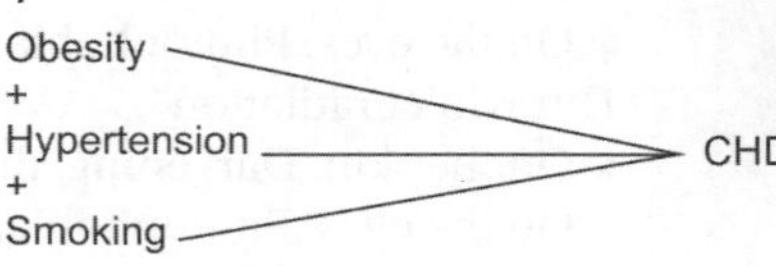

   - In some diseases, there could be additive effects of risk factors too
     - Example: In coronary heart disease, effect of smoking, obesity, hypertension results in cumulative effect.

   Significance
   - In biological phenomena, the requirement that "cause" is both "necessary" and "sufficient" condition is not easily reached, because of the existence of multiple factors in disease etiology.

SHORT ANSWERS

13. Herd immunity.

Refer Question No. 10 June 2012 (RS2) Paper I.

14. Social security.

Refer Question No. 2 December 2009 (RS2) Paper I.

15. Epidemic.

Refer Question No. 4 December 2016 (RS2) Paper I.

16. Define silicosis. How is it diagnosed?

Refer Question No. 11 December 2013 (RS2) Paper I.

17. List four micronutrient deficiency disorders in India.

- Micronutrient deficiency disorders (malnutrition) refers to a group of conditions caused by deficiency of essential vitamins and minerals such as vitamin A, calcium, iodine, iron and zinc.

Examples
- Nutritional anemia (Iron deficiency anemia)
- Vitamin A deficiency (Xerophthalmia)
- Iodine deficiency
- Rickets.

18. Occupational hazards of healthcare professionals.

- No occupation is free from occupational hazards and healthcare is no exception.

Occupational Hazards of Health Care Professionals

a. Physical hazards (Radiations)
  i. Ionizing radiation: X-rays, electromagnetic fields, radioactive isotopes like Co60, P32
    - Acute effects
      - Acute radiation syndrome
    - Chronic effects
      - Somatic effects: Leukemia, aplastic anemia, cancer, tumor induction, pancytopenia
      - Genetic effects: Stillbirths, congenital defects, neonatal deaths, sex chromosome aneuploidy, sterility
  ii. Nonionizing radiation
    - Lasers
      - On the skin: Burns, erythema, dermatitis, cancer
      - On the eyes: Photophobia, conjunctivitis, keratitis, corneal ulcer, blindness
    - Ultraviolet radiation
      - On the skin: Darkening, thickening, erythema, cancer
      - On the eyes: Photophobia, conjunctivitis, keratitis, corneal ulcer, blindness

b. Chemical hazards (Anesthetic gases)
  - Ether, chloroform, trichloroethylene

c. Biological hazards
  - Tuberculosis, hepatitis B and C, HIV
  - Other communicable diseases like respiratory infections

d. Psychological hazards (due to sleep deprivation, excessive work, failure to develop a healthy relationship co-workers, employers, management, supervisors, etc.)
  i. Psychological (Behavioral) changes
    - Hostility, aggressiveness, anxiety, depression, frustration, tardiness, alcoholism, drug addiction, sickness absenteeism, etc.
  ii. Psychosomatic ill health
    - Neurosis, fatigue, propensity to peptic ulcer, hypertension, asthma, etc.

Prevention and Control

a. Health promotion
  - Healthy, sterile working environment
  - Maintenance of personal hygiene

- Education of the support staff and others involved in health care
- Limited working works to reduce stress and fatigue

b. Specific protection
- Consists of avoiding exposure to infectious agents, radiations
- Use of protective gears like gloves, masks, eye goggles, gowns, lead aprons
- Preexposure immunization against hepatitis B
- Postexposure treatments in HIV, hepatitis B and other diseases
- Following universal precautions

c. Early diagnosis and treatment
- Periodical examinations for the detection of communicable diseases, HIV, hepatitis B, HCV
- Regular check of radiation exposure and radiation leaves at regular intervals.

19. Recommend solution for the problem of drug abuse in India.

- Drug abuse is defined as the self-administration of a drug in quantities and frequencies which may impair the ability of an individual to function normally and results in social, physical and emotional harm.

Solution for Drug Abuse in India

a. At Individual Level
  i. Deaddiction
  - Identification of drug addicts
  - Motivation for detoxication
  - Hospitalization, provide fear therapy, psychotherapy, counseling
  - Medical treatment or substitution
    - Using methadone for opioid abusers
  - Change of the environment (home, school, college, social circle)
  - Postdetoxication counseling to prevent relapse (based on clinic and home visits)
    - Drug addict is made aware of long-term hazards of the drug and he is informed about his responsibility to safeguard his health by quitting the habit
  - Rehabilitation (vocational training and placement in appropriate job)
    - Helps to prevent relapse.

b. Family Level
  i. Parents should be educated about need to shower love and affection on their children and to be neither too strict nor too lenient with them
  ii. They should be encourage to tell their children that they disapprove the drugs.

c. Community Level
  i. Educational approach
  - Public should be informed through campaigns on audio-visual media, leaflets, posters
  - Educational programs should be arranged for school children and school authorities with the help of police should make the school and surroundings a drug-free zone

  ii. Service approach
  - Establish teen centers to attract the teenagers where they are made healthy and active by participating in sports, music, athletes, gymnasium, artistic activities, etc. and prevent them from drifting into drug taking
  - Establish self-help groups consisting of ex-addicts to encourage those who want to give up the habit of taking drugs

  iii. Legal approach
  - Legislation should be directed at various levels like manufacturing, distribution, prescription, price, advertisements, consumption, etc.

Significance

- Drug abuse is a social problem which best resolved at individual level instead of legal approach since a deaddict is the best person to motivate another addict to go drug free.

20. Sample registration system in India.

- Sample registration system is a large scale demographic survey conducted in India for providing reliable annual estimates of birth rate and other fertility and mortality indicators at the national and sub-national level[Q].
- It was started in 1964-65 by Office of the Registrar—General, India on pilot basis and now covers entire nation.

Procedure

- Done once in 6 months[Q]
- A part time resident enumerator, generally a teacher does continuous field investigations regarding birth and deaths in a sample unit[Q] which is followed by a independent survey half yearly by an investigator-supervisor[Q], i.e. it is a dual record system
- The data obtained by both methods is matched and unmatched or partially matched data is re-verified in the field to obtain an unduplicated count of births and deaths
- A sample unit has population of 1500 in rural areas and 1000 in urban areas and there are currently 6671 such sample units (4436 rural and 2235 urban).

Significance

- Sample registration system is a major source of health information
- It provides reliable data for calculation of birth and death rates, age-specific fertility and mortality rates[Q], infant and adult mortality, etc. half yearly.

21. Physical quality of life index (PQLI).

Refer Question No. 16 December 2007 (RS2) Paper I.

22. Residual chlorination.

Refer Question No. 5 June 2011 (RS2) Paper I.

MBBS PHASE III EXAMINATION

DECEMBER 2017

(Revised Scheme 2 and 3)

PAPER II

LONG ESSAYS

1. **Enumerate the maternal and child health indicators. Define perinatal mortality rate. Write the causes and measures to reduce perinatal mortality rate in India.**

For maternal and child health (MCH) indicators

Refer Question No. 4 December 2009 (RS2) Paper II.

For perinatal mortality rate

Refer Question No. 2 December 2011 (RS2) Paper II.

2. **Define accident. Enumerate the types of accident. Give an account of primary factors associated with accidents.**

- Accident is an unpremeditated event resulting in recognizable damage (WHO).

Types (International Classification of Diseases)

- Motor vehicle accidents
- Suicide and self-inflicted injury
- Accidental falls
- Industrial accidents
- Accidental drowning and submersion
- Accidental poisoning
- Domestic accidents
- Other accidents include violence, homicide, suicide, air accidents, drowning, poisoning, field accidents, fire accidents, etc.

Primary Factors Associated with Accidents

For more

Refer Question No. 2 June 2016 (RS2) Paper II.

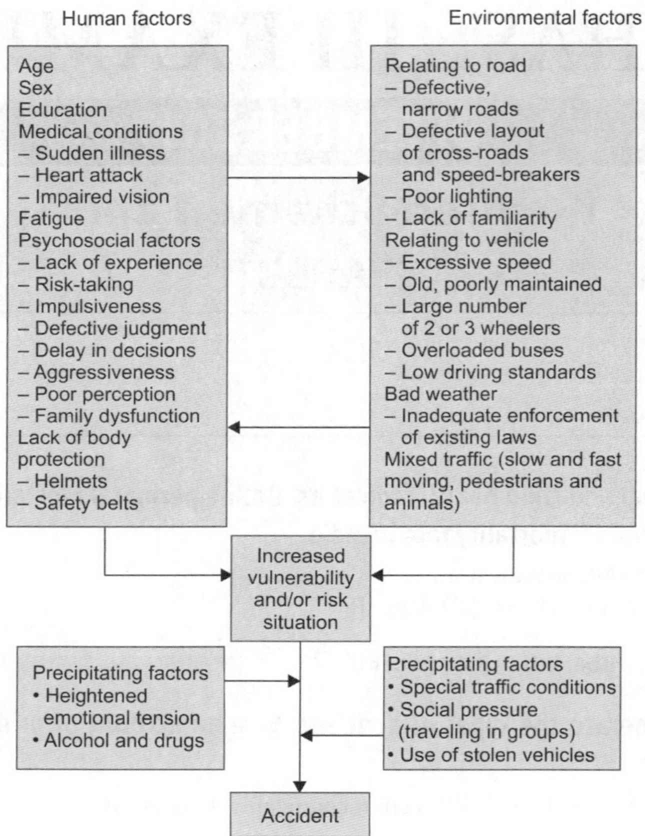

SHORT ESSAYS

3. Intrauterine device (IUD).

Refer Question No. 6 June 2009 (RS2) Paper II.

4. Prevention of industrial accidents.

- Accidents are common in many industries, more so in mines, quarries and construction works
- Accident rate in industry is about 0.14 per 1000 workers per year and every year about 7,000 workers are dying from industrial accidents.

Epidemiology

Host factors	*Agent factors*	*Environmental factors*
▪ Age—young and recently recruited workers are frequently the victims of accidents ▪ Sex—5 times more common among men than women ▪ Time—occur more frequently at end than at beginning of the shift ▪ Experience and education—lesser the experience, more the accidents	▪ Improper planning and construction of factories ▪ Machines ▪ Faulty design ▪ Lack of maintenance ▪ Entanglement of loose clothes and hair ▪ Transmission of machinery ▪ Speed of work processes ▪ Faulty planning	▪ Physical ▪ Overcrowding ▪ Defective lighting ▪ Temperature ▪ Ventilation ▪ Humidity ▪ Radiations from surroundings ▪ Pressure ▪ Noise

Contd...

Contd...

▪ Duration of work—longer the duration of work, more the accidents ▪ Concomitant disease ▪ Psychological factors—carelessness, overconfidence, lack of concentration in the work, ignorance, emotional stress and accident proneness ▪ Personality traits/emotional stability ▪ Wearing unsuitable shoes ▪ Carrying improper loads ▪ Faulty stepping ▪ Not using personal protective measures ▪ Physical defects	▪ Boiler explosion ▪ Dust explosion ▪ Corrosive materials ▪ Molten metal and hot liquids ▪ Flying solid particles ▪ Metal grinding ▪ Stone dressing ▪ Riveting ▪ Chipping metal ▪ Electricity ▪ Gassing	▪ Vibrations ▪ Ionizing radiation ▪ Slippery floors ▪ Uncovered drains ▪ Social ▪ At work place ▪ Domestic ▪ Relationship between workers and management ▪ Lack of safety policy

Prevention

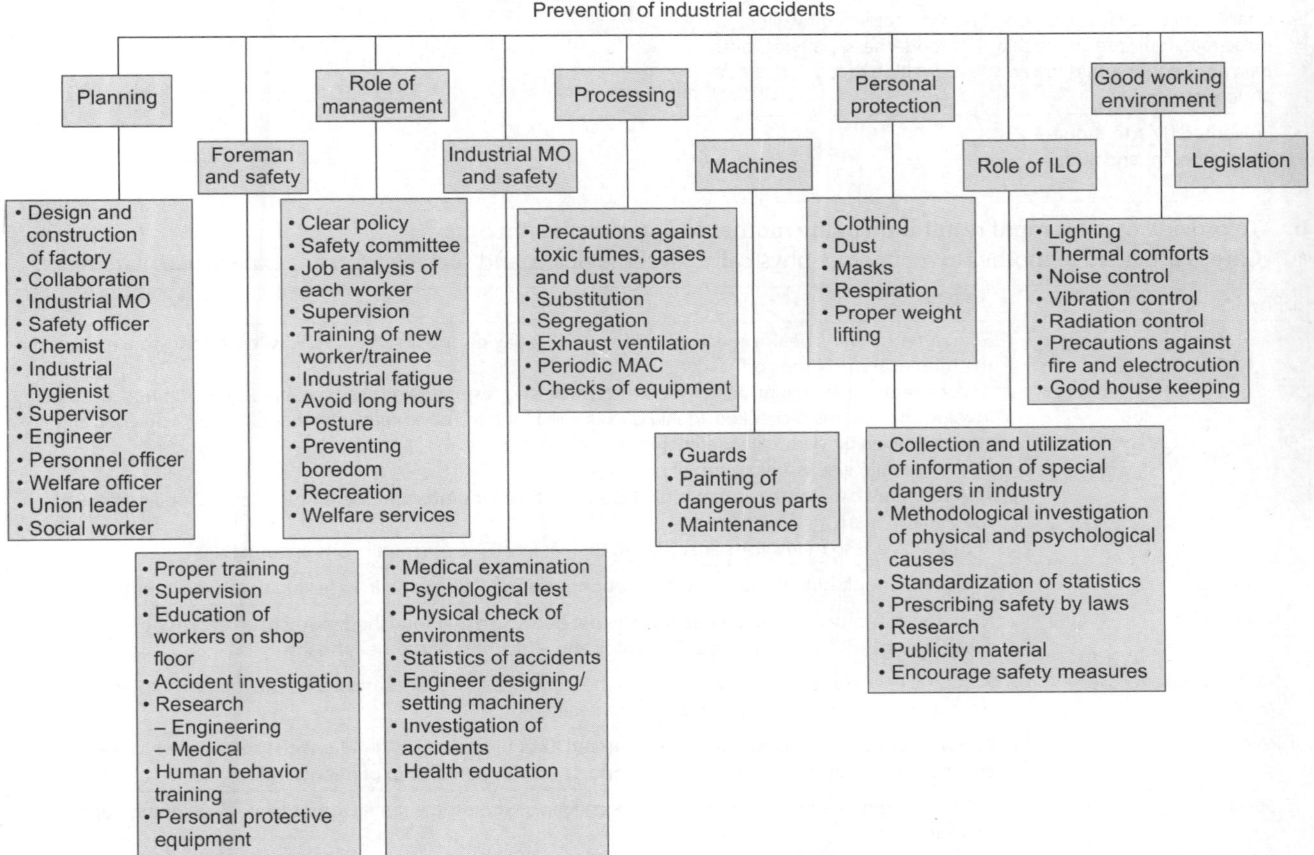

Significance

- Industrial accident causes loss to the worker, in terms of his wages apart from his sufferings, industry (or employer) suffers in terms of decreased production, provision of medical care and compensation and to the nation, it affects the progress.

5. Postnatal care.

- Care of the mother and the newborn after delivery is known as postnatal care.

Objectives	*Timing*
▪ To prevent complications of postpartal period ▪ To provide care for rapid restoration of mother to optimum health ▪ To check adequacy of breastfeeding ▪ To provide family planning services ▪ To provide basic health education to mother and family	▪ Minimum recommended postnatal visits[Q]—3 – 1st visit—<3 days – 2nd visit—1 week – 3rd visit—8 weeks

Components

a. To prevent complications of the post partal period (by early diagnosis and prompt treatment)

Puerperal sepsis	*Thrombophlebitis*	*Secondary hemorrhage*	*Others*
▪ Infection of genital tract within 3 weeks of delivery	▪ Infection of the leg veins frequently associated with varicose vein	▪ Bleeding per vaginum anytime 6 hours after delivery to the end of puerperium due to retained placenta or membranes	▪ Urinary tract infection and mastitis, etc.
▪ Characterized by fever, raised pulse rate, foul smelling lochia, pain and tenderness is lower abdomen, etc.	▪ Characterized by tenderness, paleness and swelling of leg		
▪ Prevented by attention to asepsis before and after delivery			

b. To provide case for rapid restoration of the mother to optimum health

- Care is provided to mother to recuperate physically psychologically and socially from her experience of delivery.

i. Physical	
– Postnatal examination	▪ Soon after delivery, health checkup is done twice a day during first 3 days and subsequently once a day till the umbilical cord drops off ▪ At each of these examination, temperature, pulse and respiration is checked, breast is examined, normal involution of uterus is checked, lochia is examined for any abnormality, urine and bowel is checked and advice is given on perineal toilet including care of stitches ▪ At the end of 6 weeks, involution of uterus is checked ▪ Thereafter once a month examination is done for first 6 months and thereafter once in 2 or 3 months till the end of 1 year ▪ In rural areas, if so many visits are difficult, then at least 3–6 postnatal visits are must
– Anemia	▪ Routine hemoglobin estimation is done during postnatal visits and in cases of anemia, it should be treated
– Nutrition	▪ Nutrition of mother should be adequately met because a malnourished mother secretes as much milk and a well-nourished mother but poor in quality and at the cost of mother's health
– Postnatal exercises	▪ Postnatal exercises are necessary to bring the stretched abdominal and pelvic muscles back to normal ▪ Normal house-hold duties are resumed gradually
ii. Psychological	▪ Common psychological problems encountered after birth are fear, timidity and insecurity which can be eliminated by proper instructions and support and companionship of her husband
iii. Social	▪ Mother should be encouraged to raise the child in a wholesome family atmosphere developing her own methods

c. To check adequacy of breastfeeding

- Breast milk is the main source of nourishment in the 1st year of life and in societies this may be for 1½ year or longer.
- Mothers can secrete as much as 400–600 mL of milk per day during 1st year[Q]
- Mothers are advised to breastfed the exclusively for 4–5 months followed by supplementary food rich in proteins and other nutrients from age of 4–5 months introduced gradually in small amounts (Weaning)
- Mothers should be discouraged from bottle feeding the child as they are nutritionally poor and bacteriologically dangerous.

d. Family planning
   - During postnatal visits, mothers are motivated to adopt a suitable contraceptive method for spacing the next birth or for limiting the size of family
   - In suitable candidates, postpartum sterilization is recommended on the 2nd day after delivery
   - In postpartum period, lactation offers some protection against conception and therefore cannot be relied upon, their fire
   - During the first 6 months, UD and nonhormonal contraceptive are ideal choices and hormonal contraceptives are avoided as they suppress lactation
   - However injection of medroxyprogesterone acetate after delivery is successful contraceptive as it does not suppress lactation but because of its side effects its use is limited to multiparae at ages over 35 years or those who have completed their families
e. To provide basic health education to mother/family
   - In postnatal period, mother and her family is educated in regards to
     - Hygiene—personal and environmental
     - Feeding for mother and infant
     - Pregnancy spacing
     - Importance of health check up
     - Birth registration.

6. National Leprosy Eradication Program.

Refer Question No. 12 June 2010 (RS2) Paper II.

7. Disaster management in floods.

- Floods are most common of all natural disasters, causing greater death than any other type of disaster
- Besides devastation of property, flood also affects health of individuals
- Major diseases seen after flood are water-borne diseases like diarrhea, dysentery, cholera and typhoid which affect entire population, especially poor and vulnerable, due to lack of access to safe drinking water, medicine and hygienic food
- Other diseases also seen alongside include respiratory infections, CO poisoning.

Health and Environmental Problems

a. Unsafe food
   - Floodwaters contain disease causing bacteria, dirt, oil, human and animal wastes, and farm and industrial chemicals and their contact with food items including food crops in agricultural lands during flooding can make that food unsafe to eat and hazardous to human health
   - Power failures caused by floods also damage stored food in refrigerators or cold storage
   - Foods kept inside cardboards, plastic bags, jars, bottles, and paper packaging are equally subject to disposal if contaminated by floodwaters or moulds.
b. Contaminated drinking and washing water and poor sanitation
   - Flooding impairs clean water sources with pollutants and devastates sanitary toilets
   - Direct and indirect contact with the contaminants—whether through direct food intakes, vector insects such as flies, unclean hands, or dirty plates and utensils—result in water-borne illnesses and life-threatening infection diseases
   - Pollutants also saturate into ground water and/or can infiltrate into sanitary sewer lines through ground
   - In addition, wastewater treatment plants, if flooded and malfunctioned, can be overloaded with polluted runoff waters and sewage beyond their disposal capacity, resulting into backflows of raw sewage to homes and low lying grounds
   - Private wells can be also contaminated or damaged severely by floodwaters, while private sewage disposal systems also become a cause of infection and illnesses when they are broken or overflowed
   - In this manner, unclean drinking and washing water and sanitation, coupled with lack of adequate sewage treatment, can lead to disease outbreaks, e.g. life-threatening cholera, typhoid, dysentery and some forms of hepatitis
c. Mosquitoes and animals
   - Prolonged rainfall and floods provide new breeding grounds—wet areas and stagnant pools—for mosquitoes and can lead to an increase in the number of mosquito-borne diseases such as malaria and dengue and West Nile fevers

- Contact with wild animals, rats and rodents that possibly carry viruses and diseases may also result in infection for example Leptospirosis, or Weil's disease.

d. Moulds and mildews
- Excessive exposure to moulds and mildews can cause flood victims—especially those with allergies and asthma - to contract upper respiratory diseases and to trigger cold-like symptoms, e.g. sore throat, watery eyes, wheezing and dizziness
- Molds grow in as short a period as 24 to 48 hours in wet and damp areas of the buildings and homes that have not been cleaned after flooding such as water infiltrated walls, floors, carpets, toilets and bathrooms
- Although molds exist naturally as well as in our normal life, very small mold's spores can be easily inhaled by human bodies and cause allergic reactions, asthma episodes, and other respiratory problems if a large amount of molds are inbreathed. Amongst others, infants, children, elderly people, and pregnant women are considered most vulnerable to mold induced health problems.

e. Carbon monoxide poisoning
- CO is found in combustion fumes, e.g. fumes generated by small gasoline engines, stoves, generators, lanterns, and gas ranges, or by burning charcoals and woods
- In event of power outages following floods, flood victims tend to use alternative sources of fuels or electricity for heating, cooling, or cooking inside enclosed or partly enclosed houses, garages or buildings without an adequate level of air ventilation
- CO builds up from these sources and poisons people and animals inside.

f. Other hazards when reentering and cleaning flooded homes and buildings
- Electrical power systems including fallen power lines can become hazardous during cleanup activities
- Gas leaks that may be occurring from pipelines or propane tanks can trigger another disastrous outcome, e.g. fire and explosion—when entering and cleaning damaged buildings as well as endeavoring to restore utilities services
- Flood debris—such as broken bottles, woods, stones and walls—may also cause fresh wounds and injuries when removing contaminated mud and cleaning damaged buildings.
- Containers of hazardous chemicals including pesticides, insecticides, fertilizers, car batteries, propane tanks, and other industrial chemicals may be hidden or buried under flood debris. Health hazard can also occur when hazardous dusts and molds remaining in the ducts, fans and ventilators of air-conditioning and heating equipment are circulated throughout the building and inhaled by those engaged in cleanup and restoration unless it is properly cleaned after flooding

g. Mental stress and fatigue
- A flood can cause both emotional and physical stress because of having experienced a devastating flood, seen loved ones lost or injured, and homes damaged or destroyed, flooding poses a long-term psychological impact on the flood victims
- Cost and labor required to repair flood-damaged homes places severe financial and psychological burdens on people affected, in particular the unprepared and uninsured
- Post-flood recovery commonly causes mental disorders, anxiety, anger, depression, lethargy, hyperactivity, sleeplessness, and in an extreme case, suicides amongst the flood victims
- Behavior changes may also occur in children such as an increase in bed-wetting and aggression.

Disaster Management in Floods

Disaster preparedness →	*Disaster response →*	*Disaster mitigation (Rehabilitation)*
i. Predisaster phase ▪ Identifying high-risk areas like low lying areas, areas downstream of dams, etc. and devising warning methods to people lying there ▪ Regular check on water level after heavy rain ▪ Careful analysis of past disasters ▪ Advance planning. Learning from the past ▪ Preparation of health services to take timely action	i. Impact phase ▪ Turn of off electricity to reduce risk of electrocution ▪ Protect people and property by moving to higher grounds or upper floors ▪ Beware of water contamination ▪ Comply strictly with advice issued by local authorities in terms of evacuation or warnings	▪ Wait till water is declared safe before drinking water ▪ Clean and disinfect flooded rooms ▪ Sterilize dishes and utensils by washing with boiling water ▪ Get rid of any food including canned food or food kept in refrigerators and freezers ▪ Get rid of all consumables like drinks, medicines, etc.

Contd...

Contd...

Disaster preparedness →	*Disaster response →*	*Disaster mitigation (Rehabilitation)*
▪ Integrated health care facilities. ▪ Fully-equipped hospitals with disaster response teams ▪ Linking of hospitals ▪ Good radio communications and transport facilities ii. Preimpact phase ▪ Timely forecast or issue of warning helps in early evacuation of population (fog horns for people living downstream of dams) ▪ Other techniques are building of check dams around low lying areas or river banks to prevent flooding, building channels to direct flood waters to natural water bodies	▪ Local resource utilization ▪ Community training in first aid ▪ Strengthen primary health care ▪ Decentralized predisaster planning at the community level ▪ Education of community ▪ Managing mass casualties (Triage) ii. Relief phase ▪ Information on disability and injuries ▪ Baseline data on the site of impact ▪ Detailed information on health facilities existing ▪ Survey of water and sanitation system ▪ Quick survey of food, medical and other supplies followed by its acquisition, transportation, storage and distribution	▪ Accommodation of refugees in camps and settlements ▪ Safe water supply ▪ Safe excreta disposal ▪ Vector control measures ▪ Conduct of medical camps ▪ Provision of drugs and other medical supplies ▪ Vaccination campaigns ▪ Provision of adequate nutrition

Significance

- Flood are very common in India and Government of India should formulate a disaster management protocol for it which should include health care as one of major component.

8. Categories of biomedical waste in India.

Refer Question No. 2 December 2009 (RS2) Paper II.

9. Prevention of hookworm infestation.

- Hookworm infection (Ancylostomiasis) is any infection caused by *Ancylostoma duodenale* or *Necator americanus* occurring as single or mixed infection.

Epidemiology

a. Agent factors	
i. Agent (Hookworms)	▪ *Ancylostoma duodenale* and *Necator americanus* ▪ Adult parasites lives in small intestine of humans (mainly in jejunum) by attaching themselves to villi with help of anterior end bent like a hook
ii. Reservoir	▪ Man
iii. Infective material	▪ Feces containing ova of hookworm
iv. Period of infectivity	▪ As long person harbors parasite
b. Host factors	▪ Seen in all ages (most common in 15–25 years) and both sex ▪ Malnutrition predisposes ▪ Higher prevalence in agriculture workers
c. Environmental factors (favorable factors)	▪ Damp, sandy or friable soil ▪ Temperature of 24–32°C ▪ Oxygen ▪ Moisture ▪ Rainfall over 100 cm ▪ Shade (direct sunlight kills larvae) ▪ Human habits like open air defecation, barefoot walking, untreated sewage farming, etc. ▪ Social factors like illiteracy, ignorance, low standard of living
d. Route of transmission	▪ Active penetration of skin by larvae in soil ▪ Also possible through ingestion of filariform larvae through contaminated fruits and vegetables
e. Incubation period	▪ *A. duodenale*—5 weeks to 9 months ▪ *N. americanus*—7 weeks

Clinical Features

- Hookworm infection causes iron deficiency anaemia due to chronic blood loss and depletion of body's iron stores
- Hookworms through their hooks, suck blood at rate of 0.03 ml/day (*N. americanus*) and 0.2 mL/day (*A. duodencle*)
- It manifests as
  - Children: Retarded physical growth and development
  - Mothers: Increased morbidity, LBW babies, abortion, stillbirths and impaired lactation
  - Adults: Diminished capacity for sustained hard work.

Prevention and Control

Elimination of Reservoir (Treatment)	*Breaking chain of transmission*	*Protection of susceptible*
▪ Albendazole—400 mg single dose ▪ Mebendazole—100 mg BD for 3 days ▪ Levamizole—150 mg for adults and 50 mg for children, single dose (Drug of choice) ▪ Pyrantel pamoate—10 mg per kg body weight daily for 3 days	▪ Prevent or reduce fecal contamination of soil by sanitary disposal of human excreta ▪ Provision of safe drinking water ▪ Food hygiene habits ▪ Avoid open air, indiscriminate defecation ▪ Avoiding use of untreated sewage as fertilizer	▪ Health education regarding use of sanitary latrines, personal hygiene, use of protective footwear and changing behavioral patterns ▪ Wearing footwear and making use of health facilities for diagnosis and treatment

10. Postexposure prophylaxis in rabies.

Refer Question No. 2 December 2008 (RS2) Paper II.

11. National Population Policy.

Refer Question No. 7 December 2007 (RS2) Paper II.

12. Juvenile Justice Act.

- Juvenile Justice (Care and Protection of Children) Act, 2000 (Amended in 2006) came into force on 30th December 2000.

Objectives

- To consolidate and amend the law relating to juveniles in conflict with law and children in need of care and protection by providing for proper care, protection and treatment by catering to their development needs, and by adopting a child-friendly approach in the adjudication and disposition of matters in the best interest of children and for their ultimate rehabilitation.

Salient Features

a. Definitions
   i. Juvenile (Child)
      - Juvenile/child is a person who has not completed the age of 18 years
   ii. Juvenile in conflict with law
      - Child who is alleged to have committed an offence
   iii. Children in need of care and protection
      - Children who are neglected, abused, abandoned, victim of any armed conflict or natural calamity amongst others

b. Offences against children
   - Offences committed against a child as listed in this Act
   - These offences are cognizable and punishable under the provisions of this Act.

c. Child Welfare Committee
   - Establishment of child welfare committees consisting of 5 members (one Chairperson, 1 woman, 1 expert on matter concerning children and 2 others) to be established for every district or group of districts
   - Committee has the final authority to dispose of cases for the care, protection, treatment, development and rehabilitation of the children as well as to provide for their basic needs and protection of human rights.

d. Juvenile Justice Board
   - Establishment of a 3 member Juvenile Justice Board (2 social workers of which one should be at least female both involved in child welfare activities for at least 7 years and a Principle Magistrate of first class Judicial Magistrate cadre with training in child psychology) for a district of a group of district
   - Every such bench has powers to deal with juveniles in conflict with law.
e. Children Homes
   - Establishment children's home in every district or group of districts and maintenance of these children's home by state government or in association with voluntary organizations
   - These children's home would be meant for the reception of child in need of care and protection during the investigation of any pending inquiry and subsequently for their care, treatment, education, training, development and rehabilitation.
f. Rehabilitation
   - Rehabilitation and social reintegration of a child shall be carried by
     - Stay in a children's home or special home
     - Adoption
     - Foster care
     - Sponsorship
     - Sending the child to an aftercare organization.
g. Special Juvenile Police Unit
   - Creating special juvenile police unit, to handle juveniles or children in every district and city to coordinate and to upgrade the police treatment of the juveniles and the children.

Significance

- The Juvenile Justice Act 2000 has removed all the inadequacies of its predecessor acts and has made the care more comprehensive and encompassing.

SHORT ANSWERS

13. Body mass index.

Refer Question No. 4 June 2010 (RS2) Paper II.

14. Congenital rubella.

Refer Question No. 3 June 2011 (RS2) Paper II.

15. Influenza A (H1N1).

Refer Question No. 4 June 2014 (RS2) Paper II.

16. Screening for breast cancer.

Refer Question No. 11 June 2013 (RS2) Paper II.

17. Mopping up in polio eradication.

Refer Question No. 1 June 2014 (RS2) Paper II.

18. Accredited Social Health Activist (ASHA).

Refer Question No. 2 June 2014 (RS2) Paper II.

19. Health education in schools.

Refer Question No. 4 December 2013 (RS2) Paper II.

20. Assessment of nutritional status.

Refer Question No. 2 June 2010 (RS2) Paper I.

21. Community health center.

Refer Question No. 2 December 2007 (RS2) Paper II.

22. Blocked flea.

Refer Question No. 14 June 2012 (RS2) Paper II.

Index